Mindfulness in Behavioral Health

Series Editor
Nirbhay N. Singh
Medical College of Georgia
Georgia Regents University
Augusta, Georgia, USA

More information about this series at http://www.springer.com/series/8678

Kimberly A. Schonert-Reichl
Robert W. Roeser
Editors

Handbook of Mindfulness in Education

Integrating Theory and Research into Practice

Jacqueline E. Maloney, Managing Editor

Springer

Editors
Kimberly A. Schonert-Reichl
Department of Education
and Counseling Psychology
University of British Columbia
Vancouver, BC, Canada

Robert W. Roeser
Department of Psychology
Portland State University
Portland, OR, USA

ISSN 2195-9579 ISSN 2195-9587 (electronic)
Mindfulness in Behavioral Health
ISBN 978-1-4939-3504-8 ISBN 978-1-4939-3506-2 (eBook)
DOI 10.1007/978-1-4939-3506-2

Library of Congress Control Number: 2016930835

Springer New York Heidelberg Dordrecht London

Printed on acid-free paper

Springer Science+Business Media LLC New York is part of Springer Science+Business Media (www.springer.com)

We dedicate this volume to educators everywhere who selflessly serve children and their families.

Acknowledgments

To my mom and dad for their unending love and support, and to my sweet and loving husband, Arleigh, and my amazing sons, Griffin and Gray—thank you for being my inspiration.

Kimberly A. Schonert-Reichl

To my mother and father Nancy and Richard Roeser who mindfully educated me!

Robert W. Roeser

To my dad and mom for their unwavering support and encouragement, and to my beloved husband, Brice, who is compassion personified.

Jacqueline E. Maloney

Contents

Contributors

Jeffry Beers Department of Psychology, Portland State University, Portland, OR, USA

David S. Black Keck School of Medicine, University of Southern California, Los Angeles, CA, USA

Patricia C. Broderick Bennett Pierce Prevention Research Center, The Pennsylvania State University, University Park, PA, USA

Richard C. Brown Naropa University, Boulder, CO, USA

Jennifer DeLange Metropolitan State University of Denver, Denver, CO, USA

Brian M. Galla School of Education, University of Pittsburgh, Pittsburgh, PA, USA

Gordon S. Gates Washington State University, Pullman, WA, USA

Barbara Gilbert Harvard University, Cambridge, MA, USA

Susanne Harnett Metis Associates, New York, NY, USA

Michaela Jelen BC Ministry of Children and Family Development, Victoria, BC, Canada

Patricia A. Jennings Curry School of Education, University of Virginia, Charlottesville, VA, USA

Susan Kaiser-Greenland The Inner Kids Program, Los Angeles, CA, USA

Janis B. Kupersmidt Innovation Research and Training, Durham, NC, USA

Eden Nagler Kyse Montclair State University, Montclair, NJ, USA

Linda Lantieri Inner Resilience Program, New York, NY, USA

Brooke D. Lavelle Heineberg Mind and Life Institute, Hadley, MA, USA

Molly Stewart Lawlor University of British Columbia, Vancouver, BC, Canada

Daniel P. Liston University of Colorado at Boulder, Boulder, CO, USA

Kristen E. Lyons Metropolitan State University of Denver, Denver, CO, USA

Jacqueline E. Maloney University of British Columbia, Vancouver, BC, Canada

Stacie M. Metz West Chester University of PA, West Chester, PA, USA

Madhavi Nambiar Inner Resilience Program, New York, NY, USA

Alison E. Parker Innovation Research and Training, Durham, NC, USA

Suzanne C. Parker American University, Washington, DC, USA

Daniel Rechtschaffen Executive Director of Mindful Education, San Francisco, CA, USA

Robert W. Roeser Portland State University, Portland, OR, USA

Kimberly A. Schonert-Reichl University of British Columbia, Vancouver, BC, Canada

Shauna Shapiro Santa Clara University, Santa Clara, CA, USA

Daniel J. Siegel Mindsight Institute, Santa Monica, CA, USA

UCLA School of Medicine, Los Angeles, CA, USA

Madeleine W. Siegel University of California, Berkeley, CA, USA

Genét Simone Woodring College of Education, Western Washington University, Bellingham, VA, USA

Ellen Skinner Department of Psychology, Portland State University, Portland, OR, USA

Veronica Smith Psychological Studies in Education, Department of Educational Psychology, University of Alberta, Edmonton, AB, Canada

Geoffrey B. Soloway Mindwell, Bowen Island, BC, Canada

Sarah de Sousa Santa Clara University, Santa Clara, CA, USA

Jenna Whitehead University of British Columbia, Vancouver, BC, Canada

Rona Wilensky PassageWorks Institute, Boulder, CO, USA

Lee Worley Naropa University, Boulder, CO, USA

Shinzen Young University of Vermont, Burlington, VT, USA

Arthur Zajonc Mind and Life Institute, Hadley, MA, USA

About the Editors

Robert W. Roeser is a professor of psychology and human development in the Department of Psychology at Portland State University in Portland, Oregon. He received his Ph.D. from the Combined Program in Education and Psychology at the University of Michigan (1996) and holds master's degrees in religion and psychology, developmental psychology, and clinical social work. In 2005 he was a US Fulbright Scholar in India; from 1999 to 2004 he was a William T. Grant Faculty Scholar; and from 2006 to 2010 he served as the Senior Program Coordinator for the Mind and Life Institute (Boulder, CO). Currently, Dr. Roeser's Culture and Contemplation in Education Lab (CaCiEL) at Portland State is devoted to the study of the putative effects of mindfulness and compassion training for teachers and (early childhood and early adolescent) students with regard to health and well-being and the optimization of teaching and learning.

Kimberly A. Schonert-Reichl is a professor in the Human Development, Learning, and Culture program in the Faculty of Education at the University or British Columbia (UBC) and director of the Human Early Learning Partnership, an interdisciplinary research institute in the Faculty of Medicine at UBC. She received her M.A. in educational psychology from the University of Chicago and her Ph.D. in educational psychology from the University of Iowa and was a postdoctoral National Institute of Mental Health (NIMH) Fellow in the Clinical Research Training Program in Adolescence at the University of Chicago and Northwestern University. Prior to her graduate work, Kim was a middle school teacher and a teacher at an alternative high school for "at risk" adolescents. Kim studies the social and emotional development of children and adolescents, particularly in relation to identifying the processes and mechanisms that foster positive human qualities such as empathy, compassion, altruism, and resiliency. She has won several awards, including the 2015 Joseph E. Zins Distinguished Scholar Award for Outstanding Contributions to Research in Social and Emotional Learning, given by the Collaborative for Academic, Social, and Emotional Learning (CASEL) and the Confederation of University Faculty Associations' (CUFA-BC) Paz Buttedahl Career Achievement Award for sustained contributions over the course of a career to the nonacademic community through research and scholarly activity.

About the Authors

Jeffry Beers is a former high school teacher and coach. He has a master's degree in education from the University of Portland and a master's degree in psychology from Portland State University, where he received mindfulness training. He has practiced mindfulness meditation for the past 8 years. Jeffry's main focus has been on stress and coping through mindfulness practice, and he has written seven books on the subject, four of which are now published. His most recent book, *Peace: The Art of Digesting Destructive Emotions*, is available. Three more books from *The Speed of Life* series will be published soon.

David S. Black is a tenure-track assistant professor in preventive medicine and faculty member of the Norris Comprehensive Cancer Center at USC. As the director of the American Mindfulness Research Association and editor-in-chief of Mindfulness Research Monthly, he serves as a global leader in the dissemination of meditation and mindfulness research. Dr. Black has directed or contributed to multiple National Institutes of Health-funded randomized controlled/clinical trials that stringently test the effects of meditation on disease symptomatology, neuroendocrine products, and immune parameters. These trials have focused on the psychological stress cascade linking the central nervous system, neuroendocrine activity, and immune dysregulation. He has published over 45 journal articles including those in leading journals such as *Pediatrics* and *Journal of the American Medical Association*.

Patricia C. Broderick is a research associate at the Bennett Pierce Prevention Research Center at Penn State University and founder and former director of the Stress Reduction Center at West Chester University of Pennsylvania. She holds a master's degree in counseling from Villanova University and a Ph.D. in school psychology from Temple University. She is a licensed clinical psychologist, certified school psychologist (K-12), certified school counselor (K-12), and a graduate of the Mindfulness-Based Stress Reduction (MBSR) advanced practicum at the Center for Mindfulness at UMASS. She is co-principal investigator on a recent grant from the US Department of Education to study mindfulness in public schools, an advisory board member for CASEL on the intersection of social and emotional learning and mindfulness, and a practice board member of the American Mindfulness Research Association (AMRA). She is the coauthor of a developmental text, *The Life Span: Human Development for Helping Professionals* (Broderick & Blewitt, 2014, 4th

Edition, Pearson Ed), and the author of *Learning to BREATHE: A Mindfulness Curriculum for Adolescents* (2013, New Harbinger).

Richard C. Brown founded the department of Contemplative Education at Naropa University in 1990. Early in his career he taught in public school and in a Buddhist-inspired K-12 school. He published a Buddhist view of children's spiritual development and has been involved internationally in the development of contemplative schools and contemplative parenting. Based on his experiences developing the Naropa's teacher education programs, Richard has written extensively on many areas of contemplative education, including paradigms and pedagogies utilizing awareness of sense perceptions, thoughts, and emotions. He was a founding member of the Leadership Council of Garrison Institute's Initiative on Contemplation in Education and is one of the authors of Garrison's CARE for Teachers program. Since 2009 he has been involved with the contemplative reform of the Kingdom of Bhutan's education system and with collaborative projects between Naropa' Contemplative Education program and the Royal University of Bhutan.

Jennifer DeLange is an undergraduate student at the Metropolitan State University of Denver studying psychology, neurobiology, and chemistry. In the future, she hopes to become a clinical psychologist. Her research interests include the neurobiological impacts of psychological trauma, emotion regulation, and the effectiveness of mindfulness-based modes of psychotherapy.

Brian M. Galla is assistant professor in the School of Education and Research Scientist in the Learning Research and Development Center at the University of Pittsburgh. Dr. Galla's scholarship combines laboratory and classroom field research to better understand motivational factors that support academic achievement and positive youth development. He focuses in particular on the study of self-control. Known colloquially as willpower, self-control refers to the ability to pursue long-term goals despite conflicting urges and impulses. He also has a strong interest in mindfulness-based approaches to enhancing self-control and their potential to improve health and academic achievement. Dr. Galla has received research grants from the John Templeton Foundation and the Mind and Life Institute. His work appears in a range of peer-reviewed psychology and education journals, including *Journal of Personality and Social Psychology*, *Contemporary Educational Psychology*, and *Journal of Personality*.

Gordon S. Gates is professor and academic director at Washington State University. His interests and research focus on the emotional aspects of leadership practice including educator stress and coping with conflict, change, and uncertainty; distributed and teacher leadership; and mindfulness and resilience by both individuals and organizations. He is coeditor of the *Journal of Research on Leadership Education* sponsored by the University Council for Educational Administration (UCEA) and series editor for *Research on Stress and Coping in Education* published by Information Age Publishing. Recently, he edited Volume XIII titled, *Mindfulness for*

Educational Practice: A Path to Resilience for Challenging Work (2015), in the aforementioned series.

Barb Gilbert is a project director with the Center for Education Policy Research at Harvard University, overseeing several projects related to teacher effectiveness and knowledge utilization. Barb is also co-principal investigator for the *Mathematics Teachers and Teaching Survey*, an NSF study focused on describing the current state of mathematics education in the USA. Previously, she was the senior research manager for the National Center for Teacher Effectiveness at CEPR. Barb's work incorporates an interest in Eastern philosophy and connections to high reliability organizations and the specific strategies they implement to ensure individual and organizational mindfulness. Barb is a former English teacher and taught at the middle and high school levels.

Susan Kaiser-Greenland is a former corporate attorney who developed the Inner Kids mindful awareness program for children, teens, and families. Research on the Inner Kids elementary school program was conducted at the Mindful Awareness Research Center at UCLA and is published in the *Journal of Applied School Psychology*. Susan is author of *The Mindful Child: How to Help Your Kid Manage Stress and Become Happier, Kinder, and More Compassionate* (Free Press, 2010). Her next book will be published by Shambhala Press in the Fall of 2016. She teaches children, parents, and professionals and consults with organizations on teaching mindful awareness in an age-appropriate and secular manner. She has spoken at universities, medical centers, and schools, both public and private, worldwide. Susan lives in Los Angeles with her husband Seth Greenland. They have two grown children. She can be found online at www.susankaisergreenland.com.

Susanne Harnett is a managing senior associate at Metis Associates. Dr. Harnett has more than 15 years of experience with program evaluation, research design, sampling methodology, field research, qualitative and quantitative methodology, data maintenance, and technical writing. She has substantial experience in designing and implementing randomized and quasi-experimental designs and has served as the principal researcher on several large-scale evaluations of educational programs, with a particular focus on arts education and SEL programming. Current and recent projects include the Fetzer-funded evaluation of the Inner Resilience Program, an i3-funded arts project in 80 NYC public schools, two US DOE-funded elementary school counseling grants, and evaluations of educational programs offered through Carnegie Hall's Weill Music Academy and Lincoln Center Education. She holds a Ph.D. in educational psychology from the University of Virginia.

Michaela Jelen is the coordinator for the autism outreach program for children and youth with autism spectrum disorders (ASD) for the British Columbia Ministry of Children and Family Development (MCFD) and a behavior consultant for children and youth with ASD. Her educational and research endeavors include examining programs designed to effectively support children and youth with developmental disabilities in inclusive environments. She has contributed to research reports and public policy documents in special education and services to children with developmental disabilities.

Patricia A. Jennings is an associate professor of Education at the Curry School of Education at the University of Virginia. She is an internationally recognized leader in the fields of social and emotional learning and mindfulness in education with a specific emphasis on teacher stress and how it impacts the social and emotional context of the classroom and student well-being and learning. Dr. Jennings lead the team that developed CARE for Teachers, a mindfulness-based professional development program for teachers designed to reduce stress and promote improvements in classroom climate and student academic and behavioral outcomes. She has conducted two federally funded studies of CARE. The first demonstrated that CARE improves teachers' general well-being, health, emotion regulation, efficacy, and mindfulness. A study currently underway is also examining CARE's effects on classroom climate and student academics and behavior. Her first book, *Mindfulness for Teachers: Simple Skills for Peace and Productivity in the Classroom*, is part of the Norton Series on the Social Neuroscience of Education and was released in February 2015.

Janis B. Kupersmidt is a senior research scientist at Innovation Research & Training, a behavioral sciences research organization in Durham, North Carolina. Her research program focuses on the development and evaluation of preventive intervention programs in the areas of mindfulness education, social emotional learning, mentoring and other relationship-focused approaches, media literacy education, and positive youth development focusing on reductions in risky health behaviors (e.g., substance abuse, aggression, delinquency, romantic relationship health) and enhancing protective factors. She has been the principal investigator on multiple grants awarded by federal agencies such as the National Institutes of Health and the Office of Juvenile Justice and Delinquency Prevention as well as national and local nonprofit organizations. Dr. Kupersmidt received her doctorate in clinical child psychology from Duke University, completed her clinical internship at Yale University, and served as an associate professor at the University of North Carolina at Chapel Hill.

Eden Nagler Kyse is the director of the Center for Research and Evaluation on Education and Human Services (CREEHS) at Montclair State University. She has managed dozens of large- and small-scale evaluation and applied research projects, including those focused on K-12 education, teacher education and professional development, community health, and community needs assessments. This work has been funded by grants from public agencies at the federal (e.g., US Department of Education, National Science Foundation) and state (e.g., N.J. Department of Education, N.Y. Department of Education, N.J. Department of Health) levels and by contracts with local educational agencies, community organizations, and foundations. Dr. Kyse has particular expertise in program evaluation, research design, quantitative methodology, and statistical analysis. She holds a Ph.D. in educational psychology from the Graduate Center at the City University of New York (CUNY), specializing in quantitative methods in educational and psychological research.

Linda Lantieri has been in the field in education for over 40 years in a variety of capacities: classroom teacher, assistant principal, director of a middle school in East Harlem, and faculty member at Hunter College in New York City. Currently, she serves as the director of *The Inner Resilience Program* whose mission is to cultivate the inner lives of students, teachers, and schools by integrating social and emotional learning with contemplative practice. Linda is one of the cofounders and presently a senior program advisor for the Collaborative for Academic, Social, and Emotional Learning (CASEL). She is also an adjunct assistant professor in the Psychology Department of Columbia University, Teachers College. She is the coauthor of *Waging Peace in Our Schools* (Beacon Press, 1996), editor of *Schools with Spirit: Nurturing the Inner Lives of Children and Teachers* (Beacon Press, 2001), and author of *Building Emotional Intelligence: Techniques to Cultivate Inner Strength in Children* (Sounds True, 2008, 2014).

Brooke D. Lavelle Heineberg is the cofounder and executive director of the Courage of Care Leadership Council, a nonprofit organization dedicated to providing Innate Compassion Training (ICT) programs and support to individuals and communities in education, health care, and other areas of social service. She is also senior education consultant at the Mind and Life Institute and a codeveloper of the Call to Care program for teachers and students. Brooke holds a Ph.D. in religious studies from Emory University. Her academic work focuses on the confluence of Buddhist contemplative theory and cognitive science, as well as the cultural contexts that shape the transmission, reception, and secularization of Buddhist contemplative practices in America. At Emory, she served as a lead instructor for several studies examining the efficacy of cognitively based compassion training (CBCT) and has helped to develop and adapt CBCT for school children as well as adolescents in Atlanta's foster care system. Brooke earned her B.A. in religion and psychology at Barnard College, and her M.A. degree in religion at Columbia University. While at Columbia, she worked as a research coordinator for the Columbia Integrative Medicine Program, where she developed and taught yoga and Mindfulness-Based Stress Reduction (MBSR) programs for a variety of clinical populations. Brooke serves on the Board of the Foundation for Active Compassion and now resides in the Bay Area where she works as a consultant at the Center for Compassion and Altruism Research and Education (CCARE) at Stanford University and the Greater Good Science Center (GGSC) at UC Berkeley.

Molly Stewart Lawlor has a master's degree in counseling psychology from the University of British Columbia and is a Ph.D. candidate in the Human Development, Learning, and Culture program at the University of British Columbia. She has expertise in children's social and emotional learning development and the application of mindfulness within the school context. Molly's research includes the investigation of mindfulness and psychological adjustment in children and adolescents and evaluations of social-emotional learning programs for children in school settings. In addition, Molly develops mindfulness-based programming for children and youth, is a primary author of the MindUP™ program, and is the director of Curriculum and Research for the Taxi Dog Educational Program.

Daniel P. Liston (Dan) is a Professor in the School of Education at the University of Colorado at Boulder. He utilizes philosophy, social theory, and literature to examine educational issues. His past work includes articles and books in which he explores the social and political context of schooling and examines rationales for reflective teacher education. Liston's current scholarship focuses on the role of reason and emotion in education, features of contemplative teaching, and education in film. He is past codirector of and currently a facilitator for *Colorado Courage and Renewal*, a program of professional development and renewal for the serving professions.

Kristen E. Lyons is an assistant professor of psychology at Metropolitan State University of Denver. Her research examines the development of self-awareness and self-control. As part of this research, she studies how mindfulness practice may promote emotion regulation and cognitive control in children and adolescents.

Jacqueline E. Maloney, formerly a classroom teacher, is a doctoral student in Human Development, Learning, and Culture at the University of British Columbia. Her primary area of study and research are contemplative education programs—programs that integrate yoga and mindfulness-based practices into school settings to promote the well-being of teachers and students. Jacqueline also directs the Yoga Alliance accredited Kids' Yoga Teacher Training at Semperviva Yoga in Vancouver. She has been teaching yoga and mindfulness education programs in preschools, elementary schools, and high schools since 2006.

Stacie M. Metz is an associate professor in the Department of Graduate Social Work and is cochair of the Institutional Review Board at West Chester University. She has taught public health and social work graduate courses in program evaluation, biostatistics, research methods, evidence-based programming, and human behavior. She received her doctorate in public health studies/health services research at Saint Louis University while also completing a joint MSW/MPH. She served as a data manager and a statistical analyst on a number of projects, including an AHRQ-funded R01 investigation on clinically relevant changes in health-related quality of life in persons with chronic health conditions. Dr. Metz collaborates with several community partners as an evaluation consultant and is coauthor to a number of peer-reviewed articles and conference presentations. She is currently leading the 4-year evaluation of the Brandywine Health Foundation's Youth Mental Health First Aid training in Coatesville PA, which is designed to educate the community on common mental health signs and symptoms in youth and impart a 5-step action plan in providing "first aid" support to youth experiencing a mental health challenge or crisis. She also serves the Society for Public Health Education (SOPHE) as cochair of the University Faculty Community of Practice and National Delegate for PA SOPHE. She chaired the 2014 Pennsylvania SOPHE Community Partnerships and Leadership for Health Conference. Her research interests include adolescent mental health and social-emotional learning, health promotion in young adult populations, chronic health program/treatment evaluation, and integrated service delivery.

Madhavi Nambiar is one of the cofounders of the Inner Resilience Program (IRP) and has been involved in strategic program planning and service delivery since IRP's inception in 2002. Until 2013, she served as deputy director of Programs for IRP. She continues to serve IRP as an advisor and thought partner. Madhavi has received a Ph.D. in mythological studies/depth psychology from Pacifica Graduate Institute. She has advanced certifications in Federal Contract and Grant Administration and an extensive background in extramural fund management from UCLA and Columbia University. Currently, she serves as senior project officer in the Office of Sponsored Projects Administration at Columbia University.

Suzanne C. Parker holds a B.A. in cognitive science from Dartmouth College and is currently a doctoral student in clinical psychology at American University. She studies the interpersonal effects of contemplative practice as well as shifts in cognitive style that may arise from meditation. She has studied meditation at Bodh Gaya and researched the effects of meditation with Amishi Jha, Ph.D.

Daniel Rechtschaffen, marriage and family therapist, is the author of *The Way of Mindful Education* and *The Mindful Education Workbook*. Daniel organizes the annual Mindfulness in Education conference at the Omega Institute. He leads mindfulness trainings and helps develop curricula for schools and organizations around the world, such as the South Burlington School District, Marin Preparatory School, and Phuket International Academy in Thailand. He also loves teaching mindfulness to high school basketball and baseball teams. Daniel has a private psychotherapy practice in the San Francisco Bay Area.

Robert W. Roeser is a professor of psychology and human development in the Department of Psychology at Portland State University in Portland, Oregon. He received his Ph.D. from the Combined Program in Education and Psychology at the University of Michigan (1996) and holds master's degrees in religion and psychology, developmental psychology, and clinical social work. In 2005, he was a US Fulbright Scholar in India; from 1999 to 2004 he was a William T. Grant Faculty Scholar; and from 2006 to 2010 he served as the senior program coordinator for the Mind and Life Institute (Boulder, CO). Currently, Dr. Roeser's Culture and Contemplation in Education Lab (CaCiEL) at Portland State is devoted to the study of the putative effects of mindfulness and compassion training for teachers and (early childhood and early adolescent) students with regard to health and well-being and teaching and learning.

Kimberly A. Schonert-Reichl is a professor in the Human Development, Learning, and Culture program in the Faculty of Education at the University or British Columbia (UBC) and director of the Human Early Learning Partnership, an interdisciplinary research institute in the Faculty of Medicine at UBC. She received her M.A. in educational psychology from the University of Chicago and her Ph.D. in educational psychology from the University of Iowa and was a postdoctoral National Institute of Mental Health (NIMH) Fellow in the Clinical Research Training Program in Adolescence at the University of Chicago and Northwestern University. Prior to her graduate work, Kim was a middle school teacher and a teacher at an alternative high school for "at risk" adolescents. Kim studies the social and emotional development of children and adolescents, particularly in relation to identifying the processes and mechanisms that foster positive human qualities such as empathy, compassion, altruism, and resiliency. She has won several awards, including the 2015 Joseph E. Zins Distinguished Scholar Award for Outstanding Contributions to Research in Social and Emotional Learning, given by the Collaborative for Academic, Social, and Emotional Learning (CASEL), and the Confederation of University Faculty Associations' (CUFA-BC) Paz Buttedahl Career Achievement Award for sustained contributions over the course of a career to the nonacademic community through research and scholarly activity.

Shauna Shapiro is a professor at Santa Clara University, a clinical psychologist, and an internationally recognized expert in mindfulness. Dr. Shapiro is the recipient of the American Council of Learned Societies teaching award, acknowledging her outstanding contributions to education in the area of mindfulness, and was awarded a contemplative practice fellowship by the Mind and Life Institute, cofounded by the Dalai Lama. Dr. Shapiro lectures and leads mindfulness training programs internationally and has been invited to present for the King of Thailand, the Danish Government, and the World Council for Psychotherapy, Beijing, China. She has published over 100 articles and book chapters and is coauthor of the critically acclaimed text, *The Art and Science of Mindfulness*, as well as popular parenting book, *Mindful Discipline: A Loving Approach to Raising an Emotionally Intelligent Child.* Dr. Shapiro's work has been featured in the *Wired* Magazine, *USA Today, The Yoga Journal*, and the *American Psychologist.*

Daniel J. Siegel is clinical professor at the UCLA School of Medicine, executive director of the Mindsight Institute, founding codirector of the UCLA Mindful Awareness Research Center, and author of several texts, including

The Developing Mind, Mindsight, and the *Pocket Guide to Interpersonal Neurobiology*.

Madeleine W. Siegel is an undergraduate at the University of California, Berkeley. She has worked as a co-instructor in mindfulness training for children, a teaching assistant in human development courses, and a co-therapist for adolescents in group therapy. She is currently at the College of Natural Resources focusing on the interface of well-being and the environment.

Genét Simone has been a teacher educator since 1993 and is currently academic program director and senior instructor for Western Washington University, Teacher Education Outreach Programs, in Bremerton, WA. Her program focuses on K-8 Teacher Certification with Endorsements in Elementary and Special Education. Dr. Simone teaches courses in lesson planning, assessment, and classroom management, foundations of education, and social studies methods. She oversees all aspects of school placements for 40–50 teacher candidates and trains field-experience supervisors for their role as mentors and liaisons between the university and communities spanning seven school districts on the Kitsap Peninsula. Dr. Simone works with WWU faculty and administrators to align State Certification Standards with WWU's teacher education program and develops various program-level assessments and associated curriculum. Dr. Simone also served as adjunct faculty for Naropa University's Contemplative Education program from 2000 to 2013, participating in some summer sessions and developing curriculum and then teaching online classes for their master's degree. Current research and projects involve developing contemplative curriculum for her program at WWU and creating a manual for graduate students to support their writing of thesis papers and dissertations with contemplative perspectives and practices.

Ellen Skinner is a leading expert on the development of children's motivation, coping, and academic identity in school. As part of psychology's concentration in developmental science and education, her research explores ways to promote students' constructive coping, ongoing classroom engagement (marked by hard work, interest, and enthusiasm), and perseverance in the face of obstacles and setbacks. Her research team is especially focused on two ingredients that shape motivational resilience: (1) close relationships with teachers, parents, and peers and (2) academic work that is authentic and intrinsically motivating. Recently, they have begun investigating the role that teachers' own engagement and resilience play in allowing them to support students' motivational development and cope with students who are struggling, bored, or disaffected with learning in their classrooms.

Veronica Smith is an associate professor in the Department of Educational Psychology at the University of Alberta. She has a background as a clinician and consultant in speech and language pathology in public schools, preschool, and hospital settings. In these positions she provided assessment, individual program planning, and direct intervention and participated in team problem solving for students with special needs from preschool to late adolescence.

These early career experiences piqued her interest in intervention science, prompting questions about the gaps between evidence-based practices and community practice. Much of her research has investigated the implementation fidelity of programmatic efforts to support children with developmental disabilities in community and school settings. She has published her research in national and international journals and recently coauthored a book entitled, *Getting into the Game: Sports Programs for Kids with Autism.*

Alison E. Parker is a research scientist at Innovation Research & Training, a behavioral sciences research organization in Durham, North Carolina. Dr. Parker's research program focuses on the emotional, social, and cognitive development of children and adolescents with expertise in mindfulness education, substance abuse prevention, and prevention programming for youth. She has been the principal investigator on multiple grants awarded by the National Institutes of Health and the Department of Education to develop and evaluate mindfulness education programs for children and adolescents as well as to create Web-based assessments and resources for youth. Dr. Parker received her doctorate in developmental psychology at North Carolina State University.

Geoffrey B. Soloway has been working in the area of health promotion, mindfulness, and well-being for 15 years. Geoff completed a Ph.D. on mindfulness in education at the University of Toronto, as well as a master's of education on holistic education. Geoff has worked as an instructor at University of Toronto, as health and wellness specialist at University of British Columbia (UBC), and as a consultant offering mindfulness-based workshops and programs for professionals in the workplace. Currently, Geoff is training director at MindWell Canada, an organizational coach, and instructor for UBC Continuing Studies.

Sarah de Sousa holds a B.A. in modern thought and literature from Stanford University and is a master's candidate in counseling psychology at Santa Clara University. Her academic publications include contributions to the *Oxford Handbook of Positive Psychology (3rd Ed.)* and *Mindfulness-Based Treatment Approaches: Clinician's Guide to Evidence Base and Applications* (2nd Ed.). Sarah is a dedicated student of contemplative practices, a published poet, competitive dancer, and educational consultant. Her work in education includes teaching social-emotional skills and mindfulness to adolescents in the Bay Area through a unique curriculum called LIFEPrep.

Jenna Whitehead is a doctoral student in Human, Development, Learning, and Culture at UBC. Her primary research interest is investigating the assessment and application of mindfulness and neuroscience in the context of student and teachers' social and emotional well-being.

Rona Wilensky was principal and founder of New Vista High School in Boulder from 1992 to 2009. She is currently director of Mindfulness Programs at Passageworks Institute and is responsible for growing the dissemination of SMART in Education. She is actively integrating diversity and cultural responsiveness work within the mindfulness movement through presentations and planning conferences. Rona served on the leadership council of the Initiative on Contemplative Teaching and Learning at the Garrison Institute and is a fellow of the Mind and Life Institute. A past contributor to state and national conversations on high school reform, her essays have appeared in Education Week, The Chronicle of Higher Education, Phi Delta Kappan, and Education News Colorado.

Lee Worley is a founding faculty of Naropa University. In 1976 its founder, Chogyam Trungpa Rinpoche, invited her to Boulder to develop a Theater Studies department based on contemplative principles. She has taught Trungpa's performance method, "Mudra Space Awareness" in Naropa's Religious Studies, Education, Writing, and Traditional Arts programs as well as throughout the USA, Canada, and Europe. Currently, she teaches in the contemplative education master's program. Professor Worley began her performance career as a founding member, actress, and director with Joseph Chaikin's Open Theater in NYC. While in New York, she was a member of the acting faculty at Sarah Lawrence College. Lee was the first practice director for Nalandabodhi, the Buddhist organization of Dzogchen Ponlop Rinpoche who appointed her one of four Western Buddhist teachers for that community. Her book *Coming From Nothing: The Sacred Art of Acting* outlines her philosophy of contemplative performance. Currently, she is developing a book of Trungpa's theater pedagogy and practices. A graduate of NYC's Neighborhood Playhouse, she holds a B.A. in English drama from Mount Holyoke College and an M.A. in Buddhist studies/Tibetan language from Naropa University.

Shinzen Young is an American who began his meditation career in 1970 when he ordained as a Shingon monk in Japan. He has over three decades of experience teaching meditation incorporating current scientific findings with spiritual approaches of Native Americans, Christian mysticism, as well as three traditional Buddhist vehicles: Theravada mindfulness, Mahayana Zen, and Vajrayana Shingon practice. Shinzen is known for his innovative "interactive, algorithmic approach" to mindfulness and leads meditation retreats and related programs throughout North America. He also consults widely on meditation-related research, in both the clinical and the basic science domains.

Arthur Zajonc was professor of physics at Amherst College from 1978 to 2012. He received his B.S.E. and Ph.D. in physics from the University of Michigan. He has been visiting professor and research scientist at the Ecole Normale Superieure in Paris, the Max Planck Institute for Quantum Optics, and the universities of Rochester, and Hannover. He has been Fulbright professor at the University of Innsbruck in Austria. His research has included studies in parity violation in atoms, the experimental foundations of quantum physics, and the relationship between sciences and the humanities. He has written extensively on Goethe's science. He is author or editor of eight books including *Catching the Light*, *The Quantum Challenge*, *Goethe's Way of Science*, *The Dalai Lama at MIT*, and *The New Physics and Cosmology: Dialogues with the Dalai Lama*. From 2012 to 2015 he was president of the Mind and Life Institute.

Part I

Mindfulness in Education: Historical, Contemplative, Scientific, and Educational Foundations

Mindfulness in Education: Introduction and Overview of the Handbook

1

Kimberly A. Schonert-Reichl and Robert W. Roeser

This we have now, is not imagination. This is not grief or joy. Not a judging state, or an elation, or sadness. Those come and go. This is the presence that doesn't.

—Rumi (1995)

When one door closes another door opens; but we so often look so long and so regretfully upon the closed door, that we do not see the ones which open for us.

—Alexander Graham Bell (1847–1922)

What kind of education do we need in an interconnected twenty-first century to prepare young people across the globe to flourish individually, and to contribute to solving the social and ecological challenges that confront the entire globe today? As we contemplate the future of education, it is useful, as Alexander Graham Bell reminds us, to be present and aware of the doors of opportunity that are opening before us as children grow up digitally connected to the whole world, and aware of cultures and conditions near and far in a way unprecedented in the history of the world. In a world where global awareness is just a click away—and where also stresses and distractions that new technologies bring abound, a twenty-first century education that attends to the cultivation of attention, social-emotional competencies, and systems-thinking may be particularly helpful (e.g., Goleman & Senge, 2014). One potentially effective way of re-envisioning education along these lines that is gaining increasing promise is the introduction of mindfulness in education at all levels—for administrators, teachers and students, and their families. If this is the case, then the time is particularly auspicious for this first edition of the *Handbook of Mindfulness in Education* that takes up this issue of what a renewal of education might look like—an education where the presence that is, as Rumi puts it, is central.

Mindfulness in Education

The past decade has witnessed a rapid expansion of interest in mindfulness both in the general public (see Roeser, 2014) and in educational settings (Meiklejohn et al., 2012; Mind and Life Education Research Network, 2012; Roeser, 2014). This interest is based in part on the growing body of research documenting the benefits of mindfulness practices with regard to improving attention and emotion regulation, in relieving distress and

---

Chapter to appear in K. A. Schonert-Reichl & R. W. Roeser (Eds.), *Mindfulness in Education: Emerging Theory, Research, and Programs*. New York, NY: Springer.

K.A. Schonert-Reichl (✉)
University of British Columbia,
Vancouver, BC, Canada
e-mail: kimberly.schonert-reichl@ubc.ca

R.W. Roeser
Portland State University, Portland, OR, USA
e-mail: rroeser@pdx.edu

K.A. Schonert-Reichl, R.W. Roeser (eds.), *Handbook of Mindfulness in Education*, Mindfulness in Behavioral Health, DOI 10.1007/978-1-4939-3506-2_1

cultivating well-being, and improving health in both the general population and clinical populations (see reviews and meta-analyses by Cullen, 2011; Eberth & Sedlmeier, 2012; Gotink et al., 2015; Grossman, Niemann, Schmidt, & Walach, 2004; Gu, Strauss, Bond, & Cavanagh, 2015; Hölzel et al., 2011; Khoury et al., 2013; Zoogman, Goldberg, Hoyt, & Miller, 2014). Could mindfulness training aid students in developing these same positive qualities (e.g., focused attention) and outcomes (e.g., improve learning and well being)?

The general interest in mindfulness in education today is evidenced by the sheer number of "hits" that occur in a simple Google search on the term "mindfulness in education." This yields a total of 24,000,000 "hits" as of the writing of this chapter. The term "mindfulness in schools" yields 7,870,000 "hits," and the term "mindfulness educational programs" yields 13,200,000 "hits." In order to empirically document the growth in research on mindfulness in education, we conducted a systematic search for published articles on the topic of "mindfulness in education" from 2000 to 2014 in the large "parent" database EBSCO. This database includes PubMed, PsychINFO, ERIC, and many others.

The keyword "mindfulness" was first used to search this database, which resulted in thousands of articles that were then manually reviewed for content. Titles and abstracts of papers were first reviewed and in some cases review of the full article content was conducted to insure the topic was specific to mindfulness in education. Only those articles that focused specifically on mindfulness in education were retained. To keep our scope wide, we included articles that were either theoretical, reviews of research, or reports of empirical studies. With regard to the latter, empirical studies needed to meet the following criteria to be included in our summary: (1) the focus was in a school, educational, or training setting, (2) the training or education program explicitly mentioned the utilization of mindfulness practices, (3) the participants were students (including postsecondary, or professionals-in-training) or educators, and (4) the program, training activities, or intervention was fully described and empirically investigated. Articles that investigated the use of mindfulness in therapeutic settings were excluded from our analyses (i.e., in clinical counseling, for treatment of ADHD), as were programs that did not specifically mention mindfulness practice (e.g., yoga only). Using these criteria, a total of 155 articles were retained.

As can be seen in the Fig. 1.1, there has been a steady rise in peer-reviewed publications on the topic of mindfulness in education that meet these criteria, especially since the year 2009. Furthermore, the publications have continued to increase annually, with a surge of publications in 2012. At the same time, we found that nearly half of the articles identified were either theoretical or review articles (30 % and 12 %, respectively). With regard to educational settings, 25 % of the articles were focused on postsecondary settings, 15 % in either preschool or elementary schools, and 10 % in middle or high school settings. Very few of the articles that we

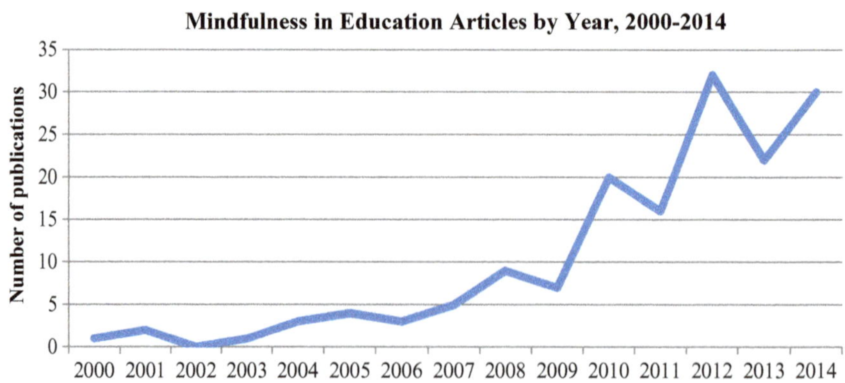

Fig. 1.1 Peer-reviewed articles on mindfulness in education, 2000–2014

found focused on teachers and/or educators (6 %), highlighting the need for more attention to the adults in school settings who "create the weather" for students.

Despite this steady increase in empirical research on mindfulness in education, the research demonstrating the benefits of mindfulness training in educational settings is still in a nascent stage (e.g., Greenberg & Harris, 2012; Roeser & Zelazo, 2012; Zelazo & Lyons, 2012). Indeed, the question of whether mindfulness training shows equivalent benefits in education compared to other sectors that have been examined (health care, mental health) remains largely unanswered at this time. A goal of many of the chapters in this Handbook is to redress this imbalance between enthusiasm for mindfulness in education and evidence showing its feasibility, efficacy, and effectiveness for educators and students alike.

Because of this nascent state of the field, this first edition handbook and its chapters represent an overview of the current state of the science that has unfolded in the field over the past decade. Each chapter summarizes a particular area of research on mindfulness in education in relation to educational leaders, teachers, and students of various ages. By bringing together various perspectives in one volume, we aim to showcase the latest multidisciplinary research on mindfulness in education from a group of world-renowned international scholars, practitioners, and educators deeply immersed in this pioneering work. We hope the volume will help readers to advance the science and practice of mindfulness in education by providing a firm foundation of this work going into the future.

Organization of Handbook

Collectively, the chapters in this volume offer a comprehensive analysis of the extant theory and research on mindfulness-based approaches in education and hence provide a foundation—conceptually, empirically, and practically—for understanding and implementing mindfulness programs and practices to promote learning, health and well-being, and social harmony. The information and knowledge included in the chapters provides fundamental information of interest to scholars, practitioners, and other professionals.

Together, the chapters in this handbook address the following aims: (1) Provide readers with scientifically tractable definitions of mindfulness and an understanding of the potential "value-added" effects of mindfulness in education from diverse perspectives; (2) Showcase emerging theory on mindfulness in education and its implications for educational outcomes and the improvement of human relationships in school settings; (3) Highlight emerging methods, measures, and rigorous designs used in research in this area; (4) Showcase emerging programs and research with children, adolescents, and emerging adults; (5) Showcase emerging programs and research with educators and educational leaders; and finally (6) Provide future directions for theory, research, and program development. This handbook is organized in three sections:

I. Mindfulness in Education: Historical, Contemplative, Scientific, and Educational Foundations
II. Mindfulness in Education: Science and Applications with Educators
III. Mindfulness in Education: Science and Applications with Students

Part I: Mindfulness in Education: Historical, Contemplative, Scientific, and Educational Foundations

The first section of the handbook includes a set of papers that provide some historical, contemplative, scientific, and educational foundations for the practice and study of mindfulness in education today. Collectively, the chapters in this first section introduce the overarching questions of this first edition of the handbook: What is the role of mindfulness and contemplation in education now and historically? How can we define mindfulness in a secular way that is both practical in the world of education and tractable in the world of science? What do we know about mindfulness in relation to the mind, the brain, and social relationships? Can mindfulness training improve the health, well-being, and educational success of educators and students? How is mindfulness similar to, but different from, social-emotional learning (SEL)?

In Chap. 2, titled "Contemplation in Education," Arthur Zajonc situates the work on mindfulness in education within a larger field called contemplative teaching and learning. He explores foundations for modern contemplative education in Asiatic and Greco-Roman traditions. Contemplative, Zajonc notes, connotes marking out a space of attentiveness to the fullness of life: inner, outer, with others. Although historically associated with the curriculum of monasteries, contemplative education today, Zajonc notes, is more frequently occurring in university settings. He describes his own work on contemplation in higher education at the Center for Contemplative Mind in Society, an organization that helped to cultivate and fund university faculty members with regard to learning how to integrate contemplation and contemplative pedagogy into their university courses. Zajonc sees the introduction of mindfulness and other forms of contemplation as a means of readdressing a growing imbalance he sees in higher education today—one wherein students' inner lives, including notions of self-reflection and altruistic purpose, are often neglected in favor of a singular focus on academic knowledge and worldly success. For Zajonc, contemplative teaching and learning, integrated within academic subject matter coursework, are means of transforming higher education *back* towards the cultivation of "whole persons." This chapter provides a unique and historical perspective on how the kinds of mindfulness practices and programs for teachers and students of all ages highlighted in sections "Organization of Handbook" and "Looking to the Future" of this handbook, can be seen as efforts at cultivating the holistic development of all persons in educational institutions, educators, and students alike.

Chapter 3 focuses specifically on the definition and operationalization of mindfulness in scientific research. Currently, there is widespread debate concerning the definition of mindfulness, perhaps especially in secular settings (see Cullen, 2011; Gethin, 2011; Grossman & Van Dam, 2011; Kabat-Zinn, 2011; Williams & Kabat-Zinn, 2011). Mindfulness has been defined, alternatively, as a mental state/trait and a practice (Roeser, 2014). For instance, Goldstein (2002) suggests "*Mindfulness is the quality of mind that notices what is present without judgment, without interference*" (*p. 89*). *Similarly*, the bulk of the current body of scientific work draws upon an early definition of mindfulness put forth by Jon Kabat-Zinn (1994) as "The awareness that emerges from paying attention in a particular way: on purpose, in the present moment, and non-judgmentally" (p. 4).

Conceived of as a practice, Kabat-Zinn (1994) also said that "*Mindfulness practice means that we commit fully in each moment to be present … inviting ourselves to interface with this moment in full awareness, with the intention to embody as best we can an orientation of calmness, mindfulness, and equanimity right here and right now*" (p. 22). The means by which one learns to practice this in daily life are formalized practices such as sitting, listening, or walking meditation in which practitioners are asked to continually bring their attention back to present moment experience, noticing their current thoughts, emotions, or body sensations with curiosity and openness, but without cognitive elaboration or emotional reactivity (Kabat-Zinn, 2003).

Given the "conceptual thicket" surrounding the definition of mindfulness in science currently, this volume begins with a chapter by renown mindfulness teacher and practitioner, Shinzen Young. In Chap. 3, titled "What is Mindfulness? A Contemplative Perspective," Shinzen Young explores various meanings of the term *mindfulness* in order to provide a secular working definition—one that can be operationalized in scientific research in ways that nonetheless maintain the integrity of mindfulness in its classical roots. He argues that the word "mindfulness" represents three separate, albeit related, concepts: a quality of awareness, a set of practices designed to foster this quality of awareness, and a path on which the application of mindful awareness may lead to greater holistic well-being. The chapter provides a unique and synthetic perspective on mindfulness that can inform the kinds of mindfulness training programs for educators and students, and research on them, that are showcased in sections "Organization of Handbook" and "Looking to the Future" of this handbook.

In Chap. 4, Siegel, Siegel, and Parker in their chapter titled "Internal Education and the Roots of Resilience: Relationships and Reflection as the New R's of Education" discuss mindfulness training in relation to resilience, reflection, and healthy relationships—their new 3Rs of social and emotional learning (SEL) that complement the traditional academic 3Rs schools focus on today. Drawing on neuroscience and attachment theory, these authors differentiate between state and trait mindfulness and discuss the developmental significance of each. The authors further distinguish between internally focused mindful awareness (intrapersonal mindfulness and reflection) and externally focused mindful awareness (interpersonal mindfulness and perspective taking) as essential and educable skills. The authors suggest that mindful awareness practices for parents, teachers, and students can foster both state and trait mindfulness directed towards self and others, thus providing a foundation for *the roots of resilience*—self-confidence, flexibility in the face of challenge, emotional resilience, and trust of others. Siegel and colleagues conclude that resilience, reflection, and healthy relationships are all supported by these various forms of mindful awareness, and mindfulness practices designed to build these SEL skills and posit that the 3Rs should be given equal importance to academic skills and learning in school settings. This chapter provides an accessible, clear framework in which to contextualize the many efforts to create such practices and programs for educators and students that are highlighted in sections "Organization of Handbook" and "Looking to the Future" of this handbook.

In Chap. 5, titled "Mindfulness and Social-Emotional Learning," Lawlor situates new research on mindfulness in relation to the longer standing SEL approach. Lawlor sees a synergy between mindfulness approaches in education and the field of SEL in which the incorporation of evidence-based programs that boost competencies such as self-awareness, self-management, social awareness, relationship skills, and responsible decision-making are focal. She provides a conceptual framework for thinking about how mindful awareness practices may foster social and emotional competencies, and may have other added value for the implementation, uptake, and effectiveness of SEL programs.

In sum, these four chapters comprise the Foundations section and are meant to provide a broader context in which to explore the science and application of mindfulness for educators and students that are described in the next two sections of the handbook. In the next section, a series of chapters on mindfulness in teacher education, teacher professional development, educational leadership development, and organizational change are presented. Each chapter explores different practical and scientific questions worthy of future investigation regarding the role of mindfulness training in the lives of educators given the various historical and social conditions of education in our times.

Part II: Mindfulness in Education: Science and Applications with Educators

The second section of the handbook focuses on a review of cutting-edge mindfulness programs, and research on them, for educators, including administrators and teachers. As noted earlier, there is very little research on the use of mindfulness with teachers and administrators at this time. Thus, these chapters all explore the potential benefits and challenges of providing direct mindfulness training to school administrators, principals, and teachers. From a stress reduction perspective, we often describe the importance of focusing on adults in one of two ways: that adults (here educators) create the "weather" in which the learning and development of children under their care occurs; and "in case of emergency, place oxygen mask on self first, then attend to those in your care." In these chapters, authors explore both the direct benefits that mindfulness training may hold for educators and the potential indirect benefits of such training for teachers (in the case of principals) or students (in the case of teachers) in terms of climate and relationship quality.

In Chap. 6, titled "Mindfulness Training for Teachers," Shapiro, Rechtschauffen, and des Sousa provide a general overview of how mindfulness may benefit teachers, teaching, and teacher development. They suggest that mindfulness training may contribute to the teachers in three main ways: self-care, mindful pedagogical practice, and skills for implementing mindfulness practices with students with higher fidelity to principle and quality. The authors also provide illustrations of some of the key mindfulness practices that comprise teacher programs. They conclude with recommendations for future studies to address current methodological limitations in the field regarding the effects of mindfulness training on teachers' well-being, pedagogy, and ability to implement mindfulness programs.

In Chap. 7, Skinner and Beers in their chapter titled "Teacher Stress and Mindfulness" provide a rich scientific account of how, specifically, mindfulness training for teachers can redress the escalating problems of teacher stress and burnout by providing teachers with new coping resources. After providing a model of stress and coping, the authors describe and delineate potential mechanisms underlying mindful awareness practices that may help teachers cope with stress and boost their resilience. They conclude by suggesting potential implications for students of having "mindful" teachers and the need for future research on these topics.

In Chap. 8 titled "Inner Resilience in Schools," continuing with the theme of mindfulness in relation to teacher stress and resilience, Lantieri, Nambiar, Harnett, and Nagler Kyse describe one of the early teacher programs in this field—the *Inner Resilience* program. Inner Resilience is a mindfulness-based social and emotional learning program initially designed for educators to address stressors related to the 9/11 crisis in New York City. In this chapter, Lantieri and colleagues outline several of the program components, including activities and practices for teachers, students, and more recently, principals. Finally, they provide an overview of research on the effectiveness and acceptability of the program, outlining findings from a randomized controlled trial as well as qualitative inquiry conducted with program participants.

In Chap. 9, Jennings describes her work with mindfulness programs for teachers in relation to her Prosocial Classroom Model in her chapter titled "Teacher Programs Overview & CARE program." This model posits that teachers' social and emotional competencies and well-being influence classroom climate, which in turn, influences student outcomes. Mindfulness training is hypothesized to be a way to cultivate social-emotional competencies in teachers, and Jennings describes efforts that she and colleagues have undertaken with the CARE program. Jennings provides examples of teacher comments on these programs and discusses how mindfulness-based programs may influence teacher–student relationships and classroom climate. A list of important suggestions for future directions for research in this largely unexamined area is provided in this chapter.

In Chap. 10, titled "Teaching, Learning, and Transfer in a Mindfulness-based Intervention for Teachers," Roeser reflects on a 7-year project of research aimed at understanding if and how a mindfulness training program (called the Stress Management and Relaxation Training (SMART) or Mindfulness-based Emotional Balance (MBEB) program) helped teachers to reduce stress and improve their classroom practice. Roeser provides a logic model describing his view of how mindfulness training may affect teachers, classrooms, and students. He then describes data from a case study that examines the ways that an experienced mindfulness instructor teaches mindfulness to teachers and fosters their learning and transfer of these skills to stress reduction initially, and changes in behavior and relationships more generally. The goal of the chapter is to focus on issues of quality and adult learning in research on mindfulness-based interventions for educators.

In Chap. 11, Smith and Jelen in their chapter titled "Mindfulness Training with Special Populations" provide an overview of research on mindfulness practices and programs designed to support special populations and their educators and professional caregivers. Although more work is needed in this area, initial research indicates that mindful awareness practices promote positive outcomes for some targeted developmental and behavioral issues in special populations, and increase stress-coping skills among educators and professional caregivers in this area.

In Chap. 12 titled "Preparing Teacher Candidates for the Present: Investigating the Value of Mindfulness-Training for Teacher Education," Soloway advocates for mindfulness training to be included in teacher-education programs in colleges and universities. He describes the results of a qualitative action study that investigated a mindfulness education course offered as an elective to teachers-in-training. Soloway goes on to suggests that mindfulness education programs offer novel and much needed skills not usually addressed in typical teacher education programs, such as the art of being present.

In Chap. 13, Brown, Simone, and Worley in their chapter titled "Embodied Presence: Contemplative Teacher Education" describe a 2-year graduate program for practicing teachers in contemplative education offered at Naropa University. They discuss the importance of *embodied presence* for effective teaching: a state of inner and outer "intelligence" that evolves from contemplative practice resulting in synchronization of body and mind. Brown and colleagues illustrate the concept of embodied presence through observations made by faculty in the Contemplative Education Department and provide examples of graduate students' writing. They also offer suggestions from the program of how teachers might cultivate embodied presence through contemplative practice.

In Chap. 14, titled "On Attentive Love in Education: The Case of Courage to Teach," Liston emphasizes the importance of love and attention in teaching and learning and how contemplative practice might facilitate these. Within the context of Parker Palmer's Courage to Teach retreats, Liston examines the interaction of love and attention and how practices involved in retreats may foster these skills that, he argues, are essential to the well-being of teachers and a caring pedagogy.

In Chap. 15, Wilensky in her chapter titled "Mindfulness and Organizational Change" theorizes that mindfulness practices may facilitate and accelerate positive individual and institutional change in education. She examines this thesis within two contexts: interventions based on Keagan and Laslow's Immunity to Change model, and interventions based on the Constructivist Listening school change model. Wilensky argues that although these models are effective on their own, they could be complemented and enhanced by integrating mindfulness practices into them.

In educational leadership literature, current discussions about high reliability organizations (HROs) for school improvement are largely focused on mindlessness. In Chap. 16, titled "Mindful School Leadership: Guidance from Eastern Philosophy on Organizing Schools for Student Success," Gates and Gilbert tackle this discussion by first examining mindfulness in Eastern philosophy and next connecting several of the identified concepts and principles to the processes advanced in research on high reliability organizing. In their discussion, they also identify the advantages and the limitations with an approach to leadership that is concerned with achieving success for all students. They conclude by delineating a number of recommendations and research on mindful school leadership that address professional responsibilities related to instructional leadership, social justice, and educator stress and coping.

Part III: Mindfulness in Education: Science and Applications with Students

The third section of the handbook focuses on a review of cutting-edge mindfulness training programs, and research on them, for students of various ages. These chapters all explore the potential benefits and challenges of providing direct mindfulness training to students in early childhood and elementary and secondary school settings. In these chapters, authors explore the direct benefits that mindfulness training may hold for students' health, well-being, and learning. Questions of who implements student programs and when, dose, implementation quality, and other challenges in this work are addressed.

This section begins with Chap. 17 titled "Developmental Social-Cognitive Neuroscience Perspective on Mindfulness in Education," in which Lyons and Delange provide an overview of research on developmental social-cognitive neuroscience, discussing how mindfulness education might contribute to healthy development in this area for children and adolescents. They contend that mindful awareness practices can easily be incorporated to elementary and high school curricula, and that doing so would improve self-regulation among students, a necessary component for academic success.

In Chap. 18, Dodson Lavelle in her chapter titled "Mindfulness and Compassion in Education" provides an overview of three contemplative education programs that have been adapted for school settings: Cognitively-Based Compassion Training, Innate Compassion Training, and adaptations of the Mindfulness-Based Stress Reduction Program. Grounded in theory on social and emotional learning, these secular programs were created for both teachers and students to cultivate self-regulation and prosocial skills. She provides preliminary evidence that these programs are generally effective and well-received, while acknowledging the many challenges of implementing and evaluating contemplative programs in schools. She provides suggestions how to approach such challenges.

In Chap. 19, Galla, Kaiser-Greenland, and Black continue the discussion on using mindful awareness practices to promote self-regulation among children and adolescents in their chapter titled "Mindfulness in Education During Early Childhood." They describe the Inner Kids program, a mindfulness training program that has been adapted for young people from ages 4–18, which emphasizes attention, emotional balance, and compassion. They review the results of a randomized controlled trial conducted with second and third grade students to evaluate children's self-regulation skills via executive functions, finding that children with initial lower executive functions scores significantly improved over children in the control group.

In Chap. 20, a discussion of mindfulness programs for children continues in the chapter by Maloney, Lawlor, Schonert-Reichl, and Whitehead titled "A Mindfulness-Based Social and Emotional Learning Curriculum for School-Aged Children: The MindUP Program." In this chapter, Maloney and colleagues describe recent research on the MindUP program, a mindfulness-based social and emotional learning (SEL) program for schools designed to be implemented by classroom teachers. The authors first describe the development of the program and then go on to describe some of the empirical research conducted over the last decade that has examined program implementation and outcomes in social and emotional competencies, executive functions, and cortisol patterns. They also present a thematic analysis of elementary-school students' responses to a consumer satisfaction survey regarding students' perceptions and experience of the program.

In Chap. 21, Kupersmidt and Parker—in their chapter titled "The Master Mind and Moment Programs: Introducing Two Universal Mindfulness Education Programs for Elementary and Middle School Students"—describe and evaluate two universal school mindfulness educations programs: the Master Mind Program that aims to prevent risky decision-making for older elementary schools students, and the Moment Program for middle school students designed to increase academic achievement. In small efficacy studies, they found that both programs significantly boosted aspects of participants' executive functions and improved behavior regulation compared to the control group. The authors also consider developmental issues surrounding introducing mindful awareness practices with youth, and offer recommendations of how they should be considered when creating mindfulness education programs.

In Chap. 22, titled "Working on the Inside: Mindfulness for Adolescents," Broderick and Metz discuss the developmental changes, challenges, and strengths among adolescents, arguing that mindful awareness practices may be especially beneficial during this time of life to promote resilience to stress and enhance academic achievement. They provide evidence for this claim by reviewing research on the Learning to BREATHE program, a school-based universal mindfulness education program designed for adolescents. In addition to decreases in perceived stress and increases in emotion regulation, the findings demonstrate that the majority of participants were satisfied with the program and applied the skills learned in the program to other areas of their lives.

Looking to the Future

The applied developmental, psychological, and educational sciences are all committed to the accurate description and truthful explanation of the processes of education and human development, as well as the compassionate use of the knowledge so-gained in optimizing learning and development for all—particularly those who are rendered most vulnerable in society due to social and economic factors (e.g., Guerra, Graham, & Tolan, 2011; Roeser, 2014). More and more, these domains of science are turning towards a consideration of innovative programs and practices that not only address problems once they have arisen, but also those that prevent problems before they begin and build strengths such as resilience, compassion, and contributions to the welfare of others that are associated with optimal human development (Durlak, Weissberg, Dymnicki, Taylor, & Schellinger, 2011; Greenberg et al., 2003; Stoolmiller, Eddy, & Reid, 2000; Weissberg, Kumpfer, & Seligman, 2003).

The emerging field of Contemplative Education, focused as it is on the creation, implementation, sustainment, and scientific study of developmentally and culturally appropriate forms of mindfulness training in schools for children, adolescents, and adults, suggests considerable promise of such training for cultivating strengths and preventing problems (Mind and Life Education Research Network, 2012; Roeser, 2013; Roeser et al., 2014; Roeser & Peck, 2009; Roeser & Pinela, 2014; Roeser & Zelazo, 2012; Schonert-Reichl et al., 2015). As the many chapters in this handbook attest, there exists preliminary evidence regarding how various programs and practices associated with mindfulness training can stabilize and clarify individuals' attention and awareness, calm the mind and body, reduce negative emotion and its personal and interpersonal sequelae, and increase positive and prosocial motivation and behavior among children, adolescents, and educators alike. In this final section, based on the chapters in this volume and our perceptions of the field as a whole, we outline several areas of practice and research that we see as meriting attention in the future to increase our knowledge and understanding of mindfulness in education.

Future Directions in Program Design and Implementation

Perhaps one of the most foundational issues in need for future attention with regard to the creation of secular programs and practices concerns the definition of mindfulness for school settings. The secular definition and practice of mindfulness is an area that has received an intensive amount of scrutiny recently (see Williams & Kabat-Zinn, 2011). How is mindfulness defined and operationalized in secular contexts, and are ethics and values included in such definitions and their derivative practices given the process of secularization? How can we incorporate attention to such issues in the creation and implementation of mindfulness-based programs in education in the future so their classical use—for the flourishing of oneself and all others, is preserved?

Culture and Context Another critical issue to address in the future, and one that has also been of concern in SEL programs, is the role of gender, race and ethnicity, and culture in the design and implementation of these programs—issues that are endemic to developing effective school programs (Bond & Carmola Hauf, 2004). What does it mean to create culturally-responsive mindfulness programs in schools? What considerations come into play in working in diverse socioeconomic and cultural settings? Such questions need to be answered to advance the field.

Related to issues of culture and context, we believe that more attention needs to be paid to how to make the concepts and language, in addition to practices, of mindfulness programs developmentally appropriate. What modifications are needed for students of different ages, from different cultural backgrounds, or with specific developmental challenges (e.g., trauma)? For instance, one key question regarding mindfulness practices is "For how long, for whom?" (Zelazo & Lyons, 2012).

Integration of Programs at Whole School Level

Schoolwide Change Integration of mindfulness training into the very DNA of the school culture is one of the most pressing topics for those who work in schools and know that "add on" programs are oftentimes burdensome to educational leaders and teachers. In addition, integration of mindfulness skills and mind-sets into subject matter teaching, rather than as stand-alone programs, may also be useful.

There is also a need to be cognizant of the problems that can arise when explicit consideration of the very culture and context in which mindfulness-based educational reform efforts are being implemented are ignored. For instance, to avoid the "predictable failure of educational reform," intentional attention must be given to understanding and addressing systemic irregularities and inherent obstacles (e.g., hierarchy of power) in the system (Sarason, 1990). Any successful reform effort needs to involve administrators, teachers, and students together in creating a high quality and respectful educational environment in which they feel motivated and supported. Indeed, we must take heed of the words of Seymour Sarason (1982) who so wisely posited: "To the extent that the effort at change identifies and meaningfully involves all those who directly or indirectly will be affected by the change, to that extent the effort stands a chance to be successful" (p. 294).

Active Ingredients Another area to investigate includes the question of which practices or combinations of practices are most effective for which individuals? For instance, movement practice has been found to be important for adults (e.g., Carmody & Baer, 2008) and students (e.g., Khalsa, Hickey-Schultz, Cohen, Steiner, & Cope, 2012). What is the added benefit of incorporating sitting meditations in addition to movement practices, and at what age are these most fruitfully introduced? Are some practices contraindicated for particular individuals or at particular times in development? These are critical issues to address.

Models of Delivery in Schools Finally, the question of the model of delivering trainings to teachers and students is important to study. Is a competent mindfulness teacher required to impart such trainings, and what defines such "competence?" (Cullen, 2011; Roeser, this volume). Can teachers be trained by competent mindfulness instructors to deliver practices in their classrooms to students? Can podcasts and web-based trainings suffice for teachers or children, or is a live person conducting the trainings desirable? Research on questions of the delivery of MBIs (direct, indirect, web-based) and the competencies of effective instructors is needed.

Future Directions for Research in Schools

Multiple-Levels-of-Analysis One direction for future research is to examine the effects of mindfulness-based educational approaches on not only intrapersonal outcomes (e.g., self-regulation, stress reduction), but also on interpersonal outcomes in teachers and students (trust, kindness, empathy, perspective-taking, generosity, altruism). In addition, examining how mindfulness-based educational approaches in education can contribute to changes in social adjustment and social relationship outcomes at systemic levels (e.g., trust and emotional support in whole classrooms and schools) will also be important. Particular chapters in this volume provide concrete suggestions in this regard (e.g., Lantieri et al., this volume, Gates & Gilbert, this volume).

Rigor of Research Designs Second, we see a need to continue to increase the rigor of research studies of mindfulness training through the use of new methods, measures, and analytic approaches. These include design features such as randomization, active control groups, blinded studies, non-self-report measures, and use of multilevel randomization and analysis strategies. Many studies in the field of mindfulness in education today are non-randomized or use waitlist control designs. In addition, there is a heavy reliance upon self-report measures in this work. Diversity in methodology and measures will continue to be important in the future. For instance, we see the use of randomization with active control groups as important. Additionally, there needs to be careful attention to documenting the implementation quality and dosage in the program being evaluated, as well as careful attention to monitoring the activities and context in control/comparison conditions (Durlak & DuPre, 2008).

At the same time, we see the use of case studies and multiple baseline designs of individual students and teachers that incorporate randomization to document mindfulness training effects as equally important (Kratochwill & Levin, 2010). Studies that use thick ethnographic descriptions, intensive measurement of individual cases over time, and other forms of qualitative and idiographic assessment of the processes and outcomes of mindfulness training, as well as those that employ longitudinal study designs to examine the long-term effects of mindfulness training on individuals are needed. The rush to randomized control trials without a period of "phenomena finding" in the field of education, we believe, is to be avoided.

Measuring Outcomes In order to upgrade the quality of the research, a third direction for future research is to consider incorporating biological, psychological, behavioral, and contextual outcome measures of the hypothesized effects of mindfulness training at the level of individuals and groups together in the same study. For instance, as noted by Cicchetti and Blender (2006), researchers should adopt a multi-method and multilevel approach and recognize that intervention effects can be manifested on several levels of functioning, such as in changes of *behaviors*, *feelings*, *attitudes*, *biological processes* (e.g., change in stress regulation), and *neuropsychological processes* (e.g., cognitive functioning). Observational measures of classrooms and schools also are important, and new observational measures of "mindful and compassionate classrooms and schools" are urgently needed. Measurement studies could do much to increase the rigor of work in this field.

Such an approach will require teams of researchers from multiple disciplines (e.g., developmental neuroscience, contemplative science, health, education, sociology) to work together (Schonert-Reichl et al., 2015) and will result in a more comprehensive and sophisticated portrayal that will serve not only to advance the science of the field, such an approach will also inform efforts to translate research on the processes that lead to positive adaptation to other settings. That is, taking a multiple-domain perspective in examining the effectiveness of mindfulness-based educational interventions will result in a more complete understanding of the ways in which biological and neurocognitive development interacts with multiple contexts (e.g., school, family, community) and inform programs and practices to be effective and result in long-lasting benefits (Roeser & Zelazo, 2012).

Developmental Timing of Trainings A third direction for future research concerns the timing of the implementation of mindfulness trainings for students and teachers. A key hypothesis in Developmental Contemplative Science is that the putative effects of mindfulness-based interventions, if delivered during different "windows of opportunity" in the lifespan such as early childhood or early adolescence, may cultivate habits and dispositions that have long-term positive effects on individuals and society (e.g., Heckman, 2007; Moffitt et al., 2011). Is it the case that the introduction of mindfulness-based interventions during such "windows of opportunity" confers more immediate and lasting benefits for individuals? In addition, at what point in teachers' professional development is the introduction of contemplative practices most effective? Do pre-service teachers benefit from the training as much as in-service teachers, or is some level of on-the-job experience necessary for maximal benefit to be received? Longitudinal research on students and teachers is needed to address this issue.

Dose–Response Relations A fourth direction to explore in future research studies concerns a determination of dose–response relationships, or how much mindfulness training is feasible and efficacious to produce effects on children, adolescents and teachers. This includes a consideration of both the amount of time of the interventions in total and the duration of time across which interventions are offered. We do not yet know, for instance, if a little practice everyday, or a lot of practice on only some days, is more effective in terms of outcomes for novices learning mindfulness. In addition, overall amount of training is very important given the time pressures characteristic of schools, families, and children's lives today.

Process Studies of Programs A fifth direction concerns a focus on teaching, learning, and mechanisms of transfer from the mindfulness training context to settings beyond. We need to delve into the "black box" of these interventions to understand basic processes of teaching, learning, and transfer (Harachi, Abbott, Catalano, Haggerty, & Fleming, 1999). In this vein, we also need to examine more specifically the factors that facilitate or impede the effective implementation of mindfulness-based programs in educational settings, including teacher buy-in so that we can uncover the processes that insure effective implementation (Reyes, Brackett, Rivers, Elbertson, & Salovey, 2012).

Conclusions

Although much work has been done in the past decade to advance our understanding of the science and practice of mindfulness in education, from our perspective, much work still needs to be done. As you read the book we hope that you are both inspired by the magnitude of the work that is being done in the field of mindfulness in education, and inspired to join the movement in education and science to seek a clearer scientific understanding of the ways in which mindfulness practice can foster the development of the skills and dispositions necessary for students and educators in the twenty-first century. We invite you to travel with us on this road to creating a world in which all individuals can experience flourishing, and where all individuals are concerned with the equal rights of all other individuals to that same flourishing.

Acknowledgments We are extremely grateful to Judy Jones, Senior Editor at Springer, for her assiduous and tireless support and encouragement of this handbook. It was Judy who instigated the notion of a handbook on mindfulness in education several years ago, and it was she who was prescient in forecasting the way the field would explode. Jacquie Maloney served as our managing editor and demonstrated unending dedication, patience, and passion for the project coupled with meticulous attention to detail and diligent organizational skills—a combination of skills rarely seen in one individual. To Jacquie we are utterly thankful for helping us bring this project to completion. We also wish to thank the wonderful contributors to this volume, who responded to the challenges of writing these chapters with unusual promptness, enthusiasm, and thoroughness and who responded to our editorial feedback so gracefully. Reading each of their thoughtful chapters and learning about the new and exciting research and innovative programs in which they are involved in the field of mindfulness-based educational approaches was a genuine pleasure!

References

Bond, L. A., & Carmola Hauf, A. M. (2004). Taking stock and putting stock in primary prevention: Characteristics of effective programs. *Journal of Primary Prevention, 24*, 199–221.

Carmody, J., & Baer, R. (2008). Relationships between mindfulness practice and levels of mindfulness, medical and psychological symptoms and well-being in a mindfulness-based stress reduction program. *Journal of Behavioral Medicine, 2*, 23–33.

Cicchetti, D., & Blender, J. A. (2006). A multiple-levels-of analysis perspective of resilience: Implications for the developing brain, neural plasticity, and preventive interventions. *Annals of the New York Academy of Sciences, 1094*, 248–258.

Cullen, M. (2011). Mindfulness-based interventions: An emerging phenomenon. *Mindfulness, 2*, 186–193. doi:10.1007/s12671-011-0058-1.
Durlak, J., & DuPre, E. (2008). Implementation matters: A review of research on the influence of implementation of program outcomes and the factors affecting implementation. *American Journal of Community Psychology, 41*, 327–350.
Durlak, J. A., Weissberg, R. P., Dymnicki, A. B., Taylor, R. D., & Schellinger, K. B. (2011). Enhancing students' social and emotional development promotes success in school: Results of a meta-analysis. *Child Development, 82*, 474–501.
Eberth, J., & Sedlmeier, P. (2012). The effects of mindfulness meditation: A meta-analysis. *Mindfulness, 3*, 174–189.
Gethin, R. (2011). On some definitions of mindfulness. *Contemporary Buddhism, 12*, 263–279.
Goldstein, J. (2002). *One dharma: The emerging western Buddhism*. San Francisco, CA: Harper.
Goleman, D., & Senge, P. (2014). *The triple focus: A new approach to education*. Florence, MA: More Than Sound.
Gotink, R. A., Chu, P., Busschbach, J. J. V., Benson, H., Fricchione, G. L., & Hunink, M. G. M. (2015). Standardised mindfulness-based interventions in healthcare: An overview of systematic reviews and meta-analyses of RCTs. *PLoS ONE, 10*(4), e0124344. doi:10.1371/journal.pone.0124344.
Greenberg, M. T., & Harris, A. R. (2012). Nurturing mindfulness in children and youth: Current state of research. *Child Development Perspectives, 6*, 161–166.
Greenberg, M. T., Weissberg, R. P., O'Brien, M. U., Zins, J. E., Fredericks, L., & Resnik, H. (2003). Enhancing school-based prevention and youth development through coordinated social, emotional, and academic learning. *American Psychologist, 58*, 466–474.
Grossman, P., Niemann, L., Schmidt, S., & Walach, H. (2004). Mindfulness-based stress reduction and health benefits: A meta-analysis. *Journal of Psychosomatic Research, 57*, 35–43.
Grossman, P., & Van Dam, N. T. (2011). Mindfulness, by any other name…: Trials and tribulations of sati in western psychology and science. *Contemporary Buddhism, 12*, 219–239.
Gu, J., Strauss, C., Bond, R., & Cavanagh, K. (2015). How do mindfulness-based cognitive therapy and mindfulness-based stress reduction improve mental health and wellbeing? A systematic review and meta-analysis of mediation studies. *Clinical Psychology Review, 37*, 1–12.
Guerra, N. G., Graham, S., & Tolan, P. H. (2011). Raising healthy children: Translating child development research into practice. *Child Development, 82*, 7–16.
Harachi, T. W., Abbott, R. D., Catalano, R. F., Haggerty, K. P., & Fleming, C. B. (1999). Opening the black box: Using process evaluation measures to assess implementation and theory building. *American Journal of Community Psychology, 27*, 711–731.
Heckman, J. J. (2007). The economics, technology, and neuroscience of human capability formation. *Proceedings of the National Academy of Sciences, 104*, 13250–13255.
Hölzel, B. K., Lazar, S. W., Gard, T., Schuman-Olivier, Z., Vago, D. R., & Ott, U. (2011). How does mindfulness meditation work? Proposing mechanisms of action from a conceptual and neural perspective. *Perspectives on Psychological Science, 6*, 537–559.
Kabat-Zinn, J. (1994). *Wherever you go, there you are: Mindfulness meditation for everyday life*. New York, NY: Hyperion.
Kabat-Zinn, J. (2003). Mindfulness-based interventions in context: Past, present, and future. *Clinical Psychology: Science and Practice, 10*, 144–156.
Kabat-Zinn, J. (2011). Some reflections on the origins of MBSR, skillful means, and the trouble with maps. *Contemporary Buddhism, 12*, 281–306.
Khalsa, S. B., Hickey-Schultz, L., Cohen, D., Steiner, N., & Cope, S. (2012). Evaluation of the mental health benefits of yoga in a secondary school: A preliminary randomized controlled trial. *Journal of Behavioral Health Services and Research, 39*, 80–90.
Khoury, B., Lecomte, T., Fortin, G., Masse, M., Therien, P., Bouchard, V., … Hofmann, S. G. (2013) Mindfulness-based therapy: A comprehensive meta-analysis. *Clinical Psychology Review, 33*, 763–771.
Kratochwill, T. R., & Levin, J. R. (2010). Enhancing the scientific credibility of single-case intervention research: Randomization to the rescue. *Psychological Methods, 15*, 124–144.
Meiklejohn, J., Phillips, C., Freedman, M. L., Griffin, M. L., Biegel, G., Roach, A., … Saltzman, A. (2012). Integrating mindfulness training into K-12 education: fostering the resilience of teachers and students. *Mindfulness, 3*, 291–307.
Mind and Life Education Research Network (MLERN). (2012). Contemplative practices and mental training: Prospects for American education. *Child Development Perspectives, 6*, 146–153. Retrieved from http://dx.doi.org/10.1111/j.1750-8606.2012.00240.x
Moffitt, T. E., Arseneault, L., Belsky, D., Dickson, N., Hancox, R. J., Harrington, H., … Caspi, A. (2011). A gradient of childhood self-control predicts health, wealth, and public safety. *Proceedings of the National Academy of Sciences, USA, 108*, 2693–2698.
Reyes, M. R., Brackett, M. A., Rivers, S. E., Elbertson, N. A., & Salovey, P. (2012). The interaction effects of program training, dosage, and implementation quality on targeted student outcomes for the RULER approach to social and emotional learning. *School Psychology Review, 41*, 82–99.
Roeser, R. W. (2013). Mindfulness and human development: A commentary on the special issue. *Research in Human Development, 10*, 273–283.
Roeser, R. W. (2014). The emergence of mindfulness-based interventions in educational settings. In T. Urdan & S. Karabenick (Eds.), *Motivational interventions* (pp. 379–419). Bingley, England: Emerald Group.
Roeser, R. W., & Peck, S. C. (2009). An education in awareness: Self, motivation, and self-regulated learning in contemplative perspective. *Educational Psychologist, 44*, 119–136.
Roeser, R. W., & Pinela, C. (2014). Mindfulness and compassion training in adolescence: A developmental

contemplative science perspective. *New Directions for Youth Development, 142*, 9–30.
Roeser, R. W., Vago, D. R., Pinela, C., Morris, L. S., Taylor, C., & Harrison, J. (2014). Contemplative education. In L. Nucci, D. Narvaez, & T. Krettenauer (Eds.), *Handbook of moral and character education* (pp. 223–247). New York, NY: Routledge.
Roeser, R. W., & Zelazo, P. D. R. (2012). Contemplative science, education and child development: Introduction to the special section. *Child Development Perspectives, 6*, 143–145.
Rumi, J. (1995). *The Essential Rumi* (C. Barks, With, J. Moyne, A. J. Arberry & R. Nicholson, Trans.). San Francisco, CA: Harper.
Sarason, S. B. (1982). *Culture of the school and the problem of change* (2nd ed.). Boston, MA: Allyn & Bacon.
Sarason, S. B. (1990). *The predictable failure of educational reform: Can we change course before it's too late?* San Francisco, CA: Jossey-Bass.
Schonert-Reichl, K. A., Oberle, E., Lawlor, M. S., Abbott, D., Thomson, K., Oberlander, T., & Diamond, A. (2015). Enhancing cognitive and social-emotional development through a simple-to-administer mindfulness-based school program for elementary school children: A Randomized Controlled Trial. *Developmental Psychology, 51*, 52–66.
Stoolmiller, M., Eddy, M. J., & Reid, J. B. (2000). Detecting and describing preventive intervention effects in a universal school-based randomized trial targeting delinquent and violent youth. *Journal of Consulting and Clinical Psychology, 68*, 296–306.
Weissberg, R. P., Kumpfer, K. L., & Seligman, M. E. P. (2003). Prevention that works for children and youth: An introduction. *American Psychologist, 58*, 425–432. doi:10.1037/0003-066X.58.6-7.425.
Williams, J. M. G., & Kabat-Zinn, J. (2011). Mindfulness: Diverse perspectives on its meaning, origins, and multiple applications at the intersection of science and dharma. *Contemporary Buddhism, 12*, 1–18.
Zelazo, P. D., & Lyons, K. E. (2012). The potential benefits of mindfulness training in early childhood: A developmental social cognitive neuroscience perspective. *Child Development Perspectives, 6*, 154–160.
Zoogman, S., Goldberg, S. B., Hoyt, W. T., & Miller, L. (2014). Mindfulness interventions with youth: A meta-analysis. *Mindfulness, 6*, 290–302.

Contemplation in Education

2

Arthur Zajonc

Introduction

The word *contemplation* is derived from Latin, meaning "to mark out a space for observation." In ancient times, a space so marked often had religious significance as a place designated for philosophical or spiritual practices. Today the space marked out for contemplation is likely to be the classroom, art studio, or science laboratory. In recent years the connection between contemplation and learning has become increasingly appreciated, and contemplative practices are finding their way into many secular educational settings from kindergarten, elementary and high schools (Wisner, Jones, & Gwin, 2010) to community colleges, universities, and professional schools (Gravois, 2005; Kroll, 2010). Perhaps we should not be surprised at this remarkable development, because the long history of contemplative practice has had as its foremost goal, the refinement of the human being, a goal which educators today surely share with those of long ago.

Submitted to
The Handbook of Mindfulness in Education: Emerging Theory, Research, and Programs

A. Zajonc (✉)
Mind and Life Institute, Hadley, MA, USA
e-mail: agzajonc@amherst.edu

The Origins of Contemplation in Education

Any attempt to trace in detail the lineage of contemplation in education would be far too ambitious for this essay, but it is important to appreciate the significant place occupied by contemplative practices in education over thousands of years in both Asia and the West.

Contemplation in the Western Tradition

Contemplation has a rich history within the Greco-Roman philosophic tradition, where it was historically understood as a process of forming the human being through education and training. The French classicist Pierre Hadot (1995, 2002) has done us a great service in looking afresh at the real ideals and purposes of ancient Greek philosophy. He has shown that we must understand that philosophy's true purpose was to educate, or better to shape, the human being through *askēsis*, which is to say through practice or training, and not simply to offer theoretical musings on abstruse topics. In Hadot's (2002) words,

> We must discern the philosopher's underlying intention, which was not to develop a discourse which had its end in itself, but to act upon souls... The point was always and above all not to communicate to them [the reader or auditor] some ready-

K.A. Schonert-Reichl, R.W. Roeser (eds.), *Handbook of Mindfulness in Education*, Mindfulness in Behavioral Health, DOI 10.1007/978-1-4939-3506-2_2

> made knowledge but to *form* them. In other words, the goal was to learn a type of know-how; to develop a *habitus*, or new capacity to judge and to criticize; and to *transform*—that is, to change people's way of living and of seeing the world. (p. 274)

This notion of practical formation through training was reflected in the words of Simplicius, who when asked, "What place shall the philosopher occupy in the city?" replied: "That of a sculptor of men" (quoted in Hadot, 2002, p. xiii). Our very way of seeing and being in the world was to be remade through ancient philosophy as a practice and a way of living; this was the ancient view of education.

With Hadot's help, we can trace the lineage of practice or askēsis through Scholasticism and the monasteries of the Middle Ages to Montaigne's *Essays* and from there to Descartes's *Meditations* (1641/1993). In the Scholasticism of the High Middle Ages, the education of the monks began with *lectio*, which was a reading or teaching by the Master with no questions permitted. The second stage was *disputatio* or dialectical reasoning, during which the particulars of the reading/teaching were vigorously debated. Extending and complementing these stages of Scholastic education was the monastic practice of *lectio divina*, which was first articulated by the Carthusian monk Guigo II in the twelfth century. Its four stages were: *lectio* (reading), *meditatio* (thinking about), *oratio* (praying), and *contemplatio* (contemplative union).

Michel Foucault viewed Descartes as the watershed figure in philosophy who substituted evidence for practice. "Before Descartes, a subject could have access to the truth only by carrying out beforehand a certain work upon himself which made him susceptible of knowing the truth… [But now] evidence has been substituted for *askēsis*" (Foucault as cited in Hadot, 2002, pp. 263–264). Contemplative exercises were the means by which one worked on and transformed oneself in a manner that was required for a new insight. After Descartes's *Meditations*, we increasingly find such practices lose their explicit place in education in favor of reasoning and evidence. Yet, even in later periods, the traditional idea of working on oneself found its voice in a number of literary and philosophical personalities.

In German, education translates as both *Erziehung* and *Bildung*. The latter word stems from the root meaning "to form," or education as formation. The German poet Goethe (1988) encapsulated this principle of education and its essential link with contemplative engagement when he wrote, "Every object, well-contemplated, opens a new organ in us" (p. 39, my translation). Giving our attention repeatedly to an object works back on the human organism in remarkable and powerful ways. The individual develops, or we could say is sculpted, through contemplative practice. Attention to an object works back on the individual as formation, and the cycle is repeated (see Fig. 2.1). It is by means of the new organ, formed through the repeated act of attending, that Goethe viewed insight as arising.

In the twentieth century, the quantum physicist Erwin Schrödinger (1967) put forward a very similar sentiment,

> And thus at every step, on every day of our life, as it were, something of the shape that we possessed until then has to change, to be overcome, to be deleted and replaced by something new. The resistance of our primitive will is the psychical correlate of the resistance of the existing shape to the transforming chisel. For we ourselves are chisel and statue, conquerors and conquered at the same time—it is a true continued 'self-conquering' (Selbstüberwindung). (p. 107)

What was for Goethe an artistic and intuitive certainty has become a field of scientific research in our time: neuroplasticity. Research in animals, and more recently using noninvasive techniques in humans, has demonstrated the scale and scope

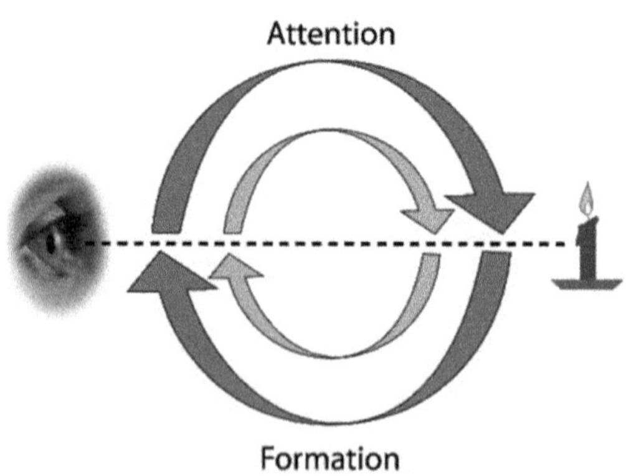

Fig. 2.1 The attention-formation cycle

of neurological changes induced by repeated practice, including by repeated contemplative exercise. For example, one set of studies, by Sara Lazar et al. (2005), have shown cortical thickening to be associated with moderate contemplative practice. The research group found that 8 weeks of contemplative practice (mindfulness training) was associated with changes in gray matter concentration in brain regions involved in learning and memory processes, emotion regulation, self-referential processing, and perspective taking. These areas of the brain are of obvious interest to educators.

Hadot's (2002) description of philosophy as a transformative contemplative practice aligns nicely with the research of Lazar and others:

> [Philosophy] is essentially an effort to become aware of ourselves, our being-in-the-world, and our being-with-others. It is also, as Maurice Merleau-Ponty used to say, an effort to "relearn how to see the world" and attain a universal vision, thanks to which we can put ourselves in the place of others and transcend our own partiality. (p. 276)

Perspective-taking, learning "how to see," empathy, and self-awareness are essential educational goals that transcend particular subject content and are central to human cognitive and affective development as described, for example, by Kegan (1982) and Mezirow (2000).

As our consideration of the Western lineage of contemplation makes clear, practice was, and is, understood as essential to the formation of the human being. This view is commensurate with that of modern developmental science and neuroscience, which also provide a means of understanding education as a process of transformation (see MLERN, 2012; Roeser, 2013).

Many contemporary researchers in the area of contemplative neuroscience and psychology see themselves as working in the tradition of William James (see The Journal of Consciousness Studies, 2010, Vol. 17). Although James's range of interests was broad, he recognized that the training of attention would have enormous educational benefit. A citation well known to contemplative scholars offered by James (1890) states the importance of attention for education in the strongest possible terms:

> ...the faculty of voluntarily bringing back a wandering attention, over and over again, is the very root of judgment, character, and will...An education which would improve this faculty would be *the* education *par excellence*. But it is easier to define this ideal than to give practical directions for bringing it about. (p. 424)[1]

One hundred and twenty years ago William James defined the ideal, but it is only now that universities and colleges are beginning to teach practices that demonstrably improve attention. We will return to this research in secular educational settings below, but for now it suffices to note that practical directions for bringing it about are now becoming available to educators.

Contemplation in the Eastern Tradition

Of equal or greater importance for the reemergence of contemplative education in recent times has been the influx of Buddhist and other Eastern spiritual traditions into the Western world. Many of those who are active today in contemplative education visited the Indian subcontinent during the 1970s and 1980s, taking up contemplative practice for personal benefit (Harrington, 2008). For many, Buddhist contemplative practice was an essentially secular activity, which facilitated the incorporation of these practices into secular settings such as health care institutions and schools. In order to better understand the role contemplation can play in modern education, it is instructive to examine the place of meditation within traditional Buddhist monastic education.

Buddhist Monastic Education The place of meditation in education in the Tibetan Buddhist monastic tradition is well described by Georges Dreyfus (2003), who went through long and arduous training to become a monk with a *Geshe* degree, which roughly corresponds to getting a Ph.D. (see also Rabten, trans. 1980). In his book *The Sound of Two Hands Clapping: The*

[1] William James, *the Principles of Psychology* (NY: Henry Holt, 1890) vol. 1, p. 424.

Education of a Tibetan Buddhist Monk, Dreyfus (2003) situates meditation within the larger curriculum of Tibetan monastic education as one of "three acumens" and points to similarities with Christian monastic education in the Middle Ages.

The first acumen is that of *listening* or *reading* for simple comprehension. This is typically accomplished by listening to a teaching or reading a text for the first time, much like the Scholastic practice of lectio. At this level, the engagement with the ideas and teachings remains quite superficial, but it provides the basis for further work.

The second acumen arises through *thinking*. At this stage, engagement is far more active intellectually: doubts are raised, questions are posed, ideas are debated, as in Scholastic disputatio. Also, at this level, one connects the ideas being studied to one's own life. The second acumen can help achieve true intellectual insight and appreciation for the relevance of the teaching to one's own life. As important as such scholarly achievement is, it lacks the transformative power of the third acumen that arises through *meditation*. In this case, that which was heard (first acumen) and grasped intellectually through thinking (the second acumen) now begins to deepen and to reshape the mind of the student through the repeated practice of meditative concentration. As Dreyfus goes on to explain:

> To effect such a transformation, the meaning must penetrate the deeper layers of the mind, an internalization that requires the power of meditative concentration. It can lead to a more direct insight into the nature of persons and other phenomena, which gradually frees an individual from the bondage of negative emotions. (p. 166)

It is important to note that meditation instruction for the young monks within Tibetan Buddhist monasteries does not begin until adolescence. At earlier ages, study and ritualistic religious practices are thought more appropriate. This timing makes sense if meditation is seen as being concerned with deepening internalization and self-reflective understanding of the meaning of contemplative practices that relies on the neural and psychological developments characteristic of adolescence (Roeser & Pinela, 2014).

Contemplation and Knowing

From these two lineages, Greco-Roman-European and Asian Indian, we can appreciate the role that contemplation has played in education in the past, and we can also begin to see the important role it can continue to play in modern, secular education. In both traditions, basic comprehension of the material at hand is viewed as a first stage in learning. This stage is followed by vigorous intellectual engagement and debate. But in both traditions, a further essential dimension of education requires that the material be internalized through contemplative engagement.[2] True mastery cannot be achieved without it.

If one would be a painter, then it is insufficient to read about or debate the art of painting. One must also practice painting, not merely to learn how to use brush and pigment, but to learn to see as a painter sees, that is to *become* an artist. In a letter to Emile Bernard, Cézanne wrote, "In order to make progress, there is only nature, and the eye is trained through contact with her. It becomes concentric through looking and working" (in Rewald, trans. 1976, pp. 45–46). One "becomes concentric" to that which is in our field of attention. If one would be a scientist, a doctor, a business leader, the principle similarly applies. "Looking and working" sets the artist on the attention-formation cycle (see Fig. 2.1). But Cézanne's insight is as true for the scientist as for the artist. To become a scientist requires that one live the discipline, not merely read about it. This connects well to the philosophy of contemplative education, which emphasizes the value of repeated attentive engagement and practice as essential to a fully integrated and embodied education.

Notice also the close connection between contemplative practice and learning. Thus, while the

[2] Dreyfus points out that only a small number of monks become committed practitioners, even if the central importance of meditation is recognized.

contemplative spiritual traditions of Asia recognize the pragmatically useful, skill- and dispositional-capacity-building effects of contemplation (e.g., increased powers of concentration and greater emotional balance), the Asian Indian practitioner ultimately views meditation as an acumen or *a path to knowledge* (Roeser, 2005). By overcoming ignorance, insight has the possibility of breaking the cycle of suffering by dispelling the false views of self and world that lead to unnecessary suffering. Knowledge that relies on external authority, or even on logical inference, is considered inferior to "direct perception," which is made possible through meditation (the Dalai Lama, as cited in Zajonc, 2004, pp. 155-159).

Contemplation in Higher Education Today

In the secular settings of today's universities, insight into self and world are still valued, but rightfully are shorn of religious associations. Education is a public service guaranteed by the government and should be entirely free of religious orientation. Because many of the practices used in contemplative pedagogy have their roots in the religious traditions of the East and West, a perennial discussion concerning decontextualization is common. There is growing evidence that the efficacy of mindfulness and secular contemplative exercises can be demonstrated independent of the religious origins of such exercises (see Lutz, Dunne, & Davidson, 2007; Lutz, Greischar, Rawlings, Ricard, & Davidson, 2004). Contemplative practices offer faculty, students, and staff tools for working productively with the mind and emotions. These tools can become an important aid to sustained reflection and capacity building. Meditation may also support the achievement of direct insight and creativity. In these ways, contemplation can play a valuable role in education at many different levels.

An integrative education is concerned with the maturation of children from their early years to adulthood, which entails cognitive, emotional, social, and moral development (Eccles & Roeser, 2014). The development of the whole human being is as much the concern of education as information and skills, insofar as education seeks to be comprehensive in executing its important task. In fact, unless and until we attend more to the social-emotional development of the student alongside his or her cognitive development, the challenging content we seek to teach (for example formal mathematics) may remain an elusive goal (Eccles & Roeser, 2014). Here too contemplative exercises can be of use, offering students a way of working with demanding content, new perspectives, and disorienting ideas and experiences (Jennings, Lantieri, & Roeser, 2012). For reasons such as these, contemplative exercises have come to play an increasingly important role in the education (Roeser, 2014).

Learning can only take place if those we teach give us their attention. This basic fact cannot be taken for granted. Factors aggravating students' ability to pay attention in school may include a wide range of stressors from family difficulties to health concerns, external distractions, or they may suffer from ADHD or other forms of learning disability (Zylowska et al., 2008). As a consequence of these and other considerations, in addition to standard pedagogical methods, contemplative exercises such as mindfulness-based stress reduction (MBSR; Kabat-Zinn, 2003) are finding an important place in education (Roeser, Skinner, Beers, & Jennings, 2012). The cultivation of emotional balance and attention is fundamental to successful learning, and an increasing body of research is showing that contemplative methods can be effective in developing these attributes (see Roeser, 2014).

Given the great autonomy of university faculty and the maturity of their students, working with young adults in colleges, universities, and professional schools raises few ethical or pedagogical issues. However, as the other chapters in this volume attest, contemplative exercises are also finding their way into numerous high schools, elementary schools, and even early childhood centers. In the face of these facts, it is essential to ask when and how to introduce contemplative exercises into the classroom for children of different ages (see Greenberg &

Harris, 2012; Zelazo & Lyons, 2012). Age-appropriate means and methods are essential to the responsible use of contemplative methods. Exercises that are suitable for adults may well not be appropriate for small children. I will not address this important issue directly, but confine the remainder of my remarks to the inclusion of contemplation in higher education where my own work has been focused for a dozen years.

Contemplation in Higher Education

The experience of higher education is, whether it be years spent in college, university, or professional school, an important and formative one. Not only does one train for a vocation during these years, but even more fundamentally, one's intellectual disposition, ethical orientation, character, and inner life are shaped in ways that can endure for decades. For these reasons, it is of special importance to offer an integrative educational experience that nurtures the whole human being, one that makes full use of the three acumens, including the reflective and contemplative. The cultivation of the mind through meditation should be as much a part of a person's education as the skills of writing, numeracy, articulate speech, and intellectual mastery of one's discipline. Good judgment, creativity, compassionate action, social-emotional intelligence, and true insight depend on the ability for balanced reflection, on sustained attention to complex situations, and equanimity in the face of difficulty. In short, a genuine, integrative education calls for the cultivation of our contemplative capacities (see Parker & Zajonc, 2010).

Contemplative exercises have been offered as part of US college instruction for decades, but this pedagogical innovation remained largely invisible until a dozen years ago. In 1997, the Center for Contemplative Mind in Society (www.contemplativemind.org) began its first academic program on contemplative practices in higher education. In collaboration with the American Council of Learned Societies, the Center initiated a Contemplative Practice Fellowship program. The intent of the program was to support faculty at colleges and universities in the USA who were interested in including a contemplative perspective or contemplative practices in their courses. We were completely uncertain at the time as to the level of interest or capacity within the Academy for contemplative education. Much to our delight and surprise, in the first year we received nearly 100 applications from institutions of every type, liberal arts colleges, public and private universities, as well as religiously affiliated colleges. Most of the applications were of high quality and submitted by faculty with many years of contemplative experience. They saw these fellowships as a way of connecting a highly valued personal practice with their classroom teaching. In the course of the 11 years during which the Contemplative Practice Fellowships were offered, 158 fellows were named from 136 colleges and universities (Craig, 2011).

Today, the Center for Contemplative Mind in Society works with over 2500 faculty and administrators in North America and beyond, who are including contemplative practices in their teaching. At the University of Michigan School of Music, students are able to get a Bachelor's in Fine Arts in Jazz and Contemplative Studies (a formal concentration in Contemplative Studies was created in 2014 by Prof. Hal Roth and colleagues). At Brown University, medical students are able to do a "Concentration in Contemplative Studies."[3]

Recognizing the importance of community in the establishment of a new form of pedagogy, since 2009 the Center has sponsored the Association for Contemplative Mind in Higher Education (www.acmhe.org). It promotes the emergence of a broad culture of contemplation in the academy by creating a network of academics, administrators, and their institutions who are interested in the recovery and development of the contemplative dimension of teaching, learning, and knowing. In 2011, the Association had 650 members. The Association serves its members by:

[3] See http://med.brown.edu/education/concentrations/contemplative.html

- Stimulating scholarship and research concerning contemplative pedagogy, methodology, and epistemology within and across disciplines.
- Sponsoring forums for the presentation of research and exchange of ideas through webinars, regional and national meetings, and an annual conference.
- Supporting the development of courses and curricula through 1-week residential summer sessions.
- Supporting the deepening of contemplative teaching through retreats for academics offering a variety of traditional and secular practices of potential value for classroom teaching.
- Distributing scholarly work and general information relating to the field of contemplative education online, including a quarterly e-newsletter.
- Providing online, social-networking resources for members to participate in discussion forums and share profiles, publications, papers, and syllabi.

The Practices and Principles of Contemplative Higher Education

A very wide range of contemplative exercises are used by faculty with their students. These include:

1. Mindfulness exercises of various types, for example, mindfulness of the breath, mindful walking, mindful reading, mindful listening, and mindful viewing. These have in common the application of moment-to-moment, nonjudgmental awareness (see other chapters in Handbook)
2. MBSR (Mindfulness-based Stress Reduction) exercises (Kabat-Zinn, 1990)
3. Concentration exercises
4. Exercises for cultivating emotional balance (CEB)[4]
5. Beholding a work of art[5]
6. Visualization
7. Silence
8. Alternation between "focused attention" and "open monitoring" (see Lutz, Slagter, Dunne, & Davidson, 2008)
9. Meditative movement: yoga, tai chi, qigong, authentic movement, eurythmy, contemplative dance, etc. (e.g., Helberg, Heyes, & Rohel, 2009)
10. Empathy, compassion, and loving kindness practices (e.g., Center for Compassion and Altruism Research and Education)
11. Analytical and settled meditation (Dalai Lama in Melrotra, 2005)

In addition to these, many professors have created contemplative exercises that are closely connected to the course content.

From the above list, it is evident that the range of contemplative exercises used is very wide, but I have come to aggregate them into three broad categories:

1. *Capacity-building exercises*, which seek to cultivate:
   (a) Equanimity, stress reduction, or emotional balance
   (b) Concentration, attention, and close observation
   (c) Memory and exact sensorial fantasy
   (d) Discernment, judgment, or relational exercises
   (e) Will or discipline
2. *Content-related exercises*, in which the material being studied (poetry, economics, art, or science) is approached through a contemplative method.
3. *Compassion and community*, in which the cultivation of empathy, compassionate concern, and altruism strengthens ethical qualities in the individual and deepens our caring relationships with others.

Capacity Building

Capacities, such as emotional balance and a stable yet flexible attention, are of value both in the classroom and throughout life. As noted above, William

[4] www.cultivatingemotionalbalance.org

[5] For example, Joel Upton, Amherst College, http://vimeo.com/9007209

James, the founder of scientific psychology, felt that the cultivation of attention would be an education *par excellence*. A wide range of contemplative exercises exist that specifically cultivate attention. Practices that promote emotional balance (e.g., loving-kindness meditation) allow one to be both empathetic yet sufficiently objective that one can hold difficult life circumstances with poise and even grace. Mindfulness practices stabilize the mind by settling attention on a simple object or process, like the breath. Focused attention and open awareness (or monitoring) are two archetypal forms of attention which can be exercised. In my own teaching and writing, these play an important role (see Zajonc, 2009). I use the lemniscate below to illustrate for my students the contrasting aspects of focused and open attention. I see the silent, patient field of open awareness as the receptive space that is required for new insights and creative initiatives to arise (Fig. 2.2).

Attention researchers have now shown that meditation leads to a range of enhancements to attention; and emotion researchers have likewise shown the benefits of meditation for emotional balance (see Hölzel et al., 2011). Shapiro, Brown, and Astin (2011) reviewed this and other research relevant to contemplation in higher education as of 2008 for the Center. This research corroborates the in-class experience of thousands of professors who are now using contemplative exercises as part of their teaching. Of course, much more research concerning the psychology and neuroscience of contemplation still needs to be done.

Content-Related Exercises: Course-Specific Contemplative Practices

In addition to generic contemplative practices for attention and emotional balance, more and more professors are developing practices that are highly relevant to their specific subject matter. For example, a number of art historians are teaching students ways of "beholding" a work of art that are based in contemplative practice. Poetry can be read in a way informed by the ancient practice of "*lectio divina*." But more technical courses such as economics are also amenable to course-specific contemplative practices.

In my own teaching with contemplative exercises for a particular content area, I have come to rely on the following design principles:

- Context: Who are you teaching? (e.g., age of students, subject matter of course).
- Intention: What is the pedagogical aim of the exercise?
- Practice: Choose a practice that suits the context and aim. Then give students a rationale, clear instructions, opportunity for questions. Gently lead the exercise.
- Process the practice afterwards by:
  1. Journaling concerning their experience
  2. Having students talk in pairs about their experience
  3. Having a class conversation

An example of this applied in the field of economics is given by Professor Daniel Barbezat of

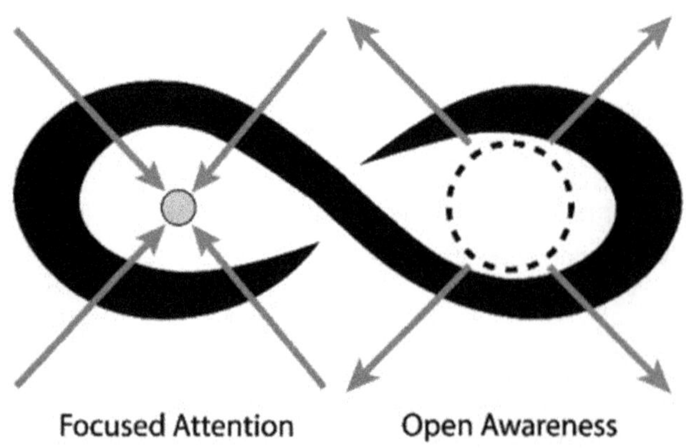

Fig. 2.2 Lemniscate of attention

the Economics Department at Amherst College who uses contemplative practices to engage students in examining their own behavior. In economics, for example, many models assume that the gains of others worsen our utility since we place our self in relation to others; by providing for others, we harm ourselves. This "relative income hypothesis" is one of the ways economists have tried to explain the rather meager gain in reported well-being that comes with overall income gains. When students first hear this, it makes sense to them. In fact, when they are asked whether they would give more to others than they would receive, more than half the class rejects the opportunity. However, after some reflection, loving-kindness meditation, and a guided introspection on gratitude, only one or two students still chose to deny the others more than they would receive; all the others gladly provide the relative gain. These exercises not only provide the students insights into the models and articles containing assumptions about relative income, they also provide an opportunity to notice that preferences are dynamic and are affected by one's relationship to the world. In fact, from these exercises, students become keenly aware of implications of the behavioral assumptions of economic models, something that they took for granted prior to these exercises.

The development of such course-specific contemplative practices is of special significance in making a strong case that contemplation enhances learning, and so contributes not only to the generic capacities of students, but also to their understanding and mastery of course material.

Compassion and Community: Cultivating Empathy Support and Compassionate Action

Finally, it is crucial that contemplative education not be misunderstood as aloof or disconnected from life. Indeed, contemplative exercises such as the one described above by Daniel Barbezat enhance empathy and compassionate connection to others, which can shape ethical action (see Hofmann, Grossman, & Hinton, 2011). The third domain of contemplative pedagogy is, therefore, directed to the cultivation of compassion and altruistic behavior (Keltner, 2009). Research on this has been recently undertaken by the Center for Compassion and Altruism Research and Education (CCARE) at Stanford University using an eight-session compassion training designed by Thupten Jinpa (Jazaieri et al., 2014). The reports on this work given at the 2010 Stanford University CCARE/Dalai Lama conference were very encouraging.[6]

Larger Implications of Contemplative Education

Inclusion of contemplative methods in higher education will, I believe, go a long way toward addressing an imbalance increasingly recognized in higher education. In short, the inner life of our students is sorely neglected. In his book *Excellence without a Soul*, Harry Lewis (2007), former dean of Harvard College, explains that "Harvard and our other great universities lost sight of the essential purpose of undergraduate education" (p. xiv). They have forgotten that they are there to help students "learn who they are, to search for a larger purpose for their lives, and to leave college as better human beings" (p. xiv). He goes on to declare that "students are not soulless, but their university is" (p. 18).

In their new book *Cultivating the Spirit: How College can Enhance Students' Inner Lives*, Alexander and Helen Astin and Jennifer Lindholm (2011) of UCLA's Higher Education Research Institute report from their research that more than eight out of ten students say "an important reason for attending college is to find my purpose in life" (p. 225 Kindle edition). The authors hold up meditation and self-reflection as a valuable means of developing direction in life as well as a sense for meaning and purpose. In other words, the laments of Lewis and others

[6]CCARE at Stanford University, http://ccare.stanford.edu/content/scientific-explorations-compassion-and-altruism. And also http://ccare.stanford.edu/programs/research-projects

concerning the soullessness of the university can be significantly addressed by a new emphasis on the contemplative and reflective in higher education.

From the Evaluation of the Contemplative Practice Fellowship Program

The Center for Contemplative Mind in Society completed a comprehensive evaluation of the Fellowship Program in early 2011. Its results are instructive beyond the specific program itself.[7] From the survey and telephone interviews, and in particular in response to a question concerning the value of using contemplative practice, a variety of views were offered by professors using contemplative pedagogy. Those interviewed described how their courses with contemplative practice had a positive reputation on campus and were recommended to other students. The value of contemplative practice was experienced, instructors said, as "self-validating." This meant that the practice itself led to such clear benefits for the students that external evidence from research studies was of secondary importance. A typical professor might begin very tentatively, but after positive student reactions, might then augment the amount of time spent with contemplative exercises.

One neuroscience researcher and professor of psychology reported that two aspects of the exercises seemed of special value to his students. The first was the training of attention, which is such a fundamental aspect of contemplative practice. He remarked, "Attention training really is a core aspect." He went on to say, "Distraction is the sea that they're swimming in." Yet even in an introductory course, with a very modest portion of time given contemplative exercise, the instructor found that students did benefit from the practice. In his opinion, a second type of contemplative practice (those directed toward compassion and altruism) was perhaps even of greater importance. The instructor noted:

> Despite all the cultural stereotypes, the current generation of college students is hungry for connecting in a meaningful way, to really find ways to make a difference in the world, and especially ways that address human suffering and enhance human portion. They don't know how best to do that, and they're often inarticulate, of course, but they seek ways to cultivate their own compassion and have it legitimized as part of higher education. It's really about caring for each other and making the world a livable place.

Toward a Theory of Contemplative Pedagogy

An essential but underdeveloped area is the theory of contemplative education. As this field develops, it will become increasingly important to have not only evidence of contemplation's efficacy, but we also will need an adequate theory of contemplative education to undergird both research and teaching. One can begin to see the broad outlines of such a theory. It will have several parts. Repetition, whether physical or mental, is known to affect brain structure. The theory of neural plasticity has become well established and is an area of active research. The practice of repetitively focusing one's attention on the breath, on a line of text, or an external object or process can be understood within this context. Neural plasticity provides a mechanism whereby not only learning can take place, but entirely new or enhanced capacities are developed within the brain. We can recall Goethe's line, "Every object, well contemplated, opens a new organ in us." Human mental faculties are not fixed or inert, but rather they are open to development by repeated practice. Neural plasticity provides a way to understand the physical foundations for this. Once one appreciates the power of repetitive mental practice, contemplative exercises as a means for the cultivation of cognitive and affective capacities make great sense (see MLERN, 2012).

I also see the stage development theories of Robert Kegan and Jack Mezirow, which I have already mentioned, as offering an important framework for a theory of contemplative pedagogy that

[7] The full report can be found at the Center website www.contemplativemind.org

views contemplative exercises as aiding students in moving from one affective, cognitive, or epistemological stage to another (see Roeser & Zelazo, 2012).

In my view, interest in the uses of contemplation in teaching, learning, and research is burgeoning for the good reason that it is a genuine aid to education at many levels, but especially in higher education. It will be critical to meet that growing interest with a wide range of programs and research of the highest quality. As the use of contemplative pedagogy increases, we can also expect that the work done will come under increasing scrutiny. It is, therefore, imperative that we not only develop program initiatives that will reach a wide audience in the academy, but that we also ensure that sound educational rationales are offered, and wherever possible that contemplative methods are backed up by high-quality scientific and social science research.

References

Astin, A. W., Astin, H. S., & Lindholm, J. A. (2011). *Cultivating the spirit: How college can enhance students' inner lives*. San Francisco, CA: Jossey-Bass.

Combs, A. editor, (2010) *Journal of Consciousness Studies*, Vol. 17. Exeter, England: Imprint Academic.

Craig, B.A. (2011). *Contemplative practice in higher education: An assessment of the Contemplative Practice Fellowship Program 1997–2009*. Retrieved from http://www.contemplativemind.org/admin/wp-content/uploads/2012/09/academic_fellowships_evaluation.pdf

Descartes, R. (1993). *Meditations on first philosophy* (D. A. Cress, Trans.). Indianapolis, IN: Hackett.

Dreyfus, G. (2003). *The sound of two hands clapping: The education of a Tibetan Buddhist monk*. Los Angeles, CA: University of California Press.

Eccles, J. S., & Roeser, R. W. (2014). School and community influences on human development. In M. H. Boorstein & M. E. Lamb (Eds.), *Developmental psychology: An advanced textbook* (7th ed.). Hillsdale, NJ: Erlbaum.

Goethe, J. W. (1988). *Scientific studies* (D. Miller, Trans.). New York, NY: Suhrkamp.

Gravois, J. (2005). Meditate on it. *Chronicle of Higher Education, 52*(9), 1–7.

Greenberg, M. T., & Harris, A. R. (2012). Nurturing mindfulness in children and youth: Current state of research. *Child Development Perspectives, 6*, 161–166.

Hadot, P. (1995). *Philosophy as a way of life: Spiritual exercises from Socrates to Foucault* (M. Chase, Trans.). New York, NY: Blackwell.

Hadot, P. (2002). *What is ancient philosophy?* (M. Chase, Trans.). Cambridge, MA: Harvard University Press.

Harrington, A. (2008). *The cure within: A history of mind-body medicine*. New York, NY: W.W. Norton.

Helberg, N., Heyes, C. J., & Rohel, J. (2009). Thinking through the body: Philosophy, yoga, and physical education. *Teaching Philosophy, 32*(3), 263–284.

Hofmann, S. G., Grossman, P., & Hinton, D. E. (2011). Loving-kindness and compassion meditation: Potential for psychological interventions. *Clinical Psychology Review, 31*, 1126–1132.

Hölzel, B. K., Lazar, S. W., Gard, T., Schuman-Olivier, Z., Vago, D. R., & Ott, U. (2011). How does mindfulness meditation work? Proposing mechanisms of action from a conceptual and neural perspective. *Perspectives on Psychological Science, 6*, 537–559.

James, W. (1890). *The principles of psychology* (Vol. 1). New York, NY: Henry Holt.

Jazaieri, H., McGonigal, K., Jinpa, T., Doty, J. R., Gross, J. J., & Goldin, P. R. (2014). A randomized controlled trial of compassion cultivation training: Effects on mindfulness, affect, and emotion regulation. *Motivation and Emotion, 38*, 23–35.

Jennings, P., Lantieri, L., & Roeser, R. W. (2012). Supporting educational goals through cultivating mindfulness: Approaches for teachers and students. In P. M. Brown, M. W. Corrigan, & A. Higgins-D'Alessandro (Eds.), *Handbook of prosocial education* (pp. 371–397). Lanham, MD: Rowan & Littlefield.

Kabat-Zinn, J. (1990). *Full Catastrophe Living*. New York: Delacorte.

Kabat-Zinn, J. (2003). Mindfulness-based interventions in context: Past, present and future. *Clinical Psychology: Science and Practice, 10*, 144–156.

Kegan, R. (1982). *The evolving self: Problem and process in human development*. Boston, MA: Harvard University Press.

Keltner, D. (2009). *Born to be good*. New York, NY: Norton.

Kroll, K. (Ed.). (2010). Special issue: Contemplative teaching and learning. *New Directions for Community Colleges, 2010*(151), 1–113.

Lazar, S.W., Kerr, C.E., Wasserman, R.H., Gray, J.R., Greve, D.N., Treadway, M.T., … Fischl, B. (2005). Meditation experience is associated with increased cortical thickness. *NeuroReport, 16*, 1893–1897.

Lewis, H. (2007). *Excellence without a soul: Does liberal education have a future?* New York, NY: PublicAffairs.

Lutz, A., Dunne, J. D., & Davidson, R. J. (2007). Meditation and the neuroscience of consciousness. In P. D. Zelazo, M. Moscovitch, & E. Thompson (Eds.), *Cambridge handbook of consciousness* (pp. 499–555). Cambridge, England: Cambridge University Press.

Lutz, A.,Slagter, H. A., Dune, J. D., & Davidson, R. J. (2008). Attention Regulation and Monitoring in Meditation. *Trends in Cognitive Science*. (4) 163–169.

Lutz, A., Greischar, L. L., Rawlings, N. B., Ricard, M., & Davidson, R. J. (2004). Long-term meditators self-induce high-amplitude gamma synchrony during mental practice. *Proceedings of the National Academy of Sciences of the United States of America, 101*, 16369–16373.

Melrotra, R. (2005) *The Essential Dalai Lama.* New York, NY: Penguin.

Mezirow, J. (2000). *Learning as transformation: Critical perspectives on a theory in progress.* San Francisco, CA: Jossey-Bass.

Mind and Life Education Research Network (MLERN). (2012). Contemplative practices and mental training: Prospects for American education. *Child Development Perspectives, 6*, 146–153.

Parker, P. J., & Zajonc, A. (2010). *The heart of higher education: A call to renewal.* San Francisco, CA: Jossey Bass.

Rabten (1980). The life and teaching of Geshé Rabten: a Tibetan Lama's search for truth (B.A. Wallace, Ed. & Trans.). Boston, MA: Allen & Unwin.

Rewald, J. (1976). Paul Cezanne. Letters (S. Hacker, Trans.). New York, NY: Da Capo Press.

Roeser, R. W. (2005). An introduction to Hindu India's contemplative spiritual views on human motivation, selfhood, and development. In M. L. Maehr & S. A. Karabenick (Eds.), *Advances in motivation and achievement* (Religion and motivation, Vol. 14, pp. 297–345). New York, NY: Elsevier.

Roeser, R. W. (2013). Mindfulness and human development: Introduction to the special issue. *Journal of Human Development, 10*, 1–11.

Roeser, R. W. (2014). The emergence of mindfulness-based interventions (MBIs) in education. In T. Urdan & S. Karabenick (Eds.), *Advances in research on motivation* (18th ed.). New York, NY: Elsevier.

Roeser, R. W., & Pinela, C. (2014). Mindfulness and compassion training in adolescence: A developmental contemplative sciences perspective. *New Directions in Youth Development, 2014*(142), 9–30. doi:10.1002/yd.20094.

Roeser, R. W., Skinner, E., Beers, J., & Jennings, P. A. (2012). Mindfulness training and teachers' professional development: An emerging area of research and practice. *Child Development Perspectives, 6*(2), 167–173.

Roeser, R. W., & Zelazo, P. D. (2012). Contemplative science, education and child development: Introduction to the special section. *Child Development Perspectives, 6*, 143–145.

Schrödinger, E. (1967). *What is life? Mind and matter.* Cambridge, England: Cambridge University Press.

Shapiro, S. L., Brown, K. W., & Astin, J. (2011). Toward the integration of meditation into higher education: A review of research evidence. *Teachers College Record, 113*(3), 493–528.

Wisner, B. L., Jones, B., & Gwin, D. (2010). School-based meditation practices for adolescents: A resource for strengthening self-regulation, emotional coping, and self-esteem. *Children & Schools, 32*, 150–159.

Zajonc, A. (2004) *The New Physics and Cosmology. Dialogues with the Dalai Lama.*Oxford, England: Oxford University Press.

Zajonc, A. G. (2009). *Meditation as contemplative inquiry.* Great Barrington, MA: Lindisfarne Books.

Zelazo, P. D., & Lyons, K. E. (2012). The potential benefits of mindfulness training in early childhood: A developmental social cognitive neuroscience perspective. *Child Development Perspectives, 6*, 154–160.

Zylowska, L., Ackerman, D. L., Yang, M. H., Futrell, J. L., Horton, N. L., Hale, T. S., … & Smalley, S. L. (2008). Mindfulness meditation training in adults and adolescents with ADHD a feasibility study. *Journal of Attention Disorders, 11*, 737–746.

3 What Is Mindfulness? A Contemplative Perspective

Shinzen Young

Quick now, here, now, always—
A condition of complete simplicity
(Costing not less than everything)
And all shall be well

—*from T.S. Eliot's* (1942) "*Little Gidding*"

Introduction

One challenge in applying a scientific lens to the effects of mindfulness is that there has been much disagreement among scientists regarding what mindful awareness actually is (see Cullen, 2011; Grossman & Van Dam, 2011; Vago & Silbersweig, 2012; Bishop et al., 2004; Gethin, 2011; Milton, 2011). From the perspective of science, the most satisfactory definition of mindful awareness would be a biophysical one—couched in the language of mathematical equations, and modeling the neurocorrelates of mindful traits. Although there has been some progress in this area (Raffone et al., 2007), we are decades, if not centuries, away from that kind of rigor. But, in order to begin research on something, we have to first define it. So, it would seem that we are in a sort of *Catch-22* situation here. One way out is to begin with a tentative definition and then refine it over time. In this chapter, I offer a candidate for that and justify it from several points of view.

Mindfulness: The Word

It's important to remember that mindfulness is merely a word in the English language. As such, its meaning has evolved through time and it may denote different things in different situations. Prior to contact with Asian culture, the English word mindfulness meant something general like "heedful" or "aware of context." After contact, it could still be used in that general way, but more and more it has come to designate a very specific type of awareness (Gethin, 2011). It is mindfulness in that specialized sense that I seek to clarify in this article.

In the nineteenth century, "mindfulness" was used to translate the Pali[1] word *sati*. In the 1960s and 1970s, Westerners began going to Southeast Asia to learn mindfulness practices. They brought those practices back to the West and began to teach them within the doctrinal framework of Buddhism. In the 1980s and 1990s, it was discovered that those practices could be extracted from the cosmology of Buddhism and the cultural matrix of Southeast Asia. Mindful awareness practices (MAPs) started to be used

S. Young (✉)
University of Vermont, Burlington, VT, USA
e-mail: shinzen@meditationtraining.com

[1] Pali is the canonical language of Theravada, a form of Buddhism found in Southeast Asia.

K.A. Schonert-Reichl, R.W. Roeser (eds.), *Handbook of Mindfulness in Education*, Mindfulness in Behavioral Health, DOI 10.1007/978-1-4939-3506-2_3

within a secular context—as systematic ways to develop and apply useful attentional skills. MAPs became ever more prevalent in clinical settings for pain management (Young, 2006), addiction recovery (Hoppes, 2006; Rogojanski, Vettese, & Antony, 2011), stress reduction (Song, Lindquist, & Choi, 2010), and as an adjunct to psychotherapy (Kabat-Zinn, 2003; Weiss, Nordlie, & Siegel, 2005). Eventually it came to be understood that mindful awareness is a cultivatable skill with broad applications through all aspects of society, including education (Lozar-Glenn, 2010), sports (Murphy, 2012), business (Hunter & McCormick, 2008), even the training of soldiers (Rochman, 2009).

Although mindfulness was originally used to translate the Pali word *sati* (Sanskrit, *smṛti*), it can more loosely refer to a number of other related terms of Indian origin, for example the terms *smṛtyupasthāna* and *vipaśyanā*[2]). It can be contentious and confusing if we try to make the English word mindfulness correspond to exactly one Asian term. Here's why: although the Asian terms are closely related, they are not quite synonyms. Moreover, Southeast Asian, East Asian, and Tibetan traditions do not necessarily agree among themselves as to how to define those terms. Indeed, even within a given cultural area, there can be disagreement among different scholars and lineages as to what a given term specifically designates.

I and some other teachers (most notably Jon Kabat-Zinn [Wilks, 2014]) would prefer to not require that mindfulness directly correspond to any specific Asian term. I think of mindfulness as any growth process that is capable of bringing a person to a state of happiness independent of conditions based on acquiring and applying three attentional skills: concentration power, sensory clarity, and equanimity.

It's useful to remember that the word mindfulness without further qualifications can refer to any one or combination of three things: (1) a form of *awareness*, (2) the *practices* that elevate that form of awareness, and (3) guidelines *for applying* that awareness to specific perceptual, behavioral, or psycho-spiritual goals. When we wish to speak with precision, we could refer to the first of these as ***mindful awareness***, the second as ***mindful awareness practices***, and the third as a ***mindfulness application*** or a mindfulness-based path. Also, it is customary to distinguish state mindfulness (how mindful a person happens to be at a given time) from trait mindfulness (how mindful a person is in general) (Shapiro, Brown, Thoresen, & Plante, 2011).

Regarding mindfulness as a path to human flourishing (Seligman, 2011), I like to group its effects into five categories which I think of as five basic dimensions of human well-being. Mindful awareness can be used to:

1. Reduce physical suffering (Zeidan et al., 2011) or emotional suffering (van Son, Nyklicek, Pop, & Pouwer, 2011).
2. Elevate physical or emotional fulfillment (Wallace, 2005).
3. Achieve deep self-knowledge (Brown & Ryan, 2003).
4. Make positive changes in objective behavior (Dutton, 2008).
5. Develop a spirit of love and service towards others (Young, 2014).

Mindfulness as a path has two sides: the theoretical side and the practical side. The *practical* side involves organizing and packaging MAPs into dedicated programs that address the interests and needs of specific populations. The *theoretical* side seeks explanatory mechanisms: by merely directing attention in a certain way, a person can dissolve intense physical pain into a kind of flowing energy—and do so consistently (Young, 2006). How do we explain this? What specific mechanisms are involved? By merely directing attention in a certain way, a person can come to an empowering "I-Thou" relationship with their world. How do we explain this? What specific mechanisms are involved? By merely directing attention in a certain way, a person can break the spell of a long-standing destructive habit. How do we explain this? What specific mechanisms are involved?

[2]The Pali version of these would be *satipa hāna and vipassanā, respectively.*

Defining Mindful Awareness

There have been many attempts to develop an operational definition of mindful awareness (Bishop et al., 2004; Gethin, 2011; Milton, 2011). But the most commonly encountered definition of mindful awareness runs something along the lines of "present-centered, non-judgmental attention." Let's begin with that.

Definitions should be unambiguous. Different people may have different ideas as to what it means to be in the Now or what it means to be non-judgmental. Perhaps by reviewing a range of examples, we'll be able to bring some clarity to the subtle issues involved. Hopefully that will allow us to refine and rigorize our formulations.

Present-Centeredness

Example #1: Sight, Sound, and Body Are Now Consider the following. You focus your attention on physical sights, physical sounds, and body sensations as they arise. If you get caught up in a thought, you let go of that thought and bring your attention back to a physical sight, physical sound, or a body experience.

Clearly, sights, sounds, and body events keep you anchored in the present. Any non-present content will come up as thought—remembering, planning, rehearsing, fantasizing, and so forth.

So the practice described above would lead to present-centeredness. Indeed some people would define present-centered in terms of a practice like this. In such formulations, present-centered means being grounded in physical senses and body experience with little or no intrusive thought.

But consider yet another possibility.

Example #2: Breath Is Now You focus your attention on the sensation of breath at your nostrils. If your attention is pulled to anything else, you return to focusing on the breath. You try to detect each in-breath and each out-breath as a distinct event. You try to detect the very instant when each in-breath begins and when it ends, and likewise for each out-breath. In addition, you try to notice any tiny fluctuations that may occur during the course of the in- or out-breath. For many people, this practice might result in a tighter experience of presentness, relative to that of Example 1.

Analysis Let's make a careful analysis of these examples.

In both cases, you're intentionally focusing on a specific type of sensory experience—sensory experience that is intrinsically free of memory, planning, or fantasy content. Clearly you need concentration to do either exercise well. Conversely, either exercise will, with time, strengthen your concentration power.

Besides concentration power, are there any other attentional skills involved in these examples?

The first example might seem to mostly involve concentration. Attention wanders into thought, bring it back to sight, sound, body! It wanders again, bring it back! Each rep strengthens your concentration muscle.

But there does seem to be a new element in the second example. Here you're also being asked to make distinctions, discriminate sensory qualities, and detect temporally fleeting events. The reason that the second example represents a tighter experience of Now is twofold: (a) your information processing channel is being saturated with data points and (b) you're trying to detect subtle events. The first factor might be thought of as resolution power or discrimination ability. The second factor might be thought of as a sensitivity or detection ability. Both of these factors could be grouped within a more general category which, for lack of a better term, I will call "sensory clarity."

Sensory clarity involves resolution power and sensitivity. By resolution power, I mean the ability to distinguish qualitative, quantitative, and spatial differences. By sensitivity, I mean the ability to detect subtle sensory signals, spot fleeting events, monitor continuous rates of change and so forth.

Evidently, both concentration power and sensory clarity are basic attentional skills associated with being present-centered.

Example #3: Everything is Now The observant reader may have noticed that there's an inherent limitation in both of the examples presented so far. They both involve selectively focusing on a certain type of sensory experience. Or, more to the point, they both involve focusing away from a certain type of sensory experience—thoughts. Now it is certainly true that, in terms of content, thoughts can be about past, future, or fantasy. But as tangible sensory events (mental image and mental talk), they occur in the present. It would be satisfying if we could be present-centered with regard *to all* sensory events, including thoughts.[3] To include thoughts as part of "Now," you need to do two things.

1. Be clearly aware when each thought begins and when it ends.
2. Not be caught in the content of the thought as it is happening.

It's the "caughtness" in the thought that pulls us out of the present and into past, future, and fantasy content.

The first point involves an attention skill we're already familiar with—sensory clarity. The second point introduces a new element—"not-caughtness." Not-caughtness is a kind of hands-off relationship, a balance point that avoids both pushing down and grasping on. Our technical term for this skill will be *equanimity* (from the Latin for "inner balance").

So it would seem that we can be present-centered without restriction with regard to sensory content as long as we have:

1. Enough clarity to detect arisings and passings, and to discriminate sensory qualities.
2. Enough equanimity to avoid getting caught up in the content of our sensory experience.

In the first and second examples of Now, you needed concentration power to focus away from thought. But in the third example, you're not focusing away from anything and there's no specified thing that you're coming back to as an anchor. You're practicing what's sometimes referred to as Choiceless Awareness or Open Presence. Does concentration have any role in such practices?

Well, it turns out that concentration comes in several types. One type is *durative*. Durative concentration involves holding attention in a restricted domain for an extended period. The domain may be qualitatively restricted (just one class of sensory experience as in Example 1). The domain may also be spatially restricted (just one location as in Example 2).

The durative type is what most people think of when they hear the word concentration. But there's also a *momentary* type of concentration. This involves briefly but intently focusing on each sensory event as it comes up. Even though your attention broadly floats within a wide range of sensory experience, you briefly "taste" a moment of high concentration with each thing as it arises.

The momentary type of concentration power is very important in traditional Southeast Asian mindfulness practice—so important that there's even a technical term for it in Pali. The term is *khaṇikasamādhi*.

So it would seem that, one way or another, concentration enters into any definition of present-centeredness. If we define present-centered as selective attention away from thought, then we need the durative type of concentration power to hold that direction. If we define present-centered so it's applicable to any type of sensory content, then momentary concentration is relevant.

We also saw that if we wish to include thoughts and emotions in our focus range, we need to utilize the equanimity skill so as not to get caught up in their content.

[3] In this chapter, the term "sensory" refers not just to sight, hearing, smell, taste, or physical touch, it also refers mental images (visual thought), mental talk (auditory thought), and emotional body sensations.

Here's a subtle question. Suppose we wish to be present-centered by focusing away from thought; is equanimity still of any relevance?

The answer is yes because equanimity aids concentration. There's a general principle at work here. Say A is your focus range and B is a distraction. To keep your focus on A, it's helpful if you can let B come and go in the background, without having to do anything about B. But that requires equanimity with B. Your concentration and clarity are going to A but your equanimity surrounds B, allowing B to "do its thing" in the background while you focus on and vividly know A.

It would seem that, to be present-centered in the broadest meaning of that term, we need three related but conceptually distinct attention skills:

1. Concentration Power
2. Sensory Clarity
3. Equanimity

Conversely, any systematic exercise that develops these three skills will allow us to be present-centered with regards to any and all sensory experiences.

Perhaps these skills are in fact the defining characteristic of mindful awareness and "present-centeredness" (as illustrated by the three examples given above) is just a consequence of applying these skills in certain ways.

Non-Judgment

Before considering that possibility, let's look carefully at what we mean by the term "non-judgment."

Example #1: No "Second Arrow" Consider the following situation. You are bombarded by the outer senses (sight, sound, physical touch), but these cause no inner reaction—no judging thoughts, no pleasant or unpleasant reactive emotions. For example, even if physical pain arises, it triggers no negative tapes, no disquieting images, no emotional body sensations of tear, fear, or irritation.

In the traditional metaphor, the physical pain is the "first arrow." The first arrow is shot at you by external circumstances, but you have, by internal volition, decided not to shoot yourself with a "second arrow" of reactive thoughts and emotions (Nyanaponika, 2000). The assumption here is that you may not always be able to prevent first arrow (caused by undesirable situations) but you can learn how not to amplify it by shooting yourselves with a second one (reactive thoughts and emotions).

This example is a candidate for what it might mean to be non-judgmental, but it immediately raises several questions.

1. Is it even possible to get to such a state of non-reactivity?
2. If we claim that non-judgment is good, then judgment must be bad. So aren't we judging judging (and hence contradicting ourselves)?
3. Even if it were possible to attain a high degree of non-reactivity, is such a state in fact even desirable?

Let's explore each of these questions.

Anyone who has looked within knows that judgments and reactions arise constantly and naturally. How could one ever get to the state of "No Second Arrow"? One possibility is to keep focusing away from judgments and reactions until the habit of reacting weakens and eventually dies off on its own. In order for that to happen, you would have to be willing to let the judging arise and pass in the background while you focused away on something else. In other words, you would need a sort of "second-order" non-judging—you don't judge the fact that you're judging. Clearly this strategy for non-judgment requires concentration power (which allows you to focus away) and equanimity (i.e., not judging the judging).

Yet another possibility would be to turn toward the judgment and deconstruct it. You could break the judgment into its components (mental image, mental talk, and emotional body sensation) and untangle them. You could then observe each component in great detail and open so fully to it that it eventually dissolves into a flow of energy.

Clearly, the turn toward approach would require a lot of clarity and equanimity.

These considerations address questions one (how to achieve a state of no second arrow) and two (judging the judging). What about question three? Judgments have a role in nature. Should we even want to be free from judgment? The answer to this question depends critically on what we mean by "free from judgment." Free could mean:

- Never experience judgment regardless of circumstance.
- Have the ability to suspend judgment when that's appropriate.
- Have the ability to not *identify* with judgments even when they arise intensely.

The first outcome is dysfunctional. The second and third are empowering.

This answers question three. What's being sought is the ability to be non-judgmental. We're not being asked to enter an eternal suspension of critical thought.

The "No Second Arrow" example above shows us that the attentional skills needed to be non-judgmental (concentration, clarity, and equanimity) are exactly the attentional skills needed to be present-centered. This lends some credence to the notion that these skills may represent the basic dimensions of mindful awareness.

Example #2: Equanimity So far we've been assuming that "judgment" is a specific type of sensory event—an arising of reactive mental images, reactive mental talk, and reactive emotional body sensations. A case could be made that the specific mental images, mental talk, and emotional body sensations that constitute the sensory experience of judgment are in fact merely the tip of a deeper, more general phenomenon.

That deeper phenomenon is a kind of pervasive subtle self-interference within our sensory systems. It's a kind of viscosity or stickiness within the nervous system itself that affects both the outer senses (physical sight, physical sound, physical-type body sensations) and the inner senses (mental images, mental talk, and emotional-type body sensations). A very loose analogy might be made with reactance and resistance in an electrical circuit. Think of sensory experience as being like a flowing current. When the current should arise, the system impedes that by pushing down. When the current should die away, the system impedes that by holding on a bit. Moreover, as the current is flowing, there is a kind of coagulating around it.

A case could be made that this microscopic push and pull within the flow of sensory experience represents a deep and pervasive reactivity—a sort of "pre-mental judging."

When we're practicing "second-order non-judgmentalness," what we are in fact doing is allowing judgmental thoughts and emotions to come and go without pushing down as they arise, without holding on as they pass, and without tightening up as they continue.

Given these considerations I would claim that equanimity is a form of non-judgment that's deeper and more general than "No Second Arrow."

Introduction to the CCE Paradigm

It would seem that three skills, concentration power, sensory clarity, and equanimity, are necessary and sufficient for a truly general theory of "present-centered, non-judgmentalness." Perhaps this core skillset could serve as a more fine-grained and quantifiable definition of mindful awareness. Let's use the acronym "CCE" as a convenient handle for this paradigm.

Let's flesh out the picture a bit.

Concentration

You can think of concentration power as the ability to attend to what you deem relevant at a given time. People often have certain assumptions around the notion of concentration.

- Spatial assumption: To concentrate means to focus on something spatially small (say, the breath sensation at the tip of your nose).
- Temporal assumption: To concentrate means to hold one experience for a long time without

interruption (maintain unbroken concentration on a mantra for, say, 20 min).

- Suppression assumption: To concentrate on a certain thing means to push everything else away.
- Effort assumption: To concentrate requires constant effort.

None of these assumptions are implied by the way I have described concentration power.

- Spatial extent of concentration may be wide as well as narrow. For example, attempting to focus on your whole body at once builds an expansive type of concentration.
- Momentarily high focus on whatever happens to call your attention can also build a taste of concentration. As mentioned previously, according to the great twentieth century mindfulness master Mahasi Sayadaw, such momentary high concentration (*khaṇikasamādhi*) is one of the defining characteristics of mindfulness. It's one of the things that makes "noting whatever comes up" different from being lost in wandering mind.
- To concentrate on a certain thing (selective attention) is not the same as trying to get rid of everything else (push distractions away). You can give the spotlight to a specific dancer without having to get the other performers off stage. Indeed, allowing distractions to come and go without push and pull is a facet of equanimity.
- It is true that learning how to concentrate may *initially* require a certain amount of effort, but once you've done enough practice, it becomes effortless and automatic. The goal is to elevate your base level of concentration—i.e., how concentrated you are in ordinary life when you're not particularly trying to be concentrated.

Clarity

There are three sides to sensory clarity:

1. Discrimination
2. Detection
3. Penetration

The first two are relatively straightforward. Appreciating the third may require some hands-on experience.

Discrimination (i.e., Resolution Power) To appreciate the utility of discrimination, you can do an experiment. Say you know that a certain situation may lead to an emotional challenge—but you're not in that situation yet, so you're still okay. As you move into that situation, emotion may begin to arise. If that happens, ask yourself:

What part of this experience involves mental images?
What part of this experience involves mental talk?
What part of this experience involves sensations in my body?
Where are those sensations located and what are their qualities?

At some point, the emotional experience may become intense. Try to keep track of it in terms of the above questions. Hopefully you won't become overwhelmed, but if you do become overwhelmed, ask yourself the following question:

At the moment of overwhelm, was I still able to distinguish:
What part of my emotion was visual thought
What part was auditory thought
And what part was body sensation

In most cases, the answer will be no. In other words, at the moment of transition between "I can handle this" to "I can't handle this," there will usually be a sudden and dramatic disappearance of sensory discrimination. The mental images, mental talk, and emotional body sensations are still there but suddenly you can no longer separate out what is what.

We can represent this compactly:

Overwhelm → Loss of sensory discrimination (read → as "implies")

This is an empirical truth. By that, I mean that it can be confirmed by repeatedly doing experiments like the one described above.

Conveniently, the reverse of the above statement is also true.

No loss of sensory discrimination $\rightarrow$ No overwhelm

Moreover, your baseline of discriminatory clarity can be strengthened by systematic practice. Baseline in this case means how clear you are when you are not particularly making an effort to be clear. Summing it up:

Systematic practice $\rightarrow$ Stronger baseline of sensory discrimination $\rightarrow$ Dramatic reduction in baseline of distress

Taken together, this leads to an extraordinary conclusion: The stresses of life are unavoidable; suffering because of them is optional.

Detection (i.e., Sensitivity) The detection dimension of clarity involves:

- An intensity-related aspect: the ability to detect subtle faint signals.
- A time-related aspect: the ability to detect the instant when a sensory event arises or the instant when it passes. (This can lead to an abiding in Absolute Now—as described in the Eliot quote at the beginning of this article.)

Penetration Burmese mindfulness masters sometimes describe awareness as being like a dart or arrow. The object of awareness (a sound, a mental image, a body sensation, and such) is like a target. According to these masters, the original meaning of the Pali word *satipaṭṭhāna* is "to penetrate with awareness":

sati—awareness, attention

paṭṭhāna—to thrust against (from *sthāna*—stand [in the transitive sense] and *upa*—upon, against)

Those who work within this paradigm hurl attention into each sensory event, giving awareness enough momentum to penetrate that target, i.e., know it through and through down to the tiniest level of detail.

Equanimity

Equanimity is a fundamental skill for self-exploration and emotional intelligence. It is a deep and subtle concept frequently misunderstood and easily confused with suppression, apathy, or inexpressiveness.

Equanimity comes from the Latin word *aequus*, meaning balanced, and *animus*, meaning spirit or internal state. As an initial step in understanding this concept, let's consider for a moment its opposite: what happens when a person loses inner balance.

In the physical world we say a person has lost their balance if they fall to one side or another. In the same way you lose inner balance if you fall into one or the other of the following contrasting reactions:

- Suppression—A (internal or external) sensory experience arises and you attempt to cope with it by stuffing it down, denying it, tightening around it, etc. This is an aspect of what in Pali is called *dosa*, often translated as aversion.
- Identification—A (internal or external) sensory experience arises and you fixate on it, hold onto it inappropriately, not letting it pass in a natural rhythm. This is an aspect of what in Pali is called *rāga*, often translated as craving.

Between suppression on one side and identification on the other lies a third possibility, the balanced state of non-self-interference—equanimity.

The Effects of Equanimity Equanimity belies the adage that you cannot "have your cake and eat it too." When you apply equanimity to unpleasant experiences, they flow more readily and as a result cause less suffering. When you apply equanimity to pleasant experiences, they also flow more readily and as a result deliver deeper fulfillment. The same skill positively affects both sides of the sensation picture. Furthermore, when inner states are experienced with equanimity, they cease to drive and distort outer behavior and instead assume their proper function of motivating and directing it. Thus equanimity plays a critical role in changing negative behaviors such as substance and alcohol abuse, compulsive eating, violence, and so forth.

You can have equanimity with thoughts as well as body sensations. You can let sense and nonsense arise and pass without suppression or identification. This will result in a new, intuitive kind of knowing (Sanskrit, *prajñā*). Equanimity with thought allows you to work through the drivenness to think. When compulsive eaters work through the drive to eat, they don't stop eating, they simply eat in a new and better way. When compulsive thinkers (i.e., just about everyone) work through the drive to think, they don't stop thinking, they just begin to think in a new and better way. This strategy for developing insight was independently discovered by three different groups: the ancient Greek Pyrrhonian Skeptics (*epoche*), medieval Christian monastics (*docta ignorantia*), and Tang Dynasty Chan masters (*kōan* practice).

Equanimity, Apathy, and Suppression Equanimity is not apathy. Equanimity involves non-interference with the natural flow of *sensory experience*. Apathy implies indifference to the controllable outcome of *objective events*. Thus, although similar sounding, equanimity and indifference are actually opposites. Equanimity frees up internal energy for responding to external situations.

Equanimity, by definition, is also the opposite of suppression, because equanimity involves giving yourself permission to fully experience your senses. What about outwardly expressing what you're feeling? This issue here is freedom. Equanimity gives you the freedom to externally express or not, depending on what is appropriate to the situation.

Physical Analogies for Equanimity Developing equanimity is in some ways analogous to:

- Reducing friction in a mechanical system (Equanimity = $1/F$).
- Reducing viscosity in a hydrodynamic system (Equanimity = $1/\mu$).
- Reducing resistance in a DC circuit (Equanimity = $1/R$).
- Reducing stiffness in a spring (Equanimity = $1/k$).

Extending these analogies, perfect equanimity would be analogous to "superconductivity" within all your sensory circuits.

A Modern Metaphor

Imagine you possess a television set with several rather undesirable features. First, it has poor tuning characteristics. It doesn't latch on to a given channel very well. Instead it skips around uncontrollably. So it's difficult to watch any program long enough to follow the story. On top of that, the screen has really low-definition—the picture is unclear and blotchy. Finally, the wires are very thin so there is a lot of electrical impedance. This wastes energy, creates heat, and occasionally blows out your fuses.

That's the bad news. Here's the good news. The manufacturer offers a free upgrade! Well, almost free. You won't have to pay any money for the upgrade but you will need to invest some time and energy in order to qualify.

If you're willing to do that, the manufacturer will provide you with a new, incomparably better system. The new system has uber-stable tuning power, a hi-def screen, and superconducting circuits.

The meaning of this analogy should be clear:

TV Set	Consciousness
Good tuning	Concentration power
Hi-Def	Sensory Clarity
Low impedance	Equanimity
Heat	Unnecessary suffering
Energy waste	Your life vitality is dissipated through subtle, subliminal self-interference
Blow fuse	You become overwhelmed by subjective suffering or behave in a way you later regret
Manufacturer	*Deus sive Natura* (as Spinoza would have said)

Does the Definition Work?

Is the CCE paradigm a good candidate for a starter definition of mindful awareness?

First let's consider what characteristics a good definition of mindful awareness should possess. Four things come to mind. I'd like a definition of mindful awareness to be intuitive, quantitative, explanatory, and historical.

1. *Intuitive.* By intuitive I mean easily understood by the average person. After all, if mindfulness is a good thing, then we want people from all educational and social backgrounds to embrace its practice. This will be easier if mindful awareness can be described in a way that is relevant to most people's experience. Stated in somewhat crass terms, we would like our definition of mindful awareness to be such that the average person will readily "buy into" it.
2. *Quantitative.* By quantitative, I mean quantifiable in a rigorous way. Something that a hard-nosed scientist would be comfortable with, something "operational"—ideally something measurable in biophysical terms.
3. *Explanatory.* By explanatory I mean convenient for forming hypotheses that explain observed effects. Previously, I listed five broad headings under which the effects of mindfulness could be classified: (1) reduced suffering; (2) elevated fulfillment; (3) deep self-knowledge; (4) fostering positive behavior; and (5) a spirit of love and service towards others. Each of those headings contain numerous subheadings. Are the mechanisms that explain this wide spectrum of effects identical or are different mechanisms at work for different effects? In either case, we would like our definition of mindful awareness to help explain, in a plausible and fine-grained way, how general attention skills can foster specific improvements.
4. *Historical.* By historical I mean historically heuristic. Something is heuristic if it is capable of providing insight. A historically heuristic definition of mindfulness would allow us to understand its relationship to other practices that have been known throughout history and across cultures.

Is the CCE Paradigm Intuitive?

Asked to reflect on their life experience, most people can recall at least one of the following: an instance of spontaneous high concentration, an instance of spontaneous sensory vividness, an instance of dropping into gentle matter-of-factness during a high-stress event, <u>or</u> they can recall suffering due to lack of concentration ability, suffering due to sensory flooding, suffering that occurred when something pleasant turned into something unpleasant due to neediness. The former three are associated with greater happiness and functionality, while the latter three are associated with the opposite of that. Once a person realizes that they have <u>already</u> experienced either the advantages associated with having mindfulness or the disadvantages associated with lacking mindfulness, they can readily appreciate the relevance of its practice. Put another way, the CCE paradigm is Socratic in that it assumes the student already knows something about the subject.

Is the CCE Paradigm Quantifiable?

It's easy to assume that mindful awareness is a scalar, a one-dimensional phenomenon. But it may be vector-like, i.e., multidimensional. In that case, several questions immediately come to mind:

- How do we capture all and only the key features of mindful awareness in a (presumably small) set of components?
- How do we measure those components?
- Can we ascribe a norm (overall size) to that vector in a natural way?

I believe that concentration, clarity, and equanimity capture the key features of mindful awareness but are they measurable by the rigorous standards of physical science? Not as things stand now. So my definition fails to be quantitative. However, I would suggest that as our knowledge of neurophysiology grows, concentration, clarity, and equanimity may be good candidates for an agreed-upon operational definition. Here's why.

Concentration power is essentially selective attention. A lot of basic science has already been done on attention (Posner, 2012). Its underlying neural networks have been somewhat classified and can be probed using standard tasks.

It should be possible to devise a battery of standard performance tasks that gauge a person's state and trait levels of concentration ability, providing an operational definition for concentration power (or at very least those aspects of concentration that are relevant to the endeavor of mindfulness).

Sensory resolution is routinely gauged through standardized tasks, i.e., somatic spatial resolution using a two-point discriminating task or temporal resolution using a flicker threshold task. Moreover, the ability to note the very instant when a sensory event arises and the very instant when it passes are important themes in mindfulness practice. It should be possible to devise operational tasks that measure that.

Admittedly, other more subtle forms of sensory discrimination power (such as distinguishing visual thought from auditory thought or detecting rates of change) may be more difficult to gauge by objective tasks, but with some imagination…?

As you'll recall, I define equanimity as a global parameter applicable to all sensory circuits—inner (visual thought, auditory thought, emotional body sensation) as well as outer (physical sight, physical sound, physical body sensation). Perhaps one way to physically measure equanimity would be to consider its opposite, a quality that some scientists call "stickiness" (Koenigsberg, 2010). Stickiness refers to moment-by-moment inappropriate holdings in the processing of sensory data. It's possible that stickiness can be monitored in terms of a physical brainwave phenomenon known as the attentional blink. If so, then equanimity could, at least in part, be measured as the reciprocal of that parameter. Another possible candidate for a quantitative measure of equanimity might be the ability to maintain global and profound physical relaxation while one is subjected to intense stimuli. Electromyography could be used to physically quantify that.

Is the CCE Paradigm Explanatory?

As I mentioned earlier, I like to think of a mindfulness-based path as having a theoretical side and a practical side. The practical side involves instruction for applying mindful awareness towards specific goals. The theoretical side involves creating an explanatory model for how mindful awareness brings about those goals.

It would be unreasonable in a short chapter such as this to attempt a detailed description for each of the five effects of mindfulness: (1) reduced suffering; (2) elevated fulfillment; (3) deep self-knowledge; (4) fostering positive behavior; and (5) a spirit of love and service towards others. Instead let's briefly explore one theme: How concentration power, sensory clarity, and equanimity working together make it possible to experience discomfort without experiencing suffering.

I posit that any experience of discomfort, whether mild or intense, involves one or a combination of four sensory elements: (1) uncomfortable physical sensations in your body, (2) uncomfortable emotional sensations in your body, (3) negative talk in your mind, and (4) negative images in your mind. For simplicity, let's say that the maximum intensity of any of these elements is represented by 10. Without loss of generality, let's assume a worst case scenario: all four elements are maximally intense. People will do anything to escape from that level of body–mind distress. And if it continues, their thoughts may move toward suicide. If the cause of the discomfort cannot be eliminated and the symptoms cannot be palliated, are you then doomed to meaningless abject suffering? Not necessarily.

Applying Sensory Clarity One factor that reduces suffering is sensory clarity. Without special training, mental image, and mental talk, physical body sensations and emotional body sensations get tangled and mutually reinforce each other. In other words, they multiply together, giving you the *impression* that you are suffering at level $10 \times 10 \times 10 \times 10$. But through training, you can learn to untangle the elements that constitute moment-to-moment experience. First, you learn to separate the body elements from the mind elements. Then, in the body, you learn to separate the purely physical sensations from the emotional sensations. Further, with regard to the mind, you also learn to separate visual thought (mental imagery) from auditory thought (mental talk). If your sensory clarity skills are good, this will dramatically reduce your suffering because the elements are no longer multiplying with each other. You're experiencing only what's *actually* going on, not what *seems* to be going on. What seems to be going on is: $10 \times 10 \times 10 \times 10 = 10{,}000$. What's actually going on is a linear combination: $10 + 10 + 10 + 10 = 40$—something incomparably smaller. In other words, untangling the sensory strands takes you from multiplicative overwhelm to additive manageability.

Applying Concentration Power If you have really good concentration power, you can focus on just your physical sensations or emotional sensations, or just your mental images or just your mental talk. That way, at any given instant, you would only have to experience a single sensory strand, resulting in a reduction in distress. If you have a high level of concentration ability, you would only have to deal with a single 10 at any given time. The other three 10s will have temporarily faded into the background due to high concentration.

Applying Equanimity Let's say that you're able to focus on just one of the 10s. There is still significant suffering because it's at maximum. Now you bring equanimity to that strand. That means you ask consciousness to open to its own creation, to stop fighting the experience it is producing. You try to greet each arising of that strand with a gentle matter-of-factness. At some point you fall into a deep altered state where consciousness stops fighting with itself, time slows down and everything gets very still.

At that point, you begin to notice yet another multiplicative effect. Each 10 is itself a product of two things: <u>actual</u> distress multiplied by <u>resistance</u> to that distress. Since resistance is the reciprocal of equanimity, as equanimity goes up, resistance goes down, and, hence, the perceived suffering goes down.

It turns out that the actual distress is often quite small relative to the size of the resistance factor i.e., the perceived 10 could be the result of actual distress at level 0.1 encountering a resistance level of 1000!

So if you can bring a lot of mindful awareness to discomfort, you're left with what was actually there all along, before the amplifying factors of tangle, tighten, and scatter kicked in. What was always there is a kind of energy flow that causes rather little real suffering.

(Please note: The math in this section is only meant to be suggestive—a sort of heuristic local linear approximation.)

Is the CCE Paradigm Historical?

I would claim that the CCE paradigm gives us a convenient framework for viewing mindfulness over time and across cultures.

Pre-History One way to characterize pre-literate tribal life might be: life was simple, life was uncomfortable, life was full of things one could not understand.

Simplicity means less to think about, which might push a person to be more focused on the moment (concentration and sensory clarity). Discomfort that cannot be removed could push one toward bodily equanimity (body stops fighting with pain, cold, fatigue, bugs, etc.). Not being able to figure out how nature works might push one toward mental equanimity (surrender to the mystery, mind stops struggling to get answers and falls into "*epoche*"—the suspension of the drivenness to know).

So the daily life of our remote ancestors had built into it certain forces that might push them in the direction of mindful awareness. Does all this mean that our remote ancestors were mindfulness adepts? Perhaps not. But it does support the notion that mindfulness is in some ways natural for humans.

History The fact that base level concentration ability could be elevated through systematic practice was probably first discovered in ancient India. Indic languages contain two commonly used words for an intentionally cultivated highly focused state: *samādhi* and *dhyāna*.

Either through diffusion or independent discovery, cultivated concentration came to be recognized within all the major civilizations of the Eastern Hemisphere. This is evidenced by the fact that those civilizations have technical terms denoting intentionally cultivated states of high focus.

- Sanskrit: *samādhi*, *dhyāna*
- Greek: *hesychia* (Eastern Orthodox Christianity)
- Latin: *recollectio* (Roman Catholic Christianity)
- Arabic: *Dhikr*/*Zikr* (Islamic Sufism)
- Hebrew: *kavana* or *devekut* (Jewish Kabbalah and Hasidut)
- Chinese: *shǒuyì* (Daoism)

In modern English, one colloquial term for a state of high concentration is to "be in the zone." Typically one hears this in the context of performance—music, sports, dance, and so forth. Also researchers within the positive psychology movement have shown that a state of high concentration is intrinsically rewarding regardless of what is being focused on. They referred to that situation being in a "flow state" (Csikszentmihalyi, 1994).

The beginnings of equanimity can be found in the widespread practices of asceticism and shamanic ordeal. It is also adumbrated in certain Greek philosophies such as Stoicism (*ataraxia*) and Skepticism (*epoche*), and the Christian practice of *apatheia*. However, these practices often conflate equanimity with non-expressiveness, white-knuckle endurance, and indifference to circumstances, and thus may fail to capture its essence.

So that's the big picture regarding concentration and equanimity across cultures. What about the sensory clarity piece? When did that enter the picture? There are hints of it in the Orthodox Christian practice of *nepsis* (sober observation). But the really big breakthrough occurred in North India with the discoveries of Prince Siddhartha Gautama, known to history as the Buddha.

The Buddha Painted in ridiculously broad strokes, the Buddha's historical contributions can be analyzed in terms of four processes: (1) he rejected certain things from his culture of birth, (2) he preserved certain things from his culture of birth, (3) he modified certain things from his culture of birth, and (4) he discovered several new and important things.

Among the things he rejected was the central role of authority as a basis of knowledge. Among the things he preserved were systematic focus exercises that develop high concentration power (the so-called "absorptions").

Among the things he modified was asceticism (Sanskrit *tapas*). Prior to the Buddha, there existed in India the belief that intentionally exposing oneself to discomfort purifies consciousness. The paradigm was: The more it hurts, the more it purifies. The Buddha both extended and refined this paradigm: The more equanimity (non-grasping) you bring to pain <u>or pleasure</u>, the more it purifies the substance of consciousness.

One of the new things he discovered is the principle of "Divide and Conquer," i.e., the liberating power of sensory clarity as described throughout this article.

So, a case could be made that the Buddha discovered mindfulness—if by mindfulness we mean the integrated package of concentration, clarity, and equanimity. As previously detailed, the value of high concentration had been widely known in human cultures. The beginnings of equanimity are adumbrated in ascetical practices, shamanic ordeals, stoic philosophy, and so forth. But it was apparently the Buddha who first realized the liberating potential of sensory clarity.

What sets mindfulness apart from other forms of meditation is its clear conceptual formulation of equanimity and its emphasis on sensory clarity. Conversely, to the extent that any growth process is capable of significantly elevating a person's concentration, clarity, and equanimity skills, to that extent it is a mindfulness awareness practice regardless of where it came from or what name it's known by.

So, is the current mindfulness movement really just crypto-Buddhism sailing under a deceptive flag? Or is it truly culturally neutral and scientifically justified? Let's address this question.

How do you think of the Buddha?

- Prophet-like? A religious figure who revealed the true nature of existence.
- Scientist-like? An extraordinary human being who made important discoveries regarding the nature of human happiness.

Let's consider in what ways the Buddha was scientist-like and in what ways he was not. Based on that, we can clarify how mainstream mindfulness differs from historical Buddhism.

Let's start with some ways in which the Buddha was scientist-like.

- He used the "divide and conquer" strategy:

The Scientist	The Buddha
Analyze physical and mathematical structures into their basic parts (atoms, primes, degrees of freedom, etc.)	Analyze selfhood into its basic parts (5 aggregates, 4 foundations, 4 elements, etc.)
Goal: Understand how true and useful properties arise from interactions among those parts	Goal: Understand how an illusory and painful property (Self as Thing) arises from interactions among those parts

- He emphasized rates of change, detachment, and evidence:

The Scientist	The Buddha
Rates of change are important: Differential equations, etc.	Rates of change are important: Impermanence
Equanimity: Humility before the facts	Equanimity: Acceptance of sensory experience
Epistemology: Knowledge comes from direct experience and logical inference; the role of authority is minimized	Epistemology: Knowledge comes from direct experience and logical inference; the role of authority is minimized

Now let's consider some ways in which he was not scientist-like:

The Scientist	The Buddha
Work is based on peer collaboration and dialogue	It is a one-man show—not based on peer collaboration and dialogue
Based on "third-person" (i.e., public) evidence	Based on "first-person" (i.e., introspective) evidence
Makes clear distinction between vivid sensory experience and objective reality	Apparently assumed his vivid experiences of gods, powers, and multiple lives were objectively real
Assumes that scientific understanding improves with time	May have assumed that human understanding deteriorates with time

Having considered all this, we are now in a position to clarify the ways in which modern mainstream mindfulness may be similar to Buddhist formulations and the ways in which it may be significantly different.

Traditional Buddhism	Mainstream Mindfulness (As I Would Have It)
Attention skills can be systematically cultivated	Yes to that
Applying those skills can completely eliminate suffering	Perhaps. But at the very least, it will significantly reduce it.
Attention skills are needed for deep self-discovery	Yes to that
We reincarnate through multiple lives	No *compelling* evidence for this
The gods and their heavens objectively exist	No *compelling* evidence for this

(continued)

(continued)

Traditional Buddhism	Mainstream Mindfulness (As I Would Have It)
There is no creator God	No *compelling* evidence for this
Psychic powers are objectively real	No *compelling* evidence for this
Developing good character and making positive behavior changes are important and mindful awareness can help with those	Yes to that
The nature of existence is suffering	$Suffering = \frac{Intensity\ of\ Discomfort}{Level\ of\ Mindful\ Awareness}$
	Since mindful awareness is relatively rare, needless suffering is a dominant theme (at this point in history)
There is no thing called a self	Mindful awareness practices can definitely lead to that insight, but some mindfulness practitioners may choose to describe that experience using different, perhaps even opposite, language: True Self, Oneness, elastic identity, spiritual nature, and so forth
Everything is impermanent	Monitoring how sensory experiences change can be liberating and empowering
Impermanence is a source of suffering (because things we hold dear eventually pass)	Yes, but the vibratory nature of one's senses can also be experienced as a pleasant flow of energy
Mindfulness lets you see reality as it is	If by reality one means philosophical or theological claims regarding the objective nature of existence, then the answer is no. Such sweeping claims are contentious and pose a barrier to mindfulness being accepted by all human societies

Conclusion

Mindfulness is currently a sizzling hot topic in many areas of mainstream culture. The downside of this is that some programs being marketed under the rubric of mindfulness have at most a tenuous connection to the practices and paradigms that are the subject of this article. Specifically, they fail to capture its potential for radical transformation and unconditional happiness. But, it's precisely this potential for radical well-being that senior practitioners like me find most exciting. I think of mindfulness as the "big guns"—something that helps when little else can (see Young, 2014—complete manuscript).

One of the convenient features of mindfulness is that is its scalability. Mindfulness Lite can calm a 6th grader. Mindfulness Mid-Strength can take the edge off of stress or dramatically improve your golf game. On the other hand, Mindfulness Classic will allow you to stride through the vicissitudes life like a Colossus—in touch with a Happiness that cannot be shaken by circumstances.

Science is currently being evoked both to confirm the clinical effects of mindfulness and to develop a theory that explains those effects. It is by no means certain that this line of research will be successful. But IF it is successful, consequences could be historic in magnitude. We would then have: a process with the potential to radically change a person for the better which is based on merely acquiring and applying a well-defined set of skills and which possesses a theory that is accepted by mainstream science. By way of contrast, previous approaches to human meaning have usually required assenting to a (potentially contentious) set of beliefs, linked to an elaborate set of communal rules and customs.

Conveniently, there is nothing intrinsic in mindfulness that directly conflicts with such faith-based approaches. Attentional skills can be thought of as lying in a dimension that is independent from personal beliefs. Mindfulness has the potential to become a sort of universal hardware platform that potentiates most forms of learning and growth, and is compatible with most commonly held worldviews.

If science is able to come up with a quantified model for what happens at the industrial strength end of mindfulness training, then innovative technologies may make those effects accessible to a significant proportion of humanity, as opposed to the current relatively small group of dedicated adepts. This would in effect democratize enlightenment. I think of this prospect as the Mindfulness Revolution.

As we have seen, aspects of mindfulness have been discovered and re-discovered across cultures and throughout the ages. Our current understanding of mindfulness is strongly influenced by the discoveries of Prince Siddhartha Gautama, known to the world by his honorific title Buddha. I think of the Buddha not as a religious figure but as the world's first proto-scientist of deep human happiness. Great scientists can be wrong about certain things and their formulations may be incomplete or in some ways lack rigor. That fact does not in the least detract from their personal greatness or the importance of their findings. If we simply think of the Buddha as an early scientist, then the fact that some of his ideas are present within modern mindfulness should offend neither the secular empiricist nor the committed theist. On the other hand, the fact that modern mindfulness significantly differs from the Buddha's worldview need not offend traditional Buddhists.

In his 1920 classic *Outline of History*, the British writer and historian H.G. Wells had this to say about the Buddha, "it is quite possible that in contact with western science, and inspired by the spirit of history, the original teaching of Gautama, revived and purified, may yet play a large part in the direction of human destiny."

Almost a century later, in addressing the first International Conference of Buddhist Geeks in Los Angeles in 2011, I found myself paraphrasing Wells thus, "It is reasonable that in contact with modern science, and inspired by the spirit of history, the original discoveries of Gautama, **rigorized and extended**, may yet play a large part in the direction of human destiny." Perhaps within this century science will establish that rigorous and extended paradigm.

Acknowledgement I would like to thank Emily Barrett, Donald W. McCormick, Todd Mertz, and Rob Roeser for their help with this chapter.

References

Bishop, S. R., Lau, M., Shapiro, S., Carlson, L., Anderson, N. D., Carmody, J., … Devins, G. (2004). Mindfulness: A proposed operational definition. *Clinical Psychology: Science and Practice, 11*(3), 230–241.

Brown, K. W., & Ryan, R. M. (2003). The benefits of being present: Mindfulness and its role in psychological well-being. *Journal of Personality and Social Psychology, 84*(4), 822–848.

Csikszentmihalyi, M. (1994). *Flow: The psychology of optimal experience*. New York, NY: Simon and Schuster.

Cullen, M. (2011). Mindfulness-based interventions: An emerging phenomenon. *Mindfulness, 2*, 186–193.

Dutton, G. R. (2008). The role of mindfulness in health behavior change. *ACSM's Health & Fitness Journal, 12*(4), 7–12.

Eliot, T. S. (1942). *Little gidding*. London, England: Faber and Faber.

Gethin, R. (2011). On some definitions of mindfulness. *Contemporary Buddhism, 12*(1), 263–279.

Grossman, P., & Van Dam, N. T. (2011). Mindfulness, by any other name…:Trials and tribulations of sati in western psychology and science. *Contemporary Buddhism, 12*, 220–239. doi:10.1080/14639947.2011.564841.

Hoppes, K. (2006). The Application of Mindfulness-Based Cognitive Interventions in the Treatment of Co-occurring Addictive and Mood Disorders. *CNS Spectrums*, 11, 829–851.

Hunter, J., & McCormick, D. W. (2008). Mindfulness in the workplace: An exploratory study. Paper presented at the *Academy of Management Annual Meeting*, Anaheim CA.

Kabat-Zinn, J. (2003). Mindfulness-based interventions in context: Past, present, and future. *Clinical Psychology: Science and Practice, 10*, 144–156. doi:10.1093/clipsy.bpg016.

Koenigsberg, H. W. (2010). Affective instability: Toward an integration of neuroscience and psychological perspectives. *Journal of Personality Disorders, 24*, 60–82.

Lozar-Glenn, J. (2010, April). The Garrison Institute: Bringing mindfulness to education. *Business Education Forum*.

Milton, I. (2011). What does mindfulness really mean? Clarifying key terms and definitions—Part I. *Psychotherapy in Australia, 17*(3), 78–81.

Murphy, S. M. (2012). *The Oxford handbook of sport and performance psychology*. New York, NY: Oxford University Press.

Nyanaponika T. (Trans.) (2000). Sallatha Sutta, "The Dart," *Samyutta Nikaya XXXVI.6,* from the Pali Canon. Retrieved from http://www.buddhismtoday.com/english/texts/samyutta/sn36-6b.html

Posner, M. (2012). *Cognitive neuroscience of attention*. New York, NY: Guilford Press.

Raffone, A., Manna, A., Perrucci, G. M., Ferretti, A., Del Gratta, C., Belardinelli, M. O., et al. (2007). Neural correlates of mindfulness and concentration in Buddhist monks: A fMRI study. *Proceedings of NFSI & ICFBI*, 242–244.

Rochman, B. (September 6, 2009). Samurai mind training for modern American warriors. *Time*.

Rogojanski, J., Vettese, L., & Antony, M. (2011). Coping with cigarette cravings: Comparison of suppression versus mindfulness-based strategies. *Mindfulness, 2*(1), 14–26.

Seligman, M. (2011). *Flourish: A visionary new understanding of happiness and well-being*. New York, NY: Free Press.

Shapiro, S. L., Brown, K. W., Thoresen, C., & Plante, T. G. (2011). The moderation of mindfulness-based stress reduction effects by trait mindfulness: Results from a randomized controlled trial. *Journal of Clinical Psychology, 67*(3), 267–277.

Song, Y., Lindquist, R., & Choi, E. J. (2010). Critical review of the effects of mindfulness-based stress reduction (MBSR) on stress and health-related quality of life (QOL). *Journal of Korean Academy of Adult Nursing, 22*(2), 121–129.

Vago, D. R., & Silbersweig, D. A. (2012). Self-awareness, self-regulation, and self-transcendence (S-ART): A framework for understanding the neurobiological mechanisms of mindfulness. *Frontiers in Human Neuroscience, 6*, 296.

van Son, J., Nyklicek, I., Pop, V. J. M., & Pouwer, F. (2011). Testing the effectiveness of a mindfulness-based intervention to reduce emotional distress in outpatients with diabetes (DiaMind): Design of a randomized controlled trial. *BMC Public Health, 11*(1), 131.

Wallace, B. A. (2005). *Genuine happiness: Meditation as the path to fulfillment*. Hoboken, N.J.: Wiley.

Weiss, M., Nordlie, J. W., & Siegel, E. P. (2005). Mindfulness-based stress reduction as an adjunct to outpatient psychotherapy. *Psychotherapy and Psychosomatics, 74*(2), 108–112.

Wilks, J. (October 8, 2014). Secular mindfulness: Potential & pitfalls. *Insight Journal*. Barre, MA: Barre Center for Buddhist Studies. Retrieved from http://www.bcbsdharma.org/insight-journal/#IJjump

Young, S. (2006). *Break through pain: A step-by-step mindfulness meditation program for transforming chronic and acute pain*. Boulder, CO: Sounds True.

Young, S. (2014). What is mindfulness? Retrieved from http://www.shinzen.org/Articles/WhatIsMindfulness_SY_Public.pdf

Zeidan, F., Martucci, K. T., Kraft, R. A., Gordon, N. S., McHaffie, J. G., & Coghill, R. C. (2011). Brain mechanisms supporting the modulation of pain by mindfulness meditation. *The Journal of Neuroscience, 31*(14), 5540–5548.

Internal Education and the Roots of Resilience: Relationships and Reflection as the New R's of Education

4

Daniel J. Siegel, Madeleine W. Siegel, and Suzanne C. Parker

Introduction

In this chapter, we will explore the fundamental nature of resilience and how educational programs at many levels can help foster emotional and social health in their students. We will examine how both internal reflection and mindfulness of our connections with one another can improve a child, adolescent, or adult's capacity for meaningful and rewarding interpersonal relationships with others. We will explore how the way in which attention is focused on the internal world of oneself and of others—a process of seeing the mind that can be termed "mindsight"—can build healthy relationships and create resilient minds (Siegel, 2012a). How these basic ideas can be applied in the educational setting will then be discussed to provide a framework for applying training in interpersonal mindfulness as a part of the "internal education" at the heart of social and emotional competencies.

Mindful States and Mindful Traits

Insight into the nature of mindfulness begins with the understanding of its states and traits. Being in a mindful *state* involves cultivating "the awareness that emerges through paying attention on purpose, in the present moment, and nonjudgmentally to the unfolding of experience moment-by-moment" (Davidson and Kabat-Zinn, 2003, pp. 145–146). Being in a mindful state can allow you and your students to be "aware of what's happening as it's happening" (Kaiser Greenland, 2006). By becoming mindfully aware of moment-to-moment experience, we can build curiosity, openness, and acceptance, allowing us to become kinder to ourselves.

We also can have mindful *traits*, enduring characteristics of an individual that are an automatic way of being, often occurring without conscious intention or effort. Ruth Baer et al. (2006) asked undergraduates to fill out a number of mindfuness trait questionnaires to assess what the distribution of mindfulness traits might be in the general population. These traits fell into four or five independent qualities: (1) Acting with Awareness, or being aware of what you are doing

D.J. Siegel (✉)
Mindsight Institute, Santa Monica, CA, USA

UCLA School of Medicine, Los Angeles, CA, USA
e-mail: drdansiegel@gmail.com

M.W. Siegel
University of California, Berkeley, CA, USA
e-mail: maddisiegel@berkeley.edu

S.C. Parker
American University, Washington, DC, USA
e-mail: suzanne.c.parker@gmail.com

K.A. Schonert-Reichl, R.W. Roeser (eds.), *Handbook of Mindfulness in Education*,
Mindfulness in Behavioral Health, DOI 10.1007/978-1-4939-3506-2_4

when you are doing it; (2) Being Non-Judgmental, or accepting what is happening and letting go of negative attitudes and reactions; (3) Non-Reactive, or being able to come back to emotional equilibrium readily; (4) Labeling the internal world, or having the capacity to describe with words the sea inside. Present as a component of other traits but existent as an independent feature only in those who'd been taught meditation is (5) Self-Observation, being able to observe oneself as if from a distance.

Mindfulness is a term used in various ways broadly to describe an intentionally created state of mind during a mindfulness practice such as mindfulness meditation, yoga, tai chi', qigong, or centering prayer. The general idea is that with repeated practice, especially if performed regularly such as on a daily basis, an intentionally created state of mind can become an automatic trait of an individual. However, some persons may have mindfulness innately as a part of their constitution without any intentional mindfulness practice. These intrinsic mindfulness traits may have their origins in genetic and temperamental make-up or in a history of secure attachment with a caregiver. A study exploring these origins has not been carried out thus far. What is interesting to note, however, is that the very traits of mindfulness greatly overlap with the outcome of secure attachment (see Siegel, 2007a).

Why would these states and traits of an individual be somehow related to the interpersonal relational experience of secure attachment? One possibility is that mindfulness is a form of attuning to oneself and secure attachment involves a similar form of interpersonal attunement. As we'll see, secure attachment and mindfulness practice may be two sides of the same coin: interpersonal mindfulness and intrapersonal mindfulness. Both experiences have been empirically demonstrated to be associated with well-being and resilience (Siegel, 2007a).

Another related term is mindful awareness, which can refer to both a state of mind as well as a trait of being. It is important to note that some researchers use the terms mindful awareness, mindfulness, and being mindful interchangeably, equating these to a focusing of attention within consciousness on the present moment. But these terms can also infer the regulation of one's emotions and compassion for both self and other (see Gilbert, 2010; Gilbert & Choden, 2013). In the way we are using the term here, mindfulness involves an internal stance of positive regard and openness to things as they are. Mindfulness is a way of being in the world with kindness and compassion toward oneself and others.

This practice of kindheartedness to ourselves can be seen as a fundamental part of what we are calling intrapersonal or internal mindfulness. Others may describe this as a part of self-compassion (Neff, 2011), loving-kindness (Salzberg, 2008) or living with a "wise heart" (Kornfield, 2008). Embedded within each of these perspectives is the notion of a way of being in the world with a non-judgmental positive regard. In this chapter, we will highlight the relationship between the internal sense of being aware of oneself in this open, receptive way with a related facet of awareness, interpersonal mindfulness. Both forms of mindfulness involve the four features of curiosity, openness, acceptance, and love, which can be readily recalled with the acronym COAL. The neural circuitry of *intra*personal attunement, we propose, overlaps with the circuitry of *inter*personal awareness, the practice of focusing one's attention on and accepting the internal state of another person. Interpersonal mindfulness is the ability to relate to another person with the same quality of awareness you have to yourself by connecting with others with kindness, openness, and acceptance. In this way, we are suggesting that interpersonal mindfulness is not only a quality of focusing attention on the here and now of another person, but also a mental stance of positive regard that honors the differentiated nature of another's internal experience.

The Science of Attuned Relationships

In reviewing the various sciences of health-promoting relationships, such as between a parent and a child or a clinician and a patient, a fundamental set of principles emerges (Cassidy

& Shaver, 2008; Norcross, 2002; Siegel, 2010a). This foundational group can be easily recalled using the acronym PART, as in "what *part* do we play in healthy relationships?". PART stands for Presence, Attunement, Resonance, and Trust (see Siegel, 2010b). We propose that these same fundamental elements are present in effective relationships between teacher and student.

Presence When we are present while interacting with another person, we give that individual our full attention and receive that person's communication back to us openly, without judgment, and with curiosity. Presence can be felt by the other person through the inner subjective sense of "feeling felt" by the other, as if our mind is seen clearly and received with openness and a receptive heart. Presence is the starting place for all interactions that enable each person to become fully engaged. With an infant and a parent, such responsiveness of the parent is called "contingent communication" in which the child's signals are (1) perceived, (2) understood in terms of their meaning for what is going on inside the child beyond the external behaviors, and (3) responded to in a timely and effective manner (Siegel, 2012a).

Attunement Attunement is the process by which we are not only open with our presence, but we also focus attention on the internal world of self or other. For interpersonal attunement there is a focusing of attention on the signals of communication—verbal and non-verbal—that are being sent to us by the other person. Attunement is the active engagement of an attentional system that tracks another's signals and takes them in as they are to facilitate the creation of a mental map of the other's internal state. In this way, attunement is the active perceptual process accompanying presence and enables the contingent communication, found in all cultures around the world, to become a part of the interpersonal experience. When we find a process as universal as contingency, it tells us something about the brain we've evolved as human beings, as we'll discuss in the next section.

Resonance Resonance is the outcome of attunement and presence. Resonance is the way our own internal state and external behaviors may become aligned with those of another person. If someone cries, we can feel sad and tears may even form on our own face. When we dance with another, we resonate with the rhythm of both the music and our partner. Resonance is the interpersonal state of joining as a "we" that enables people to feel a deep sense of belonging, of being a fundamental part of something larger than the solitary self. Resonance enables us to fulfill the neural need for connection (see Cozolino, 2014; Lieberman, 2013; Panksepp & Biven, 2012; Siegel, 2012a) that is the hallmark of our deeply social nature.

Trust When the brain perceives the presence, attunement, and resonance of another person, it activates a "social engagement system" that Steven Porges (2011) describes as the neural mechanism of being "receptive". Our muscles of the face, eardrums, and voice box relax, and we become open to receiving input from others. This is the neuroscience of trust and receptivity. With trust, our evaluative brain has determined that the interaction with another is safe, and we can let that person in. Presence, attunement, and resonance are the basic antecedents to trust and creating the receptive state of neural firing that permits both interpersonal connection and receptivity to learning to occur.

In the classroom, a teacher is faced with the challenge of bringing the PART needed for learning to a large number of students. This challenge involves being present with mindful awareness, attuning to a range of students' internal states, and being receptive enough to resonate with them so that they develop a collective sense of trust in the teacher. For example, in a study of the Garrison Institute's Curriculum for Awareness and Resilience in Education (CARE) program, findings revealed that teaching teachers how to be mindful enables them to engage with students in ways that enhance the students' academic and social and emotional learning (SEL) (Jennings,

Snowberg, Coccia, & Greenberg, 2011; Jennings, Snowberg, Frank, Coccia, & Greenberg, 2013). As we'll discuss next, intrapersonal or internal mindfulness may be one way to develop the presence and attunement that permits the creation of interpersonal resonance and trust in the classroom.

Patterns of Interpersonal Connection: The Science of Attachment

The field of attachment theory and research has demonstrated over longitudinal studies covering decades of development that internal attunement of a parent to a child enables the child's mind to become resilient (Cassidy & Shaver, 2008; Bowlby, 2003). Securely attached children can balance their emotions well, meet their intellectual potential, and have the capacity of having meaningful relationships with others. When parents do not provide such presence, attunement, and resonance on some consistent basis, allowing for repair of the inevitable ruptures as they occur, various forms of insecure attachment can result. These can lead to children's inability to trust and rely on relationships with others.

Emotionally distant parenting yields an *avoidant attachment* in which children learn to "not need others" and to be independent from a very early age. "I can go it alone" is their internal identifying feature. In many ways, this can be viewed as a lack of trusting others to meet the individuals' needs. The result with this avoidant attachment with a primary caregiver is an internal sense of a disconnected self—disconnected from others and from one's own internal experience of emotion, bodily sensation, and autobiographical identity (see Siegel, 2012a).

Emotionally inconsistent and intrusive parenting leads to an *ambivalent or resistant attachment*. Here, the child is filled with uncertainty: Will my parent be there or not? This anxiety is carried forward as a sense of ambivalence and a lack of a solid, internal core. "I am not sure if I can rely on you or not" is the identifying inner viewpoint. This would also result in hesitancy in trusting others to be consistent and accessible.

For others who have experienced terrifying interactions with their parents, a *disorganized attachment* is created. The internal conflict created with this set of frightening and disorienting experiences is that one circuit in the brain says to go away from the source of terror, while another pushes the child to move toward the attachment figure—the parent—for comfort. In this situation, there is no solution to the fear. Organized strategies of adaptation collapse, and the child's inner world fragments. These patterns of early attachment experiences do not disappear—they are carried forward into the classroom. With disorganized attachment, children not only learn to distrust others, but also to distrust their own mind to function well, especially under stress.

Here is a summary of Alan Sroufe and colleagues' Minnesota Longitudinal Study of Risk and Adaptation (MLSRA), a research project that began in 1976 (Sroufe, Carlson, & Waters, 2005) and is the longest prospective study available to date (reviewed in Sroufe & Siegel, 2011). This research study has been the source of a vast literature about the predictive power of early attachment relationships, while also distinguishing the impact of these relationships from the effects of social class and temperament. Sroufe and Siegel (2011) state:

> Those with secure histories had a greater sense of self-agency, were better emotionally regulated, and had higher self-esteem than those with histories of anxious (insecure) attachment. In general, attachment predicted engagement in the preschool peer group, the capacity for close friendships in middle childhood, the ability to coordinate friendships and group functioning in adolescence, and the capacity to form trusting, non-hostile romantic relationships in adulthood. Those with secure histories were more socially competent and likelier to be peer leaders. Each finding holds true controlling for temperament and IQ.

The findings suggest that the imprinting of interpersonal connections during the formative early attachment years impacts how a child behaves in the school setting in important ways. The findings go even further (Sroufe & Siegel, 2011):

As Bowlby's theory indicated, security of a child's attachment predicts the reactions of peers and teachers to that child. Children describe peers with avoidant histories as aggressive or "mean." They frequently victimize those with resistant or ambivalent attachment histories, who tend not to be socially competent and are the least liked by others. Those with secure histories are liked best. This finding can be best understood by recognizing that early attachments create social expectations in children, and may incline them to see the present in terms of negative past experiences. For such children, their attachment history can become a self-fulfilling prophecy as they behave toward new people in their lives—like peers or teachers—in ways that reproduce old, negative relationships.

Teachers, too, with no knowledge of the child's history, treat children in the different categories of attachment differently. Coders, who were blind to the child's history, but who watched videotapes of interactions between teachers and each child, rated teachers as treating those with secure histories in a warm, respectful manner. They set age-appropriate standards for their behavior and had high expectations for them (indicated by actions such as moving on to take care of other tasks after asking the child to do something). With those having resistant histories, the teachers were also warm, but highly controlling. They didn't expect compliance, set low standards, and were unduly nurturing (taking care of things that 5-year-olds should do for themselves). Teachers were controlling and had low expectations with the avoidant group, but displayed little nurturing and got angry at them most frequently. Thus, the reactions of teachers tended to support the attachment assessment of the children that had been made through other observations.

We can see that anyone can become "lost in familiar places" as early imprinting of patterns of adaptation to our attachment figures can be replayed as we automatically evoke similar responses from those around us. It's a self-fulfilling feedback loop that reinforces beliefs about the self and relationships with others. In this manner, peers and teachers may respond in a way that leads to distancing or infantilizing behaviors for those with insecure histories, solidifying these self-concepts and behaviors. The sad news is that the child may be vulnerable to just engage further in this familiar pattern.

Teachers' own mindfulness can enable the sensations of such interpersonal patterns to enter the foreground of their awareness, enabling them to pull out of "automatic pilot" and to attempt to engage students in a more present, attuned, and resonating manner. As children's, adolescents' and even adults' brains can, and do, change, theoretically teachers can actually become the *neurosculptors* of the next generation by simply being the PART the student needs to learn to become socially engaged and receptive, instead of the old pattern of being reactive and disconnected.

This idea that teachers can make a big difference in a student's development is revealed in the studies of resilience that suggest that even an intermittent relationship, like with a particular teacher, can create a singular sense of "feeling felt" that can last a lifetime and fuel the fire of change to awaken the mind from automatic patterns (see Sroufe et al., 2005). A recent informal survey (Siegel, personal interviews) of a dozen young, middle-aged and older adults revealed that each person had a memory of a relationship with a teacher in which he or she felt seen and accepted, and that this particular person changed the pathway of their personal and school directions. In many ways, the survey participants reflected, this relationship was the most important part of their education and what they remembered the most clearly from their experience in school.

How can teachers make such a difference? The findings from the Minnesota Study (Sroufe et al., 2005) summarized by Sroufe and Siegel (2011) may help:

> Anxious attachment doesn't directly cause later disturbance, but it initiates a developmental pathway that, without corrective experiences, increases the probability of psychopathology. In fact, anxious/resistant attachment increases the probability of anxiety disorders and avoidant attachment increases the likelihood of conduct problems. However, the strongest predictor of pathological outcomes, including dissociation, is "disorganized attachment." This "disorganized" infant attachment pattern predicts later dissociative symptoms up to age 26 (and even borderline personality symptoms at age 28).

How a teacher is present and attuned can make a huge difference for many children in helping in the path of their development. The teacher-student relationship has the potential to be a "corrective experience" for the growing child or teen, and even adult student, one that moves the individual from various forms of insecure attachment patterns toward security. The key is that these neurally encoded patterns of adaptation are open to being modified by new interpersonal experiences with peers and teachers. Naturally some individuals may require psychotherapeutic intervention, especially with histories of disorganized attachment. But the vast majority, even with insecure attachment histories, theoretically will be available for teachers to make an important and lasting impact on their developmental pathways.

What is the connection between these attachment findings, as interesting as they may be, with our topic of resilience, internal education, and interpersonal mindfulness? We are suggesting that what a parent (or teacher or friend) provides in creating a secure base of connection for a child in relating to her *internal world* is exactly what interpersonal mindfulness is. While extensive research is not yet available, a preliminary study by Amy DiNoble in 2009 found that adults with secure attachments have increased scores on mindfulness traits. We'll review these traits soon. When adults, parents or teachers are sensitive and attuned to a child, they are able to engage in a more reciprocal form of connection. This contingent communication provides the child with the *roots of resilience*: self-confidence, flexibility in the face of challenges, and emotional security.

Mindsight: Attending to the Sea Inside

The field of attachment first showed that parents' sensitivity to the child's signals enables them to engage in the contingent communication needed for the child to become securely attached. This secure base fosters the child's ability to explore the world with a sense of curiosity and confidence, to be willing to try and make mistakes, and to engage with others in collaborative ways. In short, securely attached children bring with them a teacher's ideal set of characteristics for a great student—one who is open to engagement with teachers and other students and receptive to learning.

It is important to note that Mary Ainsworth, the researching pioneer in attachment research, initially thought that it would be the warmth of the parent that would predict security. However, she found from her initial studies that warmth had no correlation with secure outcomes—only the sensitivity of the caregiver to the child that created contingent communication (Sroufe & Siegel, 2011). Ainsworth did find that this sensitivity could be seen as those parents' abilities to focus on and describe the characteristics of the child–their psychological mindedness–that seemed to be an informal predictor of the child's security of attachment (Main, 1999). Later on, Ainsworth's student Mary Main created an important instrument called the Adult Attachment Interview, a semi-structured narrative that reveals how a parent has made sense of his or her early life experiences (Main, Goldwyn, & Hesse, 2003). Part of this process is the way the parent focuses on the internal world of the mind—emotions, thoughts, memories, and beliefs—and how these mental activities influence their ongoing thoughts and behaviors. This "metacognitive monitoring" was further studied by researcher Fonagy and colleagues, who extended and quantified these observations in the formulation of a "reflective function" that reveals how a parent "mentalizes," or sees the mind behind the behaviors of self or other (Fonagy & Target, 2005; Slade, Grienenberger, Bernbach, Levy, & Locker, 2005). Mentalization is the ability to see the world through the lens of how mental life shapes our behavior, our relationships, and our inner subjective experience.

Now we know that parental sensitivity and mentalization go hand-in-hand in the development of attachment security. These lessons from developmental research can inform teachers of the ingredients necessary to foster resilience in their relationships with students. Being present and attuned to the student is a way that teachers can role model how to be sensitive to another person. Sensing the sea inside—being open to the feelings, thoughts, expectations, hopes, dreams, and memories that underlie externally observable behaviors—is the reflective function that teachers can provide that instructs students on how to articulate the inner nature of their subjective lives. This is the essence of an "internal education." As we've stated earlier and will discuss next in more detail, the ability to label and describe in words the internal world is, in fact, one of the major mindfulness traits.

Mindfulness Traits

In mindfulness studies, features of being mindfully aware can be assessed during intentionally created moments during mindfulness meditation, yoga, tai' chi' chuan, qigong, or centering prayer. The intentional practice of focusing attention on moment-to-moment experience as it unfolds cultivates the ability to create these states of mindful awareness (See Bishop et al, 2004; Brown and Ryan, 2003; and Siegel, 2007a). Research in neuroscience can focus on which areas of the brain are activated during such mindfulness practice. In general, two aspects of attention are studied (Lutz, Slagter, Dunne, & Davidson, 2008). One is focused attention whereby a subject is intensifying the focus on an object of attention, such as the breath. When attention wanders, the self-regulatory skill of redirecting attention is engaged. In another aspect of mindfulness training, "open monitoring", the subject attains a state of receptivity to whatever arises in the field of attention, allowing for openness as judgments or distractions unfold without being swept up by them. Both focused attention and open monitoring help stabilize the lens through which we see the internal workings of the mental sea.

The general saying in neuroscience is that "neurons that fire together, wire together". In this way, performing an intentional mindful awareness practice (MAP) will create repeated states that will change the brain and enable traits to develop over time. For example, ongoing studies reveal that after only 8 weeks of mindfulness practice for a little under half an hour a day, the structure of the brain in regulatory regions changes enough to be seen on a brain scan (Hölzel et al., 2011).

To give you a feeling for these remarkable findings, here is a portion of these researchers' summary:

> Therapeutic interventions that incorporate training in mindfulness meditation have become increasingly popular, but to date little is known about neural mechanisms associated with these interventions. Mindfulness-Based Stress Reduction (MBSR), one of the most widely used mindfulness training programs, has been reported to produce positive effects on psychological well-being and to ameliorate symptoms of a number of disorders. Here, we report a controlled longitudinal study to investigate pre-post changes in brain gray matter concentration attributable to participation in an MBSR program. Analyses in a priori regions of interest confirmed increases in gray matter concentration within the left hippocampus. Whole brain analyses identified increases in the posterior cingulate cortex, the temporo-parietal junction, and the cerebellum in the MBSR group compared with the controls. The results suggest that participation in MBSR is associated with changes in gray matter concentration in brain regions involved in learning and memory processes, emotion regulation, self-referential processing, and perspective taking (p. 36).

The key feature here is that the practice of focusing attention in a systematic way changes the structure of the brain. One way of focusing on this relationship between attention and neural plasticity is by stating, "Where attention goes, neural firing flows and neural connection grows." (Siegel, 2016). With repeated practice, a state can become a trait as intentionally created states during practice can create more automatic traits that arise from long-lasting alterations in the brain's structure in key regulatory areas.

Other long-term changes after mindfulness practice are seen as the outcome of MAPs. These include what Richard Davidson (2003) has shown after Jon Kabat-Zinn's Mindfulness-Based Stress Reduction (MBSR) training to be a "left-shift" in the brain that is also proportionately associated with improvements in immune function. The left-shift is thought to represent the frontal region of the brain's movement into an "approach state" tendency—to approach rather than withdraw from challenging situations (Urry et al., 2004). This can be considered the "neurosignature of resilience."

For example, practicing physicians (Spickard et al. 2002) who are at a high risk for burnout and diminished empathy can be supported to reduce these negative outcomes of their work with mindfulness training (Krasner et al, 2009; and see Shapiro et al, 2007 regarding mental health practitioners).

Consider for a moment the educational implications of what these two independent labs have found (and which are also consistent with a wide range of other scientists' findings): Regular mindfulness practice leads to changes in the structure and function of the brain that enable a teacher or student to approach challenges with resilience, improve memory, regulate emotions more effectively, have more insight into one's inner life, and have greater empathy for the experience of others. The positive benefits of mindfulness practice are found not only in our behaviors and mental life, but also in the health of our chromosomes. One study revealed that mindfulness practice improves the way our chromosomes maintain their structure by increasing an enzyme called telomerase so that we may actually be able to live longer (Jacobs et al., 2010). You may be wondering at this point, why are we waiting to put mindfulness practices into the curriculum! So, we are proposing that in addition to the first Rs of education—reading, 'riting, and 'rithmetic—we might consider adding these new Rs: Reflection and Relationships as the Roots of Resilience.

Attuning to the Internal World

Interpersonal mindfulness can be described as the way in which we have the parallel traits that Baer and colleagues assessed for intrapersonal mindfulness and can be delineated in the following manner: (1) Being aware of what is happening *with others* as it is happening; (2) Being accepting and non-judgmental of others; (3) Maintaining emotional equilibrium with others; (4) Reflecting on the internal experience of others' minds using words, and (5) Being observant of the nature of the *interactions* one is having with others. Awareness, acceptance, emotional balance, reflection, and observation are then at the heart of the traits of interpersonal mindfulness. When we examine the fundamental findings of intrapersonal mindfulness practice, we can see that the left-shift findings of approach, the core neurosignature of resilience, would support each of these functions. The few neuroscience studies of intrapersonal mindfulness outcome suggest that programs like MBSR can teach people how to distinguish ongoing sensory experience from the narrative (judging) chatter of other areas of the brain (Farb et al., 2007). This perspective suggests that we have a direct experiential set of circuits that are distinct from the more discursive regions of the brain that create our life stories and an ongoing narrator of our experience. This distinction can be illuminated when we ask someone to describe her internal experience rather than explain it. Awareness of direct experience is considered a road to being mindful in the moment. Interpersonally, such a skill would be extremely helpful in enabling a person to track their own internal reactions and not identify with those *s*ensations, *i*mages, *f*eelings or *t*houghts as the totality of who that person is (see Shapiro, Carlson, Astin, & Freedman, 2006; Siegel, 2010a). This SIFTing through the mind enables a person to achieve emotional equilibrium, to label the internal world with words, to work toward being non-judgmental, and to be fully present with intra- and interpersonal experiences as they arise, moment-by-moment.

This mindful capacity to describe the internal world is truly parallel to the reflective skill that attachment researchers suggest enables us to mentalize or have a reflective function. When we conceive and perceive the mind this way, we can also use the term, "mindsight" because it allows us to see our own and others' inner lives. Much like eyesight enables us to perceive the physical world and make three-dimensional maps, mindsight enables us to perceive the mental sea inside ourselves and others, enabling us to make maps of the mind of self and other. These are all reflections on the mind that a "psychologically-minded" or "mind-minded" person exhibits (Beitel, Ferrer, & Cecero, 2005), and ones that reveal the "theory of mind" that enables us to conceive that others, and even we as individuals, have minds.

Accordingly, it is natural as an educator to consider that if intrapersonal mindfulness produces such important and relevant changes in the brain to help learning and memory, emotion regulation, and self- and other-mind perception and understanding (reflecting on the mind, or mindsight), why not incorporate such practices into a didactic program? Further, why not focus on interpersonal mindfulness to build on these same mindsight skills? Focusing on mindsight building would cultivate such perceptual capacities on the internal and the relational worlds in which we live. In this way, internal and interpersonal mindfulness would become part of a coherent program with its bedrock in these reflective capacities. A look at the brain and how it creates mindsight and is altered by experience will help illuminate how intra- and inter- personal forms of mindfulness are like two sides of one coin. In this way, mindsight may be the common mechanism shared by mindfulness education and the development of social and emotional skills.

The Interpersonal Brain

The fundamental viewpoint we are expressing is that the neural mechanisms beneath self-awareness and other-awareness harness similar circuitries. When we focus attention on the internal world of ourselves, we use a process that can be called internal attunement. Such attunement is fundamental to mindfulness practice (see Siegel, 2007a). When we focus on the inner world of others, we call this interpersonal attunement which serves as the foundation of secure attachment (see Siegel, 2012a). What is the neural mechanism of these two forms of attunement? Let's begin focusing attention on the inner experience of another person. How do we focus on another person through our presence so that we can resonate with their states and come to know what is going on in their inner world? Some would use the word "empathy" to describe this process of connecting to another person. Studies of both internal and interpersonal mindfulness have shown that empathy increases after training (Dekeyser, Raes, Leijssen, Leysen, & Dewulf, 2008; Sawyer Cohen & Semple, 2010; Shapiro, Schwartz, & Bonner, 1998; Shapiro, Astin, Bishop, and Cordova 2005). So, what is empathy, and what does the brain have to do with it?

In the introductory chapter of an intensive research review on the social neuroscience of empathy, Daniel Batson (2009) suggests that the term empathy has at least eight different usages in the scientific literature: (1) Knowing another person's internal state, including his or her thoughts and feelings; (2) Adopting the posture or matching the neural response of an observed other; (3) Coming to feel as another person feels; (4) Intuiting or projecting oneself into another's situation; (5) Imagining how another is thinking and feeling; (6) Imagining how one would think and feel in the other's place; (7) Feeling distress at witnessing another person's suffering; and (8) Feeling for another person who is suffering.

Other terms, such as compassion, sympathy, and perhaps even morality may also come to mind for some of these various meanings of the word empathy. One useful way to make sense of this wide array of meanings is to examine a model of how the brain becomes activated during emotionally connecting communication. Below we will provide a view from the lab of Marco Iacoboni (2008; Carr, Iacoboni, Dubeau, Maziotta, & Lenzi, 2003) that explores the "insula hypothesis" of empathy. An educator knowing the rough outline of this model of the brain and interpersonal interactions will be well-prepared to understand events in the classroom. Such an understanding may also illuminate the role of mindfulness training in promoting social and emotional skills through the new three R's of education.

Our brain is the social organ of the body. In fact, the entire nervous system is distributed throughout the body to help regulate its inner functions and its interactions with the outside world. Beginning with its origins in the creation of the neural tube from the outer cells of the conceptus, this specialized set of ectoderm or skin cells actually functions to link the inner and the outer just as the skin forms the boundary between the inner world and the outer world.

When we think of the brain, it is misleading to think of this organ as just in the head. The entire nervous system functions in the body as a whole. We have neural networks around the heart and intestines, for example, that process information just like the networks up in the skull (Craig, 2003; Critchley, Wiens, Rotshtein, Öhman, & Dolan, 2004).

The nervous system provides a mechanism through which energy and information flows. The passage of an action potential, the movement of ions in and out of the membrane of the basic cell, the neuron, serves as electrical energy flow. When this flow reaches the end of the neuron, a chemical called a neurotransmitter is released and then received by the downstream neuron across their connection, called a synapse. If enough activating neurotransmitter reaches the receptors, the downstream neuron "fires off" and the sequence continues. This is the flow of electrochemical energy.

Neurons that fire together, wire together. The activation of a set of neurons that are synaptically linked will reinforce their synaptic connections with one another. This is how a circuit—a set of connected neurons—can be formed and strengthened. Because the growth of synaptic connections requires turning on genes and the subsequent production of protein, this neural growth at the heart of learning and skill-acquisition involves long-term changes in brain structure which are dependent upon protein synthesis. We can make new synapses, strengthen existing ones, make new neurons in certain regions, and even lay down an insulating sheath that makes the firing of connected neurons 3000 times more effective! We can also modify neural function and learning through changes in the epigenetic regulation of gene expression induced by experience (Meany, 2010). Learning is an art; experiences that change the brain are a form of neural sculpting (Siegel, 2012a).

When teachers encourage students to focus attention on a subject, on math for example, they are stimulating the firing of neurons in areas related to mathematical calculations. When a teacher offers students a new way to focus attention, as in mindful awareness practices, she is giving her students a chance to stimulate the neuronal activation and growth of the attention regulating circuits in the brain (Siegel, 2007). But, mindfulness is more than simply focusing attention in a stronger way. As we've seen from the first discussions of this chapter, mindfulness can be seen as a mental stance and a form of internal attunement. We can see in the findings described above that changes in the brain are *not* just in areas that regulate attention: Mindfulness induces changes in areas that are involved in memory and learning, emotion regulation, flexibility of response (impulse control), insight, and empathy (Hölzel et al., 2011). Also, as we'll soon explore, areas of the brain that are both activated during practice and that grow with continued practice are the very areas involved in both self-awareness and interpersonal attunement (Lazar et al., 2005). Our interpersonal brains are built originally from interpersonal attunement. As we grow, the focus of our attention with internal attunement harnesses similar circuitry. This finding, that self-awareness and empathy-related skills are linked, has been found in a wide array of studies, including those of mindfulness practice (Dekeyser et al., 2008; Sawyer Cohen & Semple, 2010). These studies suggest that both social connectedness and the qualities of emotional intelligence are both enhanced by mindfulness training.

Interoception and the Insula: Perceiving the Interior

In Iacoboni's lab (Iacoboni, 2009), photos of emotionally expressive faces are shown to people in functional scanners to image how the brain responds when seeing an emotionally evocative expression. Iacoboni and colleagues were interested in illuminating whether the findings from Italy of studies of monkeys exploring a set of circuits called "mirror neurons" could illuminate how human beings pick up emotional cues through empathic resonance. What follows is Iacoboni and colleagues' "insula hypothesis" about the neurobiology of empathy (Carr et al., 2003).

A set of neurons in the cortex (in the frontal and parietal—upper and side—regions) are able to process the perception of the action of others and detect if there is a predictable sequence of motion occurring. Imagine the difference if someone saw a person randomly moving his arms, in contrast to how one would feel seeing a person slowly lift a bottle of water to his lips. In the latter case, frontal and parietal neurons would detect the sequence of motion of the arm and hand *up to his lips to drink*. Once the sequence is predicted, the exciting finding was that these neurons, working closely with other neurons nearby, actually make a map of the other person's intention. One now knows that guy is going to take a sip of water! This is known because the mirror neurons "figured out the sequence" and then enabled the prediction of what was going to happen next. Much of the brain, in fact, is an anticipation machine like this. But in this case, our mirror neurons get that name because they also get us ready to act in the same way! You mirror in your behavior the intentional action you see in someone else.

The "mirror properties" of these cells involve bridging the divide between perception (seeing the person lift the water bottle) and action (you prepare to drink). This is how we align our behavior as social creatures. But Iacoboni and colleagues took this one step further. What if in addition to making maps of others' intentions and imitating their behavior, we also simulate their internal state? Could the mirror neuron system also engage our emotional processes, a kind of internal action?

A set of fascinating studies revealed that the answer is yes (Iacoboni, 2009). And here is the overall way this is thought to occur: Signals that are sent from another person, including facial expressions and tone of voice, can often reveal another's internal state. The mirror neuron and related areas detect this internal state by picking up these signals sent and then drive the neural processes down into the perceiver's own lower neural regions. For example, sadness, anger, joy, fear, surprise—any internal state—can be transmitted through our non-verbal signals of eye contact, tone of voice, posture, gestures, and the timing and intensity of responses. These signals from another person can then activate the mirror neurons to relay this information downward from the more rational cortex where they reside to the lower limbic regions where our deeper, more visceral/emotional processes arise. These limbic areas, in turn, communicate through a circuit called the insula to even lower regions such as the brainstem and the body-proper. Heart rate changes, intestines churn, lungs expand and contract, muscles tighten—these are all ways our body can "resonate" with what we perceive in the signals of another person about her inner state of being.

Next, neural signals of these shifts in the inner bodily states travel back upward to the skull, passing through Lamina I (layer one) of the spinal cord and the tenth cranial (vagus) nerve, find their way as neural firing patterns impacting the deeply situated brainstem, and then go back up through the insula to the front of the cortex. This bodily data registers itself in our prefrontal cortex, especially on the right side, where we gain awareness of our body's internal state. This is called "interoception" or perception of the interior.

Iacoboni et al. (2003) have shown that the degree of activation of these mirror neuron/right anterior insula areas is directly proportional to a person's degree of empathy. Because this circuit from mirror neurons down to the body via the insula, then back up Lamina I to the insula and other prefrontal areas enables us to resonate—to align our own internal state with that of another person—this can be called the "resonance circuit" (Siegel, 2007a). Key aspects of this resonance circuit, including the insula, are activated and grow with mindfulness practice.

When we are open to others, we turn on a "social engagement" state in which we can receive others' input. Social engagement involves our resonance circuitry. We can also shut this circuit off under conditions of threat, as Steven Porges (2009, 2011) has outlined in his important work called the Polyvagal Theory. When we become reactive, we are in the fight/flight/freeze/faint state. But, when we assess safety, we shift this reactive state to a "ventral vagal" state of being open and receptive. This state is created with interpersonal attunement, as occurs with secure attachment relationships. We propose that interpersonal mindfulness creates this receptive state so that we turn on our social engagement system in interacting with others in an attuned way. We may also see internal mindfulness as activating what can be called a "self-engagement" system when we have internal attunement. In both interpersonal and intrapersonal mindfulness, we are proposing that similar resonance circuits and states of receptivity are utilized and enhanced.

Once interoceptive data is sent upward by way of the vagus nerve and the insula, we have the ability to "know how we feel inside." These are dominant right hemisphere pieces of data about the body's state—and so they are far from the logical, linguistic, linear processing of concepts and lists of the left (McGilchrist, 2009). For a teacher, the importance of this finding is that interoception—perceiving the interior—relies on a non verbal world of sensation. These are washes of intensity of feeling, poundings of the heart, churnings of the gut, tightness in the chest, tears welling in the eyes. When students are asked to mindfully become aware of their body, such as in the body-scan practice or during the wheel of awareness practice (Siegel, 2010b, 2013), it is an instruction to sense what is arising from the body, not to think about the body in words. When the time comes to label the internal world (a basic mindfulness trait), notice how, as discussed above, the term is "describe," rather than "explain" what is going on inside. Describing may be a very different process than the explanation that requires a translation from right hemisphere representations of the body in the insula to the left side's language centers that explain what is going on through the lens of logic and linear, rational thinking. That neural translation of simply describing what one experiences is an important exercise that needs to be distinguished from the "narrative chatter" of the ever-curious left hemisphere's drive to tell a story explaining what it thinks is going on. As we've seen, at a minimum, mindfulness is about distinguishing these two streams of knowing from one another (Farb et al., 2007), and mindfulness may enable the integration of these streams by linking their differentiated components (see Siegel, 2007b; 2016).

Mindsight is comprised of insight into oneself, empathy for others, and integration that links differentiated aspects of a system into one coherent whole. Internal attunement and interpersonal attunement both harness the integrative resonance circuits that enable mindsight to flourish. These mindsight capacities are teachable by educators and learnable by students. Thus, mindsight is a skill of insight, empathy, and integration that can be systematically taught (Siegel, 2013).

Our Internal Maps: Me, You, and We and the Creation of MWe

Interoception is the gateway to both insight and empathy. Adjacent to the more lateralized insula, more toward the midline, is the medial prefrontal region. The insula hypothesis goes on to suggest that data from the insula is transferred to the medial prefrontal area where first it is used to address the question, "How am I feeling and what is going on with me?" This is the initiation of insight (Siegel, 2010b). Taken further, this state in the moment blends with other prefrontal areas in the creation of mental time travel in which we link the present to the remembered past and the imagined future (Tulving, 1993). We create a mindsight-map of "me" across time.

We can also use this insula input to the medial prefrontal area to take interoception (knowing our body's sensation) and insight (self-referential reflections) and then imagine what another person might be feeling. This is how the prefrontal regions also create empathic imagination and compassionate action. This is a mindsight-map of "you" that makes it possible for us to create an internal image of what may be going on inside of another person's subjective, inner mental life. Mindsight-maps of both you and of me permit us to envision the "sea inside" others and the self.

If we return to Batson's (2009) eight meanings of the term empathy, we can now see how this insula hypothesis and the way the resonance circuits contribute to these processes can help us explain each of them and how they correlate in the brain. Social neuroscience offers deep and helpful insights into how our interpersonal communication rides the circuits of our social brains to enable us to connect deeply with one another and with ourselves. We can also understand, from this neural view, the findings that moral reasoning emerges from these same middle prefrontal areas (Anderson, Bechara, Damasio, Tranel, & Damasio, 1999). We can imagine what is best for the larger social good and then carry out moral actions based on midline prefrontal networks of processing. This is the way we make mindsight-maps of "we" that not only connect us to people we know personally, but also create a sense of membership in a larger whole.

A range of studies of wisdom, happiness, and health suggest that when we have a sense of connection to other people and projects beyond only our personal concerns, our lives become enriched with meaning, purpose, and well-being (Christakis & Fowler, 2009; Gilbert, 2007; Haidt, 2006; Lee et al, 2001; Steger et al, 2006). The idea is not to disregard a "me," but rather to go beyond only "me" to connect with "you" and become a part of a larger "we." In many ways, an integrated identity of an internal me and an interpersonal we can be captured in the term, MWe (Siegel, 2013). The linkage of these different senses of a self may be an important part of what our prefrontal regions help us create from the inside out.

Integration and Resilience

How can this prefrontal region take part in such a wide range of important processes? When we combine the vertically and horizontally midline areas under the term "middle" prefrontal cortex, we are including the medial prefrontal, orbitofrontal, anterior cingulate, and ventrolateral regions—which includes the insula cortex. Taken as a whole interactive and integrative system (Siegel, 2007a; Siegel, 2012a), this middle prefrontal area of the cortex of the brain directly *regulates our bodily states*, influencing our heart rate, respiration, and intestinal activities through its influence on the lower brainstem. *Attuned communication* with others, the gateway to interpersonal resonance, also depends on these middle prefrontal areas. *Emotional balance*, in which we have affective states that are aroused enough so life has meaning but not too aroused so life is chaotic—and not too depleted so life becomes stagnant and rigid—is also the outcome of middle prefrontal activity. *Being flexible in responding*, controlling impulses, delaying gratification, and reflecting are carried out by the buffering these middle prefrontal areas create, permitting a pause between impulse and action. Even the *modulation of fear* is a job of this region as well. The middle prefrontal cortical areas enable both the *insight* into one's own inner life and the *empathy* essential to mapping out the mind of another (Decety & Ickes, 2009). And, as if this weren't enough, *morality* is created within these firing patterns, as is accessing *intuition* as the cortex receives the wisdom of the body and enables this important inner knowing to influence reasoning (Craig, 2003; Critchley et al., 2004).

While these discoveries come from the hard-earned investigations of neuroscientists, we also have the startling overlap from disciplines that found similar groupings in fields not primarily studying the brain. For example, the first eight of these nine middle prefrontal areas have been established as outcomes of secure parent–child attachment relationships (Cassidy & Shaver, 2010; Siegel, 2012a). Mindfulness training studies suggest that all nine middle prefrontal functions are both the outcomes, and the process, of being mindful (Siegel, 2007a). Reflections on this list by mental health practitioners (Siegel, informal interviews, 2005–2014) reveal that this is a reasonable description of mental well-being. Finally, individuals from a wide range of cultures and religions, including Inuit, Lakota, Polynesia, Buddhism, Christianity, and Hinduism have suggested that their teachings share these nine functions at the heart of how to live a wise and kind life (Siegel, informal interviews, 1999–2014).

We propose that each of these aspects of reality share a process called integration. Integration is the linkage of differentiated parts of a system. Secure attachment involves the honoring of differences between child and parent and then the cultivation of compassionate communication between the two. Mindfulness—as a form of internal attunement—cultivates the honoring by the observing self in an open and accepting way of the experiencing self, moment-by-moment. In mental health, we can see that "health" is derived from the "whole" and can emerge from integration of many parts into a functional, flexible whole at the heart of a resilient mind. And, for the wisdom traditions, we can sense that honoring others' differences with compassion is the essence of how to live a kind and meaning-filled life.

Examination of the middle prefrontal region reveals that neural integration may be the heart of how this area functions. This is a region that links the widely separated energy and information flow from distinct origins into a functional whole. The middle aspect of this prefrontal area connects input from the cortex, the limbic area, the brainstem, the body-proper, and even the neural signals from other people, other brains. This connection of the social, somatic, brainstem, limbic, and cortical is a huge process of neural integration. For this reason, it may be that the roots of resilience rest in integration. This leads to an astonishing finding: Interpersonal relationships that honor difference and promote compassionate linkages cultivate the linkage of differentiated regions of the brain. Put simply, interpersonal integration cultivates internal integration (Siegel, 2012a, 2012b). And, since the regulation of such processes as affect and mood, attention and thought, and behavior and relatedness are each dependent upon the neural integration that allows the coordination and balance of the body as a whole and the individual with the social environment, we can see how central integration is to well-being. Executive function and "self-regulation" depend upon integration (Siegel, 2012a, 2012b).

We create integration through attuned communication and stimulate the activation and growth of integrative fibers in the brain. Internal reflection in a mindful way further supports the creation of an internal stance of kindness and compassion—toward the self and toward others. The outcome of such interpersonal and internal attunement would be the reinforcement of the growth and strength of these integrative neural fibers. Mindfulness increases neural integration as revealed in recent studies of the connectome—the integrated nature of the brain (Brewer et al., 2011; Kilpatrick et al., 2011; Luders, Clark, Narr, & Toga, 2011). One of the first studies of the Human Connectome Project suggests, too, that a more linked or integrated connectome is a primary factor associated with a wide range of positive traits of living (Smith et al, 2015).

The outcome of integration is resilience and health. Integration is the heart of self-regulation, the way we modulate our internal world to create equilibrium and optimal functioning. An integrated system is flexible, adaptive, coherent, energized, and stable, one that has the vitality of harmony. When systems are not integrated, they move away from this flow of a harmonious system and toward the banks outside this "river of integration" toward chaos on one side or rigidity on the other. When things don't go well in school, chaotic behaviors or stagnant rigidity may rule the day. In contrast, when classrooms are thriving, teachers may sense the integrative flow of harmony that supports the differentiation of each member of the learning community and the subsequent linkage to one another through the compassionate and engaged communication in their shared journey of discovery (see Cozolino, 2013). Students thrive in such an environment, and the roots of resilience are reinforced and strengthened.

An Internal Education of the Mind

In a field called "interpersonal neurobiology," the development of a healthy mind is the focus emerging from the synthesis of a wide range of scientific disciplines. Despite a lack of a definition of the mind in various fields (see Siegel, 2012a, 2012b; Siegel, 2016), including that of mental health itself, a working approach to the mind from this interdisciplinary work may be useful in the field of education and our discussion of the roots of resilience. Though the mind naturally involves a sense of subjective experience and the important phenomenon of consciousness, it also entails a core function that can be defined as "an embodied and relational process that regulates the flow of energy and information" (Siegel, 1999, 2012a). We've seen already how our experience of resilience emerges from both inner attunement and interpersonal attunement. This reveals how the mind is both embodied—a part of bodily processes including those of the brain—and how it is relational—a property of how we communicate and connect with one another. Energy and information flow is simply the movement across time of the physics' property of energy, the capacity to "do stuff" such as carry out work. Sometimes that energy has symbolic value; it stands for something other than itself and thus has meaning. We call this energy pattern "information". Now we come to the regulatory aspect of this definition of the mind, which has important and practical relevance for educators.

When you regulate a car, what do you do? First, it is essential to drive well to see where you are going. This is the first part of regulation: monitoring. We monitor energy and information flow in our bodies, as in interoceptive awareness, and in our relationships, as in social communication. Next, what do we do with a car? We apply the accelerator and the brakes, we steer, we turn the car on or off. This is the modifying part of regulation. The mind modifies or modulates energy and information flow. Once we have this working definition of the mind in a teacher's toolkit, it becomes possible to very practically apply this idea to the task of helping students build a more resilient mind. We can make the mind stronger, more resilient, supple and flexible, and even healthier and happier, by building the skills of monitoring and modifying.

Mindfulness practices are one way to approach the application of these ideas to focusing on monitoring the internal world and then modifying it in a healthy way. When we build the skills of monitoring, we stabilize the mind so that we can see with more depth, clarity, and detail. The view we get is more stable and filled with more user-friendly data. We can also learn to modify energy and information flow in a positive direction. Health, in this view, emerges from modulating the internal and interpersonal world toward integration. In the brain, for example, students can learn to monitor right and left hemisphere functions and then develop the skills to link them together, rather than use only one side or the other. In interpersonal relationships, students could be taught the core values of relational health as being centered in integration: All individuals can be honored for their uniqueness and then linked in respectful and compassionate communication.

Health becomes the core value that is highlighted in this internal education approach to cultivating the roots of resilience. Instead of teaching the important but limited basic skills (e.g. reading, mathematical skills) and sets of factual knowledge, schools can offer a way to focus directly on the development of the mind itself. Building such "mindsight skills" can be done in a systematic way (see Siegel, 2013). We can build a stronger mind through reflection and relationships that build resilience as the new R's of education. These deep inner skills will allow the next generation of graduates to approach the ever-changing world prepared to create the strong minds and meaningful relationships that will help them and our global community to thrive now and in the years to come.

References

Anderson, S. W., Bechara, A., Damasio, H., Tranel, D., & Damasio, A. R. (1999). Impairment of social and moral behavior related to early damage in human prefrontal cortex. *Nature Neuroscience, 2*, 1032–1037.

Baer, R. A., Smith, G. T., Hopkins, J., Krietemeyer, J., & Toney, L. (2006). Using self-report assessment methods to explore facets of mindfulness. *Assessment, 13*(1), 27–45.

Batson, C. D. (2009). These things called empathy: Eight related but distinct phenomena. In J. Decety & W. Ickes (Eds.), *The social neuroscience of empathy* (pp. 3–15). Cambridge, MA: MIT Press.

Beitel, M., Ferrer, E., & Cecero, J. J. (2005). Psychological mindedness and awareness of self and others. *Journal of Clinical Psychology, 61*, 739–750.

Bishop, S., Lau, M., Shapiro, S., Carlson, L., Anderson, N., Carmody, J., … Devins, G. (2004). Mindfulness: A proposed operational definition. *Clinical Psychology: Science and Practice, 11*, 230–241.

Bowlby, J. (2003). *A secure base: Clinical applications of attachment theory* (7th ed.). New York, NY: Lawrence Erlbaum Associates.
Brewer, J. A., Worhunsky, P. D., Gray, J. R., Tang, Y., Weber, J., & Kober, H. (2011). Meditation experience is associated with differences in default mode network activity and connectivity. *Proceedings of the National Academy of Sciences, 108*(50), 20254–20259.
Brown, K. W., & Ryan, R. M. (2003). The benefits of being present: Mindfulness and its role in psychological well-being. *Journal of Personality and Social Psychology, 84*, 822–848.
Carr, L., Iacoboni, M., Dubeau, M. C., Maziotta, J. C., & Lenzi, L. G. (2003). Neural mechanisms of empathy in humans: A relay from neural systems for imitation to limbic areas. *Proceedings of the National Academy of Sciences USA, 100*, 5497–5502.
Carson, J. W., Carson, K. M., Gil, K. M., & Baucom, D. H. (2004). Mindfulness-based relationship enhancement. *Behavior Therapy, 35*, 471–494.
Cassidy, J., & Shaver, P. R. (2010). *Handbook of attachment: Theory, research, and clinical applications* (2nd ed.). New York, NY: Guilford Press.
Christakis, N. A., & Fowler, J. H. (2009). *Connected.* New York, NY: Little Brown.
Cozolino, L. (2013). *The social neuroscience of education: Optimizing attachment and learning in the classroom.* New York, NY: W. W. Norton.
Cozolino, L. (2014). *The neuroscience of human relationships: Attachment and the developing social brain* (2nd ed.). New York, NY: W. W. Norton.
Craig, A. D. (2003). Interoception: The sense of the physiological condition of the body. *Current Opinion in Neurobiology, 13*(4), 500–505.
Critchley, H. D., Wiens, S., Rotshtein, P., Öhman, A., & Dolan, R. J. (2004). Neural systems supporting interoceptive awareness. *Nature Neuroscience, 7*(2), 189–195.
Davidson, R. J., Kabat-Zinn, J., Schumacher, J., Rosenkranz, M., Muller, D., Santorelli, S. F., … Sheridan, J. F. (2003). Alterations in brain and immune function produced by mindfulness meditation. *Psychosomatic Medicine, 65*, 564–570.
Decety, J., & Ickes, W. (2009). *The social neuroscience of empathy.* Cambridge, MA: MIT Press.
Dekeyser, M., Raes, F., Leijssen, M., Leysen, S., & Dewulf, D. (2008). Mindfulness skills and interpersonal behavior. *Personality and Individual Differences, 44*, 1235–1245.
DiNoble, A. (2009). *Examining the relationship between adult attachment style and mindfulness traits.* A dissertation presented to the faculty of the California Graduate Institute of the Chicago School of Professional Psychology, January.
Farb, N. A. S., Segal, Z. V., Mayberg, H., Bean, J., McKeon, D., Fatima, Z., Anderson, A. K. (2007). Attending to the present: Mindfulness meditation reveals distinct neural modes of self-reference. *Social Cognitive and Affective Neuroscience*, 2(4), 313–322.
Fonagy, P., & Target, M. (2005). Bridging the transmission gap: An end to an important mystery of attachment research? *Attachment & Human Development, 7*(3), 333–343.
Gilbert, D. (2007). *Stumbling on happiness.* New York, NY: Vintage.
Gilbert, P. (2010). *The compassionate mind.* Oakland, CA: New Harbinger.
Gilbert, P., & Choden. (2013). *Mindful compassion: How the science of compassion can help you understand your emotions, live in the present, and connect deeply with others.* Oakland, CA: New Harbinger.
Haidt, J. (2006). *The happiness hypothesis.* New York, NY: Basic Books.
Hölzel, B. K., Carmody, J., Vangel, M., Congleton, C., Yerramsetti, S. M., Gard, T., & Lazar, S. W. (2011). Mindfulness practice leads to increases in regional brain gray matter density. *Psychiatry Research: Neuroimaging, 48*, 36–43.
Iacoboni, M. (2003). Understanding intentions through imitation. In S. H. Johnson-Frey (Ed.), *Taking action: Cognitive neuroscience perspective on intentional acts* (pp. 107–138). Cambridge, MA: The MIT Press.
Iacoboni, M. (2008). *Mirroring people.* New York, NY: Farar-Giroux.
Iacoboni, M. (2009). Imitation, empathy, and mirror neurons. *Annual Review of Psychology, 60*, 653–670.
Jacobs, T. L., Epel, E. S., Lin, J., Blackburn, E. H., Wolkowitz, W. M., Bridwell, D. A., … Saron, C. D. (2010). Intensive meditation training, immune cell telomerase activity, and psychological mediators. *Psychoneuroendocrinology, 36*(5), 664–681.
Jennings, P. A., Snowberg, K. E., Coccia, M. A., & Greenberg, M. T. (2011). Improving classroom learning environments by Cultivating Awareness and Resilience in Education (CARE): Results of two pilot studies. *Journal of Classroom Interactions, 46*, 27–48.
Jennings, P. A., Snowberg, K. E., Frank, J., Coccia, M. A., & Greenberg, M. T. (2013). Improving classroom learning environments by Cultivating Awareness and Resilience in Education (CARE): Results of a randomized controlled trial. *School Psychology Quarterly, 28*, 374–398.
Kaiser Greenland, S. (2006). *Information from inner kids organizational website.* www.innerkids.com
Kilpatrick, L. A., Suyenobu, B. Y., Smith, S. R., Bueller, J. A., Goodman, T., Creswell, J. D., … Naliboff, B. D. (2011). Impact of mindfulness-based stress reduction training on intrinsic brain connectivity. *Neuroimage, 56*, 290–298.
Kornfield, J. (2008). *The wise heart: A guide to the universal teachings of Buddhist psychology.* New York, NY: Bantam/Random House.
Krasner, M., Epstein, R., Beckman, H., Suchman, A., Chapman, B., Mooney, C., & Quill, T. (2009). Association of an educational program in mindful communication with burnout, empathy, and attitudes among primary care physicians. JAMA, September 23–30, 1284–1293.
Lazar, S. W., Kerr, C. E., Wasserman, R. H., Gray, J. R., Greve, D. N., Treadway, M. T., … Fischl, B. (2005). Meditation experience is associated with increased cortical thickness. *NeuroReport, 16*(17), 1893–1897.

Lee, R. M., Draper, M., & Lee, S. (2001). Social connectedness, dysfunctional interpersonal behaviors, and psychological distress: Testing a mediator model. *Journal of Counseling Psychology, 48*, 310–318.

Lieberman, M. D. (2013). *Social: Why our brains are wired to connect*. New York, NY: Crown.

Luders, E., Clark, K., Narr, K. L., & Toga, A. W. (2011). Enhanced brain connectivity in long-term meditation practitioners. *NeuroImage, 57*, 1308–1316.

Lutz, A., Slagter, H. A., Dunne, J. D., & Davidson, R. J. (2008). Attention regulation and monitoring in meditation. *Trends in Cognitive Sciences, 12*(4), 163–169.

Main, M. (1999). Mary D. Salter Ainsworth: Tribute and portrait. *Psychoanalytic Inquiry, 19*(5), 682–736.

Main, M., Goldwyn, R., & Hesse, E. (2003). *Adult attachment scoring and classification system*. Unpublished manuscript, University of California, Berkeley.

McGilchrist, I. (2009). *The master and his emissary: The divided brain and the making of the Western world*. Cambridge, MA: Cambridge University Press.

Meany, M. J. (2010). Epigenetics and the biological definition of gene×environment interactions. *Child Development, 81*(1), 41–79.

Neff, K. (2011). *Self-compassion*. New York, NY: Harper-Collins.

Norcross, J. C. (2002). *Psychotherapy relationships that work: Therapist contributions and responsiveness to patients*. New York, NY: Oxford University Press.

Panksepp, J., & Biven, L. (2012). *The archaeology of mind: Neuroevolutionary origins of human emotions*. New York, NY: W. W. Norton.

Porges, S. W. (2009). Reciprocal influences between body and brain in the perception and expression of affect: A polyvagal perspective. In D. Fosha, D. J. Siegel, & M. F. Solomon (Eds.), *The Healing Power of Emotion: Affective Neuroscience, Development & Clinical Practice* (pp. 27–54). New York, NY: W.W. Norton.

Porges, S. W. (2011). *The polyvagal system*. New York, NY: W. W. Norton.

Salzberg, S. (2008). *The kindness handbook: A practical companion*. Boulder, CO: Sounds True.

Sawyer Cohen, J., & Semple, R. (2010). Mindful parenting: A call for research. *Journal of Child and Family Studies, 19*, 145–151.

Shapiro, S. L., Astin, J. A., Bishop, S. R., & Cordova, M. (2005). Mindfulness-based stress reduction for health care professionals: Results from a randomized trial. *International Journal of Stress Management, 12*, 164–176.

Shapiro, S. L., Brown, K. W., & Biegel, G. (2007). Teaching self-care to caregivers: The effects of mindfulness-based stress reduction on the mental health of therapists in training. *Training and Education in Professional Psychology, 1*, 105–115.

Shapiro, S. L., Carlson, L. E., Astin, J. A., & Freedman, B. (2006). Mechanisms of mindfulness. *Journal of Clinical Psychology, 62*, 373–386.

Shapiro, S. L., Schwartz, G. E., & Bonner, G. (1998). Effects of mindfulness-based stress reduction on medical and premedical students. *Journal of Behavioral Medicine, 21*, 581–599.

Siegel, D. J. (1999). *The developing mind, first edition: Toward a neurobiology of interpersonal experience*. New York, NY: Guilford Press.

Siegel, D. J. (2007a). *The mindful brain: Reflection and attunement in the cultivation of well-being*. New York, NY: W. W. Norton.

Siegel, D.J. (2007b). Mindfulness training and neural integration. *Journal of Social, Cognitive, and Affective Neuroscience, 2*(4), 259–263.

Siegel, D. J. (2010a). *The mindful therapist: A clinician's guide to mindsight and neural integration*. New York, NY: WW Norton.

Siegel, D. J. (2010b). *Mindsight: The new science of personal transformation*. New York, NY: Bantam/Random House.

Siegel, D. J. (2012a). *The developing mind, second edition: How relationships and the brain interact to shape who we are*. New York, NY: Guilford Press.

Siegel, D. J. (2012b). *Pocket guide to interpersonal neurobiology: An integrative handbook of the mind*. New York, NY: W.W. Norton.

Siegel, D. J. (2013). *Brainstorm: The power and purpose of the teenage brain*. New York, NY: Penguin Putnam.

Siegel, D.J. (2016). *Mind: A journey to the heart of being human*. New York: WW Norton.

Slade, A., Grienenberger, J., Bernbach, E., Levy, D., & Locker, A. (2005). Maternal reflective functioning, attachment, and the transmission gap: A preliminary study. *Attachment & Human Development, 7*(3), 283–298.

Smith, S.M., Nichols, T.E., Vidaurre, D., Winkler, A.M., Behrens, T.E.J., Glasser, M.F., Ugurbil, K., Barch, D.M., Van Essen, D.C., & Miller, K.L. (2015). *A positive-negative mode of population co-variation links brain connectivity, demographics, and behavior. Nature Neuroscience, 18*(11), 1567–1571.

Spickard, A., Gabbe, S., & Christensen, J. (2002). Midcareer burnout in generalist and specialist physicians. *Journal of the American Medical Association, 288*, 1447–1450.

Sroufe, L. A., Carlson, E., & Waters, E. (2005). *The development of the person*. New York, NY: Guilford.

Sroufe, L. A., & Siegel, D.J. (2011, March). The verdict is in. *Psychotherapy Networker*.

Steger, M. F., Frazier, P., Oishi, S., & Kaler, M. (2006). The Meaning in Life Questionnaire: Assessing the presence of and search for meaning in life. *Journal of Counseling Psychology, 53*, 80–93.

Tulving, E. (1993). Varieties of consciousness and levels of awareness in memory. In A. Baddeley & L. Weiskrantz (Eds.), *Attention, selection, awareness, and control: A tribute to Daonald Broadbent* (pp. 283–299). London, England: Oxford University Press.

Urry, H. L., Nitschke, J. B., Dolski, I., Jackson, D. C., Dalton, K. M., & Mueller, C. J. ...Davidson, R. J. (2004). Making a life worth living: Neural correlates of well-being. *Psychological Science, 15*, 367–372.

Mindfulness and Social Emotional Learning (SEL): A Conceptual Framework

5

Molly Stewart Lawlor

Introduction

Along with teaching essential academic skills such as reading, math, and science, a fundamental mission of schooling is to educate the "whole child" which includes promoting both cognitive and noncognitive skills (Greenberg et al., 2003). Indeed, schools are a critical context in which to foster children's positive development (Masten & Motti-Stefanidi, 2009; National Research Council, 2012). Further, recent empirical evidence has shown schools to be one of the primary settings to implement primary prevention initiatives, in particular, those that promote social-emotional learning (SEL; Durlak, Weissberg, Dymnicki, Taylor, & Schellinger, 2011; Greenberg et al., 2003, Humphrey, 2013, Kress & Elias, 2006; Zins, Bloodworth, Weissberg, & Walberg, 2004). SEL involves the cultivation of five major competencies: self-awareness, self-management, social awareness, relationship skills, and responsible decision-making (Zins, Weissberg, Wang, & Walberg, 2004). Increasingly, school-based primary prevention efforts are incorporating mindfulness-based practices to foster attention, resiliency, and well-being (Garrison Institute, 2005; Greenberg & Harris, 2012; Roeser & Peck, 2009). Mindfulness is a state of consciousness that involves the direction of attention that incorporates self-awareness with a core characteristic of being open, receptive, and nonjudgmental (Brown & Ryan, 2003; Kabat-Zinn, 1990). Mindfulness-based initiatives in education are aligned with the goals of SEL, a field with an established research base supporting school-based intervention efforts. Both initiatives focus on the education of the whole child with emphasis on the development of positive self, moral, social, and emotional understanding.

Research efforts, with both clinical and non-clinical samples, evaluating the effectiveness of mindfulness-based approaches targeting children and youth have increased. In the last few years, a number of reviews have been published that summarize the findings of mindfulness-based interventions for children and youth (Burke, 2010; Harnett & Dawe, 2013; Meiklejohn et al., 2010), examining the overall effectiveness of mindfulness approaches with child and adolescent populations. What has been missing is a clear theoretical, empirical, and practical, articulation of how mindfulness-based practices align with SEL. This article puts forth a conceptual framework that describes how mindfulness practices may deepen SEL within K-12 educational contexts. First, an introduction to mindfulness and SEL is presented, followed by the proposed conceptual framework, rationale, and

M.S. Lawlor (✉)
University of British Columbia,
Vancouver, BC, Canada
e-mail: northshoremolly@gmail.com

K.A. Schonert-Reichl, R.W. Roeser (eds.), *Handbook of Mindfulness in Education*,
Mindfulness in Behavioral Health, DOI 10.1007/978-1-4939-3506-2_5

examples of practical applications in educational settings. Finally, future directions for the field of mindfulness and SEL will be discussed.

Mindfulness

A widely accepted definition of mindfulness comes from Jon Kabat-Zinn, a pioneer in the field, who defines mindfulness as "the awareness that emerges through paying attention on purpose, in the present moment, and nonjudgmentally to the unfolding of experience moment by moment" (Kabat-Zinn, 2003, p. 145). Mindfulness has been found to be associated with indicators of well-being, including optimism, positive feelings, and self-actualization and has been linked to lower rates of psychological and emotional disturbance, such as negative feelings, depression, and anxiety (Brown & Ryan, 2003; Lawlor, Schonert-Reichl, Gadermann, & Zumbo, 2014). Research examining mindfulness has also found a relationship between mindfulness and emotional intelligence (Baer, Smith, & Allen, 2004; Baer, Smith, Hopkins, Krietemeyer, & Toney, 2006; Brown & Ryan, 2003). In addition, mindfulness has been shown to promote empathy (Sahdra et al., 2011; Schonert-Reichl et al., 2014).

Mindfulness training involves the cultivation of conscious attention and awareness to the present moment. This intentional practice can take many forms and may include such practices as mindful breathing, open awareness meditation, walking meditation, and focusing on sensations in the body. Recent research on interventions that utilize training in mindfulness with adults has revealed improvements in a variety of well-being outcomes including depression, anxiety disorders, treatment for chronic pain, and range of additional mental health and medical conditions (for reviews see Baer, 2003; Grossman, Keng, Smoski, & Robins, 2011; Niemann, Schmidt, & Walach, 2004). In addition, research in the field of neuroscience has shown that mindfulness training can improve cognitive control, an important aspect of attention, and self-regulation (Jha, Krompinger, & Baime, 2007; Tang et al., 2007; Tang & Posner, 2009) in adult populations.

Social-Emotional Learning

Social-emotional learning, or SEL, encompasses the processes through which individuals attain and effectively apply the knowledge, attitudes, and skills necessary to identify and manage their emotions; understand another's perspective and show empathy for others; set and achieve positive goals; develop and sustain positive relationships; and make responsible decisions (Collaborative for Academic, Social, and Emotional Learning, 2013; Weissberg, Payton, O'Brien, & Munro, 2007). The Collaborative for Academic, Social, and Emotional Learning (CASEL; www.casel.org), a nonprofit organization in Chicago, IL, is a leader in efforts to promote SEL across the globe. Since its inception in 1994, CASEL has served as a guide to school-based SEL programming (Collaborative for Academic, Social, and Emotional Learning, 2003). Derived from extensive research, Collaborative for Academic, Social, and Emotional Learning (2013) has identified five interrelated sets of cognitive, affective, and behavioral competencies that are central to SEL: self-awareness, self-management, social awareness, relationship skills, and responsible decision-making.

The first two competencies are related to one's emotional capabilities. *Self-awareness* refers to the ability to accurately recognize one's feelings and thoughts and their influence on behaviors. This includes accurately assessing one's strengths and limitations, and possessing a well-grounded sense of confidence and optimism. *Self-management* is the ability to regulate one's emotions, thoughts, and behaviors in different situations. This includes delaying gratification, managing stress, controlling impulses, motivating oneself, and setting and working towards personal and academic goals. Although self-focused, these competencies are also fundamental for building effective social skills.

The next two competencies are linked to one's social capabilities. *Social awareness* describes the ability to take the perspective of and empathize with others from diverse backgrounds and cultures, to understand social and ethical norms for behavior, and to recognize family, school, and community resources and supports. *Relationship skills* are the ability to establish and maintain healthy and rewarding relationships with diverse individuals and groups. This includes communicating clearly, listening actively, cooperating, resisting inappropriate social pressure, negotiating conflict constructively, and seeking help when needed. Finally, *responsible decision-making* refers to the ability to make constructive choices about personal behavior, social interactions, and school and life expectations based on consideration of ethical standards, safety concerns, social norms, realistic evaluation of consequences of various actions, and the well-being of self and others.

Research on Social Emotional Learning

> Emotions can facilitate or impede children's academic engagement, work ethic, commitment, and ultimate school success.
>
> Durlak et al. (2011, p. 406)

SEL has been referred to as "the missing piece," for the reason that it embodies a part of education that is inextricably linked to school success, but historically has not been explicitly acknowledged or prioritized in public education in North America. This has changed in recent years with the increase of evidence supporting the links between SEL and student success. A 2011 meta-analysis conducted by Durlak and colleagues examined the effectiveness of SEL programs in 213 studies that included 270,034 students aged 5–18. Results revealed student improvements in *both* social-emotional skills and academics. Specifically, Durlak et al. found that well-designed and implemented SEL programs improve test-taking skills and academic performance; promote positive social behaviors; foster positive feelings and reduce behavioral problems; and decrease levels of emotional distress. Indeed, the social side of learning is explicitly linked to the academic side of learning. Further findings examined the durability of the effects of SEL interventions longitudinally. Specifically, an examination of a subgroup of 33 interventions that included follow-up data (with an average follow-up period of 92 weeks) revealed that positive effects at the time of follow-up remained statistically significant; however, the effect sizes were slighter. These findings point to the significant impact SEL has on student outcomes across social, psychological, and academic domains.

Contemplative Education

A natural bridge between SEL and mindfulness can be found in a movement described as contemplative education. Roeser and Peck (2009) describe contemplative education as an approach to education that is focused on the development of the whole person and define it as a "set of pedagogical practices designed to cultivate the potentials of mindful awareness and volition in an ethical-relational context in which the values of personal growth, learning, moral living, and caring for others are also nurtured" (p. 127). Drawing from millennia old contemplative traditions, contemplative education engages students actively with a competent teacher and a "set of experiential learning opportunities designed to help students develop clear, calm, and concentrated states of awareness in a context of personal growth and values such as humility, curiosity, open-mindedness, open-heartedness, and caring for others" (Roeser & Peck, 2009, p. 127). A fundamental component within contemplative education is the cultivation of "mindful and intentional forms of living and learning" (Roeser & Peck, 2009, p. 127). Experiential practices to promote mindful awareness include seated meditation, movement (e.g., yoga, tai chi), guided imagery, community service learning, storytelling, active witnessing, Japanese calligraphy, music, art, and literature (Greenberg, 2014; Lantieri & Nambiar, 2012; Roeser & Peck, 2009).

Research on Contemplative Education

Research in the area of contemplative education has grown in recent years with the aforementioned reviews on the topic of mindfulness interventions with children and youth presently available (Burke, 2010; Greenberg & Harris, 2012; Harnett & Dawe, 2012; Meiklejohn et al., 2012).

In addition to these reviews, a recent meta-analysis was conducted that examined 20 peer-reviewed journal articles on mindfulness interventions with children and youth under the age of 18 (Zoogman, Goldberg, Hoyt, & Miller, 2014). Findings indicated that mindfulness interventions with youth do not cause harm, or, iatrogenic effects. Omnibus analysis revealed effect sizes (*del*) in the small to moderate range (.23, $p < .001$) that suggest that mindfulness interventions provide benefits over active control comparison groups. Two moderators, sample origin (clinical versus nonclinical) and outcome type (psychological symptoms versus outcome variables), were identified. Clinical samples showed larger effects than nonclinical samples ($del = 0.500$ versus $del = 0.197$). In addition, a larger effect size was found for psychological symptoms, such as depression, compared to other outcome variables, including mindfulness-related measures (0.37 versus 0.21, $p = .028$). The authors were cautious with their interpretation of the findings due to the small sample of studies ($k = 4$) that examined clinical samples. In their discussion, the authors speculate that the mechanism underpinning the effects of mindfulness intervention is attention. This assumption follows previous research that has shown improvements in attention with mindfulness practice in adults (Brefczynski Lewis, Lutz, Schaefer, Levinson, & Davidson, 2007; Jha et al., 2007), adolescents (Baijal, Jha, Kiyonaga, Singh, & Srinivasan, 2011), and children (Flook et al., 2010).

The field of mindfulness research with children and youth is in a nascent stage (Lawlor et al. 2014; Roeser & Zelazo, 2012). Further research is needed to better understand the mechanisms of mindfulness within younger population, inclusive of both nonclinical and clinical populations (Zoogman et al., 2014). In addition, Zoogman et al. (2014) noted that there is a broad range in the application of mindfulness practices within interventions that lacks uniformity in implementation. These implementation details are not widely reported in the literature. In order to resolve these differences pertaining to implementation practices and effectively compare interventions, the authors recommend that data be collected specific to interventions, examining effectiveness rather than efficacy, and published in peer-review academic journals. Indeed, the emerging field of mindfulness with children and youth does not yet have best practices firmly established regarding implementation (Greenberg & Harris, 2012; Lawlor, 2014). To assist with the development of commonly accepted best practices in mindfulness intervention with younger populations, much can be learned from the extensive research base on SEL school-based implementation (Lawlor, 2014). To help identify the connections between mindfulness practice and SEL, the following section presents a framework delineating how mindfulness practices can deepen SEL.

Social Emotional Learning and Mindfulness: A Conceptual Framework

Greenberg proposed a conceptual framework (2014) that highlights how contemplative practices, or mindfulness, can deepen the development of social-emotional competencies. Figure 5.1, adapted from Greenberg (2014), delineates how mindfulness practices deepen each of the five components of SEL identified by Collaborative for Academic, Social, and Emotional Learning (2013). Understanding the theoretical and empirical linkages between mindfulness and SEL is valuable, but it is also important to consider the practical applications of mindfulness in K-12 education. What does mindfulness practice look like in the classroom? In light of this, the following section includes both the theoretical and empirical basis that supports the proposed framework and provides examples of practical applications of mindfulness training that are suitable for educational contexts. Table 5.1 provides select mindfulness practices that may deepen each of the five competencies of SEL.

Self-Awareness

Self-awareness includes the ability to recognize one's emotions, strengths and limitations, and values (Collaborative for Academic, Social, and

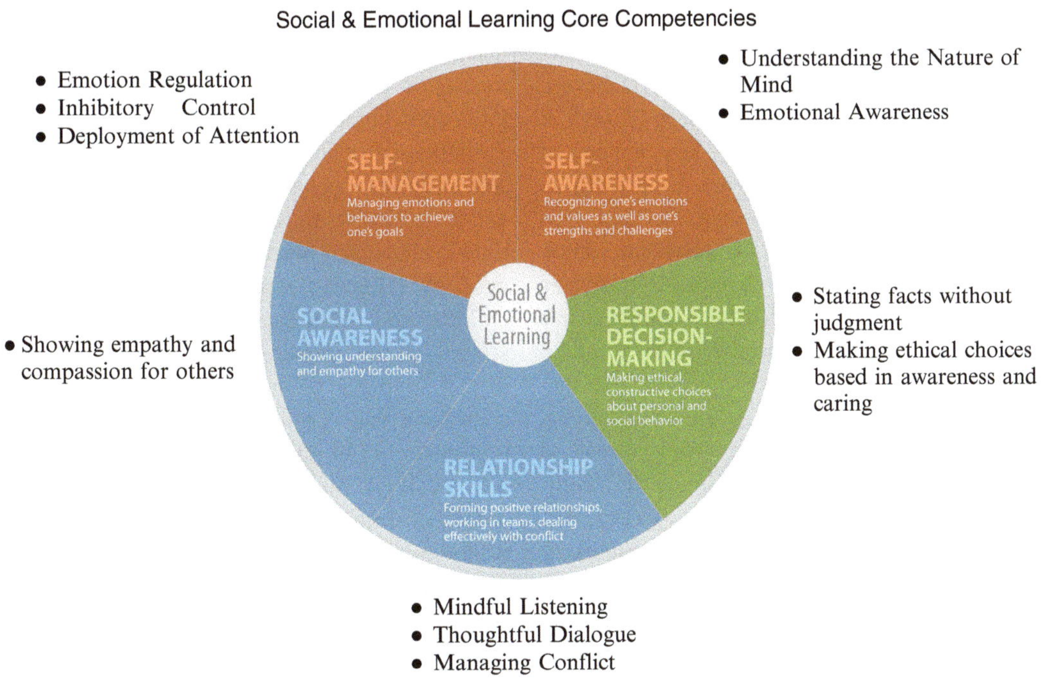

Fig. 5.1 Social emotional competencies and mindful awareness. Adapted from Collaborative for Academic, Social, and Emotional Learning (2013) and Greenberg (2014)

Table 5.1 SEL and mindfulness: select practices

SEL competency	Mindful awareness	Selected mindfulness practices
Self-awareness	• Understanding the nature of mind	• Focused mindful breathing
	• Emotional awareness	• Reflective writing
Self-management	• Emotion regulation	• Focused mindful breathing
	• Inhibitory control	• Movement (e.g., yoga, tai chi)
	• Deployment of attention	
Social awareness	• Showing empathy and compassion for others	• Literature
		• Dramatic arts
		• Compassion/loving-kindness meditation
Relationship skills	• Mindful listening	• Active listening activities
	• Thoughtful dialogue	• Cooperative activities
	• Managing conflict	
Responsible decision-making	• Stating facts without judgment	• Community service learning
	• Making ethical choices based in awareness and caring	• Active witnessing

Emotional Learning, 2013). Greenberg (2014) described the role of contemplation in self-awareness as involving emotional awareness and an understanding of the nature of mind, specifically, the fleeting nature of mind. Mindfulness can enable meaningful inner self-exploration that may aid in answering the question, "Who am I?" By facilitating the surfacing of underlying emotions, values, and motivations, mindfulness can assist in the development of self-awareness. Simple contemplative practices that foster stillness, calm, and reflection can create the necessary conditions for self-exploration and subsequent self-awareness.

Similarly, trait mindfulness has been found to be associated with an individual's ability to better describe and identify his/her emotions (Dekeyser, 2008) and intrinsic value orientation (Brown & Kasser, 2005), both of which are key elements of self-awareness. Some work has been done to understand how mindfulness may facilitate self-awareness and attunement to individual values. For instance, in their research with adults, Brown and Ryan (2003) found that trait mindfulness was associated with the fulfillment of the three fundamental needs outlined by self-determination theory (SDT: Deci & Ryan, 1985): autonomy, relatedness, and competence. They discussed how mindfulness may help facilitate the fulfillment of these fundamental needs. Specifically, mindfulness may make an individual more likely to be attuned to prompts arising from basic needs. Attunement to fundamental needs, a component of self-awareness, would then increase the likelihood of an individual engaging in autonomous action that is congruent with personal values and fulfills their fundamental needs for relatedness and competence. It is through this process that self-awareness is fostered—the ability to recognize one's values, emotions, strengths, and limitations.

Further, studies have demonstrated that adults who are more mindful embrace more intrinsic (opposed to extrinsic) values, are less materialistic, and experience less divergence between what they have and what they want (Brown & Ryan, 2004; Brown, Kasser, Ryan, Alex Linley, & Orzech, 2009). These findings suggest that individuals who are more mindful are more self-aware, in that they align themselves according to intrinsic values and goals, rather aligning themselves to external motivators, such as material wealth. The open self-awareness component of mindfulness leads to autonomous actions that align with an individual's values and goals, and subsequently leads to acquisition of fundamental needs. In short, mindfulness may enable self-awareness via a better attunement to the self.

Activities that foster a mindful state benefit this attunement by allowing inner thoughts, emotions, and motivations to come to the surface of awareness. Subsequently, individuals then develop a solid foundation of emotion and self-understanding that supports the other five competencies of SEL. In the classroom, this translates into allowing time for quiet contemplation. Examples of contemplative practices to support self-awareness include focused breath awareness and reflective writing. In a mindful state, emotions, values, and needs can surface into awareness. A reflective writing practice can offer children and youth space to explore their inner selves. Art can provide students with an opportunity to express themselves freely and create something that is guided from within. In addition, nature is an important conduit for mindfulness. A simple mindfulness practice might entail a teacher bringing the class out for a nature walk—mindful listening to bird songs, noticing the crunch of snow underfoot, noticing the fall colors on the trees. Moment-to-moment awareness when in nature, focusing attention of sights, sounds, and smells, may encourage inner stillness, contemplation, and gratitude. Taken together, these types of contemplative practices can be woven into the school day to nurture students' developing self-awareness, the building block of self-identify, and the other four competencies of SEL.

Self-Management

Self-management, as defined by Collaborative for Academic, Social, and Emotional Learning (2013), involves the ability to manage emotions and behaviors to achieve one's goals. Contemplative practices can be very beneficial in developing self-management by "helping children to better deploy their attention, to become more emotionally regulated, and to show more self-control, or inhibitory control" (Greenberg, 2014). In a mindful state, one does not attempt to change, push away, or avoid difficult emotions. This state of consciousness can foster more reflective versus reactive responses to experience. Within a more reflective state we are better able to handle difficult emotions and persevere towards our goals. A very simple example would be a child's ability to delay gratification. Although the feeling of temptation may be great, practicing mindfulness enables the child to sit with temptation, reflect on the longer-term goal in mind, and persevere to delay gratification until that specific point in time when the goal is achieved.

Mindfulness encompasses an active process to attend to the present moment that requires the ability to control attention and exercise executive functions (Zelazo & Lyons, 2012). Executive functions (EFs) are high-level functions that are central to planning behavior to achieve goals, including inhibiting impulses and responses that may derail goal-directed behavior. Core EFs include working memory, inhibition (self-control, self-regulation), and cognitive flexibility; complex executive functions include reasoning, planning, and problem-solving (Diamond, 2013; Diamond & Lee, 2011). EFs have been found to be related to myriad of positive outcomes for children and adolescents, including school readiness (Blair & Razza, 2007), academic competence (Gathercole, Pickering, Knight, & Stegmann, 2004), and mental and physical health (Moffitt et al., 2011). Research with adults in the field of neuroscience has shown that mindfulness training can improve cognitive control, an important aspect of attention, and self-regulation (Jha et al., 2007; Tang et al., 2007; Tang & Posner, 2009).

Teper, Segal, and Inzlicht (2014) have proposed a model that describes the relation of mindfulness to executive functioning and emotion regulation. The model suggests that mindfulness improves executive function because it fosters present-moment awareness, which in turn enables an individual to be attuned to subtle changes in affective states. In addition, mindfulness imparts an openness and acceptance towards these varied affective states that lends itself to effective emotion regulation. The authors posit that these functions of present awareness and acceptance work iteratively, in that "awareness facilitates acceptance by effectively detecting the affective cues that are then 'accepted,' which facilitates awareness by fostering an open mindset that allows for cue detection. Thus, mindfulness promotes executive control by enhancing experience of and attention to transient affects—the control alarms—that arise from competing goal tendencies" (p. 4). The enhanced awareness to emotional states promotes executive control, which in turn is demonstrated with effective emotion regulation.

Neuroscience provides an additional lens to help illuminate the role of mindfulness in the promotion and development of self-regulatory skills. Self-regulatory skills, often studied under the rubric of EFs, include the self-control of action, thought, and emotion (Zelazo & Lyons, 2012). EFs reside in the prefrontal cortex, the area of the brain that resides just behind the forehead. The maturation of the prefrontal cortex relates to an improvement in cognitive control and emotional regulation from childhood through early adulthood (Casey, Jones, & Hare, 2008). Research with adults has revealed that mindfulness practices develop the prefrontal region of the brain (Hölzel et al., 2011). Although there are currently no studies utilizing neuroimaging to understand how mindfulness is displayed physiologically in children and adolescents, research has found self-reported trait mindfulness to be related to EFs in a sample of early adolescents (Oberle, Schonert-Reichl, Lawlor, & Thomson, 2011). Zelazo and Lyons (2012) posited that age-appropriate mindfulness activities may support the development of self-regulatory skills. Specifically, they discussed that mindfulness may promote "top-down" processes, EFs, while lessoning "bottom-up" processes, including anxiety and stress. The result of this process stemming from mindful awareness would evoke a reflective state in both problem-solving and explorative play activities.

In their review of interventions shown to aid the development of executive functioning in children aged 4–12, Diamond and Lee (2011) noted that along with computerized training, noncomputerized games, physical activity (e.g., aerobics, marital arts, yoga), and school curricula, mindfulness training is a strategy that can improve children's executive functions. Educational programs and interventions that include mindfulness training have grown in recent years in an effort to foster resilience and prosocial behavior and thwart mental illness and antisocial behavior (Greenberg & Harris, 2012). One such program,

MindUP, a CASEL SELect program, infuses mindfulness training with SEL. Although there are many programs that support either SEL (see Collaborative for Academic, Social, and Emotional Learning, 2013) or mindfulness (see Garrison Institute, 2005), MindUP was the first program to provide explicit instruction in both mindfulness practices and SEL. A randomized controlled trial of MindUP, with fourth and fifth grade students revealed improvements in EF skills for those who participated in the program compared with students in the control group (Schonert-Reichl et al., 2014). Another randomized controlled study of 64 second- and third-grade children (ages 7–9 years) examined the effect of the 8-week mindfulness-based Inner Kids program on EF (Flook et al., 2010). The results of the study found an interaction effect between baseline EF scores and group status on posttest score of EF. Children with lower baseline levels of EF showed greater improvement in EF compared with children in the control condition. This study suggests that the mindfulness-based approaches used in Inner Kids had a stronger affect on children with EF difficulties. The research linking mindfulness to self-management, in particular, executive functions, is compelling, and highlights the malleability of these skills. Offering young people space in the day to practice contemplative deepening can promote not only cognitive skills, but also the noncognitive skills that are so vital to success in life.

Activities that help to promote self-awareness can also benefit the development self-management. A key ingredient of contemplative practices is the activation of sustained attention, which positively affects self-regulatory processes. Sustained mindful attention can be practiced through a variety of means including contemplative movement (e.g., tai chi or yoga) and meditations (sitting breath awareness or walking meditation). Transitions, such as coming in from recess or shifting activities, can be a challenging time in the classroom especially for younger students. Adding a contemplative practice at these times can be very helpful for students to help foster calmness and emotion management (see Parker & Kupersmidt, 2015). Activities such as deep belly breathing, mindful walking, or listening to quiet music can be woven into the structure of the day that provide opportunities to foster self-regulatory skills. It is within these moments that children learn, develop, and practice strategies for self-management. Regularly scheduled time for contemplative practice is beneficial not only for students, but also for teachers. As posited by Lantieri and Nambiar (2012), "one gift for ourselves and our children is that of silence and stillness. We can find times in the school day to take a quick break to pause and be still and quiet and take a few deep breaths together" (p. 32).

Social Awareness

Social Awareness includes the ability to take the perspective of others, express empathy, value diversity, and understand social and ethical norms of behavior (Collaborative for Academic, Social, and Emotional Learning, 2013). Indeed, the relation of mindfulness to social awareness has been empirically evidenced. Dekeyser, Raes, Leijssen, Leysen, and Dewulf (2008) examined the relation of mindfulness to interpersonal behavior and found mindfulness to be related to expressing oneself in a variety of social situations, and engagement in empathy. Contemplative practices, "can help children show empathy and compassion for others" (Greenberg, 2014). Mindfulness, as a state of consciousness, enables focused attention, which in turn facilitates not only attunement to the self, but also attunement to others. This awareness creates the conditions necessary to take other's perspectives, and in doing so, experience and express empathy, and engage in compassion.

Empathy and perspective-taking are key elements of social awareness and are constructs that have been identified as outcome variables for emerging mindfulness-based intervention programming for children and youth (Davidson et al., 2012). Empathy has been defined as "an affective response that stems from the apprehension or comprehension of another's emotional state or condition, and that is similar to what the other person is feeling or would be expected to feel" (Eisenberg, 2002, p 135). Recent mindfulness-based interventions with adult samples have revealed improvements in socioemotional functioning, including empathy (Sahdra et al., 2011) and prosocial responding (Kemeny et al., 2012), suggesting a connection between mindfulness practice empathy, and prosocial behavior. Similarly, research on the MindUP program with early adolescents has found improvements in prosocial behaviors as rated by peers, and self-reported improvements in empathy (Schonert-Reichl et al., 2014). Taken together, these findings with both children and adult populations reveal the link between mindfulness and social awareness; they also are encouraging regarding the potential for growth in social domains with the application of contemplative practices.

Contemplative practices that focus on others, such as compassion practices (e.g., loving-kindness meditation), can help young people develop empathy and compassion for others. Loving-kindness is a meditation practice that evokes care and compassion towards the self and others (Fredrickson, Cohn, Coffey, Pek, & Finkel 2008). An example of a developmentally appropriate loving-kindness practice for youth comes from the Learning to Breathe Program (see Broderick & Metz, 2015). In addition to compassion practices, literature, storytelling, and the dramatic arts are other ways to foster social awareness with contemplative deepening. These activities are character-based, which provides an ideal conduit for perspective-taking and empathy. Stories that include themes such as kindness, compassion, and tolerance are particularly well suited for contemplative deepening and fostering mindfulness. Open-ended questions such as "How do you think the character felt in that moment?" or "Why do you think the character behaved that way?" can facilitate thoughtful consideration of the perspective of a particular character with a story, book, or play. When an educator reads a book with an intention of completive deepening, "the reading pace becomes slower with opportunities to pause along the way. Young people experience one another's voices and can notice the various emotions that are stirring within each of them. There can be lots of unplanned moments where the story can take us to a deeper place" (Lantieri & Nambiar, 2012, p. 32).

Relationship Skills

Relationship Skills include the abilities to form and maintain positive relationships, work collaboratively with others, and resolve conflicts peacefully (Collaborative for Academic, Social, and Emotional Learning, 2013). All of these skills require effective listening. Without hearing others, we are not able to have effective or thoughtful dialogue. In the absence of thoughtful dialogue, relationship skills suffer and managing conflict becomes more difficult. Greenberg (2014) commented that listening is a "critical skill that often is not taught and not learned." Contemplative practices "can help children to really learn to listen in a different way" (Greenberg, 2014). Mindfulness provides a reflective, nonreactive state of listening and responding to others that facilitates positive relationship formation and maintenance.

Mindfulness has been linked to positive relational experience. In particular, research has found trait mindfulness to be related to, or predictive of, openness, interpersonal closeness, and relatedness (Brown & Ryan, 2003). Much of the research examining mindfulness and interpersonal relationships has been focused on marital and romantic relationships or within the medical field pertaining to patient care. Research examining romantic relationships has linked mindfulness to relationship happiness, lower relationship-specific stress (Carson, Carson, Gil, & Baucom, 2004), constructive responses to relationship stress, and better communication quality (Barnes, Brown, Krusemark, Campbell, & Rogge, 2007). Within the medical field, mindfulness practice has been encouraged for medical practitioners to enhance patient care (Connelly, 2005; Shapiro & Schwartz, 2000). Research in mindfulness interventions with physicians is promising, revealing increases in physician psychosocial orientation and empathy (Krasner et al., 2009), patient-centered pattern of communication, positive emotional tone, and higher patient ratings of clinician communication (Beach et al., 2013). These findings underline the significant function mindfulness has in relationships skills including listening and positive communication styles.

Research examining mindfulness and relationship skills is more limited in child and adolescent populations. One approach has examined the application of mindfulness in prevention interventions for parents. The Strengthening Families Program was designed with the idea that "teaching parents mindfulness skills in the context of family-focused preventive interventions may be an effective way of enhancing youth wellness and reducing youth problem behavior" (Coatsworth et al., 2014, p. 45). The program integrates brief mindfulness practices with parent skills training to help parents be more mindful in their daily interactions with their adolescents. Central to the program is a goal to strengthen parent–youth relationships. Strengthening Families includes mindful activities such as reflections (e.g., focused attention and deep breathing), cultivating kindness and compassion, and setting intentions. The program emphasizes mindful listening, seeing the whole child, and reflective versus reactive parenting practices. Results from a series of pilot studies with 65 families are promising, revealing self-reported increases in mindful parenting and improvement in parent–child relationship qualities (Coatsworth, Duncan, Greenberg, & Nix, 2010). The Strengthening Families Program and accompanying research highlight that engagement in contemplative practices is not just important for young people, but also for the adults who care for them. Adults filling many roles for children (e.g., parents, educators, coaches, and mentors) can embody the qualities of mindfulness, and in turn affect positive development in young people.

Creating opportunities for contemplative deepening specific to relationship skills often focus on listening activities. A simple mindful listening activity would include asking children to sit in stillness and listen carefully to all sounds present in the room. Listening activities can include an interpersonal aspect by engaging young people in active listening practices—truly hearing one another. Younger children can engaged in a simple game of "telephone" where an intention is set to listen mindfully. For older children, active listening can happen in dyads—students take turns being the speaker and the listener. The role of the listener is to set an intention to listen mindfully to the speaker and not interrupt. Once the speaker is finished speaking, the listening then reflects back to the speaker what they have just heard. This intentional mindful listening practice offers children the opportunity to practice the critical skill of listening and at the same time, engage in perspective-taking and empathy.

Responsible Decision-Making

Responsible decision-making includes making ethical and constructive choices about behavior (Collaborative for Academic, Social, and Emotional Learning, 2013). In his commetary, Greenberg (2014) noted that contemplative practices deepen responsible decision-making or problem solving by cultivating the ability to state facts without judgment. The ability to observe without judgment removes bias from the decision-making process and enables individuals to make ethical choices based on awareness and caring. In a mindful state an individual observes events without attempting to judge or manipulate events or experiences. Moment-to-moment mindfulness allows for "simple observation without analyzing, comparing, or otherwise evaluating events and experience" (Brown et al., 2009, p. 728). This type of consciousness lends itself to decisions and actions that are driven from awareness and compassion rather than choices based within a pro-self orientation.

Shapiro and colleagues examined the effects of mindfulness-based stress reduction (MBSR), an 8-week mindfulness intervention, developed by Kabat-Zinn (1990), on moral reasoning and decision-making with a group of adults (Shapiro, Jazaieri, & Goldin, 2012). The authors described the link between mindfulness and moral reasoning as resting on awareness—that moral reasoning requires awareness, and mindfulness practice helps cultivate this necessary awareness. Further, the authors posit that "mindfulness practice aims at transforming those automatic habits of self-grasping or self-preservation. Thus, it cultivates a more objective, less ego-centric frame of reference, and develops the capacity to consider the well-being of others in addition to oneself" (Shapiro et al., 2012, p. 505). Results from the study at 2-month follow-up included improvements in mindful attention, emotion (positive and negative affect), well-being, and moral reasoning and ethical decision-making.

Responsible decision-making (i.e., making ethical choices) concerns not only our relations to one another, but also our connection to the ecology of the very planet that sustains us. Dan Goleman (2014) discussed ecological responsibility as an important element for inclusion within SEL. Indeed, responsible decision-making extends beyond our interactions with each other. It also includes awareness and care of all creatures, and the planet that connects us all. Research suggests that mindfulness does indeed promote this type of care and awareness. Brown and Kasser (2005) investigated the question of whether psychological and ecological well-being are compatible. Their findings revealed that intrinsic value orientation and trait mindfulness were related to higher subjective well-being and ecologically responsible behavior. Analysis revealed that the compatibility of subjective well-being and ecologically responsible behavior was explained by mindfulness and intrinsic values. Empirical evidence such as this reveals the significant role mindfulness may play in ethical decision-making and actions. By fostering mindful awareness via contemplative activities, educators may develop children's appreciation for the inter-connectedness between ourselves and our environment. This awareness can promote civic responsibility, care, and compassion that extend beyond classroom walls.

Fostering responsible decision-making with mindfulness might include active witnessing, community service learning, or quiet contemplation within nature. Service learning has been found to contribute to the creation of a moral identity (Youniss & Yates, 1999), and prosocialness (cooperativeness, helpfulness, sharing and being empathic; Caprara, Barbaranelli, Pastorelli, Bandura, & Zimbardo, 2000; Scales, Benson, Leffert, & Blyth, 2000). A critical component to make service learning meaningful is the opportunity for reflection (Metz & Youniss, 2005). Connecting active witnessing or service learning with time for contemplative reflection (writing, art, sharing with others) can deepen the meaning students take from these activities and foster integration into a moral identity.

Where Are We Now and Where Do We Need to Go?

> In addition to teaching the five skills, we have to have safe, caring, well managed schools. To do that we have to have not just evidence-based programming, we have to have teachers who are aware of themselves, aware of their own social and emotional abilities and need, and are able to deliver a safe, caring, and well-managed environment in a truly genuine way, and support the development of these skills…where they model these skills…they embody them
>
> Greenberg (2014)

In their paper reviewing the potential role of contemplative practices in education, the Mind and Life Education Research Network (MLERN; Davidson et al., 2012) proposed that contemplative practices could complement and add value to SEL programming in two ways. The first highlights the complementary role mindfulness practices may have with SEL programming regarding regular practice, and the second pertains to professional development for educators. Considering regular practice, both contemplative practices and SEL require consistent opportunities to practice. With regards to SEL, best practices dictate that students are provided explicit instruction and opportunities to practice SEL skills (e.g., communication, perspective-taking activities; Collaborative for Academic, Social, and Emotional Learning, 2013). In view of mindfulness-based practices, MLERN (Davidson et al., 2012) referred to recent findings suggesting that mental training via mindfulness practices have resulted in changes in the brain (e.g. Lutz,

Brefczynski-Lewis, Johnstone, & Davidson, 2008). Specifically, "at the heart of such practices is repetition and practice to cultivate more positive habits of mind" (Davidson et al., 2012, p. 150). To date, we have limited research examining mindfulness practices in integration with SEL programming (Lawlor, 2014). Continued efforts to implement and research developmentally appropriate mindfulness practice within the framework of SEL are needed.

The second area MLERN (Davidson et al., 2012) highlighted was the role of contemplative practice in teacher professional development "to nurture the very qualities we want educators, in turn, to nurture in students" (p. 150). Successful student SEL has been found to be inextricably linked to teachers' SEL skills (see Jennings, 2015; Jennings & Greenberg, 2009). In fact, better student–teacher relationships and student outcomes are possible when teachers have stronger SEL competencies (Frank, Jennings, & Greenberg, 2013; Jennings, Snowberg, Coccia, & Greenberg, 2011). Further, research has found that better implementation of SEL curricula occurs when a teacher has robust SEL competencies (Jones, Bouffard, & Weissbourd, 2013).

Jennings and Greenberg (2009) put forth a model of teacher social emotional competence and classroom and student outcomes, called *The Prosocial Classroom* in which they posit that "socially and emotionally competent teachers set the tone of the classroom by developing supportive and encouraging relationships with their students, designing lessons that build on student strengths and abilities, establishing and implementing behavioral guidelines in ways that promote intrinsic motivation, coaching students through conflict situations, encouraging cooperation among students, and acting as a role model for respectful and appropriate communication and exhibitions of prosocial behavior" (p. 492). Extending this work, Jennings (2014) examined the relations between psychosocial characteristics, including trait mindfulness, and classroom quality and ratings of semi-structured interviews about a child the teacher identified as challenging. Mindfulness was found to be associated with emotional support. In addition, interview data revealed mindfulness to be positively related to perspective-taking and sensitivity to discipline. These findings provide support for the notion that mindfulness contributes to teachers' ability to create nurturing and supportive classroom environments.

A recent model put forth by Roeser and colleagues (see Roeser, Harrison, & Taylor, 2015; Roeser, Skinner, Beers, & Jennings, 2012) emphasizes the role of mindfulness training on teacher professional development. Specifically, the model posits that mindfulness training can promote teachers' "habits of mind," which in turn fosters their health, well-being, and ability to develop supportive relationships with students. Research investigating teacher-focused mindfulness programming has revealed benefits such as increased mindfulness, reduction in stress and burn-out (Benn, Akiva, Arel, & Roeser, 2012; Jennings et al., 2011; Roeser et al., 2013), and improvements in teacher competency (Roeser et al., 2013). A new area of investigation includes examination of whether mindfulness training for teachers leads to positive outcomes for students. Recent research indicates this may be the case; in one study with preschoolers involving a mindfulness-based intervention for the teachers, improvements were found in student behavior, including a reduction of challenging behaviors and negative interactions with peers, and increased compliance to teacher requests (Singh, Lancioni, Winton, Karazsia, & Singh, 2013). Taken together, these findings suggest that mindfulness training for teachers support can improve teacher–student interaction and teacher social-emotional competencies—two things that are critical for SEL implementation in the classroom. It is clear that the teacher is a critical piece of the puzzle regarding healthy child development. Thus, future work should place focus on supporting teachers' social and emotional awareness, and mindfulness training may be an effective approach to aid in the development of caring classroom environments.

The research demonstrating the salutary effects of mindfulness-based interventions with children, adolescents, educators, and parents is promising. Findings from the field of intervention research point to the malleability of indictors of social emotional well-being in relation to mindfulness. Nonetheless, there remains a paucity of data investigating mindfulness with younger populations (Lawlor et al., 2014). Research supporting the framework of SEL and mindfulness presented in this paper is primarily representative of research with adult populations. Future empirical explorations of mindfulness-based interventions with younger populations would benefit from the inclusion of a developmental perspective as well as an understanding of the nature of mindfulness in childhood and adolescence to inform the development of age-appropriate mindfulness-based interventions (Roeser & Zelazo, 2012). Future research directions also include longitudinal studies examining the sturdiness of the effects of mindfulness practices in integration with SEL programming. The emerging field of contemplative education in Western educational contexts complements and deepens the understanding of the development of social-emotional competencies. Prioritizing time for regular contemplative and SEL practice within the school day can provide the necessary conditions to enable young people to become healthy, compassionate, competent, and contributing citizens of tomorrow.

References

Baer, R. A. (2003). Mindfulness training as a clinical intervention: A conceptual and empirical review. Clinical Psychology: *Science and Practice, 10*, 125–143.

Baer, R. A., Smith, G. T., & Allen, K. B. (2004). Assessment of mindfulness by self-report: The Kentucky Inventory of Mindfulness Skills. *Assessment, 11*, 191–206.

Baer, R. A., Smith, G. T., Hopkins, J., Krietemeyer, J., & Toney, L. (2006). Using self-report assessment methods to explore facets of mindfulness. *Assessment, 13*, 27–45.

Baijal, S., Jha, A. P., Kiyonaga, A., Singh, R., & Srinivasan, N. (2011). The influence of concentrative meditation training on the development of attention networks during early adolescence. *Frontiers in Developmental Psychology., 2*, 1–9.

Barnes, S., Brown, K., Krusemark, E., Campbell, W., & Rogge, R. D. (2007). The role of mindfulness in romantic relationship satisfaction and responses to relationship stress. *Journal of Marital & Family Therapy, 33*, 482–500. doi:10.1111/j.1752-0606.2007.00033.x.

Beach, M., Roter, D., Korthuis, P., Epstein, R. M., Sharp, V., Ratanawongsa, N., … Saha, S. (2013). A multicenter study of physician mindfulness and health care quality. *Annals Of Family Medicine, 11*, 421–428. doi:10.1370/afm.1507.

Benn, R., Akiva, T., Arel, S., & Roeser, R. W. (2012). Mindfulness training effects for parents and educators of children with special needs. *Developmental Psychology, 48*, 1476–1487.

Blair, C., & Razza, R. P. (2007). Relating effortful control, executive function, and false belief understanding to emerging math and literacy ability in kindergarten. *Child Development, 72*, 647–663.

Brefczynski Lewis, J. A., Lutz, A., Schaefer, H. S., Levinson, D. B., & Davidson, R. J. (2007). Neural correlates of attentional expertise in long-term meditation practitioners. *Proceedings of the National Academy of Sciences of the United States of America, 104*, 11483–11488.

Broderick, P.C., & Metz, S. (2015). Working on the inside: Mindfulness for adolescents. In R.W Roeser & K.A. Schonert-Reichl (Eds.), *Handbook of mindfulness education* (Chapter 22). New York, NY: Springer.

Brown, K. W., & Kasser, T. (2005). Are psychological and ecological well-being compatible? The role of values, mindfulness, and lifestyle. *Social Indicators Research, 74*, 349–368.

Brown, K., Kasser, T., Ryan, R. M., Alex Linley, P. P., & Orzech, K. (2009). When what one has is enough: Mindfulness, financial desire discrepancy, and subjective well-being. *Journal of Research in Personality, 43*, 727–736. doi:10.1016/j.jrp.2009.07.002.

Brown, K. W., & Ryan, R. M. (2003). The benefits of being present: Mindfulness and its role in psychological well-being. *Journal of Personality and Social Psychology, 84*, 822–848.

Brown, K. W., & Ryan, R. M. (2004). Fostering healthy self-regulation from within and without: A self-determination theory perspective. In P. A. Linley & S. Joseph (Eds.), *Positive psychology in practice* (pp. 105–124). New York, NY: Wiley.

Burke, C. A. (2010). Mindfulness-based approaches with children and adolescents: A preliminary review of current research in an emergent field. *Journal of Child and Family Studies, 19*, 133–144.

Caprara, G., Barbaranelli, C., Pastorelli, C., Bandura, A., & Zimbardo, P. (2000). Prosocial foundations of children's academic achievement. *Psychological Science, 11*, 302–306.

Carson, J. W., Carson, K. M., Gil, K. M., & Baucom, D. H. (2004). Mindfulness-based relationship enhancement. *Behavior Therapy, 35*, 471–494.

Casey, B. J., Jones, R. M., & Hare, T. A. (2008). The adolescent brain. *Annals of the New York Academy of Sciences, 1124*, 111–126.

Coatsworth, J., Duncan, L. G., Berrena, E., Bamberger, K. T., Loeschinger, D., Greenberg, M. T., & Nix,

R. L. (2014). The mindfulness-enhanced strengthening families program: Integrating brief mindfulness activities and parent training within an evidence-based prevention program. *New Directions for Youth Development, 142*, 45–58. doi:10.1002/yd.20096.

Coatsworth, J. J., Duncan, L., Greenberg, M., & Nix, R. (2010). Changing parents' mindfulness, child management skills and relationship quality with their youth: Results from a randomized pilot intervention trial. *Journal of Child and Family Studies, 19*, 203–217. doi:10.1007/s10826-009-9304-8.

Collaborative for Academic, Social, and Emotional Learning. (2003). *Safe and sound: An educational leader's guide to evidence-based social and emotional learning programs*. Retrieved August 18, 2014, from http://casel.org/wp-content/uploads/1A_Safe__Sound-rev-2.pdf

Collaborative for Academic, Social, and Emotional Learning. (2013). *2013 CASEL guide: Effective social and emotional learning programs—Preschool and elementary school edition*. Chicago, IL: Author.

Connelly, J. E. (2005). Narrative possibilities: Using mindfulness in clinical practice. *Perspectives in Biology and Medicine, 48*, 84–94.

Davidson, R.J, Dunne, J., Eccles, J. S., Engle, A., Greenberg, M., Jennings, P., & ...Vago, D. (2012). Contemplative practices and mental training: Prospects for American education. *Child Development Perspectives, 6*, 146–153. doi:10.1111/j.1750-8606.2012.00240.x.

Deci, E. L., & Ryan, R. M., (1985). Intrinsic motivation and self-determination in humanbehavior. New York: Plenum.

Dekeyser, M., Raes, F., Leijssen, M., Leysen, S., & Dewulf, D. (2008). Mindfulness skills and interpersonal behavior. *Personality and Individual Differences, 44*, 1235–1245. doi:10.1016/j.paid.2007.11.018.

Diamond, A. (2013). Executive functions. *Annual Review of Psychology, 64*, 135–168.

Diamond, A., & Lee, K. (2011). Interventions shown to aid executive function development in children 4 to 12 tears old. *Science, 333*(6045), 959–964. doi:10.1126/science.1204529.

Durlak, J. A., Weissberg, R. P., Dymnicki, A. B., Taylor, R. D., & Schellinger, K. B. (2011). Enhancing students' social and emotional development promotes success in school: Results of a meta-analysis. *Child Development, 82*, 474–501.

Eisenberg, N. (2002). Empathy-related emotional responses, altruism, and their socialization. In R. J. Davidson & A. Harrington (Eds.), *Visions of compassion: Western scientists and Tibetan Buddhists examine human nature* (pp. 131–164). London, England: Oxford University Press.

Flook, L., Smalley, S. L., Kitil, J. M., Galla, B. M., Kaiser-Greenland, S., Locke, J., … Kasari, C. (2010). Effects of mindful awareness practices on executive functions in elementary school children. *Journal of Applied School Psychology, 26*, 70–95.

Frank, J. L., Jennings, P. A., & Greenberg, M. T. (2013). Mindfulness-based interventions in school settings: An introduction to the special issue. *Research in Human Development, 10*, 205–210.

Fredrickson, B. L., Cohn, M. A., Coffey, K., Pek, J., & Finkel, S. M. (2008). Open hearts build lives: Positive emotions, induced through meditation, build consequential personal resources. *Journal of Personality and Social Psychology, 95*, 1045–1062.

Garrison Institute. (2005). *Contemplation and education—A survey of programs using contemplative techniques in K-12 educational settings: A mapping report*. Garrison, NY: Author.

Gathercole, S. E., Pickering, S. J., Knight, C., & Stegmann, Z. (2004). Working memory skills and educational attainment: Evidence from National Curriculum assessments at 7 and 14 years of age. *Applied Cognitive Psychology, 18*, 1–16.

Goleman, D. (2014, May). *Focus*. Paper presented at the Dalai Lama Center for Peace and Education's Heart-Mind Conference, Vancouver, British Columbia, Canada.

Greenberg, M. T. (2014, May). *Cultivating compassion*. Paper presented at the Dalai Lama Center for Peace and Education's Heart-Mind Conference, Vancouver, British Columbia, Canada.

Greenberg, M. T., & Harris, A. R. (2012). Nurturing mindfulness in children and youth: Current state of research. *Child Development Perspectives, 6*, 161–166.

Greenberg, M. T., Weissberg, R., O'Brien, M., Zins, J., Fredericks, L., Resnik, H., & Elias, M. J. (2003). Enhancing school-based prevention and youth development through coordinated social, emotional, and academic learning. *American Psychologist, 58*, 466–474.

Grossman, P., Niemann, L., Schmidt, S., & Walach, H. (2004). Mindfulness-based stress reduction and health benefits: A meta-analysis. *Journal of Psychosomatic Research, 57*, 35–43.

Harnett, P. H., & Dawe, S. (2013). The contribution of mindfulness-based therapies for children and families and proposed conceptual integration. *Child and Adolescent Mental Health, 17*, 195–208.

Hölzel, B. K., Carmody, J., Vangel, M., Congleton, C., Yerramsetti, S. M., Gard, T., & Lazar, S. W. (2011). Mindfulness practice leads to increases in regional brain gray matter density. *Psychiatry Research, 191*, 36–43. doi:10.1016/j.pscychresns.2010.08.006.

Humphrey, N. (2013). *Social and emotional learning: A critical appraisal*. London, England: Sage.

Jennings, P. A. (2014). Early childhood teachers' well-being, mindfulness, and self-compassion in relation to classroom quality and attitudes towards challenging students. *Mindfulness, 6*(4), 732–743. doi:10.1007/s12671-014-0312-4.

Jennings, P. A. (2015). Teacher programs overview and CARE program. In R. W Roeser & K. A. Schonert-Reichl (Eds.), *Handbook of mindfulness education* (Chapter 11). New York, NY: Springer.

Jennings, P. A., & Greenberg, M. T. (2009). The prosocial classroom: Teacher social and emotional competence in relation to student and classroom outcomes. *Review of Educational Research, 79*, 491–524.

Jennings, P. A., Snowberg, K. E., Coccia, M. A., & Greenberg, M. T. (2011). Improving classroom learning environments by Cultivating Awareness and Resilience in Education (CARE): Results of two pilot studies. *Journal of Classroom Interaction, 46*, 37–48.

Jha, A. P., Krompinger, J., & Baime, M. J. (2007). Mindfulness training modifies subsystems of attention. *Cognitive, Affective, & Behavioral Neuroscience, 7*, 109–119.

Jones, S. M., Bouffard, S. M., & Weissbourd, R. (2013). Educators' social and emotional skills vital to learning. *Phi Delta Kappan, 94*, 62–65.

Kabat-Zinn, J. (1990). *Full catastrophe living: The program of the stress reduction clinic at the University of Massachusetts Medical Center*. New York, NY: Dell.

Kabat-Zinn, J. (2003). Mindfulness-based interventions in context: Past, present, and future. *Clinical Psychology: Science and Practice, 10*, 144–156.

Kemeny, M. E., Foltz, C., Cavanagh, J. F., Cullen, M., Giese-Davis, J., Jennings, P., … Ekman, P. (2012). Contemplative/emotion training reduces negative emotional behavior and promotes prosocial responses. *Emotion, 12*, 338–350. doi:10.1037/a0026118.

Krasner, M. S., Epstein, R. M., Beckman, H., Suchman, A. L., Chapman, B., Mooney, C. J., & Quill, T. E. (2009). Association of an educational program in mindful communication with burnout, empathy, and attitudes among primary care physicians. *JAMA, 302*, 1284–1293.

Kress, J. S., & Elias, M. J. (2006). School-based social and emotional learning programs. In K. A. Renninger & I. E. Sigel (Eds.), *Handbook of child psychology* (6th ed., Vol. 4, pp. 592–618). New York, NY: Wiley.

Lantieri, L., & Nambiar, M. (2012). Cultivating the social, emotional, and inner lives of children and teachers. *Reclaiming Children and Youth, 21*, 27–33.

Lawlor, M. S. (2014). Mindfulness in practice: Considerations for implementation of mindfulness-based programming for adolescents in school contexts. *New Directions for Youth Development, 142*, 83–95. doi:10.1002/yd.20098.

Lawlor, M. S., Schonert-Reichl, K. A., Gadermann, A., & Zumbo, B. D. (2014). A validation study of the mindful attention awareness scale adapted for children. *Mindfulness, 5*(6), 730–741. doi:10.1007/s12671-013-0228-4.

Lutz, A., Brefczynski-Lewis, J. A., Johnstone, T., & Davidson, R. J. (2008). Regulation of the neural circuitry of emotion by compassion meditation: Effects of meditative expertise. *PLoS One, 3*, e1897.

Masten, A. S., & Motti-Stefanidi, F. (2009). Understanding and promoting resilience in children: Promotive and protective processes in schools. In T. B. Gutkin & C. R. Reynolds (Eds.), *The handbook of school psychology* (4th ed., pp. 721–738). New York, NY: Wiley.

Meiklejohn, J., Phillips, C., Freedman, M. L., Griffin, M. L., Biegel, G., Roach, A., … Saltzman, A. (2012). Integrating mindfulness training into K-12 education: Fostering resilience of teachers and students. *Mindfulness, 3*, 291–307.

Metz, E. C., & Youniss, J. (2005). Longitudinal gains in civic development through school-based required service. *Political Psychology, 26*, 413–437. doi:10.1111/j.1467-9221.2005.00424.x.

Moffitt, T. E., Arseneault, L., Belsky, D., Dickson, N., Hancox, R. J., Harrington, H., … Caspi, A. (2011). A gradient of childhood self-control predicts health, wealth, and public safety. *Proceedings of the National Academy of Sciences, 108*, 2693–2698.

National Research Council. (2012). Education for life and work: Developing transferable knowledge and skills in the 21st century. In J. W. Pelligrino & M. L. Hilton (Eds.), *Committee on defining deeper learning and 21st century skills*. Washington, DC: The National Academic Press.

Oberle, E., Schonert-Reichl, K. A., Lawlor, M., & Thomson, K. C. (2011). Mindfulness and inhibitory control in early adolescence. *Journal of Early Adolescence, 32*, 565–588. doi:10.1177/0272431611403741.

Parker, A., & Kupersmidt, J. (2015). The master mind and moment programs: Introducing two universal mindfulness education programs for elementary and middle school students. In R. W. Roeser & K. A. Schonert-Reichl (Eds.), *Handbook of mindfulness education* (Chapter 21). New York, NY: Springer.

Roeser, R. W. (2015). Processes of teaching, learning, and transfer in mindfulness-based interventions (MBIs) for teachers: A contemplative educational perspective. In R. W. Roeser & K. A. Schonert-Reichl (Eds.), *Handbook of mindfulness education* (Chapter 10). New York, NY: Springer.

Roeser, R. W., & Peck, S. C. (2009). An education in awareness: Self, motivation, and self-regulated learning in contemplative perspective. *Educational Psychologist, 44*, 119–136.

Roeser, R., Schonert-Reichl, K. A., Jha, A., Cullen, M., Wallace, L., Wilensky, R., … Harrison, J. (2013.) Mindfulness training and reductions in teacher stress and burnout: Results from two randomized, waitlist-control field trials. *Journal of Educational Psychology, 105*, 787–804.

Roeser, R. W., Skinner, E., Beers, J., & Jennings, P. A. (2012). Mindfulness training and teachers' professional development: An emerging area of research and practice. *Child Development Perspectives, 6*, 167–173. doi:10.1111/j.1750-8606.2012.00238.x.

Roeser, R. W., & Zelazo, P. (2012). Contemplative science, education and child development: Introduction to the special section. *Child Development Perspectives, 6*, 143–145. doi:10.1111/j.1750-8606.2012.00242.x.

Sahdra, B. K., MacLean, K. A., Ferrer, E., Shaver, P. R., Rosenberg, E. L., Jacobs, T. L., … Saron, C. D. (2011). Enhanced response inhibition during intensive meditation training predicts improvements in self-reported adaptive socioemotional functioning. *Emotion, 11,* 299–312. doi:10.1037/a0022764.

Scales, P., Benson, P., Leffert, N., & Blyth, D. (2000). Contribution of developmental assets to the prediction of thriving among adolescents. *Applied Developmental Science, 4,* 27–46.

Schonert-Reichl, K. A., Oberle, E., Lawlor, M. S., Abbott, D., Thomson, K., Oberlander, T. F., & Diamond, A. (2014). *Enhancing cognitive and social-emotional development through a simple-to-administer school program.* Manuscript under review.

Shapiro, S. L., & Schwartz, G. R. (2000). Intentional systemic mindfulness: An integrative model for self-regulation and health. *Advances in Mind-Body Medicine, 16,* 128.

Shapiro, S.L., Jazaieri, H., & Goldin, P.R. (2012) Mindfulness-based stress reduction effects on moral reasoning and decision making, *The Journal of Positive Psychology 7,* 504–515, DOI: 10.1080/17439760.2012.723732

Singh, N. N., Lancioni, G. E., Winton, A. S., Karazsia, B. T., & Singh, J. (2013). Mindfulness training for teachers changes the behavior of their preschool students. *Research in Human Development, 10,* 211–233.

Tang, Y., Ma, Y., Wang, J., Fan, Y., Feng, S., Lu, Q., … Posner, M. I. (2007). Short-term meditation training improves attention and self-regulation. *PNAS, 104,* 17152–17156.

Tang, Y., & Posner, M. (2009). Attention training and attention state training. *Trends in Cognitive Sciences, 13,* 222–227.

Teper, R., Segal, Z. V., & Inzlicht, M. (2014). Inside the mindful mind: How mindfulness enhances emotion regulation through improvements in executive control. *Current Directions in Psychological Science, 23,* 1–6. doi:10.1177/0963721413495869.

Vago, D. (2012). Contemplative practices and mental training: Prospects for American education. *Child Development Perspectives, 6,* 146–153. doi:10.1111/j.1750-8606.2012.00240.x.

Weissberg, R. P., Payton, J. W., O'Brien, M. U., & Munro, S. (2007). Social and emotional learning. In F. C. Power, R. J. Nuzzi, D. Narvaez, D. K. Lapsley, & T. C. Hunt (Eds.), *Moral education: A handbook, Volume 2: M–Z* (pp. 417–418). Westport, CT: Greenwood Press.

Youniss, J., & Yates, M. (1999). Youth service and moral-civic identity: A case for everyday morality. *Educational Psychology Review, 11,* 361–376.

Zelazo, P. D., & Lyons, K. E. (2012). The potential benefits of mindfulness training in early childhood: A developmental social cognitive neuroscience perspective. *Child Development Perspectives, 6,* 154–160.

Zins, J. E., Bloodworth, M. R., Weissberg, R. P., & Walberg, H. J. (2004). The scientific base linking emotional learning to student success and academic outcomes. In J. E. Zins, R. P. Weissberg, M. C. Wang, & H. J. Walberg (Eds.), *Building academic success on social and emotional learning: What does the research say?* (pp. 3–22). New York, NY: Teachers College Press.

Zins, J. E., Weissberg, R. P., Wang, M. C., & Walberg, H. J. (2004). *Building academic success on social and emotional learning.* New York, NY: Teachers College Press.

Zoogman, S., Goldberg, S. B., Hoyt, W. T., & Miller, L. (2014). Mindfulness interventions with youth: a meta-analysis. *Mindfulness, 6*(2), 290–302. doi:10.1007/s12671-013-0260-4.

Part II

Mindfulness in Education: Science and Applications with Educators

Mindfulness Training for Teachers

6

Shauna Shapiro, Daniel Rechtschaffen, and Sarah de Sousa

In this chapter, we explore the potential benefits of integrating mindfulness training into the lives of teachers. We hypothesize that these benefits are multidimensional and far-reaching, and mindfulness training engenders three pathways of integration in teachers' lives: (1) mindfulness as a source of self-care, (2) mindfulness as a means of becoming a reflective teacher, and (3) mindfulness as a means of transforming student learning in the classroom. We consider the empirical evidence demonstrating the impact of mindfulness for teachers in these three ways, and offer an overview of applications of mindfulness in teacher trainings and curriculum.

Theoretical Foundations: What Is Mindfulness?

Mindfulness is often referred to as a consciousness discipline. It is a way of training the mind, heart, and body to be fully present with life. Although often associated with meditation, mindfulness is much more than a meditation technique. Mindfulness is fundamentally a way of being; a way of inhabiting our bodies, our minds, and our moment-by-moment experience with openness and receptivity. It is a deep awareness; a knowing and experiencing of life as it arises and passes away in each moment.

According to Shapiro and Carlson (2009), mindfulness can be defined as "the awareness that arises through intentionally attending in an open, kind, and discerning way" (p. 4). Mindfulness can be understood as both an inherent and ever-present awareness (mindful awareness), and a series of specific practices designed to enhance mindful attention and awareness (mindful practice).

Three Core Elements of Mindfulness

Mindfulness comprises three core elements: intention, attention, and attitude (Shapiro & Carlson, 2009). *Intention* involves knowing *why* we are doing what we are doing: our ultimate aim, our vision, and our aspiration. *Attention* involves attending fully to the present moment instead of allowing ourselves to become preoccupied with the past or future. *Attitude*, or *how* we pay attention, enables us to stay open, kind, and curious. These three elements are not separate—they are interwoven, each informing and nurturing the others. Mindfulness is this moment-to-moment process.

S. Shapiro (✉) • S. de Sousa
Santa Clara University, 500 El Camino Real, Santa Clara, CA 95051, USA
e-mail: slshapiro@scu.edu; sldesousa@scu.edu

D. Rechtschaffen
Executive Director of Mindful Education, San Francisco, CA, USA
e-mail: djrechtschaffen@yahoo.com

K.A. Schonert-Reichl, R.W. Roeser (eds.), *Handbook of Mindfulness in Education*, Mindfulness in Behavioral Health, DOI 10.1007/978-1-4939-3506-2_6

Intention

The first core component of mindfulness is *intention*. Intention is simply knowing why we are doing what we are doing. When we have discerned our intentions and are able to connect with them, our intentions help motivate us, reminding us of what is truly important. Discerning our intentions involves inquiring into our deepest hopes, desires, and aspirations. Mindful attention to our own intentions helps us begin to bring unconscious values to awareness and decide whether they are really the values we want to pursue. Intention, in the context of mindfulness, is not the same as (and does not include) striving or grasping for certain outcomes or goals. Rather, as meditation teacher and psychotherapist Jack Kornfield puts it, "Intention is a direction not a destination" (personal communication, 2012).

Attention

The second fundamental component of mindfulness is *attention*. Mindfulness is about seeing clearly, and if we want to see clearly, we must be able to pay attention to what is here, now, in this present moment. Paying attention involves observing and experiencing our moment-to-moment experience. And yet, this is not so easy. Recent research demonstrates that our mind wanders approximately 47 % of the time (Killingsworth & Gilbert, 2010). The human mind is often referred to as a "monkey mind," swinging from thought to thought as a monkey swings from limb to limb. Mindfulness is a tool that helps us tame and train the mind so that attention becomes stable and focused, despite our mind's inclination to wander. Therefore, attention is the component of mindfulness that facilitates a focused and clear seeing of what arises in our field of experience.

Often, as we try to pay attention, our attention becomes tense and contracted. This is because we mistakenly think we have to be stressed or vigilant to focus our attention in a rigorous way. However, the meditation traditions teach us of a different kind of attention, a "relaxed alertness" that involves clarity and precision without stress or vigilance (Wallace & Bodhi, 2006). This relaxed alertness is the kind of attention that is essential to mindfulness. Mindful attention is also deep and penetrating; as Bhikkhu Bodhi notes "…whereas a mind without mindfulness 'floats' on the surface of its object the way a gourd floats on water, mindfulness sinks into its object the way a stone placed on the surface of water sinks to the bottom" (Wallace & Bodhi, 2006, p. 7).

Attitude

Attitude, how we pay attention, is essential to mindfulness. For example, attention can have a cold, critical quality, or an openhearted, curious, and compassionate quality. Attending without bringing the attitudinal qualities of curiosity, openness, acceptance, and kindness into the practice may result in an attention that is condemning or shaming of inner (or outer) experience. This may well have consequences contrary to the intentions of the practice; for example, we may end up cultivating patterns of criticism and striving instead of equanimity, openness, and acceptance.

These attitudes of mindfulness do not alter our experience but simply contain it. For example, if while we are practicing mindfulness, impatience arises, we note the impatience with acceptance and kindness. We do not attempt to substitute these qualities for the impatience, or use them to make the impatience disappear. The attitudes are not an attempt to make things be a certain way, but an attempt to relate to whatever is in a certain way. By intentionally bringing the attitudes of mindfulness to our awareness of our own experience, we relinquish the habit of striving for pleasant experiences, or of pushing aversive experiences away. Instead, we attend to and welcome whatever is here.

It may be useful to think of mindfulness as a presence of heart as well as mind. In fact the Japanese kanji for mindfulness is composed of two symbols, the top meaning presence and the bottom translated as "heart" or "mind." Mindfulness involves bringing heartfulness to each moment—bringing our full aliveness and care to all of our experiences.

Formal and Informal Practice

What we practice becomes stronger. When we practice mindfulness, we strengthen our capacity to be present moment-by-moment in a curious, accepting, and kind way. Mindful practice can be categorized into *formal* and *informal* practice; each kind of practice supports the other. The formal practice will support the ability to practice mindfulness in day-to-day life, and informal practice is meant to generalize to everyday life what is learned during the formal practice.

Formal practices are geared towards cultivating mindfulness skills in focused and systematic ways, and emphasize the specific and purposeful training of attention with openness, acceptance, and curiosity. In mindful meditation, practitioners allow a state of "fluid attention" to emerge, rather than focusing on any specific object or sensation (Irving, Dobkin, & Park, 2009). Thoughts, emotions, and body sensations that arise during this practice are accepted as they are, without being judged or manipulated.

Informal practice involves intentionally bringing an open, accepting, and discerning attention to whatever we are engaged in, for example reading, driving, and eating. As Kabat-Zinn (2005) notes, the beauty of the informal practice is that all it requires is a rotation in consciousness. This rotation in consciousness, while subtle, is significant. And, its implications for healthcare professionals and clinical work is profound. Fundamentally, *all educational and clinical work can be considered informal mindfulness practice.* Setting the intention at the beginning of each class or therapy session to intentionally pay attention with kindness, discernment, openness, and acceptance is a powerful and effective practice that can transform the experience. This frame of education and therapy as informal mindfulness practice is, we believe, an important dimension of training the individuals who work in these professions to integrate mindfulness into their work and lives.

Why Should Teachers Practice Mindfulness?

The integration of mindfulness into the lives of teachers serves at least three broad purposes: (1) self-care, (2) becoming a more mindful, reflective teacher, and (3) developing a sound foundation for delivering mindfulness-informed or mindfulness-based instruction to students to support academic and social-emotional learning. Below, we explore each of these.

Self-Care

The increased demands placed upon teachers are associated with increased stress and burnout, which in turn negatively impact mental and physical health and have adverse consequences for the quality of care delivered to students (Jennings & Greenberg, 2009; Jennings, Lantieri, & Roeser, 2012; Roeser, Skinner, Beers, & Jennings, 2012). One of the most obvious pathways of integrating mindfulness into the training of teachers is to focus on self-care.

Self-care, for teachers, is a prerequisite to providing competent care. Lack of self-care increases risk for burnout. Self-awareness, defined in this context as an unbiased observation of one's inner experience and behavior, is thought to be foundational to self-care and important to successful teaching. Teachers who do not meet their personal needs are likely to have difficulty in providing effective instruction and care to students. Learning to take positive action when symptoms begin to appear is essential to the process of preventing and treating burnout.

It is imperative that teachers make self-care a priority so that they can attend to their own well-being and deliver appropriate and empathetic student care. Stress harms professional effectiveness by negatively impacting teachers' attention and concentration (Braunstein-Bercovitz, 2003; Mackenzie, Smith, Hasher, Leach, & Behl, 2007; Skosnik, Chatterton, Swisher, & Park, 2000), weakens decision-making and communication skills (Shanafelt, Bradley, Wipf, & Back, 2002), decreases empathy (Beddoe & Murphy, 2004; Thompson and Waltz, 2007), and reduces ability to engage in meaningful relationships (Enochs & Etzbach, 2004). This research suggests that if teachers do not care for themselves, they risk their students' health and well-being as much as their own. Being self-aware makes teachers conscious of their own physical and psychological experiences without distorting or avoiding the students' needs (Valente & Marotta, 2005).

The above literature demonstrates the importance of self-care as a prerequisite for quality student care. Yet, many in the field have difficulty integrating self-care in their everyday living. Consequently, compassion fatigue, vicarious traumatization, burnout, distress, and dissatisfaction remain problems for many teachers. It is crucial to recognize the presence of stress and to have tools to help meet the extraordinary demands placed on teachers. Training in mindfulness may be especially relevant for this purpose. Existing literature posits that the cultivation of mindfulness can enhance mental and physical health (see Baer, 2003; Grossman, Niemann, Schmidt, & Walach, 2004; Keng, Smoski, & Robins, 2011; Khoury et al., 2013, for reviews). Although most mindfulness research has focused on patient benefits, recent research has found that mindfulness training may be particularly useful for teachers as a means of managing stress and promoting self-care.

Mindfulness also teaches self-compassion, allowing teachers to accept themselves as imperfect or "perfectly human" (Shapiro & Carlson, 2009). It is important to recognize that, despite our best intentions, things will sometimes go wrong. Instead of becoming self-critical and condemning in these situations, teachers can use mindfulness to treat themselves with the same care and compassion they want to bring to their students. (Roeser et al., 2013), for instance, found that "occupational self-compassion"—taking a kind attitude towards oneself as a professional in times of difficulty, was increased through mindfulness training and was also a key mediator of the stress-reducing effects of the training compared to teachers in a waitlist-control condition.

Becoming a More Mindful Teacher

Mindfulness practice is associated with qualities that are critical to effective teaching, such as attention, empathy, emotion regulation, and affect tolerance, and several studies have shown that mindfulness training cultivates specific professional skills essential to teaching (see Shapiro & Carlson, 2009, for a review). For example, in a study by Gokhan, Meehan, and Peters (2010), undergraduate students participated in a 12-week mindfulness-based training as a part of an academic course while concurrently offering services to individuals with psychiatric and developmental disabilities as a part of an on-site field placement within a hospital setting. Students kept journals to reflect their physical, behavioral, emotional, and cognitive reactions to their field placement experience. Quantitative and qualitative findings in this study were consistent with the idea that mindfulness can increase through practice and has positive effects on characteristics associated with the provision of high-quality care. In contrast to a comparison group that did not receive mindfulness training, trained students showed increases in self-care, attention to well-being, self-awareness, empathy, compassion, and skills of directing and focusing attention.

Mindfulness practice cultivates positive qualities and skills of relating to self and others, and thus is hypothesized to improve teacher–student relationships. Below, we explore qualities of the mindful teacher that lead to enhanced student outcomes such as sustained attention, control over how attention is distributed, attunement, and self-regulation.

Attention and Presence

According to (Germer, Siegel, & Fulton, 2005), mindful practice is "like a firm handshake with one object at a time in the field of experience. Mindfulness neither squeezes the object nor is casual in its grip, but the object is distinctly perceived" (Germer et al., 2005, p. 14). It is widely accepted that successful teaching requires that teachers pay attention and sustain attention (e.g., Marzano, 2007). While the capacity to be mindfully present is inherent in all teaching, systematic practice may be required to hone this skill (Roeser et al., 2013). Existing research in adults more generally reveals that mindful presence and attention develop through formal mindfulness meditation practice.

Research supporting the impact of mindfulness on attention and presence has found greater cortical thickness in areas of the brain associated with sustained attention and awareness in practitioners experienced in mindful meditation, compared to nonmeditating participants (Lazar et al., 2005). Moreover, by measuring response times on the Attention Network Test (ANT) after 8 weeks of mindfulness meditation training for novices, and a month-long retreat for more experienced meditators, Jha, Krompinger, and Baime (2007) found improvements in overall attention. Specifically, those who participated in the 8-week training were more able to direct focused attention when required, and those who attended the 1-month retreat showed an increased ability to retain their focus when faced with distractions.

A study by McCollum and Gehart (2010) also found that graduate students trained in mindfulness meditation as a component of their coursework were better able to distinguish between what Segal, Williams, and Teasdale (2002) refer to as the *doing* and the *being* modes of mind. The doing mode focuses on planning and resolving discrepancy between our idea of how things should be versus how they actually are. In contrast, the being mode centers on simply being present with whatever is occurring in the moment, without feeling a need to change it. McCollum and Gehart point out that both modes are essential, but it is important for teachers to recognize and strengthen their capacity to shift between modes. Through the cultivation of attention and presence, mindfulness not only facilitates a being mode of mind, but also the ability to engage in the doing mode when the moment requires, as well as to shift attentional focus, capacities that are essential to teaching (e.g., Jennings & Greenberg, 2009; Roeser et al., 2012).

Research has also shown that mindfulness meditation can enhance control over how attention is distributed. For example, if too much attention is focused on one stimulus, another stimulus might be missed. Mindfulness training can help us to allocate our attention more efficiently, leading to greater clarity in information processing (see e.g., Slagter et al., 2007). This is particularly important when teachers need to deal with subtle and rapid student behavior in a class of 30 or more students.

Teacher Attitude

Although paying attention is essential, how practitioners pay attention is also critical to teaching. Attention can be cold and hard, with a critical emphasis that can hinder the establishment of a nurturing environment in which learning is enhanced. This is contrasted with the attitudes of acceptance, letting go, nonattachment, nonstriving, nonjudging, patience, trust, warmth, friendliness, and kindness, which characterize mindfulness practice (Kabat-Zinn, 1990; Segal et al., 2002; Shapiro & Schwartz, 2000). Although these attitudes are not exhaustive, they underscore the type of attention that is likely to enhance the alliance between teacher and student. Furthermore, research on acceptance-based approaches has shown an implication for neuroplasticity of the brain: When teachers allow themselves and their students to rest in experiences of acceptance and equanimity, they increase the possibility that these experiences will lead to changes in the brain (Geller & Greenberg, 2012). The teacher's accepting presence sends a message to the student that he or she is understood and is in a safe environment, and this acceptance has a neurological correlate. The nervous system evaluates the state of safety and decreases the activation of the sympathetic nervous system, followed by a physiological response of softening of facial muscles, relaxation, and perceptual openness to the teacher. In response to fear, the state of neuroception may equally trigger defensive behaviors such as fight or flight. The state of neuroception activated by a feeling of safety and acceptance releases the hormone oxytocin that creates attunement and bonding between the teacher and student (Geller & Greenberg, 2012).

Further preliminary evidence supports a relationship between the attitudes cultivated through mindfulness and enhanced skills essential for healthy relationships. Brown and Ryan (2003), for example, found that increased mindfulness is associated with "greater openness to experience," a measure of general personality characteristics measured on the NEO-Five Factor Index. Similarly, Thompson and Waltz (2007) found that higher trait mindfulness was related to less neuroticism and more agreeableness and consciousness on the same measure.

Self-Compassion and Attunement

Compassion, which is a cornerstone of effective teaching, is also enhanced through mindfulness (Condon, Desbordes, Miller, & Desteno, 2013). Compassion incorporates both the ability to empathize with the suffering of oneself or others and the desire to act upon this empathy to reduce the suffering. Attunement is a precursor to compassion, as it involves being in touch with the inner experience of oneself (self-attunement) or another. Being self-attuned entails developing a "witness consciousness," which observes the content of one's experience and accepts it without judgment or interpretation, as something that simply is. Even when teachers find themselves being self-critical, they can practice observing the thoughts without labeling them as truth or reacting to them.

Mindfulness practice is one way teachers can strengthen their self-attunement and self-compassion (e.g., Benn, Akiva, Arel, & Roeser, 2012; Roeser et al., 2013). Indeed, a central tenet of mindfulness practice is to learn to let go of self-judgment and to relate to oneself with compassion and kindness. Through mindfulness meditation, we begin to see that our personal suffering is not unique but part of the universality of being human (Shapiro & Carlson, 2009).

One mindfulness meditation that can be particularly helpful in cultivating self-compassion is the loving-kindness meditation (see Kornfield, 2009; Shapiro & Carlson, 2009). This meditation asks participants to repeat four or five phrases of well-wishing, like "May I be peaceful and happy. May I be healthy." While reciting these phrases, participants are asked to feel the quality of loving-kindness in the body and heart. After many repetitions, when love for oneself has begun to take root, the loving-kindness practice is then extended to others (family, friends, neutral people, and eventually difficult people).

Empathy and Attunement with Others

Empathy, or the ability to "sense the student's private world as if it were your own, but without losing the 'as if' quality" is essential for effective teaching (Rogers, 1957, p. 95; see also Arkowitz, 2002; Bohart, Elliott, Greenberg, & Watson, 2002). Research suggests that meditation can significantly enhance empathy (Lesh, 1970; Shapiro, Brown, & Biegel, 2007; Shapiro, Schwartz, & Bonner, 1998). Further research has shown that increases in mindfulness correlated with increases in empathy, suggesting that students may have increased their empathetic concern for others because they became more mindful (Condon, 2014).

Research from neurobiology suggests a possible mechanism by which mindfulness enhances empathy and attunement. Mirror neurons, which mirror the behavior of another, as though the observer were acting, may provide the basis for empathy and related processes within mindfulness. This line of research started with direct observation of primates (Di Pellegrino, Fadiga, Fogassi, Gallese, & Rizzolatti, 1992; Rizzolatti & Criaghero, 2004; Rizzolatti, Fadiga, Gallese, & Fogassi, 1996). Subsequently, researchers showed brain activity consistent with mirror neurons in the anterior insula, anterior cingulate cortex, and inferior parietal cortex of humans (Botvinivk et al., 2005; Cheng, Yang, Lin, Lee, & Decety, 2008).

Although research on mirror neurons in humans is less well established, and the functional significance of mirror neurons in human emotion is still being contested (e.g., Lingnau, Gesierich, & Caramazza, 2009), a large number of experiments using functional MRI, electroencephalography, and magnetoencephalography have determined that particular brain regions are active when a person experiences an emotion, and when he or she sees another person experiencing the emotion (Botvinivk et al., 2005; Cheng et al., 2008; Lamm, Batson, & Decety, 2007; Morrison, Lloyd, Di Pellegrino, & Roberts, 2004; Singer et al., 2004; Wicker et al., 2003). Jabbi, Swart, and Keysers (2006) have also demonstrated that individuals who are more empathic, based on self-report questionnaires, have stronger activations in the mirror system for emotions. This finding provides additional support for the idea that mirror neurons are associated with empathy.

Mirror neurons often fire at less intense levels in the observer than in the initial communicator of the emotion (Goleman, 2006). Mindful awareness may play a role here in enhancing one's receptivity even to small signals, somatic and emotional, thereby increasing attunement between two people.

Emotional Regulation

Positive relationships with students require that teachers know how to regulate their emotions and know when to avoid expressing their own emotions (Jennings et al., 2012). Strong emotions can often arise in the classroom. By attending to and regulating their own emotional reactions, practitioners can be more present and accepting of students across a range of emotionally charged therapy scenarios.

In a study by Christopher et al. (2010), utilizing a qualitative design to explore the long-term impact of teaching mindfulness to graduate students, many participants observed less reactivity and judgment, and the ability to better tolerate their own feelings. As one participant stated:

> I think that I can tend to get overwhelmed by other people's emotions and through the class I think I really learned to be able to separate people's emotions and be strong in my own sense of self in that moment. To be just fully aware of what I'm experiencing and being able to separate what other people are experiencing (Christopher et al., 2010, p. 333).

Because mindfulness training helps teachers become familiar with their minds and bodies, they may be better able to see their personal responses to a student's behavior and regulate their emotions, which could otherwise hamper their relationships with students.

Teachers are like the strings of a piano resonating to the music of the 20 something little pianos playing at once in their classrooms. Consciously or unconsciously, teachers' hearts strings are played by every joy and every anxiety that their students are expressing. The dysregulation that is rife in so many classrooms impacts teachers and their students in equal measure. Teachers experience the vicarious traumas and the compassion fatigue associated with their daily adventure through the emotion fields of their students. Not only are they adventuring through the emotional fields of their students, they are so often navigating the emotional demands of relating to their own colleagues and family members, and the stressors that attend all interpersonal relationships, professional and personal. One common coping strategy is to suppress or avoid emotional triggers in order to be present and available to the students. Though this is an empathic attempt, it often results in unintended consequences. When teachers have untended stress, they may have less empathy, react faster, and may find that their creativity withers. Their capacity to cultivate emotional regulation provides for a calm in the storm and allows them to be an embodiment of balance that their students can use as an anchor.

Foundations for Providing Mindfulness in the Classroom

In order to develop the foundations for a mindful classroom, the first steps, as we have already discussed, are for educators to practice self-care and embodiment of mindfulness. One's own lived presence is the most important way to teach mindfulness. From this embodied place, we propose, there are nuanced and powerful ways to offer the teachings of mindfulness to students of all ages, including those with special needs, and other diverse populations. It is helpful to consider a multistage approach when incorporating mindfulness into schools. The first stage involves creating the conditions within the school for students to learn in a mindful environment. Once a mindful learning environment has been cultivated, subsequent stages may integrate lessons, curricula, and other specific mindfulness exercises in order to help students build the same habits related to intention, attention, and attitude described above.

Mindful Classroom Climates for Student Learning

Creating Mindful Spaces Many schools and organizations weave mindfulness into the physical space of their schools. Some schools have corners of their rooms where students can practice relaxing breaths whenever they are feeling too tense. In Baltimore, the Holistic Life Foundation[1] works with many schools to set up rooms that are alternatives to suspension where students can breathe, drink a cup of tea, and receive guidance and mentoring from mindfulness coaches (see: http://hlfinc.org).

One effective practice for teachers to identify opportunities to create more mindful spaces in their schools is to simply walk through the school and observe how the environment affects their mood. When teachers are able to notice how certain lighting, artwork, and layouts impact their own mood, they can then learn how to set up the space in such a way that students will likely feel more comfortable, happy, and inspired. Setting up a room with plants, art, lighting that is not too harsh, and couches, and introducing other creative ideas creates a mindful space for students to relax into. Simply by attuning to the needs of the students' space, teachers are practicing mindfulness and supporting their students' practice as well. There is evidence that features of the physical setting are important to student engagement and learning (Roeser & Eccles, 2014).

In addition to creating a safe and nurturing environment for students, it is also crucial to create a safe space for teachers. The stress and conflict in so many faculty rooms can have an adverse effect on the faculty themselves and indeed on the whole atmosphere of the school. In an effort to address this common concern, many schools have begun offering weekly sitting groups, mindfulness book clubs, or a yoga class for teachers before school. In an academic setting, scheduling often presents an obstacle in coordinating these kinds of group activities, but the power of coming together and practicing, even for 15 min, is profoundly supportive. Creating an opportunity for teachers to share what is really going on for them inside can create a teaching atmosphere of compassion and connectedness that can then be a foundation on which bringing the teaching to the students can build.

Practicing Mindful Communication An important way that teachers weave mindfulness into their schools is by practicing mindful communication. As teachers developing a greater language for their inner worlds, they likely can begin to communicate with students in more attuned and empathic ways. Further, through developing their own language for the interior, teachers will model for students this emotional intelligence. Teachers can also incorporate specific practices to help students develop this language, for example, by inviting students to begin the day by naming what they are aware of in the present moment. Students learn how often they can get lost in future worries and past concerns and gain the capacity to name what they are noticing in their hearts, bodies, and minds in the present moment. This practice supports students in feeling seen, as well as developing empathy towards the experiences of others. Through this practice, teachers also gain the opportunity to track the inner experiences of the students so they can be attuned to their learning needs. When teachers engage in these practices, it is essential to create a safe sharing space for students. The vulnerability associated with sharing one's inner experience must be met with kindness and nonjudgment in order to promote the positive feedback loop afforded by mindfulness practice in a group setting, particularly with children whose developmental needs are different than those of adults.

Creating Mindful Moments As teachers begin to incorporate mindfulness into schools, they often start by thinking of how to structure moments of reflection and connection into the fabric of the day. Some schools have a minute of silent breathing over the loudspeaker every morning. Some teachers begin and end every class with the ring of a bell, a few mindful movements, or a mindful sharing.

It is imperative to teach mindfulness in such a way that teachers are not forcing the students to practice for longer or more intensively then will feel enjoyable and within their capability. If

[1] See: http://hlfinc.org

teachers began by telling students to sit quietly for 30 min, students would begin to equate mindfulness with a frustrating punishment. Short intervals of stillness throughout the day are ideal. When these moments of mindfulness are integrated skillfully during transitions and in moments of stress, teachers may find that students come to thirst for mindfulness as a way of self-regulating. They ideally will ask for mindfulness knowing that it is a nourishing inner tool rather than a boring imposition.

Teaching Mindfulness Curricula to Students

We hypothesize that teachers who have learned mindfulness practices and how to embody them in classrooms are in the best position to explore the potential of offering mindfulness-based lessons to students. There are various mindfulness-based education curricula available today for every age group (see Part III in this volume). Some of these curricula are readily available for sale and do not require any particular training from those who would wish to utilize the curricula in their classrooms. Other curricula are only provided after thorough training and with requirement of a certain level of commitment to a personal mindfulness practice.

As an example of the readily available curricula, the MindUp curricula, from the Hawn Foundation, can be purchased and implemented without any additional requirements, though training and implementation support are available. This curriculum was developed with great focus on neuroscience and supporting the students to be able to understand the dynamics of their own minds (see Maloney, Lawlor, Schonert-Reichl, & Whitehead, this volume). Readily available curricula offer wonderful resources for teachers who are already committed to a personal practice so they can complement their own embodied experience of mindfulness with specific age-appropriate lessons and exercises in their classrooms.

The danger with these readily accessible curricula is that it is easy for teachers to begin teaching these lessons without the understanding and embodiment of the larger paradigm of mindful teaching that comes from a personal practice. One concern here is that mindfulness practices might be used as behavioral modification tools and a way to force calm and quiet on difficult or challenging students. In one school, for instance, students were made to sit in the corner on the "mindfulness chair" if they had misbehaved so they could be "mindful" of what they had done. This is not the way of mindfulness that we are interested in. We want to compassionately invite students and teachers to gain greater self-understanding and mastery, not to use mindfulness as another instrumental means of externally controlling students and their behavior.

Examples of Mindfulness Curricula There are many exemplary curriculum trainings that offer teachers manuals, PowerPoints, and apps that they can incorporate into their teaching. Most of these trainings require previous practice of mindfulness, either having completed a Mindfulness-Based Stress Reduction course or an equivalent amount of personal contemplative practice time. These trainings last from several days to an entire year.

As an example of a curriculum training, the *.b Curriculum* is a wonderful training developed by the Mindfulness in Schools Project. The *.b Curriculum* is fun, adaptable, and built upon the fundamentals of mindfulness. The .b stands for developing the capacity to "pause and be" or to "stop and breathe." Before mindfulness trainers lead these trainings with teachers, they are committed to making sure that the participants who will be receiving their manuals are steeped in the paradigm of mindful teaching and have learned to stop and breathe themselves. The Mindfulness in Schools Project requires participants to have taken a Mindfulness-Based Stress Reduction training or an equivalent personal mindfulness practice as a prerequisite for their course.

Having a prerequisite mindfulness practice makes it harder to bring these types of curricula into entire schools. Although it is wonderful to offer the opportunity of mindfulness to an entire school, it is not possible to force anyone to be mindful. The problem with mandatory mindfulness training across entire schools and school districts is that introspection cannot be enforced. The heart is a vulnerable terrain, and any true mindfulness training is an invitation out of the usual comfort zone of one's sense of self into a larger experience of who one really is. When people are ready to look within, it is the greatest of human journeys. However, until they are ready, the journey cannot begin. The journey of self-realization is exactly that, a realizing of who one truly is, and no one else can provide that answer. Mindfulness offers teachers a safe space in which to explore their hearts and minds, but if there is too much resistance to that invitation there is no realizing that can unfold. In any mindfulness training program, it is the program facilitator's job to use language that is the most accessible, culturally appropriate, and scientifically validated to encourage, engage, and support people in mindfulness practice, but at the end of the day if the teacher is still uninterested it is also the trainer's job to honor that person's resistance. Likewise, even the most committed teachers, who are well trained and well intentioned in sharing the benefits of mindfulness practice with their students, can at best offer the invitation for students to engage in mindfulness practice; it cannot be forced.

Mindful-Based Curriculum

The majority of available mindful education curricula share the same basic ingredients. Each curriculum focuses on a slightly different population of students and on different facets of mindfulness-based education, but all of them incorporate the fundamentals of breath awareness, generating compassion, mindfully eating a raisin, and many other crossovers. It is ideal for teachers to peruse these curricula and to seek training with experienced mindfulness practitioners, but perhaps more essential is developing one's own lessons and approaches to teaching mindfulness as is appropriate in each moment.

In the book, *The Way of Mindful Education* there is a curriculum offered in a toolbox format in which teachers are encouraged to learn how to become comfortable with each lesson so that eventually they can be utilized in a fluid and skillful manner. If the class is stressed about a test, then the teacher will instinctively gravitate towards relaxation and focusing practices. If the students are riled up from the playground then movement and stillness practices may represent the more skillful response to what the moment requires. Rather than adhering to a prescribed lesson order, the mindful teaching paradigm invites the teacher to be attuned to the needs of the class in the moment and to respond with a toolbox of mindfulness practices.

As a whole, the mindfulness lessons can be broken into four types, including embodiment, attention, heartfulness, and interconnection. The program offers a progression of lessons that help to build certain foundational capacities before moving on to others, but it also offers flexibility in how one organizes the journey from here to there. Here we lay out the four basic forms of mindfulness practice and the general progression that is recommended.

Embodiment Teachers begin by teaching the language of the body. When they teach mindfulness to students, teachers need to remember to learn to "play mindfulness," rather than "practicing" or "doing" mindfulness. They need to help students to feel comfortable, connected, and relaxed in their bodies before introducing them to the more introspective arts of mindfulness.

Sometimes teachers may play fun movement games that incorporate breath and awareness before they even say the word mindfulness. Especially with students who experience significant stress and trauma, it is crucial to begin by teaching them within the range of their capacity to be present. Before teachers invite students to be aware of what is happening in their minds and hearts, it is crucial to give the students some tools to orient their awareness and to engage a relaxing and enjoyable experience in their bodies. Teachers may have them shake their bodies and then freeze, tense, and relax, or lead students through various progressive relaxation exercises. These types of body explorations empower students to feel more comfortable in their bodies and give them the capacity to witness and regulate their sensory field.

Focused Attention Once students learn the language of their bodies, they can begin cultivating their attention. Teachers work with various sensory phenomena, such as the breath and sound to anchor and stabilize attention. These practices cultivate the capacity to focus on schoolwork and other activities, but this attention is also the key building block for emotional regulation and responsible decision-making.

Attention lessons are taught through focusing exercises as well as distraction games. Teachers learn to have students pay attention to a spot on a wall and then try to distract their eyes by waving their arms. Another distraction exercise is to instruct students to focus clearly on their breathing while the teacher walks around the room making distracting noises. Students engage easily when focus and distraction is turned into a game where the whole class can examine the dynamics of distraction in real time, learning how to build attention "muscles" and work with the very real distractions of everyday life.

Heartfulness Once students have an understanding of the language of their bodies and how to anchor their awareness, they can learn how to identify and feel emotions in their bodies. Students learn to regulate difficult emotions by bringing kind awareness to these feelings. Students also learn to feel and strengthen beneficial emotions such as joy and compassion.

Teachers build upon the awareness of body sensations and attention by inviting students to be aware of a real frustration in their lives, teaching them to witness the thoughts correlated with the frustration, and then showing them how to feel the emotion as a sensation within the body. The capacity to witness the physical root of an emotion is the missing link in supporting students to truly work with impulse control. When students can slow down the impulse process enough to be able to experience a trigger, take a pause, untangle from the thoughts, and breath into the uncomfortable corresponding feelings in the body, they gain a life-transforming skill.

Interconnection Once students have built their awareness of their bodies, minds, and hearts, they can integrate their mindfulness into everyday life. They can learn to work with everyday distraction, frustrations, discomforts in the body, and other inevitable difficulties. Students can also bring compassion, forgiveness, and gratitude into action.

Often teachers offer students the opportunity to create mindful service projects, having them decide how they will show their compassion in the world. This is where teachers can get creative in facilitating classroom or school-wide mindfulness projects. For example, teachers might take their students on field trips to become aware of real environmental problems where students can develop empathy for the frogs in a polluted stream, and then feel the empowerment of making a difference. Compassion in action is the end goal.

Above, we have explored recommended strategies and curricula geared to incorporating mindfulness in the classroom and into the broader school community. Once a teacher has learned their own mindfulness practice then they can begin embodying the teachings with their students and eventually teachers can directly offer these priceless lessons to their students.

Directions for Future Research

Mindfulness appears to have the potential to enhance and deepen our educational system (Mind and Life Education Research Network (MLERN), 2012). However, we need research to continue to refine and expand our knowledge of the possible applications of mindfulness to education. To move forward we must develop broader paradigms for the field, which include specific directions for future studies. Below we discuss seven key potential directions for the field with specific suggestions for future study designs.

Specific Suggestions for Future Research

The results of past research are qualified by their limitations in methodology. We offer the following seven criteria as a platform for future research:

1. Differentiation between types of mindfulness practices. There are many types of mindfulness, both informal and formal meditation practice. This is crucial to recognize for theoretical, practical, and research reasons. Yet researchers often implicitly assume that different meditations have equivalent effects. This is an assumption to be empirically tested. Most likely, different techniques have been overlapping but by no means equal effects. Therefore, it is essential that researchers clearly define the type of mindfulness practice being studied.
2. Temporal effects. Frequency and duration of mindfulness practice must be recorded (e.g., meditation journals) to determine if greater amounts/frequency of practice induces greater effects and if so, is the relationship linear, curvilinear, or some other more intricate pattern.
3. Follow-up assessment. Follow-up should include long-term as well as short-term assessment.
4. Component analysis. Mindfulness is now recognized to be a multifaceted process with multiple potentially potent components. These range from nonspecific factors such as belief and expectancy through postural, somatic, attentional, cognitive, and other factors. Research can attempt to differentiate the effects and interactions of various components. This is a kind of component analysis.
5. Mediating variables. Development of subjective and objective measures to determine the mediating variables that account for the most variance in predicting change.
6. Qualitative data. The subtlety and depth of mindfulness experiences do not easily lend themselves to quantification. Further, the interplay between subjective and objective is essential to understanding mindfulness. Qualitative data provides a means to access the subjective experience of the practitioner.
7. The value of practice. Several lines of evidence suggest that personal practice of mindfulness may enhance one's understanding of meditative and transpersonal experiences, states, and stages. Without direct experience, concepts (and especially transpersonal concepts) remain what Immanuel Kant calls "empty" and devoid of experiential grounding. Without this grounding we lack *adequatio*: the capacity to comprehend the deeper "grades of significance" of phenomena, which Aldous Huxley (1945) summarized in The Perennial Philosophy, as "knowledge is a function of being." Therefore, for research to progress, optimally it may be helpful for researchers themselves to have a personal mindfulness practice. Without direct practice and experience we may be in part blind to the deeper shades of significance of mindfulness experiences, and blind to our blindness.

Conclusion

The progression of this paper corresponds with our recommendation for the process in which teachers and administrators can weave mindfulness into their schools. Teachers can begin with their own mindfulness practice, learning self-care, and basic introspective and interpersonal capacities. Mindfulness supports the development of universal positive qualities, such as compassion, attention, and emotional balance. With the development of these qualities, teachers can teach more mindfully, modeling these virtues to their students. From an embodied mindful presence, teachers can begin to teach mindfulness to their students from a variety of curricula and eventually with creative and spontaneous skills. There are countless examples of inspiring ways teachers and whole schools are integrating mindfulness (see chapters in this volume). As we continue to grow in this movement, we must simultaneously stay rooted in validated research. During the past four decades, research in mindfulness has developed a strong foundation, demonstrating significant psychological, physiological, and therapeutic effects. And yet, the integration of mindfulness into education is in its infancy and its exploration requires great sensitivity and a range of methodological glasses (see Roeser et al., 2012). Future research could benefit by looking through all of them, thereby illuminating the richness and complexity of mindfulness, and deepening our understanding of its applications to education and teaching.

References

Arkowitz, H. (2002). Empathy, psychotherapy integration, and meditation: A Buddhist contribution to the common factors movement. *Journal of Humanistic Psychology, 45*, 483–502.

Baer, R. A. (2003). Mindfulness training as clinical intervention: A conceptual and empirical review. *Clinical Psychology: Science and Practice, 10*, 125–143.

Beddoe, A. E., & Murphy, S. O. (2004). Does mindfulness decreases stress and foster empathy among nursing students? *Journal of Nursing Education, 43*, 305–312.

Benn, R., Akiva, T., Arel, S., & Roeser, R. W. (2012). Mindfulness training effects for parents and educators of children with special needs. *Developmental Psychology, 48*, 1476–1487.

Bohart, A. C., Elliott, R., Greenberg, L. S., & Watson, J. C. (2002). Empathy. In J. C. Norcross (Ed.), *Psychotherapy relationships that work: Therapist contributions and responsiveness to patients* (pp. 89–108). New York, NY: Oxford University Press.

Botvinivk, M., Jha, A. P., Bylsma, L. M., Fabian, S. A., Solomon, P. E., & Prkachin, K. M. (2005). Viewing the facial expressions of pain engages cortical areas involved in the direct experience of pain. *NeuroImage, 25*, 312–319.

Braunstein-Bercovitz, H. (2003). Does stress enhance or impair selective attention? The effects of stress and perceptual load on negative priming. *Anxiety, Stress and Coping, 16*, 345–357.

Brown, K., & Ryan, R. (2003). The benefits of being present. Mindfulness and its role in psychological well-being. *Journal of Personality and Social Psychology, 84*, 822–848.

Cheng, Y., Yang, C. Y., Lin, C. P., Lee, P. R., & Decety, J. (2008). The perception of pain in others suppresses somatosensory oscillations: A magnetoencephalography study. *NeuroImage, 40*, 1833–1840.

Christopher, J. C., Chrisman, J. A., Trotter-Mathison, M. J., Shure, M. B., Dahlen, P., & Christopher, S. B. (2010). Perceptions of long-term influence of mindfulness training on counselors and psychotherapists: A qualitative inquiry. *Journal of Humanistic Psychology, 51*, 318–349.

Condon, P. (2014). *Cultivating compassion: The effects of compassion-and mindfulness-based meditation on pro-social mental states and behavior.*

Condon, P., Desbordes, G., Miller, W., & Desteno, D. (2013). Meditation increases compassionate responses to suffering. *Psychological Science, 24*(10), 2125–2127.

Di Pellegrino, G., Fadiga, L., Fogassi, L., Gallese, V., & Rizzolatti, G. (1992). Understanding motor events: A neurophysical study. *Experimental Brain Research, 91*, 176–180.

Enochs, W. K., & Etzbach, C. A. (2004). Impaired student counselors: Ethical and legal considerations for the family. *The Family Journal, 12*, 396–400.

Geller, S. M., & Greenberg, L. S. (2012). *Therapeutic presence: A mindful approach to effective therapy.* Washington, DC: American Psychological Association.

Germer, C. K., Siegel, R. D., & Fulton, P. R. (Eds.). (2005). *Mindfulness and psychotherapy.* New York, NY: Guilford Press.

Gokhan, N., Meehan, E. F., & Peters, K. (2010). The value of mindfulness-based methods in teaching at a clinical field placement. *Psychological Reports, 106*, 455–466.

Goleman, D. (2006). *Emotional intelligence: Why it can matter more than IQ* (10th ed.). New York, NY: Bantam Books.

Grossman, P., Niemann, L., Schmidt, S., & Walach, H. (2004). Mindfulness-based stress reduction and health benefits. A metaanalysis. *Journal of Psychosomatic Research, 57*, 35–43.

Huxley, A. (1945). *The perennial philosophy.* New York, NY: Harper.

Irving, J. A., Dobkin, P. L., & Park, J. (2009). Cultivating mindfulness in health care professionals: A review of empirical studies of mindfulness-based stress reduction. *Complementary Therapies in Clinical Practice, 15*, 61–66.

Jabbi, M., Swart, M., & Keysers, C. (2006). Empathy for positive and negative emotions in the gustatory cortex. *NeuroImage, 34*, 1744–1753.

Jennings, P., & Greenberg, M. (2009). The prosocial classroom: Teacher social and emotional competence in relation to student and classroom outcomes. *Review of Educational Research, 79*(1), 491–525.

Jennings, P., Lantieri, L., & Roeser, R. W. (2012). Supporting educational goals through cultivating mindfulness: Approaches for teachers and students. In P. M. Brown, M. W. Corrigan, & A. Higgins-D'Alessandro (Eds.), *Handbook of prosocial education.* Lanham, MD: Rowan & Littlefield.

Jha, A. P., Krompinger, J., & Baime, M. J. (2007). Mindfulness training modifies subsystems of attention. *Cognitive, Affective and Behavioral Neuroscience, 7*, 109–119.

Kabat-Zinn, J. (1990). *Full catastrophe living: Using the wisdom of your body and mind to face stress, pain and illness*. New York, NY: Dell.

Kabat-Zinn, J. (2005). *Coming to our senses: Healing ourselves and the world through mindfulness*. New York, NY: Hyperion.

Keng, S. L., Smoski, M. J., & Robins, C. J. (2011). Effects of mindfulness on psychological health: A review of empirical studies. *Clinical Psychology Review, 31*, 1041–1056.

Khoury, B., Lecomte, T., Fortin, G., Masse, M., Therien, P., Bouchard, V., … Hofmann, SG. (2013). Mindfulness-based therapy: A comprehensive meta-analysis. *Clinical Psychology Review, 33*, 763–771.

Killingsworth, M. A., & Gilbert, D. T. (2010). A wandering mind is an unhappy mind. *Science, 12*, 932.

Kornfield, J. (2009). *The wise heart: A guide to the universal teachings of Buddhist psychology*. New York, NY: Bantam Books.

Lamm, C., Batson, C. D., & Decety, J. (2007). The neural substrate of human empathy: Effects of perspective-taking and cognitive appraisal. *Journal of Cognitive Neuroscience, 19*, 42–58.

Lazar, S. W., Kerr, C. E., Wasserman, R. H., Gray, J. R., Greve, D. N., Treadway, M. T., … Fischld, B. (2005). Meditation experience is associated with increased cortical thickness. *Neuroreport, 16*, 1893–1897.

Lesh, T. V. (1970). Zen meditation and the development of empathy in counselors. *Journal of Humanistic Psychology, 10*, 39–74.

Lingnau, A., Gesierich, B., & Caramazza, A. (2009). Asymmetric fMRI adaptation reveals no evidence for mirror neurons in humans. *Proceedings of the National Academy of Sciences, 106*, 9925–9930.

Mackenzie, C. S., Smith, M. C., Hasher, L., Leach, L., & Behl, P. (2007). Cognitive functioning under stress: Evidence from informal caregivers of palliative patients. *Journal of Palliative Medicine, 10*, 749–758.

Marzano, R. J. (2007). *The art and science of teaching: A comprehensive framework for effective instruction*. Alexandria, VA: Association for Supervision and Curriculum Development.

McCollum, E. E., & Gehart, D. R. (2010). Mindfulness meditation to teach beginning therapists' therapeutic presence: A qualitative study. *Journal of Marital and Family Therapy, 36*, 347–360.

Mind and Life Education Research Network. (2012). Contemplative practices and mental training: Prospects for American education. *Child Development Perspectives, 6*, 146–153.

Morrison, I., Lloyd, D., Di Pellegrino, G., & Roberts, N. (2004). Vicarious responses to pain in anterior cingulate cortex: Is empathy a multisensory issue? *Cognitive and Affective Behavioral Neuroscience, 4*, 270–278.

Rizzolatti, G., & Criaghero, L. (2004). The mirror neuron system. *Annual Review of Neuroscience, 27*, 169–192.

Rizzolatti, G., Fadiga, L., Gallese, V., & Fogassi, L. (1996). Premotor cortex and the recognition of motor actions. *Cognitive Brain Research, 3*, 131–141.

Roeser, R. W., & Eccles, J. S. (2014). Schooling and the mental health of children and adolescents in the United States. In M. Lewis & K. D. Rudolph (Eds.), *Handbook of developmental psychopathology* (3rd ed., pp. 163–184). New York, NY: Springer.

Roeser, R. W., Schonert-Reichl, K. A., Jha, A., Cullen, M., Wallace, L., Wilensky, R., … Harrison, J. (2013). Mindfulness training and reductions in teacher stress and burnout: Results from two randomized, waitlist-control field trials. *Journal of Educational Psychology*. doi:10.1037/a0032093.

Roeser, R. W., Skinner, E., Beers, J., & Jennings, P. A. (2012). Mindfulness training and teachers' professional development: An emerging area of research and practice. *Child Development Perspectives, 6*, 167–173.

Rogers, C. R. (1957). The necessary and sufficient conditions of therapeutic personality change. *Journal of Consulting Psychology, 21*, 95–103.

Segal, Z. V., Williams, M. G., & Teasdale, J. D. (2002). *Mindfulness-based cognitive therapy for depression: A new approach to preventing relapse*. New York, NY: Guilford Press.

Shanafelt, T. D., Bradley, K. A., Wipf, J. E., & Back, A. L. (2002). Burnout and self-reported patient care in an internal medicine residency program. *Annals of Internal Medicine, 136*, 358–367.

Shapiro, S. L., Brown, K., & Biegel, G. M. (2007). Teaching self-care to caregivers: Effects of mindfulness-based stress reduction on the mental health of therapists in training. *Training and Education in Professional Psychology, 1*, 105–115.

Shapiro, S. L., & Carlson, L. E. (2009). *The art and science of mindfulness: Integrating mindfulness into psychology and the helping professions*. Washington, DC: American Psychological Association.

Shapiro, S. L., & Schwartz, G. E. (2000). Intentional systemic mindfulness: An integrative model for self-regulation and health. *Advances in Mind Body Medicine, 16*, 128–134.

Shapiro, S. L., Schwartz, G. E., & Bonner, G. (1998). Effects of mindfulness-based stress reduction on medical and pre-medical students. *Journal of Behavioral Medicine, 21*, 581–599.

Singer, T., Seymour, B., O'Doherty, J., Kaube, H., Dolan, R. J., & Firth, C. D. (2004). Empathy for pain involves the affective but not sensory components of pain. *Science, 303*, 1157–1162.

Skosnik, P. D., Chatterton, R. T., Swisher, T., & Park, S. (2000). Modulation of attentional inhibition by norepinephrine and cortisol after psychological stress. *International Journal of Psychophysiology, 36*, 59–68.

Slagter, H. A., Lutz, A., Greischar, L. L., Francis, A. D., Nieuwenhuis, S., Davis, J. M., & Davidson, R. J. (2007). Mental training affects distribution of limited brain resources. *PLoS Biology, 5*, e138.

Thompson, B. L., & Waltz, J. (2007). Everyday mindfulness and mindfulness meditation: Overlapping constructs or not? *Personality and Individual Differences, 43*, 1875–1885.

Valente, V., & Marotta, A. (2005). The impact of yoga on the professional and personal life of the psychotherapist. *Contemporary Family Therapy: An International Journal, 27*, 65–80.

Wallace, A. B., & Bodhi, B. (2006). *The nature of mindfulness and its role in Buddhist meditation: A correspondence between B. Alan Wallace and the venerable Bhikkhu Bodhi.* Unpublished manuscript, Santa Barbara Institute for Consciousness Studies, Santa Barbara, CA.

Wicker, B., Keysers, C., Plailly, J., Royet, J. P., Gallese, V., & Rizzolatti, G. (2003). Both of us disgusted in my insula: The common neural basis of seeing and feeling disgust. *Neuron, 40*, 655–664.

Mindfulness and Teachers' Coping in the Classroom: A Developmental Model of Teacher Stress, Coping, and Everyday Resilience

7

Ellen Skinner and Jeffry Beers

Introduction

Teaching can be a stressful occupation. Twenty-five to thirty percent of teachers rate their jobs as either very or extremely stressful (Borg, 2001; Kyriacou, 2001) and teaching is consistently ranked as one of the top jobs in terms of stress-related health problems (Johnson et al., 2005). Reviews of research on the causes of stress for teachers suggest that it stems from many sources, chief among them student disciplinary and motivational problems; friction with administrators, colleagues, and parents; instructional and administrative demands; time and evaluation pressures; and poor working conditions (Kyriacou, 1987, 2001; Montgomery & Rupp, 2005). Moreover, teachers' occupational stress has likely been on the rise over the last decade: Ongoing educational reform efforts that involve high stakes testing have resulted in increased evaluation pressure, scrutiny, and criticism of teachers' job performance (Lambert & McCarthy, 2006; Nichols & Berliner, 2007).

E. Skinner (✉)
Department of Psychology, Portland State University, P.O. Box 751, Portland, OR 97207-0751, USA
e-mail: ellen.skinner@pdx.edu

J. Beers
Department of Psychology, Portland State University, Portland, OR, USA
e-mail: jeffrybeers@gmail.com

Recent conceptualizations of human service occupations, like teaching, suggest that one reason such jobs are stressful is that they require high levels of emotional work (Chang, 2009; Hargreaves, 2000; Roeser, Skinner, Beers, & Jennings, 2012; Schutz & Zembylas, 2009; Sutton & Wheatley, 2003; Zapf et al. 2001). As explained by Klassen, Perry, and Frenzel (2012), "Teaching is a unique occupation in its emphasis on establishing long-term meaningful connections with the 'clients' of the work environment (i.e., students) at a depth that may not be found in other professions" (p. 151). Working with students, as individuals or in groups, is likely to be emotionally taxing. Students' behavioral and motivational issues, coupled with their inherent immaturity, often make them challenging interaction partners. Moreover, teaching involves the potential burden of "emotional labor," in which teachers are required to display professionally appropriate emotions, even in the face of distressing interactions with students who may show disrespectful, disruptive, disinterested, or dismissive behavior in the classroom (Hargreaves, 2000; Zapf, 2002). In fact, open-ended interviews with teachers (e.g., Blase, 1986) suggest that "problems with students" are among the most stressful events in teachers' daily lives, with issues such as student misbehavior, apathy, absences, and failure to learn cited as common and upsetting, especially when motivational and disciplinary problems interfere with teachers'

K.A. Schonert-Reichl, R.W. Roeser (eds.), *Handbook of Mindfulness in Education*, Mindfulness in Behavioral Health, DOI 10.1007/978-1-4939-3506-2_7

effectiveness in delivering instruction to the rest of the class (Chang, 2009; Friedman, 1995; Kyriacou, 2001).

It seems to be the continual repetition of these seemingly minor events, rather than isolated severe incidents, that cumulatively create the "unpleasant, negative emotions, such as anger, anxiety, tension, frustration, or depression" characteristic of stress (Kyriacou, 2001, p. 28). Recent discussions of emotion in the classroom suggest that the cumulative chronic activation of negative emotions saps teachers' energy and enjoyment, and poses a risk factor for burnout (Chang, 2009), described as the erosion of engagement in which "[w]hat started out as important, meaningful, and challenging work becomes unpleasant, unfulfilling, and meaningless. Energy turns into exhaustion, involvement turns into cynicism, and efficacy turns into ineffectiveness" (Maslach, Schaufeli, & Leiter, 2001, p. 416). The primary symptoms of burnout, namely, emotional exhaustion, diminished sense of accomplishment, and depersonalization, pose a risk to teachers as well as to the schools and students they serve. Elevated symptoms of burnout can fuel teachers' physical absence from work or psychological absence while at work (Jennings & Greenberg, 2009). Especially pernicious is "depersonalization," in which teachers begin to develop a negative callous, cynical, and detached attitude toward students (Evers, Tomic, & Brouwers, 2004).

The consequences of chronic occupational stress can be seen in teachers' mental and physical health and well-being (Litt & Turk, 1985; Mearns & Cain, 2003). Research on teacher burnout reveals that about 20 % of teachers fall above the standardized cut-off score (Bauer et al., 2005), indicating significant stress with psychological and physical symptoms (Unterbrink et al., 2007). Effects are also likely to be apparent in student outcomes as well: Chronic stress can interfere with teachers' ability to create the supportive, challenging, and well-managed classrooms that students need in order to learn (Briner & Dewberry, 2007; Jennings & Greenberg, 2009). Occupational stress seems especially taxing for teachers just starting their careers, with desistence rates estimated to be as high as 46 % within the first 5 years (Jalongo & Heider, 2006).

Teacher Stress and Coping

Because of the toll chronic stress takes on teachers' mental and physical functioning, an important focus of research on occupational health has been to identify the factors that minimize or mitigate its effects (Boekaerts, 2002; Klusmann, Kunter, Trautwein, Luktke, & Baumert, 2008; Sutton & Wheatley, 2003). Among the most important of these candidate processes is teacher *coping*, which refers to how teachers actually react to and deal with the challenges and problems they face everyday (Parker & Martin, 2009). Adaptive coping, such as problem-focused coping or support-seeking, may buffer the effects of teachers' occupational stress. In fact, teachers themselves report both problem-focused coping and support-seeking to be among the most effective coping strategies (Litt & Turk, 1985). Problem-solving is associated with a stronger sense of personal accomplishment and higher levels of job satisfaction as well as lower levels of psychological distress, disengagement, and depersonalization, and fewer somatic complaints and physical symptoms related to burnout (Chan, 1998; Griffith et al., 1999; Griva & Joekes, 2003; Innes & Kitto, 1989; Pascual et al., 2003; Pomaki & Anagnostopoulou, 2003; Rasku & Kinnunen, 2003). In a similar vein, the availability of social support is associated with higher levels of active coping, positive thinking, and self-reported health, and lower levels of negative affect and disengagement (both mental and behavioral; Griffith et al., 1999; Schweitzer & Dobrich, 2003).

In contrast, maladaptive ways of coping, like avoidance, escape, or emotion-focused coping are associated with more distress and burnout among teachers. Teachers who use more avoidant coping are less satisfied with the outcome and tend to view problems as recurrent (Green & Ross, 1996). Both avoidant coping and emotion-focused coping are associated with higher levels of psychological distress, somatic complaints, emotional exhaustion, depersonalization, physical symptoms and burnout, and lower levels of personal accomplishment and job satisfaction (Chan, 1998; Griva & Joekes, 2003; Innes & Kitto, 1989; Pascual et al., 2003; Pomaki &

Anagnostopoulou, 2003; Rasku & Kinnunen, 2003; Verhoeven et al., 2003). Taken together, these findings suggest that adaptive coping may act as a protective factor and maladaptive coping as a risk factor when teachers are dealing with stress. At the same time, since most of these studies are correlational in nature, findings are also consistent with the notion that poor coping is not only a *cause* but also a *symptom* of stress and burnout for teachers.

Mindfulness, Developmental Models of Coping, and Everyday Resilience

Recent developmental models suggest that coping can do more than ward off the deleterious effects of stress (Compas, 2009; Skinner & Zimmer-Gembeck, 2007). It is possible that constructive coping can transform previously stressful interactions into opportunities for learning and development, contributing to higher quality engagement in teaching and greater levels of teacher professional satisfaction and well-being (Parker & Martin, 2009). Teachers' engagement and satisfaction may, in turn, contribute to higher quality instruction in the classroom and thus provide a learning context that nurtures students' own motivation, engagement, and achievement. In fact, constructive coping is hypothesized to be a mechanism of "everyday resilience" defined as the "ability to successfully deal with setbacks and challenges that are typical of the course of ordinary life" (Parker & Martin, 2009, p. 69). In such models, coping is characterized as an adaptive process that can make a physiological, psychological, and behavioral difference to the effects of daily adversities and is one determinant of whether stress will play a positive or negative role in teachers' professional and personal development.

Despite the potential for growth depicted in models of everyday resilience, research on the harmful effects of stress on teachers (e.g., Chang, 2009; Montgomery & Rupp, 2005) provides ample evidence that most educators do not have the resources to deal with daily problems in ways that convert stressors to learning experiences (e.g., Jennings & Greenberg, 2009; Roeser et al., 2012). Consistent with the goals of this volume, however, we have become interested in the promise of *mindfulness* practices and interventions to aid teachers in developing the kinds of personal resources that would help them cope more constructively with the demands of their profession, and thereby provide a pathway toward more everyday resilience and satisfying engagement in the classroom.

Hence, this chapter has two goals. The first is to present a developmental model of stress and coping that includes a description of the kinds of constructive coping that promote engagement and learning. The second goal is to provide our working definition of mindfulness and to identify multiple points in the process of coping where we think mindfulness could make an important difference, focusing especially on the mechanisms through which mindfulness could have its salutary effects on dealing with stress. The research base on this topic, although growing, is limited, so many of our ideas are frankly speculative. We conclude with a few suggestions for how mindful coping might change students' experiences in the classroom, since better coping may improve educators' engagement in teaching, and the quality of their relationships with students and classroom management (Roeser et al., 2012). As subtext throughout, the chapter is the hope that the developmental model might provide a framework useful for guiding future studies on mindfulness and teachers' everyday resilience.

A Developmental Model of Stress and Coping

Consistent with dominant models in the field today, we view coping as a transactional process that unfolds over time (Lazarus & Folkman, 1984). As depicted in Fig. 7.1, coping episodes typically begin when an individual engaged in ongoing goal-directed interactions begins to experience *resistance* to his or her efforts and realizes that a relevant personal goal is (or may

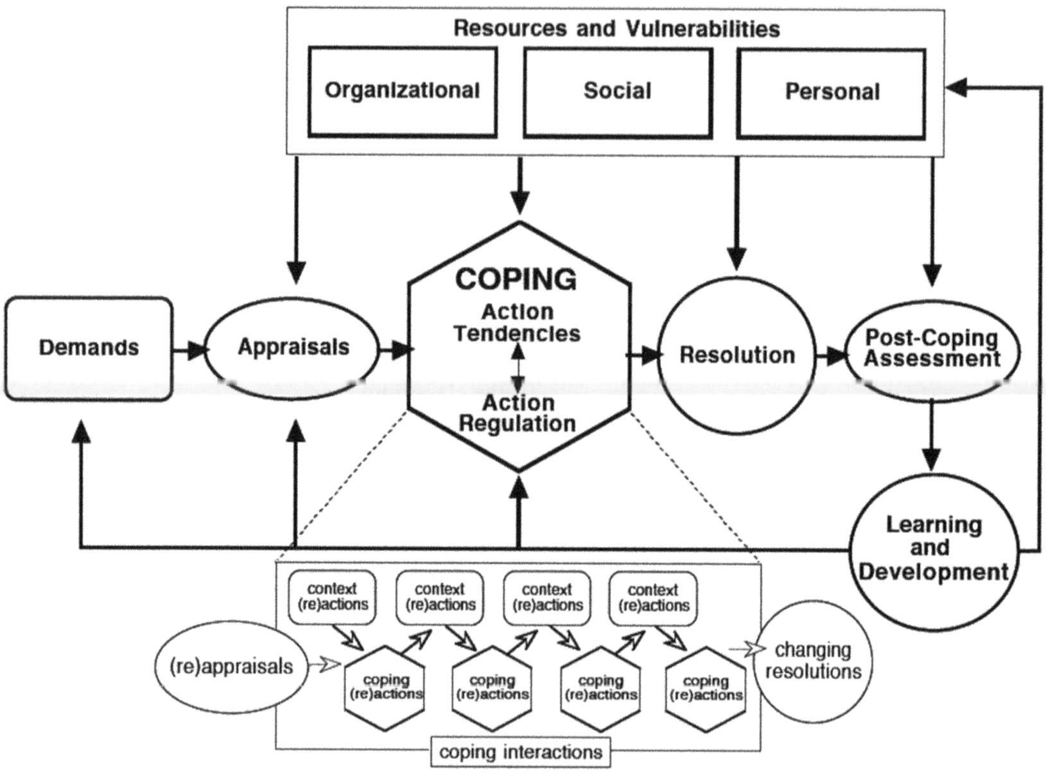

Fig. 7.1 A developmental model of the stress and coping process

be) blocked. This resistance has been variously labeled as the objective or environmental stressor or the stressful event or encounter. We label it as a "demand" to show that challenging interactions with the environment are not necessarily stressful. They signal that an individual's automatic responses are ineffective, and that more effort, different actions, or help may be needed.

Appraisals

The next step in the coping process is "appraisal" in which the individual appreciates the significance of the demand. According to Lazarus and Folkman (1984), two types of appraisals are critical: (1) primary appraisals, which evaluate what is at stake for the person in the stressful encounter by asking "Am I in trouble or being benefited, now or in the future, and in what way?" and (2) secondary appraisals, which evaluate "What if anything can be done about it?" (p. 31). When, through primary appraisal, an encounter is evaluated as "stressful" (as opposed to irrelevant or benign-positive), the event can be further appraised as: *harm/loss,* in which damage has already been sustained and cannot be reversed; *threat*, characterized by fear and anxiety, in which harm/loss is anticipated but has not yet occurred; and/or *challenge*, characterized by eagerness and excitement, in which potentials for gain are anticipated. Secondary appraisals focus on evaluations of possibilities for control—coping options, their expected efficacy, and the likelihood that one can enact the strategy effectively (Folkman, 1984). These (re)appraisals can be experienced sequentially or simultaneously, are repeatedly updated during stressful transactions, and are key in shaping emotional reactions to the stressor, action tendencies, and the kinds of coping that are expressed.

Coping as "Regulation under Stress"

The next step in the process is coping itself. Over the last decade, developmental conceptualizations have focused on coping as an adaptive self-regulatory process, by defining it as "self-regulation under stress" (Compas, 2009; Eisenberg, Fabes, & Guthrie, 1997; Skinner & Zimmer-Gembeck, 2007). Dual-process models of coping (like other dual-process models of emotion, attention, and behavior regulation) distinguish between *reactivity* and *regulation*. Stress *reactivity* refers to relatively automatic and non-conscious physiological, attentional, emotional, and behavioral reactions to stressful encounters (such as increased heart rate, shallow breathing, or emotional outbursts). From an action theoretical perspective (Brandtstädter, 2006), these stress reactions can be thought of as *action tendencies* (Skinner, 1999), which are triggered by the individual's appreciation of the significance of an interaction with the context, and reflect the organism's history of learning and experiences.

Action tendencies are emotionally colored goal-directed motor programs that create an "urge" or "impulse" that is redundantly experienced as a desire to move (or freeze), an emotion, and a goal orientation or attentional focus. They are part of fast, reactive, impulsive "hot" systems that appraise and react to external situations relatively automatically and with little conscious control (Metcalfe & Mischel, 1999). Action tendencies bring the organism into a state of *readiness* to respond to external conditions, and are adaptive because they organize readiness and speed up response time while still remaining more flexible than reflexes (Case & Griffin, 1990).

In contrast, *action regulation* refers to relatively intentional and conscious efforts to coordinate or modulate these responses (through strategies such as information seeking, strategizing, or distraction; Compas, Connor, Saltzman, Thomsen, & Wadsworth, 1999; Skinner, 1999). A focus on *action* as the target of regulation highlights the notion that coping requires the coordination of many, sometimes competing, subsystems. Encounters with stressful conditions activate physiology, attention, emotion, behavior, volition, and motivation. The function of regulation is to work with the multiple (sometimes opposing) action tendencies that are generated under stress in order to guide, organize, sequence, redirect, or block them. Although the strategies studied most often are cognitive and deliberate, a wide variety of regulatory processes seem to operate at multiple levels, starting with hormonal and neurological, already in infancy (Campos, Frankel, & Camras, 2004). Regulatory processes are also adaptive because they allow actions to be more informed and flexible, and less determined by current conditions.

A focus on coping as an adaptive self-regulatory process emphasizes that coping actions reflect the (im)balance between stress reactivity and action regulation. Adaptive coping reflects low stress reactivity and/or strong regulatory capacities, whereas maladaptive coping reflects overwhelming reactions to stress and/or a regulatory system that is weak, immature, or disabled. A central challenge to interventionists focused on coping and regulation is presented by the neurophysiological and behavioral effects of chronic stress on these systems: Prolonged exposure to stressful experiences appears to increase bottom-up psychobiological stress reactivity and, at the same time, to disrupt functions in the brain regions that underlie top-down self-regulation (Compas, 2006).

As can be seen in Fig. 7.1, coping actions are considered to be the outcomes of action tendencies (reactivity) and action regulation. According to this perspective, the study of coping subsumes the regulation of emotion, attention, behavior, physiology, motivation, and cognition, to focus on how people organize or coordinate these features of action under stress (or fail to do so; Compas, 2009; Skinner, 1999). However, coping researchers do not see the primary goal of regulation as calming or downregulating emotion. Although it is clear that high emotional reactivity can overwhelm regulatory resources, it is also clear that rigid suppression of negative emotion both uses up regulatory energy (Baumeister, Bratslavsky, Muraven, & Tice, 1998) and blocks important information needed for adaptive coping (Cole, Michel, & Teti, 1994). From a functionalist perspective, "negative" emotions, like distress, anger, and sadness, signal interactions of adaptive significance, where goals are at stake (Barrett & Campos, 1991; Williams, 2010). This is why they attract the organism's attention. Hence, coping can benefit from access to the entire range of genuine emotions as long as they are expressed in ways that allow them to be integrated with other coping subsystems like motivation and behavior (Ekman, Davidson, Ricard, & Wallace, 2005).

Coping Transactions

As depicted in Fig. 7.1, coping episodes actually consist of a sequence of interactions between the person and the demand or context, which reciprocally shape each other over an extended period of time (Folkman & Lazarus, 1985). The actual actions people show in dealing with stressors, such as problem-solving, support-seeking, venting, or escape, are called "ways of coping." They are the building blocks of the area, distinguishing research on coping from other strands of work that focus on the effects of stress or adversity without an explicit account of how people interact with specific stressful events on the ground. Individual instances of coping are virtually infinite in their variety because coping responses are calibrated to the particular set of stressors, the person's current capacities, and the social resources and contexts in which events are unfolding. As a result, hundreds of ways of coping, and corresponding systems to categorize them, have been suggested by researchers (Skinner, Edge, Altman, & Sherwood, 2003).

However, categories of coping are more than a list of things people can do when they run into trouble. If coping is an adaptive process, then its categories reflect a conceptualization of how particular responses to stress improve the fit between an organism and its environment when the demands on the organism exceed (or are expected to exceed) its resources. From this perspective, higher order coping categories can be discriminated by the set of adaptive functions they serve. Researchers following this line of reasoning have converged on about a dozen higher-order coping *families* which can accommodate most of the lower order ways of coping identified in previous research (see Table 7.1; Skinner et al., 2003). Each family subsumes all the lower order ways of coping that serve the same set of functions. For example, the "*problem-solving*" family includes not only generating solutions to a problem, but other ways of fitting actions to contingencies, such as effort exertion, experimentation or trying out different instrumental actions, planning, and repair. These families include adaptive responses to stress, such as problem-solving, seeking information or support, self-reliance, accommodation (e.g., positive restructuring or distraction), and negotiation, as well as maladaptive reactions, such as helplessness, escape, isolation, delegation, opposition (e.g., blaming others), and submission (e.g., rumination, self-blame, or resignation).

Coping, Learning, and Development

Developmental views of coping encourage researchers to reconceptualize "stressful" interactions as opportunities for learning and for developing robust personal and social resources for dealing with challenges and threats (Aldwin, 2007; Compas, 1993; Skinner & Zimmer-Gembeck, 2007). From this perspective, "adaptive" ways of coping prolong the individual's constructive engagement with stressful situations, allowing the individual to learn as much as possible from the encounter and to bounce back more quickly from any actual loss or harm. The stance taken toward the stressor—as a challenge—combined with the active learning that takes place should contribute to the development of actual coping resources. These, in turn, should promote resilience and a willingness to reengage with challenging tasks in the future (Skinner & Wellborn, 1994, 1997). The "adaptive" significance of these ways of coping both evolutionarily and developmentally is self-evident.

Table 7.1 A hierarchical model of adaptive processes and families of coping

Adaptive process #1: Coordinate actions and contingencies in the environment				
Family of coping:	1. Problem-solving	2. Information Seeking	3. Helplessness	4. Escape
Family function in adaptive process:	Adjust actions to be effective	Find additional contingencies	Find limits of actions	Escape noncontingent environments
Ways of coping:	Strategizing	Reading	Confusion	Behavioral avoidance
	Instrumental action	Observation	Cognitive interference	Mental withdrawal
	Planning	Asking others	Cognitive exhaustion	Flight
	Mastery		Passivity	Denial
				Wishful thinking
Adaptive process #2: Coordinate reliance and social resources available				
Family of coping:	5. Self-reliance	6. Support-Seeking	7. Delegation	8. Social isolation
Family function in adaptive process:	Protect available social resources	Use available social resources	Find limits of resources	Withdraw from unsupportive contexts
Ways of coping:	Emotion regulation	Contact seeking	Maladaptive help-seeking	Social withdrawal
	Behavior regulation	Comfort seeking		Concealment
	Emotional expression	Instrumental aid	Complaining	Avoiding others
		Social referencing	Whining	Freeze
	Emotion approach		Self-pity	
Adaptive process #3: Coordinate preferences and available options				
Family of coping:	9. Accommodation	10. Negotiation	11. Submission	12. Opposition
Family function in adaptive process:	Flexibly adjust preferences to options	Find new options	Give up preferences	Remove constraints
Ways of coping:	Distraction	Bargaining	Rumination	Other-blame
	Cognitive restructuring	Persuasion	Rigid perseveration	Projection
		Priority-setting	Intrusive thoughts	Aggression
	Minimization			Defiance
	Acceptance			

Post-Coping Assessment

Hence, for researchers and interventionists interested in the development of coping, the goal is not to eliminate stressful experiences but to convert them to occasions for growth. Especially interesting are opportunities after a coping episode to reflect on what has happened in order to determine what can be learned for future encounters (Howard & Johnson, 2004). We refer to these processes as "post-coping assessments." Such reflections should be opportunities to use stressful encounters (even in the face of "failures") to improve future coping. As can be seen in Fig. 7.1, post-coping assessments can feed back into the resources available for future coping, especially personal resources, or they can feed forward into subsequent stressful encounters by influencing future demands, as described by "proactive" or "preventative" coping and "anticipatory" or "antecedent-focused" self-regulation (Aspinwall

& Taylor, 1997; Diamond & Aspinwall, 2003). They can also shape subsequent appraisals, action tendencies, action regulation, or coping interactions themselves.

Resources

As can be seen in Fig. 7.1, processes of stress and coping are influenced by the resources and vulnerabilities brought into transactions by the person, their social partners, and the organizational contexts in which they operate. Although coping is often portrayed as an individual affair, it is actually highly social in nature (Berg, Meegan, & Deviney, 1998) and fully embedded in the institutional and societal contexts in which it takes place (Tolan & Grant, 2009). Studies of coping typically focus on *personal* resources; those most commonly studied are self-efficacy, sense of control, optimism, hardiness, and negative emotionality. The *social* resources examined most often are instrumental and emotional social support.

Mindfulness and Coping

A developmental conceptualization of coping provides traction for an analysis of the effects of mindfulness in at least three ways. First, it deconstructs processes of coping, expanding on standard models that focus largely on appraisals and ways of coping, to incorporate additional steps, like stress reactivity or action tendencies, action regulation, families of coping, and coping interactions. Such elaborated models identify more entry points for analyzing how mindfulness could influence coping. Second, developmental conceptualizations by definition link the processes of dealing with stress to the potential for growth, focusing researchers on what can be learned through struggles and how adversity can act as a "teacher." In the current model, processes captured in the concept of "post-coping assessments" explicitly identify a location in the coping process, namely, after an episode has been resolved, for reflection and learning, and hence, specify a potential pathway toward development.

Perhaps most importantly, such conceptualizations remind researchers that, at its core, coping is an adaptive process (Lazarus & Folkman, 1984; White, 1974). Its primary function is to monitor and detect threats, and to calibrate responses to deal effectively with actual problems as they evolve on the ground. Good coping is not easy. It requires clear and accurate information about current internal and external conditions with continued access to strategies used during past episodes, selected based on their anticipated effects on future outcomes. It requires individuals to maintain their internal organization or composure, so they are able to carry out difficult actions in the face of threat, and to flexibly adjust as conditions change, recovering from setbacks and keeping options open. Individuals require the capacity to access and benefit from additional resources and the ability to coordinate their coping with others, sometimes many others. Moreover, to boost speed and preserve energy, coping should be accomplished as automatically as possible. A focus on coping as an adaptive self-regulatory process reminds researchers about the complex nature of "good" coping (Skinner & Zimmer-Gembeck, 2007).

Tenets of Mindfulness

To explore the effects of mindfulness on coping, it is necessary to have a clear conceptualization, not only of coping, but also of mindfulness. The vigor and enthusiasm with which psychology has embraced the ideas and practices of mindfulness over the last 25 years, has produced a host of definitions (Bishop et al., 2004). Because much of the research is based on clinical work that combines psychotherapies with selected practices (e.g., Coelho, Canter, & Ernst, 2007; Hofmann, Sawywe, Witt, & Oh, 2010; Melbourne Academic Interest Group, 2006), the specific defining characteristics of mindfulness itself have not always been clearly identified (Brown, Ryan, & Creswell, 2007; Kabat-Zinn, 2003). However, as the pace of this work has accelerated, definitions of mindfulness have been clarified and the mechanisms through which it operates, both neurophysiological and psychological, have become increasingly clear (Hölzel et al., 2011).

Table 7.2 Working definition of mindfulness

Mindfulness is a natural mode of consciousness, awareness, and attention that has the following characteristics:
1. **Present-oriented.** Focus of awareness and attention to the direct and immediate experience of present events as they arise and unfold from moment to moment, without distraction by past or future concerns.
2. **Receptivity.** Openhearted, friendly, affectionate, compassionate, and accepting awareness and acknowledgement of experience, that is nonjudgmental and nonevaluative, without the chatter of self-centered thoughts ("quiet ego").
3. **Clarity.** Dispassionate clear seeing of internal and external phenomena (including thoughts, emotions, sensations, actions, or surroundings) as they are, and not as distorted by conceptual filters or habitual ways of seeing.
4. **Empirical stance.** Explorative, interested, and curious observation of the full objective facts of life, without preferring self-enhancing or shying away from distressing or threatening information and experiences.
5. **Flexibility.** Voluntary fluid regulation of states of attention and awareness from narrow focus to broad vista, without confusion or loss of contact to present moment experience.
6. **Steadiness.** Composed intentional continuity of sustained awareness and attention, without distraction or fixation.
7. **Presence.** "Integrative awareness" as the agent of action. The integrated "I" is actively engaged with, has direct contact with, and ownership of experience while also being immersed in it.

Note. From Bishop et al. (2004), Brown et al. (2007), Kabat-Zinn (2003), and Chambers et al. (2009).

As summarized in Table 7.2, we rely on conceptualizations that not only identify core characteristics of mindfulness as a mode of consciousness, awareness, and attention (Bishop et al., 2004), but also include qualities that emerge from prolonged experiences of these states, as suggested by Buddhist psychology (Brown et al., 2007; Chambers, Gullone, & Allen, 2009; Kabat-Zinn, 2003). Mindfulness refers to a receptive attention to and an awareness of present events and experience that has two components: (1) the intentional sustained focus of awareness and attention on the direct and immediate experience of present events as they arise and unfold from moment to moment (Bishop et al., 2004), and (2) an orientation toward that experience which is accepting, openhearted, compassionate, and nonjudgmental (Kabat-Zinn, 2003).

Such an explorative, interested, and curious stance facilitates the full and clear observation of the objective facts of inner and outer life (including thoughts, emotions, sensations, actions, and surroundings) as they are, and not as distorted by conceptual filters, aroused emotions, or habitual ways of seeing. Prolonged involvement in this mode is considered to contribute to the capacity for intentional regulation of states of sustained attention and awareness from narrow focus to broad overview, without confusion or loss of contact with present moment experience (Brown et al., 2007). Eventually, the experience of the separation of the field of awareness from the contents of thought and feeling is postulated to lead to a fundamental shift in perspective (Shapiro, Carlson, Astin, & Freeman, 2006) that gives rise to the meta-awareness of the "integrated I" as the agent of action who is actively engaged with, has direct contact with, and ownership of experience while also being immersed in it (Brown et al., 2007). Greater levels of expertise and practice allow this meta-awareness to be transcended, leading to the realization that the "integrated I" is an illusory experience, created by a series of temporary states of awareness (Ekman et al., 2005).

Mindfulness and the Processes of Stress and Coping

The central question of this chapter is how mindfulness, thus conceived, could influence the processes of stress and coping for teachers. Reviews of the benefits of mindfulness consistently posit that mindfulness reduces distress and its physical and psychological costs (e.g., Greeson, 2009). In fact, one of the earliest programs to promote mindfulness, Mindfulness-based Stress Reduction (MBSR; Kabat-Zinn, 1990), is named for this desired effect, and subjective experiences of distress are one of the most common targets of both naturalistic and intervention studies. Many of the beneficial consequences of mindfulness are hypothesized to accrue through improved coping (Garland, 2007). In fact, an overarching goal of mindfulness interventions is to help people "cope" more effectively with a broad range of clinical and nonclinical problems (Anderson, Lau, Segal, & Bishop, 2007; Grossman, Niemann, Schmidt, & Walach, 2004; Klatt, Buckworth, & Malarkey, 2009, p. 609).

Theoreticians, researchers, and practitioners are all struggling with the same questions: Does mindfulness reduce distress, improve coping, and ameliorate the deleterious consequences of stress? And if so, *how* does it accomplish this? Some specific mechanisms have been hypothesized and documented (Brown et al., 2007; Chambers et al., 2009; Hölzel et al., 2011; Shapiro et al., 2006; Williams, 2010). As summarized by Greeson (2009),

> It has specifically been postulated that mindfulness may preempt stress-related illness through a number of psychological, biological, and behavioral pathways, including (a) clarifying primary appraisal of stressors, (b) facilitating accurate secondary appraisal of stressor demands and coping resources, (c) mitigating dysfunctional coping styles, such as catastrophizing and ruminating, (d) enhancing adaptive coping processes, such as positive reappraisal, and (e) reducing distress and psychophysiological activation (Garland, 2007). (pp. 13–14)

Building on this work in the following sections, we explore a variety of mechanisms explaining how mindfulness might shape appraisals of stress and coping in nonclinical populations, using the developmental model to identify multiple entry points into the process.

The overarching framework posits that mindfulness facilitates changes in teachers' stance toward teaching, converting it from one focused on chronic stress, coping, and self-protection, to one organized around broaden-and-build goals of long-term professional development (Roeser et al., 2012). From this perspective, mindfulness promotes resilience and effectiveness in the classroom by allowing teachers (a) to conserve and recoup personal resources, by reducing stress, emotional reactivity, and distressing appraisals of self and others, including students; and (2) to intentionally nurture personal resources, such as skills and dispositions involved in effective classroom teaching and healthy relationships with students and colleagues. Mindfulness training as a novel form of professional development is hypothesized to assist teachers in conserving and cultivating self-regulatory resources that are then available for investment in classroom relationships, classroom management, and classroom instruction (Roeser et al., 2012). The specific mechanisms are summarized in Table 7.3.

Appraisals of Stressful Demands

An important way in which mindfulness supports teacher coping is by encouraging teachers to rework their appraisals of stressful incidents in the classroom (Chambers et al., 2009; Garland, 2007), especially interactions involving students' disaffected and disruptive behaviors (Spilt, Koomen, & Thijs, 2011). Teachers experience more emotional reactivity when they view student misbehavior as important (self-relevant), goal incongruent, and uncontrollable (Spilt, Koomen, Thijs, & van der Leij, 2012). Mindfulness encourages teachers to rethink these habitual appraisals. For example, it is possible for teachers to see student misbehaviors as goal-congruent, that is, as providing useful information about students' underlying psychological or motivational states (Tsouloupas et al., 2010). Likewise, mindfulness, with its focus on self-compassion and compassion for others, also encourages teachers to rework their habitual patterns of blame (self-blame or blaming students) when things go wrong in the classroom. Instead, teachers can come to view "failures" as essential steps in a larger arc of learning and progress (Furrer, Skinner, & Pitzer, 2014).

Moreover, the receptive orientation which is part of mindfulness should help teachers feel more sanguine about maintaining contact with the genuinely painful aspects of the current situation (sometimes referred to as exposure; Shapiro et al., 2006). Such sensations might be more likely to be viewed as informative and, based on an improved capacity to release attention from distressing events (Ortner, Kilner, & Zelazo, 2007; Slagter et al., 2007), also as temporary. Perhaps most importantly, mindfulness has the potential to help teachers recognize their appraisals for what they actually are: not reality, but "mental commentary" on reality. This can help teachers see that part of

Table 7.3 Possible ways in which mindfulness could influence coping

Potential to reduce maladaptive processes	Potential to promote adaptive processes
1. Reactivity and appraisals of stressful events.	
Reduces evaluations of what is at stake for the self. Reduces evaluations of events as "good" or "bad". Reduces cognitive distortions. Reduces catastrophizing. Reduces sense of threat and coercion. Reduces distress.	Promotes awareness of appraisal as a mental construction, and not reality. Promotes curiosity, openness, and interest about the actual nature of events, including uncertainty about how they will unfold. Promotes comfort with experiences of distress. Maintains awareness of the appraisal's and the event's temporary nature.
2. Action tendencies in the face of threat appraisals.	
Reduces reactivity to apparent reality created by threat appraisals. Reduces impulsivity. Reduces experiential avoidance.	Appreciates the information value of a feeling of threat. Maintains awareness of the temporary nature of urges to react. Creates a readiness to engage authentically and constructively with the stressor.
3. Action regulation in the face of strong action tendencies.	
Reduces tendency to automatically follow impulses. Reduces tendency to automatically suppress impulses. Reduces disorganized, rigid, or punitive regulation.	Creates a "gap" for regulation. Creates space for information from all subsystems to register. Maintains access to deepest and most genuine values. Promotes regulation that is organized, flexible, and benevolent. Allows self to choose or spontaneously act out of integrated autonomous awareness.
4. During coping interactions.	
Reduces disengagement or disaffection from genuinely experiencing the stressor and everything surrounding it. Reduces misguided or ignorant actions	Promotes "right action," all things considered. Allows full engagement with the actual stressful events and the social partners that are part of them. Promotes composure while acting and while not acting Allows full access to all capacities. Allows experience of all genuine emotions. Allows full range of actions. Allows flexible adjustment of actions to changing conditions.
5. Post-coping assessment of stressful episodes.	
Reduces evaluation of coping interactions as good or bad, "success" or "failure" Reduces inclination to avoid thinking about stressful events Reduces inclination to brood about stressful events	Allows sorrow for losses and suffering. Allows clear reflection on actual coping interactions. Promotes compassionate understanding of all participants. Allows acknowledgement of weakness and mistakes. Promotes gratitude for the right actions of others. Promotes focus on future "right action" and service.
6. Learning, growth, and development following coping.	
Reduces blame of self and others. Reduces anger and bitterness. Reduces sense of futility and helplessness.	Promotes openness to change. Allows learning to be fully incorporated. Promotes gratitude for the opportunity to learn. Allows new knowledge to be applied and practiced. Promotes sense of purpose and direction. Promotes curiosity about what else could be learned.

the destructive power of appraisals is based on their self-focus, which tends to exaggerate concern for the self, as captured by questions like, "What is at stake here for me? What do I stand to lose?" Distress may be reduced if appraisals can be seen as temporary open-ended mental models that will need to be updated and revised, and if the focus of appraisals can shift to a set of more inquisitive nonevaluative open-ended questions, such as "What is going on here? Where is this feeling of threat coming from?" Together, these mindful processes might make it more likely for stressful events to be appraised as challenges, rather than threats, and thus reduce the sense of panic, pressure, fear, and coercion that accompany the experience of threat, and promote a sense of ease, equanimity, and curiosity about current events as they unfold.

Stress Reactivity or Action Tendencies in the Face of Threat One of the primary goals of mindfulness is to lower reactivity, or automatic habitual patterns of thought and action (Brown et al., 2007; Chambers et al., 2009). Mindfulness practices (such as meditation, deep breathing, focusing on the current moment, and intentional relaxation) are designed to reduce distress under demanding circumstances by downregulating neurophysiological stress reactivity systems (i.e., the sympathetic nervous system and hypothalamic–pituitary–adrenal axis) at the same time that they boost safety signals and the relaxation response (via the parasympathetic nervous system) (Greeson, 2009; Hofmann et al., 2010; Hölzel et al., 2011).

In the face of threat, mindfulness seems to help desensitize individuals so they can tolerate the experience of fear and discomfort without the need to shut it down through escape or striking out. It also allows people to explore these sensations and become more aware of their temporary nature. Most importantly, mindfulness seems to shift this phase of the coping process from one of reactivity to one guided by habitual action tendencies that are characterized by a willingness to face and accept threatening thoughts and emotions, and thereby create a readiness to engage authentically, fully, and constructively with stressful events, whatever they may turn out to be (Hölzel et al., 2011).

Action Regulation in the Face of Strong Action Tendencies

Mindfulness is thought to foster more adaptive regulation through several channels (Baer, 2003; Chambers et al., 2009; Shapiro et al., 2006). First, by helping people distinguish the field of awareness from the contents of experience (a process called "defusion," "decoupling," or "disidentification"), mindfulness inserts a "mental gap" between the stimulus and response relations of automatic behavior, and so creates a space for intentional regulation of action. This "increases the range and adaptability of responses to challenges, or *cognitive flexibility*, allowing challenges to be addressed consciously rather than merely reacted to" (Chambers et al., 2009, p. 562). As a result, mindfulness should decrease underregulation of impulses because it promotes the ability to interrupt or override undesired behavioral tendencies. At the same time, because it decreases aversion to "negative" emotions, it should also reduce overregulation or the tendency to rigidly suppress responses that are considered unacceptable (Feldman, Hayes, Kumar, Greeson, & Laurenceau, 2007; Ostafin & Marlatt, 2008).

In fact, the practice of mindfulness, by repeatedly exercising attentional control, is thought to enhance executive functioning and monitoring (Tang & Posner, 2009), which is central to action regulation more generally, but would be especially important under stressful conditions when executive capacities are taxed (e.g., Blair & Diamond, 2008). Moreover, because mindfulness reduces preoccupation with self-relevant thoughts, anxiety, and future worry (see Hölzel et al., 2011), executive capacity would not be diverted to these concerns, and as a result, mindful regulation should require less energy, thus preventing the depletion of self-regulatory energy resources and freeing up more resources for constructive engagement with the stressor (Leary, Adams, & Tate, 2006; Masicampo & Baumeister, 2007; Ortner et al., 2007).

Coping Interactions

Most important to adaptive coping are the capacities mindfulness brings to individuals during coping interactions themselves, that is, as people actively deal with stressors from moment to moment. A goal of mindfulness is to provide the individual with ongoing access to the full range of accurate information about current internal and external realities as they unfold, as well as "unhindered access to all of one's relevant knowledge (e.g., intellectual, emotional, and physical/intuitive) to aid in negotiating life situations" (Brown et al., 2007, p. 213). To be effective, coping actions have to be exquisitely tuned to the full range of factors that shape how stressful interactions will be resolved, including external contingencies, individuals' capacities, contextual conditions, and other resources available (Williams, 2010). In addition, coping actions have to be continuously recalibrated with each iteration of the ongoing interaction. As explained by Garland (2007), "Mindfulness may be conceptualized as a self-regulatory feedback mechanism through which the individual's cognitive processing is informed by undistorted perceptions, thereby calibrating behavior to function adaptively to present conditions" (p. 21).

Above all, mindfulness may aid in the search for "right action" during the process of coping. As explained by Brown and Ryan (2003), "a person acting in an integrated mindful way seeks not self-esteem, but rather, right action, all things considered" (p. 75). When important outcomes are at stake, the pressures and confusion of stress make "right action" more important, but at the same time harder to find. Mindfulness may allow people to be "more capable of acting in ways that are more choiceful and more openly attentive to and aware of themselves and the situations in which they find themselves 'all things considered'" (Brown et al., 2007, p. 227). A key contribution of mindfulness may be to provide an opportunity, in the midst of chaos and fear, for "all things" to be considered.

An important part of the "all things" that mindful coping allows people to experience is the myriad beautiful and tender events that are taking place all the time, even in the midst of genuine suffering and sorrow. The capacity to remain aware of them, and to experience them clearly and vividly, seems to be an important protective factor in dealing with stress (Folkman, 2008; Folkman & Moskowitz, 2000), perhaps in part because of the respite positive emotions such as love, gratitude, and joy offer to both the physiological and psychological systems (Fredrickson, Cohn, Coffey, Pek, & Finkel, 2008).

Ways of Coping

A theme running through discussions of mindfulness is that it should help reduce reliance on harmful coping strategies (Feldman et al., 2007; Garland, 2007; Jacob & Blustein, 2008). For example, through the development of increased tolerance of discomfort, mindfulness should diminish "experiential avoidance," as expressed through ways of coping, such as denial, thought suppression, or escape, that are used to avoid (real or anticipated) experiences of pain (Hayes et al., 2004). By promoting an attitude of acceptance, mindfulness is also thought to reduce rumination, which seems to result from an inability to disengage from desired but unobtainable goals (Coffey & Hartman, 2008; Feldman et al., 2007; Shapiro, Oman, Thoresen, Plante, & Flinders, 2008).

In general, mindfulness should reduce ways of regulating actions that are rigid, disorganized, and derogatory, such as the maladaptive ways of coping described previously, namely, escape, helplessness, social isolation, delegation, opposition, and submission. At the same time, mindfulness should promote ways of regulating actions that are flexible, organized, and constructive, such as the adaptive ways of coping described previously, like problem-solving, information seeking, comfort seeking, self-reliance, negotiation, and accommodation (Feldman et al., 2007; Walach et al., 2007). Research on the effects of mindfulness training provide some evidence that such training can indeed shift teachers' reliance on different families of coping with stressors at work (Roeser et al., 2013; Taylor et al., 2014).

Although it should promote adaptive ways of coping, mindful coping does not imply that individuals are more likely to use one or the other of these specific strategies in a particular situation. Based on general descriptions of mindfulness, it is easy to assume that, when acting mindfully, individuals are more likely to use positive reappraisal (Garland, 2007), to accommodate to (rather than attempt to change) negative events, to remain passive (rather than "fight back"), or to fully engage all of life's harsh realities all of the time (rather than to withdraw). However, this is likely not the case. Positive reappraisal often implies "a process of cognitively reevaluating certain situations in such a way as to negate the generation of potentially distressing emotions" (Chambers et al., 2009, p. 566), which is fundamentally different from mindful emotion regulation which is focused on learning to accept "all emotional experience, regardless of its apparent valence, intensity, or perceived utility" (Chambers et al., 2009, p. 556). Mindful appraisals imply accuracy—which may involve a positive reappraisal if one has been previously catastrophizing, or it may involve a more "negative" reappraisal if one has been previously avoiding painful realizations through denial (Hölzel et al., 2011).

By the same token, mindfulness does not imply coping through passivity or accommodation to the current state of affairs. Acceptance refers to an attitude brought to awareness, but seeing things as they are does not mean leaving things as they are. Mindfulness contributes to a "full engagement" mode of coping (Feldman et al., 2007). As explained by Brown et al. (2007), mindfulness "is not a form of escape that results in passivity or disconnection from life; rather it is thought to bring one into closer contact with life by helping to circumvent the self-generated accounts *about* life that act to pull one away from it" (p. 227). At the same time, Brown et al. (2007) point out that the compassion inherent in mindful coping can also allow people to intentionally take a break from stressful interactions when they state, "A mindfully chosen turning away from what appears to be overwhelming facts may foster more peace of mind and greater success in later opening up to, and thereby integrating those facts, than a defensive flight that is driven by fear and despair" (p. 230).

Post-Coping Assessment and Learning

Mindful awareness would seem to offer several advantages when reviewing stressful episodes after they are resolved. First, the clarity, accuracy, and fullness of mindful processing would give the individual the most complete account of what actually took place, which is the best springboard for analysis and learning. Especially important are opportunities to learn from one's own mistakes and maladaptive ways of coping, which are usually either edited out or fixated upon in retrospective descriptions of stressful episodes.

Second, the friendly and receptive attitude inherent in mindfulness would be likely to move an assessment away from evaluating the episode as a "success" or "failure," or labeling the participants as "winners" or "losers." This should allow the assessment to proceed without the distractions of self- or other-blame, second-guessing, and rumination that often follow stressful interactions (Roeser & Pinela, 2014). This might also minimize the secondary fall-out from stressful events, in which the participants often argue and blame each other for the ways in which they coped with them. By curtailing preoccupation and friction, resources are freed up for reflection and learning (Masicampo & Baumeister, 2007; Slagter et al., 2007).

Third, mindfulness might hasten restoration and recovery from stressful interactions. A present-centered orientation reminds people that the stressful episode is over and helps them stop bringing the past trauma with them into present experiences. Mindfulness also seems to produce a variety of physiological effects that aid in recovery, including downregulation of the stress reactivity systems and upregulation of the rest and recovery systems (Greeson, 2009; Hofmann et al., 2010; Hölzel et al., 2011). These effects are likely accomplished through both physiological (e.g., deep breathing, relaxation, lowered heart rate) and psychological (e.g., direct relief from stress, contact with positive experiences) means of restoring or creating energetic resources (Kabat-Zinn, 2003).

Fourth, in the face of actual losses, the loosening of attachments that is central to mindfulness may "enhance efforts to reflectively process the accompanying challenges to individuals' previous understandings of themselves and the world, permit an easier disengagement from previous goals that are no longer adaptive, and facilitate the process of developing new life goals and meaning based on present life realities" (Brown et al., 2007, p. 230). Taken together, the qualities of these assessment processes should allow the individual to completely "let go" of the stressful interaction. However it was resolved in the short-term, the episode can then be left behind psychologically and physically, and what is carried forward into the present moment is gratitude for its service in the important purpose of helping one learn how to deal with adversity (Benn, Akiva, Arel, & Roeser, 2012; Jennings, Frank, Snowberg, Coccia, & Greenberg, 2013; Winzelberg & Luskin, 1999).

Development of "Wise" Coping

A consideration of coping from a mindfulness perspective opens up interesting (and as yet unanswered) questions about whether one of the lifelong lessons of mindful coping involves learning more about how to engage in ethical action under increasingly stressful circumstances (see Roeser et al., 2014 for hypotheses on mindfulness training and ethical behavior). Such a goal focuses individuals on a clear-eyed and compassionate assessment of the thoughts and conditions that pull people toward and away from ethical action. It may also facilitate gratitude for the ethical actions of others and help generate next steps to be taken to allow oneself to engage in such actions in future stressful encounters.

What is "right action" under stress? A focus on coping as an adaptive process can easily lead to the criteria of "effectiveness," that is, efficacy at producing a desired or preventing an undesired outcome. At a deeper level, however, it is clear that determining what is ethical is always more difficult than just deploying the most effective means at one's disposal. Such actions may hurt others, disturb relationships, consume too many resources, interfere with prior commitments, or jeopardize other more important goals. Ethical coping involves a wise moral judgment that requires perspective and insight into one's deepest most genuine principles, values, and intentions, as well as the courage and strength to act on them.

Mindful Coping and Everyday Resilience in the Classroom

If interventions or training programs for teachers can promote the kinds of mindful responses to stress and coping just described, they have the potential to transform teachers' experiences of dealing with unexpected and challenging events so that descriptors such as "stressor," "appraisal," and "coping" may no longer seem as applicable. Perhaps the most fundamental change would be teachers' appraisals of the stressfulness of their classroom experiences. If the disciplinary, motivational, and learning issues that students present are no longer viewed as problems, but instead are seen as informative feedback that provide opportunities for teachers to learn more about their own teaching, management, and motivational practices, then teachers' appraisals of them as distressing should decrease (Roeser et al., 2012).

Studies examining the effects of mindfulness training for teachers find evidence for the operation of many of the processes depicted in this chapter, in that such training reduces teachers' exhaustion, discouragement, disaffection, and other symptoms of occupational burnout, and increases their well-being and satisfaction with teaching (Benn et al., 2012; Kemeny et al., 2011; Roeser et al., 2013; Taylor et al., 2014). It is also possible that teachers' mindful coping in the classroom might make a noticeable difference to students, by shaping the quality of instruction teachers provide, their classroom management, the interpersonal climate in the classroom, and the nature of teacher–student relationships (Roeser et al., 2012). The key idea is that, since coping is an action, students would experience teachers' mindful coping in their daily interactions with teachers. In this last section, we suggest a few ways that mindful coping could change the typical experiences of students.

Less Stress Reactivity

One significant change that students would likely notice is that their teachers are not as stressed out. Teachers would appear less nervous, irritable, or easily set off by student behavior. Teachers would not fly off the handle, or take it personally if a student is distracted from a lesson or conversing with their neighbor. Therefore, teachers' responses to infractions would be experienced as measured and in proportion to the situation, even under potentially threatening conditions. At the same time, however, students would likely experience teachers as on top of things: Teachers would not be as liable to miss things, to let things slide, or to be intimidated by student (mis)behaviors. As a result, students might also see their teachers as setting high expectations for them and not letting them get away with anything. Such a combination could lead students to see teachers as challenging but fair.

Full Engagement Coping

During stressful encounters with mindful teachers, students should experience them as fully focused and present in interactions, instead of pulling up past business or threatening dire future consequences. Because teachers would be interacting with them based on the facts on the ground, and not operating on reputations or stereotypes, students would be apt to feel that teachers are fair, and not arbitrary or picky. At the same time, teachers would not be easy to hoodwink because they would be tracking what is actually happening, and not relying on any self-serving version of events that students might be tempted to provide. Even during arguments, teachers would likely appear as responsive listeners because they would actually be open-minded, asking students for their perspectives, accepting students' emotions, and tuning their reactions to what students are actually saying and intending with their actions.

Speedier Recovery

Mindful coping on the part of teachers could also result in less time spent on behavioral or motivational management. Teachers should be able to more quickly and accurately discriminate snags and problems that need attention from those that do not. Teachers' concentrated attention should produce fair and constructive solutions, which in turn would be hypothesized to result in less pushback from students, as well as less lingering friction once problems are solved. When teachers can bounce back from even distressing interactions, letting them go, so can students, and more of everyone's time and mental energy would be freed up for learning.

More Supportive Classroom Climate

In general then, through mindful coping, teachers should be able to contribute to a more positive classroom climate. Teachers would not only be more calm and centered, but they would also be more likely to experience and express the full range of positive emotions toward their students, including affection, gratitude, and happiness. They would also be prone to experience and express more positive emotions toward teaching itself, through their interest, curiosity, and enthusiasm. Hence, students might experience teachers as enjoying teaching and having more fun in the classroom, which is likely to make the classroom a more lively place where learning is more fun.

Less Stressful Behavior from Students

As a result of all of these potentially beneficial effects of mindfulness on teachers, students themselves might actually improve as interaction partners for teachers. Students would get used to being straight with teachers, listening to them, and owning their own mistakes because teachers would be doing the same. Students would be more communicative because teachers are listening carefully. Teachers' investment, commitment, and full engagement in the classroom would be likely to elicit fuller engagement from students as well. By the same token, the fact that teachers aren't letting students get away with anything should also discourage students from trying to do so. The climate created by teachers' openness, kind curiosity, and acceptance may eventually convince even "problem" students that they are not "problems," but partners in learning and achievement.

Higher Quality of Instruction, Engagement, and Learning

Taken together, these teacher and student actions should result in higher quality teaching and learning in the classroom. Both teachers and students would have better access to their cognitive capacities because less working memory capacity would be occupied by self-concerns, worries, frustrations, or rumination about negative events. More time and energy in the classroom would be spent on academic instruction, and student "problems" with academic material would become opportunities for focused discussion and learning. Overall, both teachers and students would be more fully engaged in the hard work of teaching and learning, in ways that create synergistically positive effects.

Conclusion

Teaching can be a stressful profession. But, it can also be a source of joyous, rewarding, and satisfying experiences—ones that remind teachers everyday why they went into teaching in the first place. If, by bringing mindfulness into their daily lives, teachers can realize some of the changes described in this chapter, then interventions to promote mindfulness may help to reduce the wear and tear, burnout, and physical and mental health problems so prevalent among teachers today. In fact, mindfulness holds the promise of transforming stressful experiences into opportunities for teachers to learn and grow, thus promoting the development of robust personal resources for everyday resilience. These benefits, if they are realized by teachers in the classroom, may also transform the daily experiences of their students, allowing them to experience the kind of warm and supportive instructional and motivational climate that nurtures their own engagement, achievement, and healthy development.

References

Aldwin, C. M. (2007). *Stress, coping, and development: An integrative perspective* (2nd ed.). New York, NY: Guilford Press.

Anderson, N. D., Lau, M. A., Segal, Z. V., & Bishop, S. R. (2007). Mindfulness-based stress reduction and attentional control. *Clinical Psychology and Psychotherapy, 14*, 449–463.

Aspinwall, L. G., & Taylor, S. E. (1997). A stitch in time: Self-regulation and proactive coping. *Psychological Bulletin, 121*, 417–436.

Baer, R. A. (2003). Mindfulness training as a clinical intervention: A conceptual and empirical review. *Clinical Psychology: Science and Practice, 10*(2), 125–143.

Barrett, K. C., & Campos, J. J. (1991). A diacritical function approach to emotions and coping. In E. M. Cummings, A. L. Greene, & K. H. Karraker (Eds.), *Life-span developmental psychology: Perspectives on stress and coping* (pp. 21–41). Hillsdale, NJ: Erlbaum.

Bauer, J., Stamm, A., Virnich, K., Wissing, K., Muller, U., Wirsching, M., & Schaarschmidt, U. (2005). Correlation between burnout syndrome and psychological and psychosomatic symptoms among teachers. *International Archives of Occupational and Environmental Health, 79*, 199–204.

Baumeister, R. F., Bratslavsky, E., Muraven, M., & Tice, D. M. (1998). Ego depletion: Is the active self a limited resource? *Journal of Personality and Social Psychology, 74*, 1252–1265.

Baumeister, R. F., Heatherton, T. F., & Tice, D. M. (1994). *Losing control: How and why people fail at self-regulation*. San Diego, CA: Academic Press.

Benn, R., Akiva, T., Arel, S., & Roeser, R. W. (2012). Mindfulness training effects for parents and educators of children with special needs. *Developmental Psychology, 48*(5), 1476–1487.

Berg, C., Meegan, S., & Deviney, F. (1998). A social-contextual model of coping with everyday problems across the life span. *International Journal of Behavioural Development, 22*, 239–261.

Bishop, S. R., Lau, M., Shapiro, S., Carlson, L., Anderson, N., Carmody, J., … Devins, G. (2004). Mindfulness: A proposed operational definition. *Clinical Psychology: Science and Practice, 11*, 230–241.

Blair, C., & Diamond, A. (2008). Biological processes in prevention and intervention: The promotion of selfregulation as a means of preventing school failure. *Development and Psychopathology, 20*(03), 899–911.

Blase, J. J. (1986). A qualitative analysis of sources of teacher stress: Consequences for performance. *American Educational Research Journal, 23*, 13–40.

Boekaerts, M. (2002). Coping with challenge. *Anxiety, Stress and Coping, 15*, 321–326.

Borg, M. G. (1990). Occupational stress in British educational settings: A review. *Educational Psychology, 10*, 103–126.

Brandtstädter, J. (2006). Action perspectives on human development. In R. M. Lerner (Ed.), *Handbook of child psychology* (6th ed.), Vol. 1: *Theoretical models of human development.* (pp. 516-568). W. Damon & R. M. Lerner ((Eds.-in-Chief). Hoboken, NJ: Wiley.

Briner, R., & Dewberry, C. (2007). *Staff well-being is key to school success*. London, England: Worklife Support/Hamilton House.

Brown, K. W., & Ryan, R. M. (2003). The benefits of being present: Mindfulness and its role in psychological well-being. *Journal of Personality and Social Psychology, 84*, 822–848.

Brown, K. W., Ryan, R. M., & Creswell, J. D. (2007). Mindfulness: Theoretical foundations and evidence for its salutary effects. *Psychological Inquiry, 18*, 211–237.

Campos, J. J., Frankel, C. B., & Camras, L. (2004). On the nature of emotion regulation. *Child Development, 75*, 377–394.

Carmody, J., & Baer, R. A. (2008). Relationships between mindfulness practice and levels of mindfulness, medical and psychological symptoms and well-being in a mindfulness-based stress reduction program. *Journal of Behavioral Medicine, 31*, 23–33.

Case, R., & Griffin, S. (1990). Child cognitive development: The role of central conceptual structures in the development of scientific and social thought. *Advances in Psychology, 64*, 193–230.

Chambers, R., Gullone, E., & Allen, N. B. (2009). Mindful emotion regulation. An integrative review. *Clinical Psychology Review, 29*, 560–572.

Chan, D. W. (1998). Stress coping strategies, and psychological distress among secondary school teachers in Hong Kong. *American Educational Research Journal, 35*, 145–163.
Chang, M.-L. (2009). An appraisal perspective of teacher burnout: Examining the emotional work of teachers. *Educational Psychology Review, 21*, 193–218.
Coelho, H. F., Canter, P. H., & Ernst, E. (2007). Mindfulness-based cognitive therapy: Evaluating current evidence and informing future research. *Journal of Consulting and Clinical Psychology, 75*, 1000–1005.
Coffey, K. A., & Hartman, M. (2008). Mechanisms of action in the inverse relationship between mindfulness and psychological distress. *Complementary Health Practice Review, 13*(2), 79–91.
Cole, P. M., Michel, M. K., & Teti, L. O. (1994). The development of emotion regulation and dysregulation: A clinical view. In N. A. Fox (Ed.), *Monographs of the society for research in child development* (Vol. 59, pp. 73–100).
Compas, B. E. (1993, April). *An analysis of "good" stress and coping in adolescence*. Paper presented at the 60th meeting of the Society for Research in Child Development, New Orleans.
Compas, B. E. (2006). Psychobiological processes of stress and coping: Implications for resilience in children and adolescents. *Annals of the New York Academy of Sciences, 1094*, 226–234.
Compas, B. E. (2009). Coping, regulation, and development during childhood and adolescence. In E. A. Skinner & M. J. Zimmer-Gembeck (Eds.). *Coping and the development of regulation. A volume for the series*, R. W. Larson & L. A. Jensen (Eds.-in-Chief), *New directions in child and adolescent development*, San Francisco, CA: Jossey-Bass.
Compas, B. E., Connor, J. K., Saltzman, H., Thomsen, A. H., & Wadsworth, M. (1999). Getting specific about coping: Effortful and involuntary responses to stress in development. In M. Lewis & D. Ramsey (Eds.), *Soothing and stress* (pp. 229–256). New York, NY: Cambridge University Press.
Diamond, L. M., & Aspinwall, L. G. (2003). Emotion regulation across the life span: An integrative perspective emphasizing self-regulation, positive affect, and dyadic processes. *Motivation and Emotion, 27*, 125–156.
Eisenberg, N., Fabes, R. A., & Guthrie, I. K. (1997). Coping with stress: The roles of regulation and development. In S. A. Wolchik & I. N. Sandler (Eds.), *Handbook of children's coping: Linking theory and intervention* (pp. 41–70). New York, NY: Plenum Press.
Ekman, P., Davidson, R. J., Ricard, M., & Wallace, B. A. (2005). Buddhist and psychological perspectives on emotions and well-being. *Current Directions in Psychological Science, 14*(2), 59–63.
Evers, W. J. G., Tomic, W., & Brouwers, A. (2004). Burnout among teachers. *School Psychology International, 25*(2), 131–148.
Feldman, G., Hayes, A., Kumar, S., Greeson, J., & Laurenceau, J. P. (2007). Mindfulness and emotion regulation: The development and initial validation of the Cognitive and Affective Mindfulness Scale-Revised (CAMS-R). *Journal of Psychopathology and Behavioral Assessment, 29*(3), 177–190.
Folkman, S. (1984). Personal control and stress and coping processes: A theoretical analysis. *Journal of Personality and Social Psychology, 46*(4), 839–852.
Folkman, S. (2008). The case for positive emotions in the stress process. *Anxiety, Stress, and Coping: An International Journal, 21*(1), 3–14.
Folkman, S., & Lazarus, R. S. (1985). If it changes it must be a process: Study of emotion and coping during three stages of a college examination. *Journal of Personality and Social Psychology, 48*, 150–170.
Folkman, S., & Moskowitz, J. T. (2000). Positive affect and the other side of coping. *American Psychologist, 55*, 647–654.
Fredrickson, B. L., Cohn, M. A., Coffey, K. A., Pek, J., & Finkel, S. M. (2008). Open hearts build lives: Positive emotions, induced through loving-kindness meditation, build consequential personal resources. *Journal of Personality and Social Psychology, 95*(5), 1045.
Friedman, I. A. (1995). Student behavior patterns contributing to teacher burnout. *Journal of Educational Research, 88*(5), 281–289.
Furrer, C. J., Skinner, E. A., & Pitzer, J. R. (2014). The influence of teacher and peer relationships on students' classroom engagement and everyday resilience. In D. J. Shernoff & J. Bempechat (Eds.), *National society for the study of education yearbook. Engaging youth in schools: Empirically-based models to guide future innovations* (Vol. 113, pp. 101–123). New York, NY: Teachers's College, Columbia University.
Garland, E. L. (2007). The meaning of mindfulness: A second-order cybernetics of stress, meta-cognition, and coping. *Complementary Health Practice Review, 12*(1), 15–30.
Green, S. B., & Ross, M. E. (1996). A theory-based measure of coping strategies used by teachers: The problems in teaching scale. *Teaching & Teacher Education, 12*, 315–325.
Greeson, J. M. (2009). Mindfulness research update: 2008. *Complementary Health Practice Review, 14*, 10–18.
Griffith, J., Steptoe, A., & Cropley, M. (1999). An investigation of coping strategies associated with job stress in teachers. *British Journal of Educational Psychology, 69*, 517–531.
Griva, K., & Joekes, K. (2003). UK teachers under stress: Can we predict wellness on the basis of characteristics of the teaching job? *Psychology and Health, 18*, 457–471.
Grossman, P., Niemann, L., Schmidt, S., & Walach, H. (2004). Mindfulness-based stress reduction and health benefits: A meta-analysis. *Journal of Psychosomatic Research, 57*, 35–43.
Hargreaves, A. (2000). Mixed emotions: Teachers' perceptions of their interactions with students. *Teaching and Teacher Education, 16*, 811–826.
Hofmann, S. G., Sawyer, A. T., Witt, A. A., & Oh, D. (2010). The effect of mindfulness-based therapy on anxiety and depression: A meta-analytic review. *Journal of Consulting and Clinical Psychology, 78*(2), 169.
Hölzel, B. K., Lazar, S. W., Gard, T., Schuman-Olivier, Z., Vago, D. R., & Ott, U. (2011). How does mindfulness

meditation work? Proposing mechanisms of action from a conceptual and neural perspective. *Perspectives on Psychological Science, 6*(6), 537–559.
Howard, S., & Johnson, B. (2004). Resilient teachers: Resisting stress and burnout. *Social Psychology of Education, 7*, 399–420.
Innes, J. M., & Kitto, S. (1989). Neuroticism, self-consciousness and coping strategies, and occupational stress in high school teachers. *Personal and Individual Differences, 10*, 303–312.
Jacobs, S. J., & Blustein, D. L. (2008). Mindfulness as a coping mechanism for employment uncertainty. *The Career Development Quarterly, 57*(2), 174–180.
Jalongo, M. R., & Heider, K. (2006). Editorial teacher attrition: An issue of national concern. *Early Childhood Education Journal, 33*, 379–380.
Jennings, P. A., Frank, J. L., Snowberg, K. E., Coccia, M. A., & Greenberg, M. T. (2013). Improving classroom learning environments by Cultivating Awareness and Resilience in Education (CARE): Results of a randomized controlled trial. *School Psychology Quarterly, 28*, 374–390.
Jennings, P. A., & Greenberg, M. (2009). The prosocial classroom: Teacher social and emotional competence in relation to child and classroom outcomes. *Review of Educational Research, 79*, 491–525.
Johnson, S., Cooper, C., Cartwright, S., Donald, I., Taylor, P., & Millet, C. (2005). The experience of work-related stress across occupations. *Journal of Managerial Psychology, 20*, 178–187.
Kabat-Zinn, J. (1990). *Full catastrophe living: Using the wisdom of your body and mind to face stress, pain, and illness*. New York, NY: Bantam Doubleday Dell.
Kabat-Zinn, J. (2003). Mindfulness-based interventions in context: Past, present, and future. *Clinical psychology: Science and practice, 10*(2), 144–156.
Kemeny, M. E., Foltz, C., Cavanagh, J. F., Cullen, M., Giese-Davis, J., Jennings, P., ... Ekman, P. (2012). Contemplative/emotion training reduces negative emotional behavior and promotes prosocial responses. *Emotion, 12*(2), 338–350.
Klassen, R. M., Perry, N. E., & Frenzel, A. C. (2012). Teachers' relatedness with students: An underemphasized component of teachers' basic psychological needs. *Journal of Educational Psychology, 104*, 150–165.
Klatt, M. D., Buckworth, J., & Malarkey, W. B. (2009). Effects of low-dose mindfulness-based stress reduction (MBSR-ld) on working adults. *Health Education & Behavior, 36*, 601–614.
Klusmann, U., Kunter, M., Trautwein, U., Luktke, O., & Baumert, J. (2008). Teachers' occupational well-being and the quality of instruction: The important role of self-regulatory patterns. *Journal of Educational Psychology, 100*, 702–715.
Kyriacou, C. (1987). Teacher stress and burnout: An international review. *Educational Research, 29*, 146–152.
Kyriacou, C. (2001). Teacher stress: Directions for future research. *Educational Review, 53*, 27–35.
Lambert, R. G., & McCarthy, C. J. (Eds.). (2006). *Understanding teacher stress in an era of accountability* (Vol. III). Greenwich, CT: Information Age.
Lazarus, R. S., & Folkman, S. (1984). *Stress, appraisal, and coping*. New York, NY: Springer.
Leary, M. R., Adams, C. E., & Tate, E. B. (2006). Hypo-egoic self-regulation: Exercising self-control by diminishing the influence of the self. *Journal of Personality, 74*, 1803–1831.
Litt, M. D., & Turk, D. C. (1985). Sources of stress and dissatisfaction in experienced high school teachers. *The Journal of Educational Research, 78*, 178–185.
Masicampo, E. J., & Baumeister, R. F. (2007). Relating mindfulness and self-regulatory processes. *Psychological Inquiry, 18*(4), 255–258.
Maslach, C., Schaufeli, W. B., & Leiter, M. P. (2001). Job burnout. *Annual Review of Psychology, 52*(1), 397–422.
McCurry, S. M., Hayes, S. C., Strosahl, K., Wilson, K. G., Bissett, R. T., Pistorello, J., ... Stewart, S. H. (2004). Measuring experiential avoidance: A preliminary test of a working model. *The Psychological Record, 54*, 553–578.
Mearns, J., & Cain, J. E. (2003). Relationships between teachers' occupational stress and their burnout and distress: Roles of coping and negative mood regulation expectancies. *Anxiety, Stress, and Coping, 16*, 71–82.
Melbourne Academic Mindfulness Interest Group. (2006). Mindfulness-based psychotherapies: A review of conceptual foundations, empirical evidence and practical considerations. *Australian and New Zealand Journal of Psychiatry, 40*(4), 285–294.
Metcalfe, J., & Mischel, W. (1999). A hot/cool-system analysis of delay of gratification: Dynamics of willpower. *Psychological Review, 106*, 3–19.
Montgomery, C., & Rupp, A. A. (2005). A meta-analysis exploring the diverse causes and effects of stress in teachers. *Canadian Journal of Education, 28*, 458–486.
Nichols, S. L., & Berliner, D. C. (2007). *Collateral damage: How high stakes testing corrupts America's schools*. Cambridge, MA: Harvard Education Press.
Ortner, C. N., Kilner, S. J., & Zelazo, P. D. (2007). Mindfulness meditation and reduced emotional interference on a cognitive task. *Motivation and Emotion, 31*(4), 271–283.
Ostafin, B. D., & Marlatt, G. A. (2008). Surfing the urge: Experiential acceptance moderates the relation between automatic alcohol motivation and hazardous drinking. *Journal of Social and Clinical Psychology, 27*(4), 404–418.
Parker, P. D., & Martin, A. J. (2009). Coping and buoyancy in the workplace: Understanding their effects on teachers' work-related well-being and engagement. *Teaching and Teacher Education, 25*, 68–75.
Pascual, E., Perez-Jover, V., Mirambell, E., Ivanez, G., & Terol, M. C. (2003). Job conditions, coping and wellness/health outcomes in Spanish secondary school teachers. *Psychology and Health, 18*, 511–521.
Pomaki, G., & Anagnostopoulou, T. (2003). A test and expansion of the demand/control/social support model: Prediction of wellness/health outcomes in Greek teachers. *Psychology and Health, 18*, 537–550.
Rasku, A., & Kinnunen, U. (2003). Job conditions and wellness among Finnish upper secondary school teachers. *Psychology and Health, 18*, 441–456.

Roeser, R. W., & Pinela, C. (2014). Mindfulness and compassion training in adolescence: A developmental contemplative sciences perspective. *New Directions in Youth Development, 2014*(142), 9–30.

Roeser, R. W., Schonert-Reichl, K. A., Jha, A., Cullen, M., Wallace, L., Wilensky, R., … Harrison, J. (2013). Mindfulness training and reductions in teacher stress and burnout: Results from two randomized, waitlist-control field trials. *Journal of Educational Psychology, 105*, 787–804. doi:10.1037/a0032093.

Roeser, R. W., Skinner, E. A., Beers, J., & Jennings, P. A. (2012). Mindfulness training and teachers' professional development: An emerging area of research and practice. *Child Development Perspectives, 6*, 146–153.

Roeser, R. W., Vago, D. R., Pinela, C., Morris, L. S., Taylor, C., & Harrison, J. (2014). Contemplative education. In L. Nucci, T. Krettenauer, & D. Narvaez (Eds.), *Handbook of moral and character education* (pp. 223–247). New York, NY: Routledge.

Schutz, P. A., & Zembylas, M. (Eds.). (2009). *Advances in teacher emotion research: The impact on teachers' lives*. New York, NY: Springer.

Schweizer, K., & Dobrich, P. (2003). Self-reported health, appraisal, coping, and stress in teachers. *Psychology Science, 45*, 92–105.

Shapiro, S. L., Carlson, L. E., Astin, J. A., & Freeman, B. (2006). Mechanisms of mindfulness. *Journal of Clinical Psychology, 62*(3), 373–386.

Shapiro, S. L., Oman, D., Thoresen, C. E., Plante, T. G., & Flinders, T. (2008). Cultivating mindfulness: Effects on well-being. *Journal of Clinical Psychology, 64*(7), 840–862.

Skinner, E. A. (1999). Action regulation, coping, and development. In J. B. Brandstradter & R. M. Lerner (Eds.), *Action and self-development* (pp. 465–503). Thousand Oaks, CA: Sage.

Skinner, E. A., Edge, K., Altman, J., & Sherwood, H. (2003). Searching for the structure of coping: A review and critique of category systems for classifying ways of coping. *Psychological Bulletin, 129*, 216–269.

Skinner, E. A., & Wellborn, J. G. (1994). Coping during childhood and adolescence: A motivational perspective. In D. Featherman, R. Lerner, & M. Perlumutter (Eds.), *Life-span development and behavior* (Vol. 12, pp. 91–133). Hillsdale, NJ: Erlbaum.

Skinner, E. A., & Wellborn, J. G. (1997). Children's coping in the academic domain. In S. A. Wolchik & I. N. Sandler (Eds.), *Handbook of children's coping with common stressors: Linking theory and intervention* (pp. 387–422). New York, NY: Plenum Press.

Skinner, E. A., & Zimmer-Gembeck, M. J. (2007). The development of coping. *Annual Review of Psychology, 58*, 119–144.

Slagter, H. A., Giesbrecht, B., Kok, A., Weissman, D. H., Kenemans, J. L., Woldorff, M. G., & Mangun G. R. (2007). fMRI evidence for both generalized and specialized components of attentional control. *Brain Research, 1177*, 90–102.

Spilt, J. L., Koomen, H. M., Thijs, J. T., & van der Leij, A. (2012). Supporting teachers' relationships with disruptive children: The potential of relationship-focused reflection. *Attachment & Human Development, 14*(3), 305–318.

Spilt, J. L., Koomen, H. M. Y., & Thijs, J. T. (2011). Teacher wellbeing: The importance of student-teacher relationships. *Educational Psychology Review, 23*, 457–477.

Sutton, R. E., & Wheatley, K. (2003). Teachers' emotions and teaching: A review of the literature and directions for future research. *Educational Psychology Review, 15*, 327–358.

Tang, Y. Y., & Posner, M. I. (2009). Attention training and attention state training. *Trends in Cognitive Sciences, 13*(5), 222–227.

Taylor, B. L., Strauss, C., Cavanagh, K., & Jones, F. (2014). The effectiveness of self-help mindfulness-based cognitive therapy in a student sample: A randomised controlled trial. *Behaviour Research and Therapy, 63*, 63–69.

Tolan, P., & Grant, K. (2009). How social and cultural contexts shape the development of coping: Youth in the inner-city as an example. In E. A. Skinner & M. J. Zimmer-Gembeck (Eds.). *Coping and the development of regulation*. A volume for the series, R. W. Larson & L. A. Jensen (Eds.-in-Chief), *New directions in child and adolescent development*. San Francisco, CA: Jossey-Bass.

Tsouloupas, C. N., Carson, R. L., Matthews, R., Grawitch, M. J., & Barber, L. K. (2010). Exploring the association between teachers' perceived student misbehavior and emotional exhaustion: The importance of teacher efficacy beliefs and emotion regulation. *Educational Psychology: An International Journal of Experimental Educational Psychology, 30*, 173–189.

Unterbrink, T., Hack, A., Pfeifer, R., Buhl-Griehaber, V., Müller, U., Wesche, H., … Bauer, J. (2007). Burnout and effort-reward-imbalance in a sample of 949 German teachers. *International Archives of Occupational and Environmental Health, 80*, 433–441.

Verhoeven, C., Kraaij, V., Joekes, K., & Maes, S. (2003). Job conditions and wellness/health outcomes in Dutch secondary school teachers. *Psychology and Health, 18*, 473–487.

Walach, H., Nord, E., Zier, C., Dietz-Waschkowski, B., Kersig, S., & Schüpbach, H. (2007). Mindfulness-based stress reduction as a method for personnel development: A pilot evaluation. *International Journal of Stress Management, 14*(2), 188.

White, R. W. (1974). Strategies of adaptation: An attempt at systematic description. In G. V. Coelho, D. A. Hamburg, & J. E. Adams (Eds.), *Coping and adaptation* (pp. 47–68). New York, NY: Basic Books.

Williams, M. (2010). Mindfulness and psychological process. *American Psychological Association, 10*, 1–7.

Winzelberg, A. J., & Luskin, F. M. (1999). The effect of a meditation training in stress levels in secondary school teachers. *Stress and Health, 15*, 69–77.

Zapf, D., Seifert, C., Schmutte, B., Mertini, H., & Holz, M. (2001). Emotion work and job stressors and their effects on burnout. *Psychology & Health, 16*(5), 527–545.

Zapf, D. (2002). Emotion work and psychological well-being: A review of the literature and some conceptual considerations. *Human Resource Management Review, 12*, 1–32.

Cultivating Inner Resilience in Educators and Students: The Inner Resilience Program

8

Linda Lantieri, Madhavi Nambiar, Susanne Harnett, and Eden Nagler Kyse

Introduction

On the morning of September 11, 2011, more than 5000 students and nearly 200 teachers ran for their lives from schools in downtown Manhattan. In the following days, an additional 9000 students were evacuated from nearby schools. These displaced students and teachers were sheltered as disaster refugees in other NYC classrooms. Overall, 20,000 students were directly impacted by the events of that historic day. Due to the inner resourcefulness of educators in the area, every teacher and student in lower Manhattan survived. For those who witnessed these events first-hand, two fundamental questions arose: What resources did those students, teachers, and administrators draw upon in order to respond the way they did? Could we cultivate "ways of being" that helped them remain calm in the face of profound uncertainty?

Unfortunately, for many downtown teachers and students, the sense of crisis did not end with that terrifying day almost 15 years ago. In the wake of September 11th, students found themselves displaced and temporarily housed in other schools for several months. This situation created a tremendous strain on teachers and students throughout lower Manhattan. In the quest to maintain normalcy, months elapsed before some teachers realized they had not spoken about these issues with their peers and colleagues. Clearly, there was a need to address the long-term recovery of both youth and adults in Lower Manhattan. However, it also seemed clear that people were healing at different rates and in different ways. As a result, the challenge was to create long-term approaches that not only addressed teachers' and children's basic psychological needs, but also broader aspects of their "inner life" as well. These efforts had to be flexible and inclusive enough to address differing needs of teachers and their students in a subtle and respectful, yet profound manner.

The events of September 11, 2001 presented a crisis that led to the founding of the *Inner Resilience Program* (*IRP*) to address the diverse needs of teachers and students affected by that fateful day. This chapter profiles *IRP* and the research that has examined its effectiveness.

L. Lantieri (✉)
Inner Resilience Program, New York, NY, USA
e-mail: llantieri@att.net

M. Nambiar
Inner Resilience Program, New York, NY, USA
e-mail: madhavinambiar@hotmail.com

S. Harnett
Metis Associates, New York, NY, USA
e-mail: sharnett@metisassociates.com

E.N. Kyse
Montclair State University, Montclair, NJ, USA
e-mail: kysee@mail.montclair.edu

K.A. Schonert-Reichl, R.W. Roeser (eds.), *Handbook of Mindfulness in Education*,
Mindfulness in Behavioral Health, DOI 10.1007/978-1-4939-3506-2_8

We begin this chapter by providing the case for a focus on teacher risk and resilience, and provide the foundation of *IRP* in which social and emotional learning (SEL) is integrated with contemplative practices. In the next section, we describe in detail the core components of *IRP* and highlight the ways in which *IRP* can promote teacher and student well-being. Following, we provide a description of research examining the effectiveness of *IRP* via a randomized controlled trial that investigated impacts on teachers and students and qualitative research examining the impact of the program through the lens of school principals. The chapter ends with a discussion of how an understanding of *IRP* has implications for our thinking about promoting teacher and student well-being, along with thoughts on future directions for work in this area.

The Need to Address Teacher Risk and Resilience

The work of a teacher can be perceived as never-ending in its expectations: the scheduling demands of the work day, the consecutive hours spent in their own classrooms, and the task of addressing both the academic and social-emotional needs of so many students. Humphrey (1992) attributes the increased stress level of teachers to several additional factors: the large numbers of important decisions teachers must make on a single day, the great level of public scrutiny that teachers face, the high risk of violence in many schools, and the level of emotional sensitivity needed to respond to the emotional needs of students.

Given the stresses that teachers face and the little support that they receive to address these challenges, it is not surprising that teachers respond with common physiological, emotional, and behavioral manifestations of stress or by leaving the profession altogether (see Ingersoll, Merrill, & Stuckey, 2014 for a recent review). Those who stay are at risk of developing another serious problem: teacher burnout—a multidimensional construct that consists of emotional exhaustion, depersonalization, and reduced personal accomplishment (Maslach, Jackson, & Leiter, 1997). Burnout occurs when teachers have attempted unsuccessfully to cope with stress over long periods of time (Kyriacou, 2001). Teacher burnout can be tremendously destructive to teacher–student relationships, classroom management, and the classroom environment, as well as to the health of individual students (Jennings & Greenberg, 2009).

Bringing Together Social and Emotional Learning and Mindfulness Practices

A new movement in mainstream education supports an integration of SEL with contemplative, mindfulness-based approaches to teaching and learning as a way in which to reduce stress in both teachers and their students and promote their well-being (Lantieri & Nambiar, 2012; Lawlor, this volume). SEL involves the processes through which individuals acquire and effectively apply the knowledge, attitudes, and skills necessary to understand and manage their emotions, feel and show empathy for others, establish and achieve positive goals, develop and maintain positive relationships, and make responsible decisions (Weissberg, Payton, O'Brien, & Munro, 2007). Often called the "missing piece" in school improvement efforts, the field of SEL reflects the growing recognition that healthy social-emotional development advances children's success in school and life (Weissberg & Cascarino, 2013). The field of SEL builds from work in child development, classroom management, prevention of problem behavior, and new knowledge about the role of the brain in social and cognitive growth. It is informed by scholarly research demonstrating that all children can have a school experience that helps them to be not just academically competent, but also supports them in being engaged lifelong learners who are self-aware, caring, connected to others, and active contributors to a more just, peaceful, productive, and sustainable world (Durlak, Weissberg, Dymnicki, Taylor, & Schellinger, 2011; Schonert-Reichl & Weissberg, 2014). Most research-based SEL programming in schools focuses on five core components of SEL as espoused by the Collaborative for Academic, Social, and Emotional Learning (CASEL)—an organization at the forefront of the SEL movement—and includes: self-awareness, self-management, social awareness, relationship skills, and responsible decision-making (CASEL, 2013).

As Roeser and Zelazo (2012) posit "Contemplative practices are conceptualized as specialized forms of mental and physical training that, when engaged in over time for extended periods under the guidance of experienced practitioners, lead to the development of particular skills" (p. 143). Secularized contemplative practices generally fall under the labels of mindfulness, meditation, and yoga, and provide examples of structured and socially scaffolded activities that teach skills by imposing some discipline on a normally unregulated mental or physical habit. Mindfulness, often defined as "paying attention in a particular way, on purpose, in the present moment, and nonjudgmentally" (Kabat-Zinn, 2004, p. 4), refers to an ability to focus on thoughts, feelings, or perceptions that arise moment to moment in a cognitively nonelaborative and emotionally nonreactive way (Roeser, 2014). With sustained effortful practice, complex skills such as mindfulness and empathy are hypothesized to become routinized at neural/mental levels and, subsequently, to regulate behavior in relatively automatic ways by being highly accessible and available (Jennings, Lantieri, & Roeser, 2011).

Drawing upon evidence-based research, there is growing support that mindfulness practices can strengthen the brain functions that are responsible for emotion and attention regulation, empathy and compassion, and resilience in the face of life stress (Davidson, Kabat-Zinn, Schumacher et al., 2003; Davidson & Harrington, 2002; Davidson et al., 2003; Lutz, Brefczynski-Lewis, Johnstone, & Davidson, 2008; Lutz & Davidson, 2008; Lutz, Slagter, Dunne, & Davidson, 2008; Singer & Lamm, 2009). Moreover, studies of stress reduction across multiple sectors have suggested that some mindfulness programs can be effective in reducing participants' perceived and demonstrated stress and can break cycles, such as the "burnout cascade" (e.g., Kemeny et al., 2012; Roeser et al., 2013). Research also has shown that mindfulness is associated with more positive affect, reduced anxiety and depression, and better relationships with others (Barnes, Brown, Krusemark, Campbell, & Rogge, 2007; Brown & Ryan, 2003). With regard to education, changes in teachers' mindsets due to mindfulness training may have a positive impact on classroom climate, although more research is needed to support this conjecture at this time (Jennings, this volume; Roeser, Skinner, Beers, & Jennings, 2012). There is however research demonstrating that teachers' mindsets do influence students' behaviors. For instance, Marzano, Marzano, and Pickering (2003) conducted a meta-analysis of more than 100 studies of classroom management and found that a teacher's "mental set" had the greatest effect on reducing student misbehavior. Teachers who were able to remain objective and calm under pressure were the most effective.

Benefits for children have also been found for children who practice mindfulness. Indeed, the more children can begin to experience quiet and stillness, the more they can feel an inner balance and sense of purpose, which can offset the overstimulation that is so abundant in most of our lives (Lantieri, 2008, 2010).

The benefits of such a regular practice can include:

- Increased self-awareness and self-understanding
- Greater ability to relax the body and release physical tension
- Improved concentration
- Improved ability to deal with stressful situations more effectively by creating a more relaxed way of responding to stressors
- Greater control over one's thoughts with less domination by unwelcome thoughts
- Greater opportunity for deeper communication and understanding between adults and children because thoughts and feelings are being shared on a regular basis.

Accordingly, an integration of SEL with contemplative teaching and learning can become powerful enhancement to the SEL field. This enhancement acknowledges that the field of education must not only pay attention to the inner lives of teachers and students but also give them pedagogical tools to cultivate skills that foster calm and resilience. Such practices may be designed to cultivate the potential of mindful awareness in an ethical-relational context in which the values of personal growth, learning, moral living, and caring for others are also nurtured (Jennings, this volume; Roeser & Peck, 2009).

The Inner Resilience Program

IRP's mission is to cultivate the inner lives of students, teachers, and schools by integrating SEL with contemplative practices. As described above, *IRP* was created in response to the needs of teachers and students impacted by the September 11th attacks. Linda Lantieri, whose experiences include work as a former school administrator in a middle school in East Harlem and a co-founder of the Resolving Conflict Creatively Program—a research-based SEL program (see Aber, Brown, & Jones, 2003 for a description of RCCP), became the founding director of *IRP* after a small group of NYC educators and mental health professionals began to shape the particular intervention that was needed in the eleven schools in Lower Manhattan that were most deeply affected by September 11, 2011. In taking on her new role, Lantieri drew on her three-year experience as a Senior Scholar at the Fetzer Institute in Kalamazoo, Michigan—a privately endowed foundation whose mission is to help individuals make a deeper connection between "their inner life of mind and spirit and their outer life of action and service"—which she had completed immediately prior to September 11, 2001. During her time at the Fetzer Institute, Lantieri was part of a group of 18 individuals from diverse backgrounds who had been brought together to reflect with each other about how to bring a more holistic perspective to their various fields of work. This work would become foundational for Lantieri's creation of the *IRP* to respond to the educators and students impacted by the September 11th attack.

As Lantieri visited schools in the aftermath of the September 11th attack, she saw educators struggling to cope with their feelings of helplessness and despair without any personal support. As a result of the attack, countless educators had been transformed overnight into grief counselors, recovery coordinators, and crisis intervention experts for their students. "I saw how much listening they had to do—to experts, students, parents, and administrators. But who was listening to their stories?" Lantieri asked. "Many displayed the classic signs of 'compassion fatigue.' In all the listening, they had not yet had the chance to check in with their own feelings and tell their stories. It was clear to me that teachers were running out of the emotional support and inner resilience they needed to sustain those they were serving."

New York City's educators needed help in strengthening their inner resources and supporting one another in contexts where they would be able to be reflective about their experiences. Who was taking care of the caregivers? Where would they get the space to rejuvenate their spirits and feed their resiliency? To help answer some of these questions, The September 11th Fund provided a generous seed grant for Lantieri to create and implement *IRP*.

Grounded in evidence-based research, *IRP* recognizes that teachers often face a variety of stresses such as: heavy workloads, relative isolation from their colleagues, time constraints, emphasis on academic achievement testing, low decision-making power, and frequent lack of support from administrators and colleagues (Byrne, 1993; Murray, 2005; Winzelberg & Luskin, 1999). Indeed, given the varied levels of stress and the challenge of meeting the social-emotional needs of their students, often the educator is unable to take the time necessary to cultivate key personal and interpersonal skills as well as sustain a contemplative practice that may help them remain focused, calm, and strong in the midst of constant demands. As a result of the current reality for teachers, *IRP* works mostly with adults at the beginning, helping them develop competency in their own emotional regulation and focus. They are first introduced to a mindfulness approach themselves before they are offered training to prepare them to teach children similar strategies.

IRP's core programs help parents and educators balance their inner and outer lives. Since its inception, *IRP*'s approach has been to bring contemplative practices into the school environment by integrating developments occurring in the field of SEL. By integrating the skills of SEL with contemplative practices, such as mindfulness or focused attention meditation, SEL competencies, such as self-awareness, take on a new depth of inner exploration. Managing emotions becomes self-discipline and empathy becomes a basis for altruism, caring, and compassion.

IRP offers caregivers a comprehensive understanding of how stress affects health and performance, along with relaxation and self-care techniques to effectively manage stress. *IRP* creates opportunities for educators to reflect on the meaning of their work in the company of like-minded colleagues. It also brings contemplative practices to children by implementing a K-8 curriculum entitled *Building Resilience from the Inside Out,* which is based on the book, *Building Emotional Intelligence: Techniques to Cultivate Inner Strength in Children* (Lantieri, 2008). When *IRP* is fully embraced by a school district, it includes the components discussed below.

Residential Retreats

IRP conducts weekend residential retreats in order to introduce teachers and administrators to contemplative strategies for staying calm, strong, and creative amidst the stresses of work and life. At these retreats, participants are introduced to and take home practical tools for keeping a sense of purpose alive in their work. They have an opportunity to begin experiencing the inward journey in the company of a like-minded community of trust. Since the start of the program, *IRP* has conducted more than 35 residential retreats.

Professional Development Workshops

In addition to residential retreats, *IRP* offers a wide range of professional development workshops at schools on topics such as: "Self-Care Techniques for Stress Management;" "Educating the Heart: The Concepts and Skills of Emotional Intelligence;" "Stress Reduction through Gentle Stretching and Creative Movement" among others. Schools participating in the program are encouraged to devote their required professional development time to continue work with their staff to increase adult social-emotional competencies as well as to offer time for self-reflection.

Stress Reduction Days

Stress reduction days provide 20-min bodywork sessions (incorporated into the school day during teachers' free periods) offering the powerful effects of massage and healing touch. Typically, one to three bodywork practitioners work within the school setting during the school day. This bodywork takes place fully clothed and, depending on the circumstances and the clients' preference, may occur seated on a chair or lying on a table or mat. *IRP* has delivered over 4000 stress reduction sessions to school personnel in more than 30 NYC schools since 2002.

Monthly Nurturing the Inner Life Series

Through interactive exercises, individual reflection, and small group discussion, *IRP* features a series of monthly workshops where educators explore the skills associated with mindfulness practices, which include strategies to strengthen focused attention, emotional regulation, empathy, and compassion. This four-part monthly after-school group is hosted by *IRP* in an atmosphere of safety and relaxation.

Parent Workshops

IRP offers individual parent workshops and a series of five group workshops entitled *Skills for Life for Families* that help caregivers strengthen their own resilience and understand better the stresses affecting today's children. Parents are introduced to contemplative practices and encouraged to offer their children a regular "quiet time" at home using the book *Building Emotional Intelligence: Techniques to Cultivate Inner Strength in Children* (Lantieri, 2008). There is a Trainer of Trainer component of the parent workshops and trainers in the Warren and Youngstown City Schools in Ohio, and trainers from the Oakland Unified School District in California have been trained to carry out these workshops which are available in both English and Spanish and can complement any SEL or mindfulness program.

K-8 Curriculum: Building Resilience from the Inside Out

IRP's K-8 curriculum helps teachers create the optimal learning environment in their classrooms by teaching students how to calm themselves when upset, relax their bodies and minds, and enhance their attention skills. Techniques such as progressive muscle relaxation and mindfulness meditation practices are used. *IRP* offers teachers a 10-hour training in curriculum implementation and follow-up, including continued support for teachers and counselors through classroom visits and coaching sessions. This aspect of the work has been implemented in many school districts across the United States and a pilot project in Spain.

Effectiveness of the Inner Resilience Program on Teacher and Student Wellness and Classroom Climate

In the spring of 2006, the Fetzer Institute provided funding to conduct an evaluation of the *IRP* on teacher and student well-being and classroom climate via a randomized controlled trial (RCT)—the gold standard in evaluation in which groups are randomly assigned to receive a treatment or serve as controls. The study was conducted during the 2007–2008 school year (from September 2007 through May 2008) by Metis Associates, an independent research and evaluation firm (Simon, Harnett, Nagler, & Thomas, 2009), It was theorized that the IRP intervention would positively impact teachers' attention, well-being, and social relationships, which, in turn, would have a positive impact on the climate of their classrooms and on their students' attention and well-being. It was further theorized that students' well-being would be positively impacted from their teachers' implementation of lessons and activities from the *Building Resilience from the Inside Out* curriculum module for students.

The study took place in 3rd–5th grade classrooms from schools across New York City. Participants in the study included 57 classroom teachers, with 29 teachers randomly assigned to the *IRP* (treatment) group and 28 teachers to the control group. A total of 855 students of these teachers also participated in the study, with 471 in the treatment group and 384 in the control. The 57 participating teachers worked in 33 different NYC public schools. Because randomization was conducted at the teacher level, there were instances of multiple teachers participating from the same school.

Teachers in the *IRP* group participated in activities intended to reduce teacher stress and increase their concentration, attention, and job satisfaction, as well as improve relationships with their colleagues. Specifically, the *IRP* group participated in a series of weekly yoga classes, monthly *Nurturing the Inner Life* meetings, a weekend residential retreat, and training and support in the use of a curriculum module—*Building Resilience from the Inside Out*—for students.

To test the hypotheses, teachers and students from both the treatment and control groups completed a battery of self-report measures in the fall, prior to the commencement of *IRP* and again in late spring, after the program had ended. Wherever possible, published instruments with established reliability and validity were utilized.

Teachers completed measures assessing the following constructs: attention and awareness (e.g., focused attention, mindfulness); well-being (e.g., stress, burnout, coping skills); occupational health (e.g., job satisfaction) and social relationships (e.g., trust of colleagues). Students completed measures assessing constructs similar to those of teachers, including: attention and awareness (e.g., focused attention, perceptual awareness); well-being (e.g., fear, frustration, depressed mood), and behavior (e.g., aggression). Student wellness was measured through a set of scales from the Early Adolescent Temperament Questionnaire-Revised, Short Form (EATQ-R SF) (Ellis & Rothbart, 2001). Scales from the EATQ-R SF for 5th-grade participants included subscales measuring aggression, attention, depressive mood, fear, frustration, pleasure sensitivity, and perceptual sensitivity. This survey was modified for 3rd- and 4th-grade students to be more developmentally appropriate for these younger children. The modifications included fewer overall items and a change in the response scale from five-points to three-points. Moreover, the specific questions for the 3rd- and 4th-grade wellness survey were modified by the researchers in collaboration with program personnel from six of the original EATQ-R SF scales, including: aggression, attention, depressive mood, fear, frustration, and perceptual sensitivity.

Classroom climate was examined with regard to teacher's leadership and management style and the supportiveness of the environment for implementing the *IRP*. To assess the extent to which the classroom climate was positively influenced, treatment and control group teachers and their students completed appropriate versions of the Classroom Climate Inventory (Developmental Studies Center, 2005) in the fall and again in late spring.

Analyses examining differences between the treatment group and comparison classrooms revealed several significant results. With regard to changes in teachers' well-being, repeated measures analyses indicated that the program led to statistically significant improvements for treatment teachers on three of the teacher wellness areas that were assessed. More specifically, in contrast to controls, *IRP* teachers reported significantly decreased stress ($F=6.59$, $p=.013$; Cohen's $d=.71$), increased attention and mindfulness ($F=8.88$, $p=.004$; Cohen's $d=.81$), and increased relational trust with colleagues ($F=4.37$, $p=.041$; Cohen's $d=.57$). Additional analyses examining differences between treatment and control teachers on body awareness ($F=1.65$, $p=.205$; Cohen's $d=.35$), emotion-oriented coping ($F=3.80$, $p=.056$; Cohen's $d=.53$), avoidance-oriented coping ($F=1.76$, $p=.190$; Cohen's $d=.36$), and burnout ($F=2.15$, $p=.149$; Cohen's $d=.40$) were not statistically significant, although they were in the expected direction and had moderate effect sizes (Cohen's $d \geq 0.33$). With regard to changes in student wellness, repeated measures analyses indicated that 3rd- and 4th-grade in the treatment group, in contrast to students in the control group, experienced significant reductions in their frustration levels from pre- to post-test ($F=4.85$, $p=.028$; Cohen's $d=.28$). No other statistically significant differences were found between treatment and control students on any other of the wellness dimensions.

Changes in classroom climate were assessed through self-reports of participating teachers and their students on the Classroom Climate Inventory. Repeated measures analysis results indicated that 3rd and 4th grade treatment students' perceptions of autonomy and influence in the classroom increased significantly from pre to post-test in comparison to 3rd- and 4th-grade control students ($F=24.31$, $p<.001$; Cohen's $d=.41$). Significant differences in classroom climate were not found for any of the teacher measures or for 5th grade students.

In addition to examining differences between treatment and control groups, variations *within* the treatment group were examined in order to determine differential impacts of the intervention, on "high-risk" students (i.e., students particularly high or low on measured wellness factors as defined below) in comparison to the rest of the treatment sample. For all negative wellness factors (e.g., aggression, frustration, depressive mood), a cutoff score of one standard deviation above the mean pretest score was established. All treatment students with pretest scores above this cutoff were identified as "high-risk" on that particular factor. For all positive wellness factors (e.g., attention, perceptual sensitivity, pleasure sensitivity), a cutoff score of one standard deviation below the mean presurvey score was established. All treatment students with pretest scores below this cutoff were identified as "high-risk" on that particular factor.

Repeated measures analyses conducted to examine the equality of means across "high-risk" status groups and time revealed that in almost all cases, significantly greater treatment effects were observed for the "high-risk" treatment students than for students in the non "high-risk" group. Specifically, in contrast to those students in the non "high-risk" group, significant improvements for 3rd- and 4th-grade students identified as "high risk" were found for all six dimensions of student wellness: Attention ($F=84.43$, $p=<001$; Cohen's $d=1.03$), Aggression ($F=44.97, p<.001$; Cohen's $d=.75$), Depressed Mood ($F=52.79$, $p<.001$; Cohen's $d=.81$), Fear ($F=23.95$, $p<.001$; Cohen's $d=.55$), Frustration ($F=45.95, p<.001$; Cohen's $d=.1.41$), and Perceptual Sensitivity ($F=67.55$, $p<.001$; Cohen's $d=.1.59$). Grade 5 "high-risk" treatment students were found to have made significantly greater gains from pre- to post-test on six of the seven student wellness dimensions—namely Attention ($F=24.17$, $p<.001$; Cohen's $d=.67$), Aggression ($F=36.19, p<.001$; Cohen's $d=1.68$), Depressed Mood ($F=6.03$, $p=.015$; Cohen's $d=.42$), Frustration ($F=10.29, p=.002$; Cohen's $d=.54$), Pleasure Sensitivity ($F=20.04$, $p<.001$; Cohen's $d=.76$), and Perceptual Sensitivity ($F=30.61$, $p<.001$; Cohen's $d=.94$)—in comparison to their non "high-risk" treatment student counterparts.

It is important to consider two statistical phenomena that may potentially limit the extent of findings in the high-risk group: *regression to the mean* and *restriction of range*. The statistical phenomenon known as *regression to the mean* states that if participants are assessed on two successive occasions, samples far from the mean on the first occasion will tend to be closer to the mean on the second occasion. In addition, at least some of the found difference must be attributed to the issue of *restriction of range* associated with intentionally selecting out teachers or students with high or low scores, as the restricted range of scores allows little room to change in one direction.

The *IRP* Pilot Schools Program: Principals' Perspectives

Encouraged by the findings of the experimental study on *IRP*'s impact, the program launched its second year of the pilot, widening the scope to include administrators. We hypothesized that the positive effects would be even greater if program activities focused on the principal (who is both the instructional leader and sets the emotional tone for the school) and if multiple staff members from a school participated in the program together (Lantieri, Kyse, Harnett, & Malkmus, 2011). Thus, the *IRP* Pilot Schools Program was initiated in 2009 in 10 schools in NYC Public Schools.

Reasons for Participating in *IRP* Pilot Schools Program

A monthly focus group was conducted with principal group participants ($N=10$) in March 2011. In focus groups, respondents indicated a number of reasons why they were interested in the *IRP* Pilot Schools Program. One key reason they elected to participate was that they hoped to develop their own emotional intelligence and to have time to take care of themselves. For example, one participant indicated the following:

> The idea of carving out time to attend to emotional/mental health was very appealing. Too often in my work I am busy taking care of everyone and their needs. Seldom do I get the chance to pause to be revitalized in this way, while also being in the presence of colleagues who have similar work experiences.

Respondents also recognized the need for this work in their schools. For example, one respondent wrote, "Stress reduction and self-care are essential in a profession where the threat of burnout is constant. The IRP program sounded like it would address these issues."

A third key reason that respondents gave as to why they chose to participate, related to them having the opportunity to build their school communities. One principal wrote that he/she chose to participate because the program promotes "the philosophical framework and understanding that all (work) organizations, particularly those that impact on youngsters, should be reflective, humane, supportive and nurturing and that all members need to 'take care' of each other and of themselves in order to maximize their effectiveness and the effectiveness of the organization (and positively impact the youngsters)." Another respondent wrote that he/she was interested in the program because it "would provide an enormous amount of support for the school's community. It also focused on an area in which a great need existed but nothing was really in place to address it." This respondent went on to say, "We knew that this program would help everyone in the school's community—personally and professionally."

Perceptions of *IRP* Pilot Schools Program Activities

Principals reported participating in various *IRP* Program activities over the course of the two project years. These included activities that they personally participated in and those in which their staff participated. Principals attended a monthly "principals' meeting" where they learned mindfulness practices and also went on an *IRP Residential Retreat for Educational Leaders*. Their schools actively participated in stress reduction days, professional development workshops for their school staff, and parent workshops. Principals and their staff participated in *Nurturing the Inner Life* meetings, yoga classes, and curriculum trainings.

Principals were asked to participate in research on the pilot schools project, also conducted by Metis Associates. Participating principals completed online surveys and participated in a focus group. They answered a series of questions regarding the impact of the program on their personal lives, their professional practices, and on the climate of their schools.

Principals' Perceptions of *IRP*'s Impact on their Personal and Professional Capacities

Principals' responses to the perceived impact of the *IRP* activities on themselves were examined across five dimensions: stress level, mindfulness, coping skills, and body awareness. Principals were asked to respond to a series of questions on a five-point scale ranging from "Don't Know" to "A Great Extent." Findings revealed that 100 % of principals perceived that the program impacted them either "to some extent" or "to a great extent" on each dimension examined.

Principals' open-ended responses to questions about the impact of *IRP* supported their responses to the closed-ended questions. Overall, they reported that they found the work extremely valuable in helping them to keep balance in their lives and to cope with everyday stresses. They also reported that they found the interaction with other principals exceedingly valuable. Below is a sample of responses that they provided in an open-ended section of the survey:

> This has made a significant impact on me personally. I now handle stress better and I have learned strategies to reduce stress. The principal meetings are very powerful and I have learned a lot from my colleagues. It is a safe place for all of us.
>
> Participation in this principal group has had a tremendous impact on me personally. It has provided a safe haven for me. It has introduced me to other school leaders and allowed me to interact with them on a personal level rather than just on a professional level. It's difficult to leave a building, especially when so many things are happening. However, this principal group has taught me that it's necessary to take time for myself to recharge and try to give myself what I need to go on before I can support others.
>
> This was a wonderfully profound experience for me, which allowed me to see things in perspective when I would have otherwise made different decisions about my job. In a more personal way, I am more cognizant of the emotional needs of the staff around me and try to find balance between the academic and the emotional.

Table 8.1 displays principals' responses to the perceived impact of the *IRP* activities on themselves *professionally*. As the table shows, principals were extremely positive about the program's impact in these areas as well.

Again, the open-ended responses corroborated findings from principals' closed-ended responses. Principals indicated that the program assisted them professionally by helping them to be calmer, more focused, and to deepen their relationships with staff in their schools. Following

Table 8.1 Respondents' perceptions of *IRP*'s impact on their professional skills

Impact area	*N*	Don't know	Not at all	A little	To some extent	To a great extent
Job satisfaction	10	0 (0 %)	0 (0 %)	0 (0 %)	3 (30 %)	7 (70 %)
Staff management style	10	0 (0 %)	0 (0 %)	1(10 %)	1 (10 %)	8 (80 %)
Relationships with staff	10	0 (0 %)	0 (0 %)	0 (0 %)	2 (20 %)	8 (80 %)
Relationships with students	10	0 (0 %)	0 (0 %)	0 (0 %)	2 (20 %)	8 (80 %)

is a sample of their open-ended responses to the question regarding their perception of the impact of the program on them professionally:

> My [participation in] the retreats and in the principal group has enhanced my leadership skills—I have learned how to be more direct AND more compassionate.
>
> I am calmer, more relaxed and I am able to handle stress better.
>
> It helps me develop skills and postures that enhance my ability to be a nurturing, supportive, and understanding leader. It helps me prioritize.

Principals' Perception of on the Impact *IRP* on their School Community

Principals indicated that, due to their participation in the program, they had made a number of changes to their schedules and routines in their schools, as well as to their leadership approach. For example, some principals indicated that they made changes to their regular staff meetings, such as starting the meetings with ice-breakers, breathing and relaxation techniques, and acknowledgements. Additionally, one principal indicated that he now has "agenda-less" monthly meetings (with snacks, watercolors, etc.). Other principals indicated that they added activities to their schedules. For example, one respondent noted that she instituted a day of meditation and relaxation for the staff during an already set professional development day. Another reported that she supported (logistically and financially) a social skills study group that was started by teachers. Yet another pointed adding yoga and other calming/focus-building activities in his school.

Overall, most principals indicated that the key impact on their approach to the work in their buildings is the program's enabling of them to be more supportive and encouraging of their staff. For example, one respondent wrote that as a result of her participation:

> I think that I approach every interaction with the hope of being positive, supportive and encouraging. I try to listen and manage conflict in the community as best as I can. When situations are difficult and stressful, I am more able to step back, learn from the situation and hopefully not take things personally.

Principals' responses to the perceptions of the program's impact on their schools' culture were also assessed. Five of the principals (50 %) reported that *IRP* had an influence on school culture "*to a great extent*," three indicated that *IRP* had an influence on school culture "*to some extent*," and only two reported that *IRP* had an influence on school culture "*a little.*"

Again, open-ended comments corroborated the closed-ended responses, and principals elaborated on ways that the program has impacted their school climate, including, among other differences, changes in teachers' practices and ways that staff and students relate to each other. A sample of their responses to an open-ended question asking them to elaborate on changes in their school culture is below:

> We have lots of visitors coming to [our school]. They all comment on the calmness of the school and how students are nurtured and cared for. I think the teacher stress reduction days acknowledge how hard the teachers work and that we care about their well-being.
>
> Teachers are more peaceful and include some of the practices in their own classrooms. For example yoga, using a chime to call the group to meeting.
>
> The main success that I've observed is that members of the staff have seen the importance in addressing the children's social-emotional needs in the same way that we address their academic needs.

> Sometimes we focus so much on the children's academics. However, unless we meet their social-emotional needs as well, they will not make the progress that we need them to make. This program has given staff members the strategies that can be implemented and incorporated into our daily program to support the children in this manner.

Challenges and Lessons Learned

In both studies, participants had the opportunity to discuss the challenges that they faced in the implementation of the program in their schools by responding to an online survey and to focus group questions. During the focus group, the principals passionately described their frustration in trying to include this work in their schools. They perceived the work as eminently valuable to themselves and to their staff; however, they struggled to find the time to implement it in the context of other demands that they faced on a day-to-day basis. Although "time" might be considered the basic challenge expressed, the principals described a more fundamental issue: The value of this work seems to be at odds with the current overall educational context. The emphasis on testing is dominating education to the point that there is little time left to address any other student or teacher needs. Paradoxically, the current climate is making the work more necessary than ever, adding to the principals' frustration over the situation. This problem extended even to the teacher level. A couple of participants indicated that it was difficult to get teachers to see the value of the program activities when they felt so pressured by other instructional demands and the seemingly impossible expectations for their time.

Discussion and Future Directions in Theory, Research, and Practice

Results from both the quantitative and qualitative studies (Metis Associates, 2011; Simon et al., 2009) suggest that *IRP* had the intended effect of helping teachers and principals focus on their inner selves and to improve their own wellness. Through work with *IRP* and research on similar programs, it appears that teaching these practices to students is increasing not only their social-emotional skills, but their resilience as well: the capacity to not only cope, but thrive in the face of adversity.

These results are extremely important considering the research on teacher stress and burnout. It is now well documented that teachers have highly stressful jobs and are at risk of leaving the teaching profession or—equally problematic—staying and burning out. The results produced by *IRP*, including stress reduction, increased mindfulness, and improved relationships with colleagues, have the potential to break the negative cycle whereby teacher and student actions play off of each other, leading to increased teacher stress, poor classroom climate, and continued student misbehaviors (Jennings & Greenberg, 2009; Marzano et al., 2003). These studies also found that *IRP* can improve teachers' perceptions of relational trust with their colleagues. These results are particularly important considering the work of Bryk and Schneider (2002), who contended that schools that are high in relational trust are more likely to make improvements in student achievement. Specifically, according to Murray (2005), the ability of new teachers to foster positive relationships with their students and their colleagues can "make or break" their teaching careers, and the most important factor for schools to consider with regard to retention is the quality of the relationships between new teachers and their colleagues.

There is evidence that changes in the wellness of teachers and principals can create classroom and school contexts where students are viewed more as individuals and have more student autonomy and influence. There may also be a greater feeling of community in treated teachers' classrooms. Furthermore, changes in the teachers, along with direct intervention through the use of the curriculum, can reduce students' levels of frustration. Although these results are interesting and important to note, the brief nature of the intervention may have impacted the strength of the results. Impact on the classrooms and on the students' wellness decreased in strength compared to the effects of the intervention on proximal teacher outcomes. Increasing the strength and, importantly, the duration of the intervention would likely increase the impact that the program would have on teachers' classroom climates and their students' wellness.

The within-treatment analyses from the quantitative study also provide useful results, suggesting that the most vulnerable students may see the greatest benefit from the program. These results are important considering the needs of these students and the potential benefits of breaking negative cycles and treating such problems before they escalate.

Furthermore, in the qualitative study of pilot implementation across ten NYC public schools, participating principals reported that they made a number of changes to the way they lead their schools, including changes to their school meetings to include time for staff to relax, reflect, and connect with their colleagues. Some also added activities that promote inner resilience work and reflection to their school programming for both teachers and students. Moreover, most respondents indicated that they felt more equipped to support and encourage their staff members since they began participating in the program.

These findings provide important preliminary evidence that school-wide implementation of *IRP* works as hypothesized. When principals participate in the program, they can be catalysts for change that occurs beyond the individual classroom to affect the culture of the entire school. Additionally, when multiple members of the school participate in the program, the result can be more powerful than when only one or a small number of teachers participate. Interestingly, the findings also suggest that the logic of the impact follows as one might predict as well. That is, as results from this preliminary examination of the pilot program suggest that the strongest impact is on individuals personally, followed by professional changes, followed by changes in school culture. It is extremely encouraging that in the relatively short time that administrators have participated in this program, they have made the kind of changes in their leadership routines and styles that can lead to deep change, and, indeed, many reported observing cultural changes in their schools already.

Future Directions

Currently, the *Inner Resilience Program* is being implemented in ten pilot schools in the NYC Public Schools, all six schools in the South Burlington School District in Vermont (since 2007), in Warren and Youngstown City School Districts (11 schools in Ohio since 2009), in the Mamaroneck School District (since 2012) and in six schools in Madrid, Spain (since 2009). The *IRP* of today remains actively involved in disseminating lessons learned and in shaping the burgeoning field of SEL and Contemplative Teaching and Learning (e.g., Jennings et al., 2011). *IRP* plans to produce key program resources that offer sustainable and concrete ways in which school staff, parents, and students can continue to strengthen their inner resources. The program is actively involved in its largest initiative with the *Collaborative for Academic, Social and Emotional Learning* and *Morningside Center for Teaching Social Responsibility*. This initiative continues to work in conjunction with Youngstown and Warren City School Districts to develop a sustainable district-wide implementation of SEL integrated with a contemplative focus on nurturing the inner lives of principals, teachers, parents, and students.

Since *IRP* began, over 6200 school staff, 3200 parents and over 30,000 students have been directly served. Adults and students alike are helping to reclaim schools as caring and mindful communities of learning. As a program, *IRP* will remain focused on advocating for a broader vision of education—one that includes the integration of SEL and mindfulness-based contemplative educational practices.

References

Aber, J. L., Brown, J. L., & Jones, S. M. (2003). Developmental trajectories toward violence in middle childhood: Course, demographic differences, and response to school-based intervention. *Developmental Psychology, 39*, 324–348.

Barnes, S., Brown, K. W., Krusemark, E., Campbell, W. K., & Rogge, R. D. (2007). The role of mindfulness in romantic relationship satisfaction and responses to relationship stress. *Journal of Marital and Family Therapy, 33*, 482–500.

Brown, K. W., & Ryan, R. M. (2003). The benefits of being present: Mindfulness and its role in psychological well-being. *Journal of Personality and Social Psychology, 84*, 822–848.

Byrk, A. S., & Schneider, B. (2002). *Trust in schools: A core resource for improvement*. New York, NY: Russel Sage.

Byrne, B. M. (1993). Burnout: Testing for the validity, replication, and invariance of causal structure across elementary, intermediate, and secondary teachers. *American Educational Research Journal, 31*, 645–673.

Collaborative for Academic, Social, and Emotional Learning. (2013). *CASEL schoolkit: A guide for implementing schoolwide academic, social, and emotional learning*. Chicago, IL: Author.

Davidson, R. J., & Harrington, A. (Eds.). (2002). *Visions of compassion: Western scientists and Tibetan Buddhists examine human nature*. New York, NY: Oxford University Press.

Davidson, R. J., Kabat-Zinn, J., Schumacher, J., Rosenkranz, M., Muller, D., Santorelli, S.F., … Sheridan, J. F. (2003). Alterations in brain and immune function produced by mindfulness meditation.*Psychosomatic Medicine, 65*, 564–570.

Developmental Studies Center. (2005). *Scales from student questionnaire, child development project for elementary school students (grades 3–6)*. Oakland, CA: Developmental Studies Center.

Durlak, J. A., Weissberg, R. P., Dymnicki, A. B., Taylor, R. D., & Schellinger, K. B. (2011). Enhancing students' social and emotional development promotes success in school: Results of a meta-analysis. *Child Development, 82*, 474–501.

Ellis, L. K., & Rothbart, M. K. (2001). *Revision of the adolescent temperament questionnaire*. Poster presented at the 2001 biennial meeting of the Society for Research in Child Development, Minneapolis, MN.

Humphrey, J. H. (1992). *Stress among women in modern society*. Springfield, IL: Charles C. Thomas.

Ingersoll, R., Merrill, L., & Stuckey, D. (2014). *Seven trends: The transformation of the teaching force, CPRE Report (#RR-80)*. Philadelphia, PA: Consortium for Policy Research in Education, University of Pennsylvania.

Jennings, P. A., & Greenberg, M. T. (2009). The prosocial classroom: Teacher social and emotional competence in relation to student and classroom outcomes. *Review of Educational Research, 79*, 491–525.

Jennings, P. A., Lantieri, L., & Roser, R. (2012). Chapter 12: Supporting educational goals through cultivating mindfulness approaches for teachers and students. In P. M. Brown, M. Corrigan, & A. Higgins-D'Alessandro (Eds.), Handbook of prosocial education. New York: Rowman & Littlefield.

Kabat-Zinn, J. (2004). Wherever you go, there you are: Mindfulness meditation for everyday life (p. 4). London: Piatkus.

Kemeny, M. E., Foltz, C., Cavanagh, J. F., Cullen, M., Giese-Davis, J., Jennings, P. A., et al. (2012). Contemplative/emotion training reduces negative emotional behavior and promotes prosocial responses. *Emotion, 12*, 338–350.

Kyriacou, C. (2001). Teacher stress: Directions for future research. *Educational Review, 53*, 27–35.

Lantieri, L. (2008). *Building emotional intelligence: Techniques to cultivate inner strength in children*. Boulder, CO: Sounds True.

Lantieri, L., & Nambiar, M. (2012). Cultivating the social, emotional and inner lives of children and teachers. *Reclaiming Children and Youth, 21*(2), 27–33.

Lantieri, L., Kyse, E. N., Harnett, S., & Malkmus, C. (2011). Building inner resilience in teachers and students. In G. M. Reevy & E. Frydenberg (Eds.), *Personality, stress and coping: Implications for education* (pp. 267–292). Charlotte, NC: Information Age.

Lutz, A., Brefczynski-Lewis, J., Johnstone, T., & Davidson, R. J. (2008). Regulation of the neural circuitry of emotion by compassion meditation: Effects of meditative expertise. *PLoS ONE, 3*(3), e1897.

Lutz, A., Slagter, H., Dunne, J., & Davidson, R. (2008). Attention regulation and monitoring in meditation. *Trends in Cognitive Science, 12*, 163–169.

Marzano, R. J., Marzano, J. S., & Pickering, D. J. (2003). *Classroom management that works*. Alexandria, VA: ASCD.

Maslach, C., Jackson, S. E., & Leiter, M. P. (1997). Maslach Burnout Inventory. In C. P. Zalaquett & R. J. Wood (Eds.), *Evaluating stress: A book of resources* (pp. 191–218). Lanham, MD: Scarecrow Education.

Metis Associates. (2011). *Building inner resilience in teachers and their students: Results of the Inner Resilience Pilot Program*. Unpublished evaluation report.

Murray, J. (2005). *Social-emotional climate and the success of new teachers: A new look at the ongoing challenge of new teacher retention (Wellesley Centers for Women, Report WCW 9)*. Wellesley, MA: Wellesley Centers for Women.

Roeser, R. W. (2014). The emergence of mindfulness-based interventions in educational settings. In S. Karabenick & T. Urdan (Eds.), *Advances in motivation and achievement* (Interventions, Vol. 18, pp. 379–419). Greenwich, CT: Emerald.

Roeser, R. W., & Zelazo, P. D. R. (2012). Contemplative science, education and child development: Introduction to the special section. *Child Development Perspectives, 6*, 143–145. doi:10.1111/j.1750-8606.2012.00242.x.

Roeser, R. W., Schonert-Reichl, K. A., Jha, A., Cullen, M., Wallace, L., Wilensky, R., et al. (2013). Mindfulness training and reduction in teacher stress and burnout: Results from two randomized, waitlist-control field trials. *Journal of Educational Psychology, 105*, 787–804.

Schonert-Reichl, K. A., & Weissberg, R. P. (2014). Social and emotional learning during childhood. In T. P. Gullotta & M. Bloom (Eds.), *Encyclopedia of primary prevention and health promotion* (2nd ed., pp. 936–949). New York, NY: Springer Press.

Simon, A., Harnett, S., Nagler, E., & Thomas, L. (2009). *Research on the effect of the Inner Resilience Program on teacher and student wellness and classroom culture*. Unpublished evaluation report.

Singer, T., & Lamm, C. (2009). The social neuroscience of empathy. *Annals of the New York Academy of Sciences, 1156*, 81–96.

Weissberg, R. P., & Cascarino, J. (2013). Academic learning + social-emotional learning = national priority. *Phi Delta Kappan, 95*, 8–13.

Weissberg, R. P., Payton, J. W., O'Brien, M. U., & Munro, S. (2007). Social and emotional learning. In F. C. Power, R. J. Nuzzi, D. Narvaez, D. K. Lapsley, & T. C. Hunt (Eds.), *Moral education: A handbook* (Vol. 2: M-Z, pp. 417–418). Westport, CT: Greenwood Press.

Winzelberg, A. J., & Luskin, F. M. (1999). The effect of a meditation training in stress levels in secondary school teachers. *Stress Medicine, 15*, 69–77.

CARE for Teachers: A Mindfulness-Based Approach to Promoting Teachers' Social and Emotional Competence and Well-Being

9

Patricia A. Jennings

Introduction

Teacher quality has grown to become a top priority of our national policy agenda of improving student academic achievement (Wilson et al., 2008). One important dimension of teacher quality involves psychological qualities such as kindness, patience, and flexibility associated with teachers' ability to provide emotional support to their students (Strong, 2011). Especially relevant to this section of this handbook is the mounting evidence that teachers' emotional support adds value to instructional support in narrowing the achievement gap among children at risk of school failure (Crosnoe et al., 2010; Hamre & Pianta, 2005; Howes et al., 2008; Pianta, Belsky, Vandergrift, Houts, & Morrison, 2008).

Emotional support encompasses classroom warmth and child-centeredness as well as teachers' responsivity towards specific children (NICHD-ECCRN, 2002, 2004). High-quality instructional support is characterized by interactions with students that are direct, intentional, focused, and characterized by feedback linked to student achievement (Hamre & Pianta, 2005). Teachers' skillful application of instructional and emotional support contributes to a classroom environment that promotes both prosocial behavior and academic success (Oliver & Reschly, 2007). Furthermore, student attachment to school predicts school success, especially among high-risk students, and teachers play a critical role in helping such students feel connected to their school by way of the emotional climate they create in the classroom (Bergin & Bergin, 2009).

However, teachers face challenges that undermine their ability to provide instructional and emotional support to their students. Growing numbers of children come to school unprepared, many with serious behavior problems (Gilliam, 2005; U.S. Department of Health and Human Services, 2000). Disruptive behavior is a problem particularly in classrooms of economically disadvantaged students (Oliver & Reschly, 2007), and the advent of accountability linked to high stakes testing may intensify teacher distress, especially among those who serve children at most risk of school failure (Darling-Hammond & Sykes, 2003).

Indeed, regulating negative emotional reactivity in response to challenging student behaviors is a major stressor for classroom teachers (Carson, Weiss, & Templin, 2010; Montgomery & Rupp, 2005; Sutton & Wheatley, 2003). Experiencing frequent negative emotions may reduce teachers' intrinsic motivation and teaching efficacy (Kavanagh & Bower, 1985). Over time, high levels of emotional stress can affect teachers' performance, may lead to burnout (Tsouloupas,

P.A. Jennings (✉)
Curry School of Education, University of Virginia, Charlottesville, VA, USA
e-mail: tishjennings@virginia.edu

K.A. Schonert-Reichl, R.W. Roeser (eds.), *Handbook of Mindfulness in Education*,
Mindfulness in Behavioral Health, DOI 10.1007/978-1-4939-3506-2_9

Carson, Matthews, Grawitch, & Barber, 2010), and may increase the likelihood of a downward spiral of deteriorating teacher performance and student behavior (Osher et al., 2007). In contrast, teachers who regularly experience more positive emotions may experience more resilience (Cohn, Brown, Fredrickson, Milkels, & Conway, 2009; Gu & Day, 2007).

Supporting teachers' well-being and their social and emotional competence (SEC) to manage stress and emotion reactivity in the context of the classroom may be key to optimizing their teaching effectiveness. Managing the social and emotional dynamics of the classroom in a manner that promotes a warm and caring emotional climate most conducive to learning requires that teachers regulate their emotional reactivity in response to student disruptions. Teachers function best when they can both downregulate intense negative emotions, such as anger and frustration, and upregulate positive emotions, such as enthusiasm and interest, in ways that do not threaten their health (Jennings, 2015).

Evidence supports the need for specialized professional development that promotes teachers' well-being and SEC to improve teachers' resilience and reduce their occupational stress, burnout, and attrition thereby improving teachers' capacity to provide well-organized and instructionally and emotionally supportive classrooms, especially in high-risk settings where the most beneficial impacts of such classrooms, as discussed above, are found for the most educationally vulnerable students (Jennings & Greenberg, 2009).

The Prosocial Classroom Model

We developed the Prosocial Classroom theoretical model to explicate the systemic importance of teachers' SEC and well-being for classroom and student impacts (Jennings & Greenberg, 2009; see Fig. 9.1). The model presents an organizational framework proposing that a teacher's well-being and SEC influence the classroom climate and student outcomes. This effect is mediated by the quality of teacher–student relationships, classroom management, and social and emotional learning (SEL) instruction. We used this model as a guide in the development and researching of professional development programs aimed at cultivating teachers SEC and well-being.

The Collaborative for Academic, Social, and Emotional Learning (CASEL) defines SEC in terms of five competencies: self-awareness, self-regulation, relationship skills, responsible decision-making, and social awareness (Zins, Weissberg, Wang, & Walberg, 2004). Two of these competencies, self-awareness and self-management, are intrapersonal skills. Self-awareness involves the ability to notice and monitor one's emotions, and the thoughts and physical sensations associated with them. It also involves the ability to accurately assess and accept one's strengths and weaknesses with self-compassion. Self-management involves the ability to self-regulate emotional reactivity and associated cognitions and behavior, even in the midst of emotionally provocative situations. Relationship skills, responsible decision-making, and social awareness are intrapersonal skills. Relationship skills include perspective-taking, empathy, and compassion, and facilitate the development and maintenance of supportive interpersonal relationships. The competency of responsible decision-making is the ability to apply relationships skills, self-regulation, and self-responsibility to considering situations and making decisions that take into account multiple needs and perspectives. Finally, the competency of social awareness involves the understanding of how social groups function.

The Prosocial Classroom model proposes that teachers with higher levels of SEC have more supportive relationships with their students, utilize more effective classroom management strategies and more effectively teach social and emotional skills to their students. Teachers who recognize and understand students' emotions and their associated cognitive appraisals are more able to understand their motivations and respond to their needs accordingly. For example, if a teacher understands that her student's disruptive behavior and emotional reactivity results from problems at home, she is better prepared to

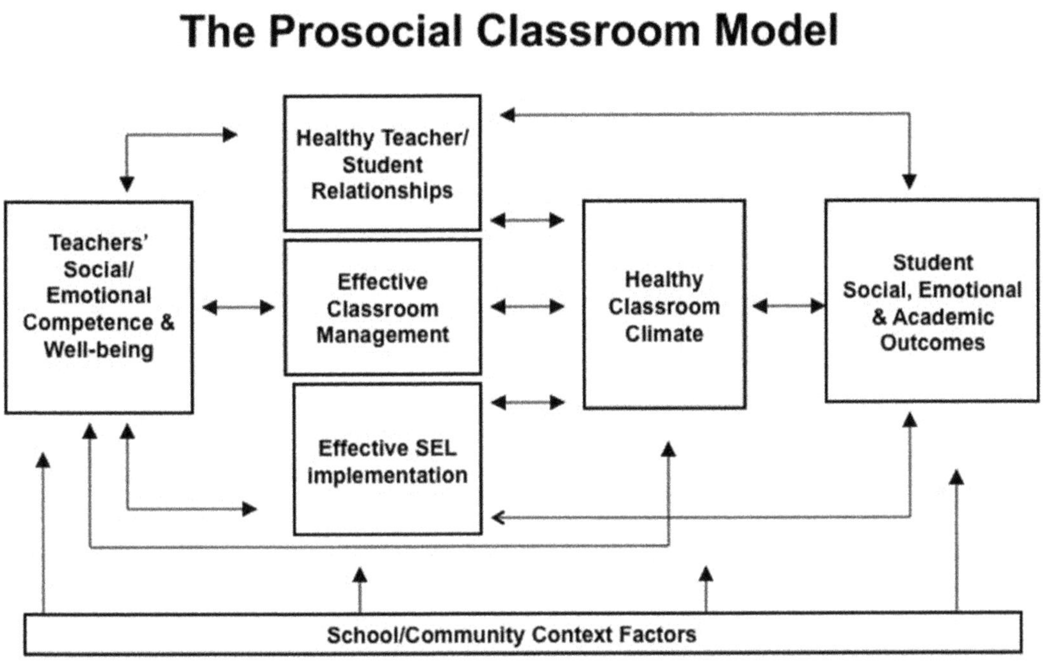

Fig. 9.1 A model of teacher well-being and social and emotional competence, support and classroom and student outcomes. From: Jennings, P.A. & Greenberg, M.T. (2009). The Prosocial classroom: Teacher social and emotional competence in relation to student and classroom outcomes. *Review of Educational Research, 79*: 491–525. Reprinted with permission from SAGE Publications, Inc.

express empathy and help him self-regulate rather than resort to punitive or coercive methods of discipline.

Teachers with higher levels of SEC can better manage their classrooms. These teachers are more authoritative and proactive, monitoring changes in children's engagement and skillfully using their expressions of positive affect and verbal support to promote enthusiasm for learning and to guide student behavior with positive reinforcement. Finally, teachers' SEC supports their ability to successfully teach SEL curriculum. They act as role models and coaches as they apply extensive process-based SEL learning activities in everyday situations as they naturally occur in the classroom.

The Prosocial Classroom model hypothesizes a transactional relationship between these three elements (teacher–child relationships, classroom management, and SEL) and a healthy classroom climate. Accordingly, a healthy classroom climate directly contributes to students' social, emotional, and academic outcomes. The healthy classroom climate may also reinforce a teacher's enjoyment of teaching, efficacy, and commitment to the profession thereby generating a positive feedback loop that may prevent teacher burnout.

Finally, the model hypothesizes that SEC is context dependent; the SEC of the average adult may not be adequate to successfully manage the specific social and emotional demands of the classroom. However, we propose that the SEC required for the classroom context can be developed through specific training (Jennings & Greenberg, 2009).

In line with the Prosocial Classroom model, teachers' SEC and well-being are hypothesized to be reflected in teachers' classroom behavior (e.g., teaching and management style, interactions with students). These interactions are a primary mechanism through which classroom experiences affect development; for example, teachers with higher levels of SEC may provide higher levels of classroom organization and emotional and instructional support associated with quality classroom climate (Hamre & Pianta, 2001).

Results of our research have begun to confirm the hypothesized relationships between teachers' SEC and well-being and quality classroom climate. In a study involving a sample of 35 preschool teachers, we found correlations between teachers' SEC and well-being, and dimensions of supportive classroom climate (Jennings, 2015). For this study, we operationalized SEC as high levels of self-reported mindfulness, self-compassion, and efficacy and well-being as high levels of self-reported positive affect and low levels of self-reported negative affect, depressive symptoms, and burnout.

To measure classroom climate, we used the pre-K version of the *Classroom Assessment Scoring System* (CLASS) observational measure of classroom climate (Pianta, La Paro, & Hamre, 2008). The pre-K CLASS rating system assesses three domains of classroom climate: (a) *emotional support*, (b) *classroom organization*, and (c) *instructional support*. Each domain is composed of dimensions that operationalize teacher–student and student–student interactions. *Emotional support* consists of the dimensions: *positive climate, negative climate, teacher sensitivity*, and *regard for student perspectives. Classroom organization* consists of the dimensions: *behavior management, productivity,* and *instructional learning formats. Instructional support* is composed of the dimensions: *concept development, quality of feedback,* and *language modeling.*

We conducted Pearson correlation analyses comparing scores on the self-report measures and scores on the three domains of the CLASS. Three of the five factors of the *Five Facet Mindfulness Questionnaire* (FFMQ; Baer, Smith, Hopkins, Krietemeyer, & Toney, 2006) and *self-compassion* as measured by the *Self-Compassion Scale* (SCS; Neff, 2003) were significantly correlated with the *emotional support* domain of the CLASS: *describe* ($r=.52$, $p<.01$), *aware* ($r=.50$, $p<.01$), *non-judge* ($r=.59$, $p<.01$), and *self-compassion* ($r=.38$, $p<.05$). None of the correlations between the FFMQ factors and *self-compassion* and the CLASS domains of *classroom organization* and *instructional support* were significant.

Personal efficacy, as measured by the *Teacher Efficacy Scale* (TES; Hoy & Woolfolk, 1990), and *positive affect* as measured by the *Positive and Negative Affect Schedule* (PANAS; Watson, Clark, & Tellegen, 1988), were significantly correlated with the *emotional support* domain of the CLASS ($r=.39$, $p<.05$ and $r=.40$, $p<.05$, respectively).

Two factors of burnout as measured by the *Maslach Burnout Inventory* (MBI; Maslach, Jackson, & Leiter, 1996) *emotional exhaustion* and *depersonalization* were significantly negatively correlated with *emotional support* ($r=-.35$, $p<.05$ and $r=-.46$, $p<.01$, respectively).

Depression as measured by the *Beck Depression Inventory* (BDI; Beck, Ward, Mendelson, Mock, & Erbaugh, 1961) was significantly negatively correlated with all three dimensions of the CLASS: *emotional support* ($r=-.42$, $p<.05$), *classroom organization* ($r=-.45$, $p<.01$), and *instructional support* ($r=-51$, $p<.01$).

These findings suggest that teachers who are happy, mindful and self-compassionate and who feel efficacious are more likely to create and maintain an emotionally supportive classroom climate. They also suggest that teacher burnout and depression may have adverse effects on classroom climate.

In the same study, we also found support for the hypothesized relationship between teachers' SEC and well-being, and teachers' attitudes associated with supportive teacher–student relationship quality. The same sample of teachers responded to interview questions about a student who they felt exhibited challenging behavior. These responses were coded to reflect patterns or internal working models of expectations, feelings, and beliefs that are reflected in teacher–student relationships following the interview and coding protocol from the *Teacher Relationship Interview* (TRI; Stuhlman & Pianta, 2001). The study focused on two dimensions of relationship quality: *perspective taking* and *sensitivity of discipline*.

The *observe* factor of the FFMQ was significantly correlated with *perspective taking* ($r = .37$, $p < .05$) and the *aware* factor of the FFMQ was significantly correlated with *sensitivity of discipline* ($r = .41$, $p < .05$). Both *personal efficacy* and *teaching efficacy* were significantly correlated with *sensitivity of discipline* ($r = .40$, $p < .05$, and $r = .35$, $p < .05$, respectively). The *depersonalization factor* of the MBI was significantly negatively correlated with *sensitivity of discipline* ($r = -.46$, $p < .01$). These results suggest that teachers who are more mindful and efficacious demonstrate more supportive attitudes towards those students whose behavior they find challenging. They also suggest that teachers who report high levels of *depersonalization* demonstrate less sensitivity in their attitudes towards the discipline of challenging students.

Mindful Awareness Practices May Promote SEC

Considering the high social and emotional demands of teaching, and the importance of teachers' SEC and well-being for high-quality classroom climates, it is surprising that teachers rarely receive instruction in SEC (Sutton & Wheatley, 2003). Although much intervention work has focused on the social–emotional skill development of students, little has focused on teachers' development in this area.

A promising approach for cultivating teachers' SEC and well-being is through mindfulness-based contemplative practices (Brown, Ryan, & Creswell, 2007; Grossman, Niemann, Schmidt, & Walach, 2004; Jennings, Lantieri, & Roeser, 2012; Kabat-Zinn, 1990). Consistent with our conceptualization of SEC, *mindful awareness practices* (MAPs) engage and promote self-awareness and self-regulation through a "non-elaborative, nonjudgmental, present-centered awareness in which each thought, feeling, or sensation that arises in the attentional field is acknowledged and accepted as it is" (Bishop et al., 2004, p. 232). This practice involves two primary mechanisms: *self-regulation of attention* and *non-judgmental awareness. Self-regulation of attention* promotes awareness of one's emotional and cognitive experience as it occurs moment-to-moment. *Non-judgmental awareness* is characterized by curiosity, openness, and acceptance of one's moment-to-moment experience.

Practicing mindfulness enhances self-regulatory processes that promote well-being and buffer against psychological distress (Jimenez, Niles, & Park, 2010). A recent study found that contemplative practice results in changes to the brain associated with more effective stress management. MRI brain scans taken before and after an 8-week Mindfulness-Based Stress Reduction (MBSR) program found increased gray matter in the hippocampus, an area important for learning and memory and a reduction of gray matter in the amygdala, a region associated with anxiety and stress. The control group participants who did not practice mindfulness showed no such changes (Hölzel et al., 2011).

Mindfulness may facilitate emotional self-awareness (Brown & Ryan, 2003) and contribute to engagement or *psychological presence*, defined as "feeling open to oneself and others, connected to work and others, complete rather than fragmented, and within rather than without the boundaries of a given role" (Kahn, 1992, p. 322). Thus, MAPs may support the ability to reflect upon one's internal and external experience from a broader perspective, one that allows for a wider variety of interpretations of and responses to stressful situations (Zelazo & Cunningham, 2007). As a result, mindfulness-based interventions (MBIs) may be ideally suited to the promotion of the teachers' SEC and well-being.

Since MBIs promote cognitive flexibility (Kashdan & Rottenberg, 2010) and self-reflection, they may help teachers overcome the tendency to make automatic, reactive appraisals of students' behavior that contribute to emotional exhaustion (Chang, 2009) and that may negatively impact the classroom emotional climate. In this way, developing greater mindful awareness may support both effective classroom management and caring.

Indeed his kind of *mental set* has been associated with effective classroom management (Marzano, Marzano, & Pickering, 2003).

Mindfulness-Based Approaches to Promoting Teachers' Well-Being and SEC

Over the past decade, several MBIs have been developed and tested with samples of teachers (Jennings et al., 2012). The Cultivating Emotional Balance (CEB) program was tested on a sample of teachers in 2005 and 2006 involving MAPs in combination with emotion skills training. CEB utilizes Ekman's (2004) Emotion Awareness Training system for teaching emotion awareness and mindfulness training developed by Wallace (2005). This hybrid intervention model involves 8 weeks (42 h) of training designed to reduce destructive enactment of the emotions and enhance empathy and compassion.

Tested on a sample of 82 female teachers (preK–12) utilizing a randomized, controlled trial design, the training significantly reduced self-reported depressive symptoms and rumination and increased emotional self-awareness (Kemeny et al., 2012). Female teachers were chosen for the study because measures of cortisol reactivity were included and there can be differential effects by sex. Since it would be difficult to recruit equal numbers of men and women teachers the researchers excluded men.

While the results of CEB have been promising, the intervention was not specifically designed for teachers or focused on improving their performance in the classroom: CEB is a generic model designed for use with any group of healthy adults. To examine whether changes in teachers' well-being found in the original CEB trial translate into improvements in teachers' classroom behavior and classroom climate, we performed a pilot randomized controlled trial examining classroom climate, attitudes towards challenging students, and teachers' SEC and well-being. Results replicated the previous findings that CEB improved teachers' well-being and demonstrated significant improvements in teachers' attitudes about students they reported as difficult. However, it did not demonstrate effects on teachers' classroom behavior or classroom climate, suggesting that MBIs and emotion skills training may need to be tailored to specifically address the particular challenges of teaching in order for them to change teaching behavior (Jennings, 2007).

CARE for Teachers

Building upon the CEB study and other research (Brown et al., 2007), the Garrison Institute in Garrison, New York began the development of a new intervention directed towards supporting teacher SEC and well-being as a means of improving classroom climate and student academic and social–emotional outcomes. Cultivating Awareness and Resilience in Education™ (CARE) was designed by a team of educators and scientific advisors to promote SEC and well-being to help teachers manage classroom stress and enliven their teaching in order to promote improvements in relationships with students, classroom management, and social–emotional learning.

The CARE program blends didactic instruction in the neuroscience of emotion with related experiential activities including time for group discussion and individual reflection. As a field-based in-service professional development program, CARE is typically presented during the school year in five daylong sessions. The first 4 days are spread out over 4–5 weeks, and a booster session is offered several months later. Facilitators coach teachers by phone and email between sessions to help them practice and apply new skills to their teaching. CARE is also offered to the public every summer in the form of a 5-day intensive retreat at the Garrison Institute.

The CARE Program Model

The CARE intervention aims to build teachers' SEC and well-being utilizing three primary instructional components: (a) emotion skills instruction, (b) mindfulness and stress reduction practices, and (c) listening and compassion exercises (Jennings, 2011). Each component is described in detail below.

Emotion Skills Instruction Emotional exhaustion is a major contributor to teacher burnout and often interferes with teachers' functioning (Byrne, 1994). To address this problem, CARE introduces emotion skills instruction drawn from the neuroscience of emotion involving a combination of didactic instruction and experiential activities (e.g., reflective practices and role-plays) to support teachers' recognition of emotional states and exploration of their *emotional landscapes*—their habitual emotional patterns. CARE aims to help teachers to be more sensitive to students' needs, more aware of classroom emotional climate, and more able to regulate their emotions while managing provocative behavior. To promote resilience and the ability to reappraise emotionally challenging situations, CARE introduces the practice of self-induction of positive emotions (Cohn et al., 2009).

Mindfulness/Stress Reduction Practices CARE introduces a series of MAPs, beginning with short periods of silent reflection and extending to activities that bring mindfulness into aspects of daily living such as standing, walking, being present in front of a group, and listening to others. This series of activities culminates in mindful role-plays where teachers apply CARE skills to challenging situations that they face in their work settings. Through these activities, teachers learn to bring mindful awareness to their classroom management and their relationships with students, parents, and colleagues.

Caring and Listening Practices To promote empathy and compassion, CARE introduces *caring practice* and *mindful listening*. A secularized adaptation of the Buddhist *loving-kindness practice* or *metta*, caring practice involves silent reflection focused on generating feelings of care for self and others. Practiced over time this activity produces increases in daily experiences of positive emotions and decreased illness and depressive symptoms (Fredrickson, Coffey, Pek, Cohn, & Finkel, 2008). Mindful listening exercises develop the skill to simply listen to another and apply mindful awareness to emotional reactions, such as urges to offer advice or judge, without acting upon them. These exercises are designed to help teachers listen more effectively to students and respond with greater sensitivity, especially during conflict situations where a calm, supportive presence can support conflict resolution.

CARE Logic Model The CARE program was designed to promote teachers' social and emotional development and well-being as hypothesized in the project logic model (Fig. 9.2). The CARE program elements are designed to improve teachers' well-being, efficacy, mindfulness, and to improve the classroom climate (e.g., classroom organization, instructional support, and emotional support). The model proposes that these teacher and classroom improvements reinforce each other and contribute to improvements in students' academic and social and emotional skills. Finally, it is expected that CARE will have a direct effect on student outcomes.

Research

Development and Evaluation Research In response to ongoing program evaluation, teachers overwhelmingly report that they enjoy CARE and find that it helps them deal with the emotions of teaching, resulting in improvements in classroom management and relationships with their students. The first pilot program was offered to a group of 17 public school teachers in Denver, CO. All the participants reported that the program benefited their professional lives. In response to open-ended questions about how the program had affected them, one teacher shared that CARE was "the most valuable, personally rewarding and important class that [she has] ever

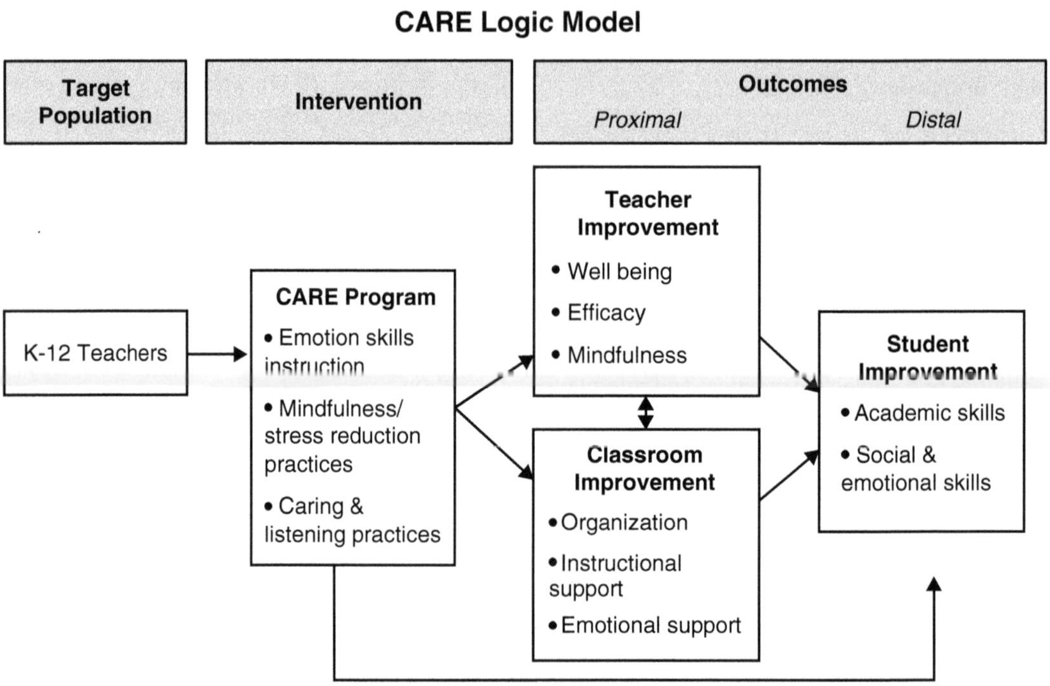

Fig. 9.2 CARE logic model

taken." Another teacher commented, "I am more grounded and focused and able to deal better with uncomfortable situations that arise in my classroom." According to another, "Now I have the tools to stay calm, reflective, appreciative, joyful and grateful every day, which will help me interact positively with my students and colleagues." Another wrote, "I am learning to slow down, wait and respond rather than react. I am also taking better care of myself."

A middle school teacher from this sample applied the caring practice to help him deal with his frustration and uncomfortable feelings in response to a difficult class. He wrote:

> I am amazed at how the exploration of caring practice has changed my relationship with students. After focusing on the most challenging students in my "bad" class, things have started to change. This was the class that I used to dislike, grudgingly waiting for it to come every day, hoping that the challenging students may be absent. These feelings began to diminish as I used the caring practice in private, and I think the students noticed the subtle change. I have been in a much better mood when this class arrives, instead of immediately being on the defensive and anticipating a problem. This has increased my use of humor and personal talk with the students.

In April 2009, Wellspring conducted an evaluation of a series of summer retreats at the Garrison Institute in New York and a program offered to teachers at a private school outside of Philadelphia. Eighty-five participants with valid email addresses (out of 93 total participants) were invited to take the online evaluation survey (Jennings, 2011).

Most of the responding participants found CARE to be valuable and reported being highly likely or likely to recommend CARE to a colleague. Eighty-four percent said that CARE was highly important or important for their professional development, and 87 % strongly agreed or agreed that all teachers should receive this training. Comments included the following:

> I now have a calm and unshakable feeling that is deep within me, and this helps me to stay present, grounded, focused, creative, and thankful for each of the little miracles that I experience each and every day!
>
> I found the time to be some of the best spent time on training that I have had. I have implemented the strategies that I learned throughout a very difficult year and have offered some of the ideas to my colleagues and my student teachers.

> The interpersonal (listening) work was very powerful. Most professional trainings lack this type of experiential component, which is the type of learning that stays with me.
>
> I am much more present with my students throughout the day. I'm aware when emotions start to take over in a positive or negative way. This awareness helps me respond rather than react to a situation.

One teacher explained how CARE helped her be more responsive to a disruptive student:

> CARE has given me the tools and skills to be more calm and centered. In a particular situation, I can act in response to what is needed in the moment rather than reacting to it. Taking deep breaths, I can calm myself down and notice what feelings his comments are triggering in me. I can see beyond his behavior (shouting, swearing, interrupting the class) into his feelings and the needs behind those feelings which triggered his reaction. This way of relating to myself and others is a more compassionate way that leads to open and honest communication. This provides a model to the student of how to relate to himself and to others with compassion. It creates an atmosphere of confidence, trust, and more joy in the classroom. (Jennings, 2011, p. 40)

In 2008, the U.S. Department of Education Institute of Educational Sciences (IES) awarded Pennsylvania State University and the Garrison Institute funding to complete the development and preliminary evaluation of CARE. A series of studies were conducted to examine whether CARE improves teachers' and student teachers' well-being and SEC and consequently whether it improves their ability to create and maintain a well-managed learning environment and provide optimal emotional and instructional support to their students (for full details of these studies see Jennings, Snowberg, Coccia, & Greenberg, 2011; Jennings, Frank, Snowberg, Coccia, & Greenberg, 2013; Schussler, Jennings, Sharp, & Frank, 2015).

The studies involved three samples: two samples of urban teachers working in high poverty schools ($N=39$ and 50) and one sample of student teachers and some of their mentors working in more affluent suburban and semi-rural schools ($N=43$). For these studies, we utilized most of the same measures reported above (Jennings, 2014), but we added a measure of time urgency to operationalize well-being (e.g., we hypothesized that lower levels of time urgency would be evidence of well-being).

Studies 1 and 2 are reported in Jennings et al. (2011). In Study 1, we examined pre-post CARE changes among a sample of 31 teachers working in the urban setting. Two factors on the *Time Urgency Scale* (TUS; Landy, Rastegary, Thayer, & Colvin, 1991) showed significant ($p<.10$) change: *task-related hurry* ($d=.24$) and *general hurry* ($d=.27$), suggesting that teachers felt reduced stress associated with time demands. The most consistent significant effects were found among measures of mindfulness. We found significant ($p<.10$) improvement at post-test for the five facets of the FFMQ ranging in effect size from $d=.21$ to .94 and the *Mindfulness in Teaching Scale* (MTS; Frank, Jennings, & Greenberg, 2015) scores improved at post-test with an effect size of $d=.48$.

As expected, urban teachers found CARE to be enjoyable and beneficial to their teaching. Overall, participants reported high levels of satisfaction with the program and found it helpful in improving their classroom management and relationships with students. A majority reported improvements in their students' behavior and academic performance as a result of participating in CARE. Focus group data supported the program satisfaction findings and revealed that as a result of CARE, teachers developed a greater awareness of their stress and emotional reactivity and cultivated skills to better self-regulate in the midst of their busy working lives.

Study 2 involved a sample of student teachers and their mentors from a suburban/semi-rural district. This sub-study included random assignment to CARE or a wait-list control condition. At the pretest period, two groups were created from 43 subjects: a treatment group consisting of 16 students and five mentors and a control group consisting of 16 students and six mentors. In addition to the self-report measures used with the urban sample, the classrooms of these student teachers and their mentors were observed and rated using the CLASS measure (Pianta, La Paro & Hamre, 2008).

In this study, we hypothesized that CARE student teachers and their mentors would report higher levels of autonomy supportiveness than controls. To test this hypothesis, we utilized the *Problems in Schools Questionnaire* (PIS; Deci, Schwartz, Sheinman, & Ryan, 1981). The PIS is based on Ryan and Deci's (2000) self-determination theory and assesses whether teachers are oriented towards controlling their students' behavior versus supporting their autonomy as it relates to promoting intrinsic motivation. In support of our hypothesis, we found a significant treatment effect on the PIS motivating total score ($p < .05$; $d = .63$).

However, contrary to our expectations, we found no significant treatment effects on measures of mindfulness or the dimensions of the CLASS. These student teachers and mentors did not report the same high level of satisfaction as found among the urban sample. Furthermore, the student teachers and mentors did not report high levels of engagement with the program nor the same beneficial personal or professional outcomes.

Several factors may elucidate the differences in findings across the two samples. The urban and suburban/semi-rural school environments are enormously different. The urban schools serve high-poverty neighborhoods with large numbers of children with behavioral and academic difficulties that put them at risk of school failure. These teachers reported that they had marginal institutional support. In contrast, student teachers and mentors worked in suburban/semi-rural school environments with lower numbers of children at-risk and stronger institutional support. The district was stable and well funded by a high local tax rate and had very low teacher turnover. Indeed, the mentor teachers were chosen to become mentors based upon their exceptional performance, and they reported that CARE did not provide new information but served as a reminder of an orientation that was familiar to them.

Although student teachers reported having high levels of stress associated with the pressure of academic performance (lesson plans, coursework, and performance evaluations), it is notable that CARE did not appear to be as relevant to their current needs as it did to the urban sample. Sharing the program with mentors may have inhibited the uptake of the material by the student teachers, who may have been reluctant to openly express their concerns about classroom difficulties in the presence of their mentors. It may be especially important to take social hierarchies into account when planning and delivering such programs, as the presence of supervisors may inhibit participation. Furthermore, mentors, chosen for their superior teaching, may have provided a buffer for the student teachers, protecting them from the occupational stress that the urban sample of teachers reported. These contrasting results suggest that CARE may need modification to be helpful to student teachers.

During the second year of the IES-funded project, we conducted a pilot randomized, controlled trial involving 50 teachers from the same urban setting as Study 1 (Study 3) (Jennings et al., 2013). We randomly assigned teachers to receive CARE ($n = 23$) or become part of a wait-list control group ($n = 27$). To operationalize and measure well-being, we added the *Emotion Regulation Questionnaire* (Gross & John, 2003), the *Maslach Burnout Inventory* (MBI; Maslach et al., 1996), and *Daily Physical Symptoms* (DPS; Larsen & Kasimatis, 1997) to our self-report battery. A series of ANCOVAs, controlling for baseline measures, indicated that significant intervention effects were found on the *reappraisal* subscale of the ERQ ($F(1, 47) = 10.9$, $p = .002$; $d = .80$), and the DPS ($F(1, 47) = 10.2$, $p = .002$; $d = -.32$). Contrary to our hypothesis, we did not find intervention effects on the PANAS or a measure of depression, the *Center for Epidemiologic Studies Depression Scale* (CES-D-20; Radloff, 1977).

Significant and positive intervention effects were found for the total score on the *Teachers' Sense of Efficacy Questionnaire* (TSES; Tschannen-Moran & Woolfolk Hoy, 2001) ($F(1, 47) = 10.6$, $p = .002$; $d = .60$), efficacy in *student engagement* ($F(1, 47) = 10.3$, $p = .002$; $d = .56$), and sense of efficacy in *instruction* ($F(1, 47) = 11.6$, $p = .001$; $d = .59$). However, no significant intervention effects were found on the efficacy in *classroom management* subscale ($F(1, 47) = 2.3$, $p = .13$; $d = .24$).

Significant intervention effects were found on the *general hurry* subscale of the TUS ($F(1, 47)=5.4$, $p=.025$; $d=-.42$) and the *personal accomplishment* subscale of the MBI ($F(1, 47)=3.9$, $p=.05$; $d=.40$). Significant intervention effects were found for the *observe* ($F(1, 47)=9.8$, $p=.003$; $d=.69$) and *non-react* ($F(1, 47)=8.4$, $p=.006$; $d=.73$) subscales of the FFMQ. Significant intervention effects were also found on the FFMQ summary mindfulness score (average of all items) ($F(1, 47)=4.29$, $p=.044$, $d=.56$).

As in Study 1, CARE was well received by the participants. Most (93 %) reported that they "strongly agreed" or "agreed" that this type of program should be integrated into preparation and in-service training for all teachers. Participants reported that CARE improved their self-awareness (97 %, $n=28$) and well-being (93 %, $n=27$). Most "strongly agreed" or "agreed" that as a result of CARE they are "better able to manage classroom behaviors effectively and compassionately" (83 %, $n=24$) and are "better able to establish and maintain supportive relationships" with their students (79 %, $n=23$). Finally, participants noticed improvements in their students' ("much better" or "better") prosocial behavior (74 %, $n=20$), on-task behavior (74 %, $n=20$), and academic performance (65 %, $n=17$) as a result of their participation in CARE.

To better understand the mechanisms through which the CARE program affected teachers' self-awareness, self-regulation, and aspects of their physical and emotional health, we conducted focus groups with the teachers who received CARE after the last quantitative data collection period was complete. There were four focus groups with 5–8 members each. These data were analyzed using explanatory design (McMillan, 2004).

In the focus groups, teachers described becoming more aware of how they physically held stress and also how they could alleviate it. For example, one participant said, "It has made me more aware of my posture before it gets to the headache. I better do some shoulder rolls or take some breaths."

Some participants expressed recognition of the connection between their awareness of their physical stress and their awareness of their mental state of being. For example, one participant said, "I think [CARE] helps you make that connection between your physical feelings and your mental state of being.... When you feel tired, to realize that that's affecting how you are going to think about things and how you are going to react to things in turn. I think it heightens the awareness of that."

Teachers described how they became more aware of how they responded to others, especially their students. For example one teacher said, "I'm quicker to catch things coming out of my mouth or quicker to not react as fast which helps in the classroom.... I think it has helped me work through some of my ADHD tendencies of wanting to jump all the time, to think and be mindful of what and how I'm feeling and reacting."

Participants reported that CARE helped them to become more aware of their emotions which then helped them to regulate their negative emotions. They reported that being able to maintain a more neutral, less emotionally charged state helped them relate to their students more effectively (Schussler et al., 2015).

Although further research is necessary to fully understand CARE's effects for teachers working under various conditions, the results of Study 3 suggest that CARE is a promising intervention to support teachers experiencing the emotional stress of working in challenging settings. In this way, CARE may begin to address an important professional development need that has been long ignored by the education research community.

CARE's Affect on Classroom Climate and Student Outcomes To examine whether CARE's affect on teachers' SEC and well-being might translate into improvements in classroom climates and student behavioral and academic outcomes as suggested by the Prosocial Classroom model, we were awarded a second grant from IES to conduct a large efficacy trial of

CARE in the context of 36 schools across two cohorts of teachers located in high poverty neighborhoods of a large city located on the East Coast of the United States. Teachers were randomly assigned within schools to receive CARE or be part of a wait-list control group.

During the first year of this study (Cohort 1), we collected data from 51 teachers from 8 schools randomly assigned within schools to CARE ($n=25$) or a wait list control condition ($n=28$). Participants completed a battery of self-report measures at pre- and post-intervention to assess the impact of the CARE program on well-being, efficacy, burnout/time pressure, and mindfulness. ANCOVAs were computed between the CARE group and control group for each outcome, and the pretest scores served as a covariate.

Considering the limited sample size of Cohort 1, the preliminary results showed promise. Compared to teachers assigned to the control group, CARE participants were significantly ($p<.05$) less anxious ($d=-.77$) as measured by the *Generalized Anxiety Disorder* scale (Spitzer, Kroenke, Williams, & Lowe, 2006). They also reported a significantly ($p<.01$) reduced sense of *task-related hurry* ($d=-.40$) as measured by the TUS. We found significant ($p<.05$) increases in the *non-react* factor ($d=.44$) of the FFMQ and *total efficacy score* on the TES ($d=.27$).

There were trends towards improvements in *positive affect* as measured by the PANAS ($p=.12$, $d=.26$), *depression* ($p=.12$, $d=-.77$), as measured by the *Patient Health Questionnaire* (Kroenke & Spitzer, 2002), *emotional exhaustion* ($p=.15$, $d=-.59$), and *depersonalization* ($p=.12$, $d=-.26$) factors of the MBI, *sleep* as measured by the *Perceived Sleep Scale* ($p=.15$, $d=.55$), the *non-react* dimension of FFMQ and the *interpersonal awareness* dimension of MTS ($p=.08$, $d=.77$) (Jennings et al., 2014).

At the time of this writing, we had completed the collection of pre-post data on all 226 teachers (117 assigned to the intervention group and 107 assigned to the control group), their classrooms, and 5036 of their students. One more wave of follow-up data collection is scheduled for the fall of 2014 and preliminary data analyses are currently underway. These data will allow us to test our hypotheses that teachers' participation in CARE has intervention effects on teachers, classrooms, and students and whether levels of risk among students moderate the effects of CARE on student outcomes.

Evaluation of Fidelity Fidelity measures were developed and piloted in preparation for Cohort 2 of the study described above which required two CARE programs delivered concurrently, only one of which was presented by a program developer. The *CARE Daily Session Fidelity Rating Form* was created to evaluate the percentage of core intervention components covered during the training, the degree to which participant objectives were achieved, and the time spent on each activity of the program. Quality of delivery was assessed with the *CARE Facilitator Skill Rating Form*. Participant engagement, knowledge of concepts, and satisfaction with the program were also assessed. Two project staff who helped develop the fidelity measures observed and rated the Cohort 1 CARE program with high interrater reliability (>80 %).

The Cohort 1 CARE program was presented with a high degree of fidelity to the intervention model. Ninety percent of the core components were covered and most participant objectives were met each day of training. As expected, of the 30 h spent in training, 6.5 were spent engaging in experiential and mindfulness practices. Participant engagement was high. Participating teachers attended an average of 4.22 (out of 5) days and scored high on the knowledge assessments ($M=95$ %). The overall mean facilitator rating for the entire program was 3.66 out of 4 (Doyle, Jennings, DeWeese, & Frank, 2014). Results from the second cohort are being analyzed at the time of this writing.

Future Directions

Given the high social and emotional demands of teaching, plus the high costs of teacher attrition, it is surprising that little work has explored teacher stress and burnout and how to prevent it. Indeed, it is surprising that there has never been a large longitudinal study of teacher career development in the USA.

While there is strong evidence that nearly 50 % of teachers leave the profession within their first 5 years of teaching (Ingersoll, 2003; National Commission on Teaching and America's Future, 1996), there is little understanding regarding what factors contribute to this high level of attrition and what types of interventions might reduce it. Furthermore, evidence suggests that job satisfaction among teachers is in steep decline. In 2013, MetLife Survey of the American Teacher reported:

> Teachers are less satisfied with their careers; in the past two years there has been a significant decline in teachers' satisfaction with their profession. In one of the most dramatic findings of the report, teacher satisfaction has decreased by 15 points since the MetLife Survey of the American Teacher measured job satisfaction two years ago, now reaching the lowest level of job satisfaction seen in the survey series in more than two decades. This decline in teacher satisfaction is coupled with large increases in the number of teachers who indicate that they are likely to leave teaching for another occupation and in the number who do not feel their jobs are secure. (MetLife, 2013, p. 3)

These data are alarming and point to the urgent need for larger and more comprehensive studies of teacher development and occupational stress. Research is needed to better understand the development and nature of teacher stress and burnout and to find the appropriate means for providing the skills to teachers to help them develop the resilience to maintain their commitment to the profession. Both longitudinal and intervention studies are required to better understand the personal characteristics associated with burnout and teacher performance and to explore what interventions may be most helpful to teachers at various stages in their careers, including pre-service teacher education.

While more research is needed to explore the mechanisms of teacher stress and how MAPs may help reduce stress and improve teachers' performance, preliminary research has demonstrated that MBIs show promise. The growing body of research pointing to the effectiveness of mindfulness in reducing stress and promoting well-being supports the movement to apply a mindfulness-based approach to teacher professional development. Mindfulness-based approaches are also being applied to supporting students' stress reduction and learning. Indeed, mindfulness may be key to helping both teachers and students develop the resilience they need to maintain optimal affective and cognitive states for teaching and learning.

References

Baer, R. A., Smith, G. T., Hopkins, J., Krietemeyer, J., & Toney, L. (2006). Using self-report assessment methods to explore facets of mindfulness. *Assessment, 13*, 27–45.

Beck, A. T., Ward, C. H., Mendelson, M., Mock, J., & Erbaugh, J. (1961). An inventory for measuring depression. *Archives of General Psychiatry, 4*, 561–571.

Bergin, C., & Bergin, D. (2009). Attachment in the classroom. *Educational Psychology Review, 21*, 141–170.

Bishop, S. R., Lau, M., Shapiro, S., Carlson, L., Anderson, N., Carmody, J., ... Devins, G. (2004). Mindfulness: A proposed operational definition. *Clinical Psychology: Science and Practice, 11*, 230–241.

Brown, K. W., & Ryan, R. M. (2003). The benefits of being present: Mindfulness and its role in psychological wellbeing. *Journal of Personality and Social Psychology, 84*, 822–848.

Brown, K. W., Ryan, R. M., & Creswell, J. D. (2007). Mindfulness: Theoretical foundations and evidence for its salutary effects. *Psychological Inquiry, 18*, 211–237.

Byrne, B. M. (1994). Burnout: Testing for the validity, replication, and invariance of causal structure across elementary, intermediate, and secondary teachers. *American Educational Research Journal, 31*, 645–673.

Carson, R. L., Weiss, H. M., & Templin, T. J. (2010). Ecological momentary assessment: A research method for studying the daily lives of teachers. *International Journal of Research & Method in Education, 33*, 165–182.

Chang, M. L. (2009). An appraisal perspective of teacher burnout: Examining the emotional work of teachers. *Educational Psychology Review, 21*, 193–218.

Cohn, M. A., Brown, S. L., Fredrickson, B. L., Milkels, J. A., & Conway, A. M. (2009). Happiness unpacked: Positive emotions increase life satisfaction by building resilience. *Emotion, 9*, 361–368.

Crosnoe, R., Morrison, F., Burchinal, M., Pianta, R. C., Keating, D., Friedman, S. L., & Clarke-Stewart, K. A. (2010). Instruction, teacher-student relations, and math achievement trajectories in elementary school. *Journal of Educational Psychology, 102*(2), 407–417.

Darling-Hammond, L., & Sykes, G. (2003). Wanted: A national teacher supply policy for education: The right way to meet the "highly qualified teacher" challenge. *Education Policy Analysis Archives, 11*(33), 1–55.

Deci, E. L., Schwartz, A. J., Sheinman, L., & Ryan, R. M. (1981). An instrument to assess adults' orientations toward control versus autonomy with children: Reflections on intrinsic motivation and perceived competence. *Journal of Educational Psychology, 73*, 642–650.

Doyle, S., Jennings, P. A., DeWeese, A., & Frank, J. (2014, May). *Evaluating the fidelity of the Cultivating Awareness and Resilience in Education (CARE) program.* Poster presented at the Society for Prevention Research 2014 annual meeting, Washington, DC.

Ekman, P. (2004). *Emotions revealed* (2nd ed.). New York, NY: Times Books.

Frank, J. L., Jennings, P. A., & Greenberg, M. T. (2015). Validation of the mindfulness in teaching scale Published online: doi: 10.1007/s12671-015-0461-0.

Fredrickson, B. L., Coffey, K. A., Pek, J., Cohn, M. A., & Finkel, S. M. (2008). Open hearts build lives: Positive emotions, induced through loving-kindness meditation, build consequential personal resources. *Journal of Personality and Social Psychology, 95*, 1045–1062.

Gilliam, W. S. (2005). *Prekindergarteners left behind: Expulsion rates in state prekindergarten programs.* New York, NY: Foundation for Child Development.

Gross, J. J., & John, O. P. (2003). Individual differences in two emotion regulation processes: Implications for affect, relationships, and well-being. *Journal of Personality and Social Psychology, 85*, 348–362.

Grossman, P., Niemann, L., Schmidt, S., & Walach, H. (2004). Mindfulness-based stress reduction and health benefits: A meta-analysis. *Journal of Psychosomatic Research, 57*, 35–43.

Gu, Q., & Day, C. (2007). Teachers' resilience: A necessary condition for effectiveness. *Teaching and Teacher Education, 23*, 1302–1316.

Hamre, B., & Pianta, R. C. (2001). Early teacher-child relationships and trajectory of school outcomes through eighth grade. *Child Development, 72*, 625–638.

Hamre, B. K., & Pianta, R. C. (2005). Can instructional and emotional support in the first-grade classroom make a difference for children at risk of school failure? *Child Development, 76*, 949–967.

Hölzel, B. K., Carmody, J., Vangela, M., Congletona, C., Yerramsettia, S. M., Garda, T., & Lazar, S. W. (2011). Mindfulness practice leads to increases in regional brain gray matter density. *Psychiatry Research: Neuroimaging, 191*, 36–43.

Howes, C., Burchinal, M., Pianta, R. C., Bryant, D., Early, D., Clifford, R., & Barbarin, O. (2008). Ready to learn? Children's pre-academic achievement in pre-Kindergarten programs. *Early Childhood Research Quarterly, 23*, 27–50.

Hoy, W. K., & Woolfolk, A. E. (1990). Organizational socialization of student teachers. *American Educational Research Journal, 27*, 279–300.

Ingersoll, R. M. (2003). *Is there really a teacher shortage?* Seattle, WA: University of Washington Center for the Study of Teaching and Policy.

Jennings, P. A. (2007). Cultivating emotional balance in the classroom. In M. Utne O'Brien, Chair. *Supporting school-based prevention programs by promoting teacher social-emotional competence.* Symposium presented at the 115th annual convention of the American Psychological Association, San Francisco, CA.

Jennings, P. A. (2011). Promoting teachers' social and emotional competencies to support performance and reduce burnout. In A. Cohan & A. Honigsfeld (Eds.), *Breaking the mold of pre-service and in-service teacher education: Innovative and successful practices for the 21st century* (pp. 133–143). New York, NY: Rowman and Littlefield.

Jennings, P. A. (2015). Early childhood teachers' well-being, mindfulness and self-compassion in relation to classroom quality and attitudes towards challenging students. *Mindfulness, 6*(4), 732–743. doi:10.1007/s12671-014-0312-4.

Jennings, P. A. (2015). *Mindfulness for teachers: Simple skills for peace and productivity in the classroom.* New York, NY: W. W. Norton.

Jennings, P. A., Brown, J. L., Frank, J. L., Doyle, S. L., Tanler, R., Rasheed, D., … Greenberg, M. T. (2014, March). Promoting teachers' social and emotional competence: The Cultivating Awareness and Resilience in Education (CARE) program. In A. R. Harris (Chair), *Mindfulness-based approaches for supporting teachers' social and emotional skills and dispositions.* Symposium presented at the American Education Research Association 2014 annual meeting, Philadelphia, PA.

Jennings, P. A., Frank, J. L., Snowberg, K. E., Coccia, M. A., & Greenberg, M. T. (2013). Improving classroom learning environments by Cultivating Awareness and Resilience in Education (CARE): Results of a randomized controlled trial. *School Psychology Quarterly, 28*, 374–390. doi:10.1037/spq0000035.

Jennings, P. A., & Greenberg, M. T. (2009). The prosocial classroom: Teacher social and emotional competence in relation to student and classroom outcomes. *Review of Educational Research, 79*, 491–525.

Jennings, P. A., Lantieri, L., & Roeser, R. (2012). Supporting educational goals through cultivating mindfulness: Approaches for teachers and students. In A. Higgins-D'Alessandro, M. Corrigan, & P. M. Brown (Eds.), *The handbook of prosocial education* (pp. 371–397). New York, NY: Rowman and Littlefield.

Jennings, P. A., Snowberg, K. E., Coccia, M. A., & Greenberg, M. T. (2011). Improving classroom learning environments by Cultivating Awareness and Resilience in Education (CARE): Results of two pilot studies. *Journal of Classroom Interaction, 46*, 37–48.

Jimenez, S. S., Niles, B. L., & Park, C. L. (2010). A mindfulness model of affect regulation and depressive symptoms: Positive emotions, mood regulation expectancies, and self-acceptance as regulatory

mechanisms. *Personality and Individual Differences, 49*, 645–650.
Kabat-Zinn, J. (1990). *Full catastrophe living: Using the wisdom of your body and mind to face stress, pain, and illness*. New York, NY: Bantam Doubleday Dell.
Kahn, W. A. (1992). To be fully there: Psychological presence at work. *Human Relations, 45*, 321–349.
Kashdan, T. B., & Rottenberg, J. (2010). Psychological flexibility as a fundamental aspect of health. *Clinical Psychology Review, 30*, 865–878.
Kavanagh, D. J., & Bower, G. (1985). Mood and self-efficacy: Impact of joy and sadness on perceived capabilities. *Cognitive Therapy and Research, 9*, 507–525.
Kemeny, M. E., Foltz, C., Ekman, P., Jennings, P. A., Rosenberg, E., Gillath, O., ... Wallace, A. (2012). Contemplative/emotion training improves emotional life. *Emotion, 12*, 338–350.
Kroenke, K., & Spitzer, R. L. (2002). The PHQ-9: A new depression diagnostic and severity measure. *Psychiatric Annals, 32*, 1–7.
Landy, F. J., Rastegary, H., Thayer, J., & Colvin, C. (1991). Time urgency: The construct and its measurement. *Journal of Applied Psychology, 76*, 644–657.
Larsen, R. J., & Kasimatis, M. (1997). Day-to-day physical symptoms: Individual differences in the occurrence, duration, and emotional concomitants of minor daily illnesses. *Journal of Personality, 59*, 387–423.
Marzano, R. J., Marzano, J. S., & Pickering, D. J. (2003). *Classroom management that works*. Alexandra, VA: Association for Supervision and Curriculum Development.
Maslach, C., Jackson, S. E., & Leiter, M. P. (1996). Maslach burnout inventory. In C. P. Zalaquett & R. J. Wood (Eds.), *Evaluating stress: A book of resources* (pp. 191–218). Lanham, MD: Scarecrow Education.
McMillan, J. H. (2004). *Educational research: Fundamentals for the consumer* (4th ed.). Boston, MA: Pearson.
MetLife. (2013). *The MetLife survey of the American teacher*. New York, NY: MetLife.
Montgomery, C., & Rupp, A. A. (2005). A meta-analysis for exploring the diverse causes and effects of stress in teachers. *Canadian Journal of Education, 28*, 458–486.
National Commission on Teaching and America's Future. (1996). *What matters most: Teaching for America's future*. New York, NY: Author.
Neff, K. D. (2003). Development and validation of a scale to measure self-compassion. *Self and Identity, 2*, 223–250.
NICHD-ECCRN. (2002). The relation of first grade classroom environment to structural classroom features, teacher, and student behaviors. *Elementary School Journal, 102*, 367–387.
NICHD-ECCRN. (2004). Does class size in first grade relate to changes in child academic and social performance or observed classroom processes? *Developmental Psychology, 40*, 651–664.
Oliver, R. M., & Reschly, D. J. (2007). *Effective classroom management: Teacher preparation and professional development*. Washington, DC: National Comprehensive Center for Teacher Quality.
Osher, D., Sprague, J., Weissberg, R. P., Axelrod, J., Keenan, S., & Kendziora, K. T. (2007). A comprehensive approach to promoting social, emotional, and academic growth in contemporary schools. In A. Thomas & J. Grimes (Eds.), *Best practices in school psychology* (5th ed., Vol. 4). Bethesda, MD: National Association of School Psychologists.
Pianta, R. C., Belsky, J., Vandergrift, N., Houts, R., & Morrison, F. (2008). Classroom effects on children's achievement trajectories in elementary school. *American Educational Research Journal, 45*, 365–397.
Pianta, R. C., La Paro, K. M., & Hamre, B. (2008). *Classroom assessment scoring system*. Baltimore, MD: Brooks.
Radloff, L. S. (1977). The CES-D scale: A self report depression scale for research in the general population. *Applied Psychological Measurement, 1*, 385–401.
Ryan, R. M., & Deci, E. L. (2000). Self-determination theory and the facilitation of intrinsic motivation, social development, and well-being. *American Psychologist, 55*, 68–78.
Schussler, D. L., Jennings, P. A., Sharp, J., & Frank, J. (2015). Improving teacher awareness and well-being through CARE: A qualitative analysis of the underlying mechanisms mindfulness. Published online: doi: 10.1007/s12671-015-0422-7.
Spitzer, R. L., Kroenke, K., Williams, J. B. W., & Lowe, B. (2006). A brief measure for assessing generalized anxiety disorder. *Archives of Internal Medicine, 166*, 1092–1097.
Strong, M. (2011). *The highly qualified teacher: What is teacher quality and how do we measure it?* New York, NY: Teachers College, Columbia University.
Stuhlman, M., & Pianta, R. C. (2001). Teachers' narratives about their relationships with children: Associations with behavior in classrooms. *School Psychology Review, 31*, 148–163.
Sutton, R. E., & Wheatley, K. E. (2003). Teachers' emotions and teaching: A review of the literature and directions for future research. *Educational Psychology Review, 15*, 327–358.
Tschannen-Moran, M., & Woolfolk Hoy, A. (2001). Teacher efficacy: Capturing an elusive construct. *Teaching and Teacher Education, 17*, 783–805.
Tsouloupas, C. N., Carson, R. L., Matthews, R., Grawitch, M. J., & Barber, L. K. (2010). Exploring the association between teachers' perceived student misbehaviour and emotional exhaustion: The importance of teacher efficacy beliefs and emotion regulation. *Educational Psychology, 30*, 173–189.
U.S. Department of Health and Human Services. (2000). Report of the Surgeon's General's conference on Children's Mental Health: A national action agenda. Retrieved September 1, 2014, from http://www.surgeongeneral.gov/topics/cmh/childreport.html
Wallace, B. A. (2005). *Genuine happiness: Meditation as a path to fulfillment*. Hoboken, NJ: Wiley.

Watson, D., Clark, L. A., & Tellegen, A. (1988). Development and validation of brief measures of positive and negative affect: The PANAS. *Journal of Personality and Social Psychology, 54*, 1063–1070.

Wilson, S., Ball, D. L., Bryk, A. S., Figlio, D., Grossman, P., … Porter, A. (2008). *Teacher quality: Education white paper*. Washington, DC: National Academy of Education.

Zelazo, P. D., & Cunningham, W. (2007). Executive function: Mechanisms underlying emotion regulation. In J. Gross (Ed.), *Handbook of emotion regulation* (pp. 135–158). New York, NY: Guilford.

Zins, J. E., Weissberg, R. P., Wang, M. C., & Walberg, H. J. (2004). *Building academic success on social and emotional learning*. New York, NY: Teachers College Press.

Processes of Teaching, Learning, and Transfer in Mindfulness-Based Interventions (MBIs) for Teachers: A Contemplative Educational Perspective

10

Robert W. Roeser

Chapter Aims

It is a secret hidden in plain sight: Well-designed educational curricula and school-based interventions are effective in large measure due to the quality of their implementation by skillful, knowledgeable, and authentic teachers (Palmer, 1998). Thus, it is ironic that in the history of scientific research on teaching and learning in schools, the person of the teacher, with his or her qualities, has remained largely in the shadows while a focus on disembodied curricular content, content standards, and educational practices have taken up a disproportionate share of the limelight (e.g., Roeser, Marachi, & Gelhbach, 2002; Tharp & Gallimore, 1988). This absence of a focus on the teacher in educational research is even harder to comprehend when one considers the essentially relational nature of teaching and learning (Palmer, 1998). In fact, a focus on the disembodied aspects of education rather than the person of the teacher has been viewed by some as a key reason for the "predictable failure of educational reform" over the decades (Sarason, 1998).

The same critique, I argue in this chapter, can be leveled at the emerging field of contemplative science generally and the study of mindfulness-based interventions (MBIs) in applied settings like schools in particular (see Roeser, 2014 for overview). In this work, one discerns a rather narrow focus on mindfulness programs and their efficacy in terms of affected brain regions and individual outcomes, with little consideration of the quality of program implementation, the dose or exposure of participants to curricula, and the embodied presence of instructors with their unique qualities, pedagogical practices, and background (see Hölzel et al., 2011). As one indication of this singular focus on outcomes, a meta-review of three recent literature reviews of research on the effectiveness of MBIs (Chiesa & Serretti, 2009; Grossman, Niemann, Schmidt, & Walach, 2004; Virgili, 2013) showed that very few of the studies reviewed even considered how the amount of mindfulness training an individual underwent (e.g., "dose") might have related to outcomes. Specifically, only between 11 and 29 % of the highest quality studies in the field on mindfulness training (those that met rigorous criteria of validity) examined the question of whether or not program dose (e.g., the length of the program and the amount of home practice participants engaged in) was associated with the outcomes of training (Harrison, 2014). Granted, the notion of dose, which is often conceptualized as the amount of time individuals spend in and out of class practicing mindfulness, is a rather gross proxy measure for the quality of teaching

R.W. Roeser (✉)
Portland State University, Portland, OR, USA
e-mail: rroeser@pdx.edu

K.A. Schonert-Reichl, R.W. Roeser (eds.), *Handbook of Mindfulness in Education*, Mindfulness in Behavioral Health, DOI 10.1007/978-1-4939-3506-2_10

and learning that goes on in MBIs. Nonetheless, this statistic is quite telling. It suggests that as a field, scientists who study mindfulness interventions are currently primarily focused on how such interventions, of unknown length and uptake, with unspecified qualities of instructors and practices of teaching, produce "program effects." From an educational perspective, the fact that the person of the mindfulness instructor and the quality of his or her implementation of the training has remained in the shadows of the research limits our knowledge in fundamental ways, and may adversely affect the translation of these programs to schools.

In this chapter, I argue we need to know more about what is inside the so-called black box of MBIs in applied settings like schools. But, just how might an investigation into the processes of teaching and learning in MBIs be important for the field of education in particular? For applied researchers who work in schools, a pragmatic and compelling question often asked by administrators and school leaders who are considering such programs is this: "Will the introduction of MBIs for teachers or students improve the practice, and the outcomes, of teaching and learning in the classroom?" To adequately answer this question and to give a theory of how this is possible, practical knowledge concerning how mindfulness training for teachers works, and how such training may "transfer" to the classroom and affect the way teachers' approach teaching, and by extension the way their students might approach learning, seems primary. Furthermore, given the history of desultory results with regard to teacher professional development in changing basic teaching practices in the classroom, the question of the quality of professional development activities seems especially important to address in the field of education (Birman, Desimone, Porter, & Garet, 2000; Garet, Porter, Andrew, & Desimone, 2001).

In this chapter, I hypothesize that the quality of teaching and learning that goes on within MBIs is a key factor in adequately answering basic questions of how and why mindfulness skills "transfer" from the training context to schools in ways that may improve teaching, teacher–student relationships, and student engagement in classroom learning. The purpose of this chapter is to explore this thesis from a Contemplative Educational perspective, using case study data obtained from an expert mindfulness instructor who has worked with educators for almost 10 years. The central questions I take up in this chapter include: (1) What is the ***definition of mindfulness*** and the ***theory of change*** that might explain how mindfulness training impacts teacher, classroom, and student outcomes?; (2) What is the ***extant research evidence*** for this proposed theory of change?; (3) What are ***key aspects of the implementation*** of mindfulness trainings (e.g., pedagogical strategies and practices) that highly effective mindfulness instructors may use within the "black box of MBIs" to engage and teach teachers mindfulness-based skills and dispositions in the most effective manner?; (4) How do highly effective instructors ***scaffold and support teachers' transfer of mindfulness skills*** from the training context to their classrooms in ways that plausibly impact the quality of teaching, relationships, and learning that occur there?; and (5) What are important ***future directions for research*** on mindfulness training for teachers? Before turning to these questions, I provide a brief overview of some of the underlying assumptions of Contemplative Education as an applied domain of Contemplative Science.

Assumptive Framework of Contemplative Education

Contemplative Education is an emerging field of applied science devoted to carefully and rigorously describing and explaining the putative effects of MBIs in educational settings on educational leaders and schools, teachers and classrooms, and students (see Roeser, 2014; Roeser & Peck, 2009). Furthermore, Contemplative Education aims to apply the knowledge so-gained to optimize the development, implementation, and scaling of such programs if they prove feasible and efficacious.

As an applied scientific endeavor, Contemplative Education is a subfield of the Contemplative Science Project (CSP—see Roeser & Zelazo, 2012; Wallace, 2007). The CSP is a transdisciplinary effort to explore the effects of engagement with contemplative practices on the mind, brain, body, behavior, and social relationships within and across different periods in the lifespan. Contemplative practices refer to specialized mental and physical exercises that aim, through discipline and repeated practice, to train various forms of attention and prosocial emotions (e.g., kindness, generosity). For instance, many forms of contemplative practice involve the conscious focusing of attention in three ways: (1) as one-pointed concentration on an intentionally chosen object (e.g., the breath, sounds, physical movement, an image of a person who is kind to oneself) to focus, quiet, and calm the mind and body; (2) as an open and receptive manner on whatever arises in the mind, the body or one's environment to gain insight and clarity into the nature of sensory and mental phenomena, and (3) as one-pointed way on particular images, thoughts, and feelings involving expressions of care and compassion for oneself, others, or nature (Lutz, Dunne, & Davidson, 2007). There exist myriad practices that train these basic habits mind and body, including forms of sitting meditation, visualizations, movement activities such as yoga and tai chi, and conscious, calm and concentrated engagement in the arts or with nature.

According to Roeser and Zelazo (2012), the scientific goals of the CSP, from an explicitly *developmental* perspective, are threefold: (a) to **describe** the beneficial or contraindicated developmental effects of engagement in contemplative practices on body, brain, mind, and social relationships; (2) to **explain** contemplative practice effects at neurophysiological, psychological, behavioral, and social levels of analysis; and (3) to use descriptive and explanatory findings to **optimize** human development through the introduction of MBIs and related secular practices in families, schools, clinics, and communities in developmentally and culturally appropriate ways.

Two key assumptions of the CSP are that (a) the brain is an inherently adaptive organ, evolved to change in response to experience and intentional training and education (e.g., mindfulness training) through the processes of neuroplasticity (see MLERN, 2012); and (b) that contemplative practices ***such as focused attention or mindfulness meditation*** are specialized forms of mental training that, when practiced for an extended period of time with appropriate scaffolding, mentorship, and levels of challenge, significantly alter "default" cognitive, emotional, and motor processes and their underlying neural substrates. These alterations are associated with the development of new skills and habits related to the particular training undertaken (e.g., Bransford, Brown, & Cocking, 1999; Ericsson & Charness, 1994).

Defining Mindfulness

What exactly is mindfulness (see Lutz, Jha, Dunne & Saron, 2015)? Substantive, consensual definitions of what mindfulness *is* at the level of individuals remain elusive in science and applied secular approaches to mindfulness training, today (see Cullen, 2011; Kabat-Zinn, 2011). An early definition of mindfulness offered by Jon Kabat-Zinn (1994) was "Paying attention, on purpose, in the present moment, non-judgmentally" (p. 2). A key element in this definition, according to Cullen (2011), is a disposition of compassion, kindness, and curiosity towards all facets of experience—inner, outer, and others. In a similar vein, Shinzen Young (2011, 2015) proposed a definition of mindful awareness as a threefold attentional skill set encompassing *concentration*, the ability to focus on what one considers to be relevant at a given time; *sensory clarity*, the ability to keep track of what one is actually experiencing in the moment; and *equanimity*, the ability to allow sensory experiences to come and go moment by moment without pushing them away as in suppression or avoidance, or identifying with them as in personalization or attachment. These definitions have proven important for guiding the science on the putative effects of mindfulness training.

For example, Kabat-Zinn's definition of mindfulness was conceptualized by Bishop et al. (2004) as consisting of two facets: (1) the self-regulation of attention, "so that it is maintained on immediate experience, thereby allowing for increased recognition of mental events in the present moment" (p. 232); and (2) an orientation towards experience in the present moment "that is characterized by curiosity, openness, and acceptance" (p. 232). To assess this operational definition of mindfulness, scientists have developed and used both third-person (objective), as well as first-person (subjective), indicators of mindfulness-based skills and dispositions outlined in Table 10.1. Third-person measures of mindfulness, for instance, include the use of neuro-imaging techniques and behavioral tasks assessing the kinds of specific skills and dispositions listed in Table 10.1 before and after mindfulness training—those such as attention regulation and working memory, emotion regulation, and a nonreactive, non-judgmental awareness of somatic, emotional, self-related, and social experience (Hofmann, Grossman, & Hinton, 2011; Hölzel et al., 2011; Vago & Silbersweig, 2012). First-person, subjective measures of mindfulness have also been developed. Baer, Smith, Hopkins, Krietemeyer, and Toney (2006) and Baer et al. (2008), for instance, pursued a series of measurement studies to create, refine, and validate indicators of these dimensions of mindfulness. The resultant self-report measure, derived from input from Buddhist meditation teachers, clinical psychologists, and other practitioners, is called the "Five Facets of Mindfulness Questionnaire" (FFMQ). The five factors, measured by 39 items, include:

1. Mindful awareness of mental states—including sensations, feelings, and thoughts (e.g., "I pay attention to how my emotions affect my thoughts and behavior.")
2. Mindful awareness of behavior rather than acting in automatic, non-conscious ways (e.g., "I do jobs or tasks automatically without being aware of what I am doing."—item reversed)
3. Ability to verbally note and label experience (e.g., "I can easily put my beliefs, opinions, and expectations into words.")
4. Attitude of non-judgment towards moment-to-moment experience (e.g., "I tell myself that I shouldn't be feeling the way that I'm feeling."—item reversed)
5. Attitude of non-reactivity towards moment-to-moment experience (e.g., "In difficult situations I can pause without immediately reacting.")

The FFMQ scale is used as both an omnibus factor as well as in terms of the five separate subscales, and has demonstrated convergent and predictive validity in studies with adults (Baer, 2011). In addition, there is some evidence of dose–response relations between increases on self-reported mindfulness and individuals' amount of mindfulness practice (Carmody & Baer, 2008). In our own work with teachers, we often add another scale to complement this one—that of "occupational self-compassion"—the ability to adopt an attitude of kindness and compassion towards oneself as a teacher, especially during times of setback or difficulties on the job (see Roeser et al., 2013). In the research studies involving teachers done by my lab, as I discuss

Table 10.1 Lines of skill and disposition development hypothetically cultivated by mindfulness training

Domains of training	Default skills/dispositions	Cultivated skills/dispositions
Self-regulation	Mind-wandering	Focused attention
	Mindlessness	Mindfulness
	Emotional reactivity	Emotion regulation
Self-evaluation	Self-stereotyping	Experiential self-awareness
	Self-judgment	Self-kindness and self-compassion
Motivation	Confirmation bias	Curiosity and uncertainty-orientation
	Self-interest	Generosity
	In-group favoritism	Altruism
Social cognition	Singular perspective	Social perspective-taking
	Social-stereotyping	Empathic curiosity
	Social-judgment	Kindness and Compassion
	Social fear/distrust	Social connection/trust

below, teachers randomly assigned to receive training report increases in the skills and dispositions associated with mindfulness and occupational self-compassion following training compared to teachers randomly assigned to a waitlist who have yet to undergo training.

In summary, mindfulness can be defined in relation to attention, openness to experience, and a compassionate stance towards present moment experience (Kabat-Zinn, 1994). It can be measured both objectively and subjectively in terms of skills and dispositions associated in the science of psychology with self-regulation, self-evaluation, motivation, and social cognition (see Table 10.1). At the same time, vigorous debates regarding the conceptualization and measurement of mindfulness are ongoing (e.g., Lutz et al., 2015; Grossman & Van Dam, 2011; Williams & Kabat-Zinn, 2011).

Theory of Change: Mindfulness Training Effects on Teachers

Given this definition of mindfulness, what theory of change might plausibly account for the effects of mindfulness training on teachers, classrooms, and students? What is the functional significance of these cultivated skills and dispositions (see Table 10.1) for educationally relevant outcomes? For the last 7 years, I have been working closely with Margaret Cullen on a mindfulness training program she created specifically for teachers (see Cullen & Pons, 2015). The program has been called both the SMART-in-Education program (**S**tress **M**anagement **a**nd **R**esiliency **T**raining) and the Mindfulness-based Emotional Balance program (MBEB). It is a fully manualized professional development (PD) program designed to help educators (a) develop mindfulness, (i.e., the skills of present-centered awareness, focused attention, working memory, and emotion regulation); (b) apply mindfulness to reduce occupational stress and increase resilience and engagement in teaching; (c) apply mindfulness to interpersonal relationships in order to create well-managed and caring classroom climates.

The program incorporates approximately 50 % of the components from Kabat-Zinn's (2003) widely used Mindfulness-based Stress Reduction (MBSR) program, including many of the same mindfulness exercises, contemplative movement practices, and focus on setting intentions and clarifying values. Differing from MBSR, about 30% of the program is devoted to mindfulness-based emotion skills and theory, and the remaining 20 % to mindfulness-based prosocial dispositions like kindness, compassion, and forgiveness. The main program components fall into three categories: (a) group activities, (b) mindfulness practices, and (c) homework assignments. Group activities include visualizations, experiential exercises, dyads, small and large group discussions of practice, didactic lectures on topics like stress and forgiveness, and guided mindfulness and "heart" practices. Mindfulness practices include specific mental training exercises like an attentional focus on the body, the breath, or the ongoing flow of experience that aim to develop concentration, clarity of perception, and non-reactivity. Homework includes things like daily mindfulness practice, keeping a meditation journal, and engaging in weekly homework assignments (e.g., doing loving-kindness practice for a challenging student for one week and writing about the experience).

To help teachers to reduce stress and foster their resilience, the program focuses particular attention on how mindfulness can be used to regulate emotion and cope with stress through greater awareness of one's emotional habits and triggers (an antecedent-focused form of mindful emotion regulation or ER); and new skills for dealing with emotion once it is activated (a response-focused form of mindful ER). The program aims to do this through components such as (a) lectures on emotion and how mindfulness can help regulate emotion and reduce stress, rumination, and fatigue; (b) practices such as mindfulness of emotions and other mental states; (c) guided visualizations to explore the "inner geography" of emotions such as fear and anger; and (d) weekly discussions about how practices are working for teachers in their lives. The home practices and "practice in life" dimensions of the program are hypothesized to be essential for teachers' learning and transfer of mindfulness skills to the classroom (Carmody & Baer, 2009). For purposes of this chapter, I summarize three pathways of influence by which my colleagues and I hypothesize this particular mindfulness program affects teacher outcomes and related downstream classroom and student consequences (see Roeser, Skinner, Beers, & Jennings, 2012; Skinner & Beers, 2015).

First, there is considerable evidence that mindfulness training reduces individuals' stress and distress (Chiesa & Serretti, 2009; Grossman et al., 2004; Virgili, 2013). Based on theories of stress and coping (Lazarus & Folkman, 1984), mindfulness training (MT) is predicted to promote teachers' *resilience* by reducing stress reactivity through the cultivation of self-regulatory (e.g., executive functions) and coping resources. MT reduces stress reactivity by helping teachers to refine their attention and awareness to what is occurring moment by moment. Improved attention and awareness affords the necessary conditions for teachers to utilize other tangible skills they are taught for down-regulating stress (e.g., stopping and breathing), and for affording teachers the presence of mind to be aware of and rework their habitual appraisals of negative incidents in the classroom that tend to amplify stress reactions. With its focus on self-compassion and compassion for others, MT not only reduces habitual patterns of blame (self-blame or blaming students) when the processes of teaching and learning are challenging in the classroom, but also provides strategies for coping constructively with stress once such challenges arise. These strategies can include simple non-judgmental awareness, acceptance, reappraisal, and self-calming or refocusing techniques (e.g., stop, breathe). Together, the resources for coping with stress that MT is hypothesized to cultivate are thought to allow teachers to feel (and appear) less reactive or "stressed out" and more mentally present in the classroom, maintaining their emotional equanimity even under challenging situations. As stress is reduced, the energy teachers previously expressed or used to suppress negative emotion is freed up and is available to be dedicated to instruction, classroom management, and building relationships with students. Such calm, focused energy may thus contribute to creating an open and caring classroom climate, managed by a teacher who is psychologically available and who makes good use of instructional time.

The second pathway through which MT is hypothesized to improve teaching is based on "broaden and build" theory of emotion (Frederickson, 2013). From this perspective, MT helps teachers to generate an additional set of resources beyond coping with stress by recognizing and amplifying positive emotional experiences—for instance, teachers' original motives and ethical purposes for joining the profession. By reducing stress, the theory goes, one is able to better perceive and amplify positive work-related emotional experiences more readily and regain a sense of energy and vitality in teaching. Thus, the cultivation of positive psychological resources (e.g., a sense of professional accomplishment, joy in teaching) generated by mindfulness training are thought to help teachers to engage more fully, and with greater vigor and zest, in teaching and relationships in school. When teachers appear happier and more engaged in teaching, and this creates a positive classroom climate for learning, students might be more likely to engage in and enjoy learning.

The third pathway through which MT is hypothesized to affect teachers' classroom practices is by cultivating pro-social dispositions such as empathy, perspective taking, and a loving and kind attitude towards self and others (Fredrickson, Cohn, Coffey, Pek, & Finkel, 2008). MT helps teachers to feel feelings more fully and clearly, and to adopt a witness-stance on one's own mental states (see Hölzel et al., 2011). These skills, in turn, support the skills of empathizing and cognitively interpreting the mental states of others (e.g., Singer & Lamm, 2009). In addition, MT involves the intentional cultivation of an attitude of compassion for self and others. By learning a disposition of self-compassion, teachers can begin to "let go" of some of the unnecessary evaluation pressures placed upon them by self and others. Similarly, by learning an attitude of kindness towards their students, especially challenging students, teachers can begin to "let go" of appraisals that generate stress and reactive cycles of interaction with such students in favor of kinder and calmer approaches. Over time, such prosocial dispositions are thought to contribute to the creation of an emotionally supportive climate for student learning, one in which the capacity to see students in their own right, with their unique gifts, may be more likely.

In sum, by enhancing the mindfulness-related skills and dispositions outlined in Table 10.1, our Theory of Change (see Fig. 10.1) posits increases in teacher resilience to stress, in engagement with teaching, and in a prosocial and autonomy-supportive approach to interactions with students (the three pathways). Such personal changes, in turn, are hypothesized to manifest behaviorally in teachers in terms of **classroom effects**.

For instance, when teachers are less exhausted, more resilient, and enthusiastically engaged in teaching, they should be able to create more emotionally supportive classrooms. Mindful teachers should be more emotionally available and trustworthy sources of support, and create a safe and responsive atmosphere. Such teachers care about and want to hear what students are actually thinking, even if this includes "negative" emotions. They are able to take students' perspectives and help students listen to each other with acceptance and appreciation. As a result, we predict that mindfulness cultivated by training allows teachers to create (and students to report) a warmer, more caring, and more emotionally supportive climate in their classrooms for student learning.

In addition, we hypothesize that teachers who are more resilient and engaged are also more likely to minimize motivational and disciplinary issues in the classroom; and when they arise, to handle them fairly and effectively. Mindful teachers remain more calm and fully present, showing measured and fair discipline that is appropriate to the transgression. They are especially notable for autonomy support, in which they remain open to each student's version of events, reach fair conclusions about culpability, and mete out appropriate consequences, emphasizing responsibility and repair. Hence, we hypothesize that teachers who benefit from MT will pass those benefits on to their students through the creation of better-managed, more consistent classroom climates for learning that students also perceive as fair, organized, and predictable.

In the final stage of our Theory of Change, we postulate that students will be more motivated and engaged in classrooms that they perceive as emotionally-supportive, safe, and well-managed; and where they have emotionally closer relationships with their teachers, because such classrooms address their needs for autonomy, belonging, and competence (Eccles & Roeser, 2015). Decades of naturalistic, observational, and intervention studies have documented that teacher practices and relationships that address students' stage-relevant needs also promote students' (1) motivational beliefs, including their self-efficacy, valuing of learning, and mastery goals; (2) feelings of belonging or relatedness; and (3) levels of academic engagement in the classroom (Wigfield, Eccles, Schiefele, Roeser, & Kean, 2006.)

In sum, the Theory of Change in Fig. 10.1 proposed that mindfulness training assists teachers in realizing a calmer, clearer, and kinder frame of mind with which to perceive and respond to students' autonomy-, belonging- and competence-related needs in the classroom. By being more available and attuned to students' needs and perspectives, we predict students will feel safer, a greater sense of belonging, and thus, more likely to engage in learning. In the next section, I briefly discuss the evidence for this Theory of Change.

Evidence for Effects of MBIs on Teachers, Classrooms, and Students

Teacher Mindfulness Skills and Self-Compassion To the extent that teachers' engagement with MBIs is high, the Theory of Change we developed predicts that teachers will develop mindfulness and self-compassion as assessed by first-person reports, and the related capacities for focused attention and working memory capacity and emotion recognition and

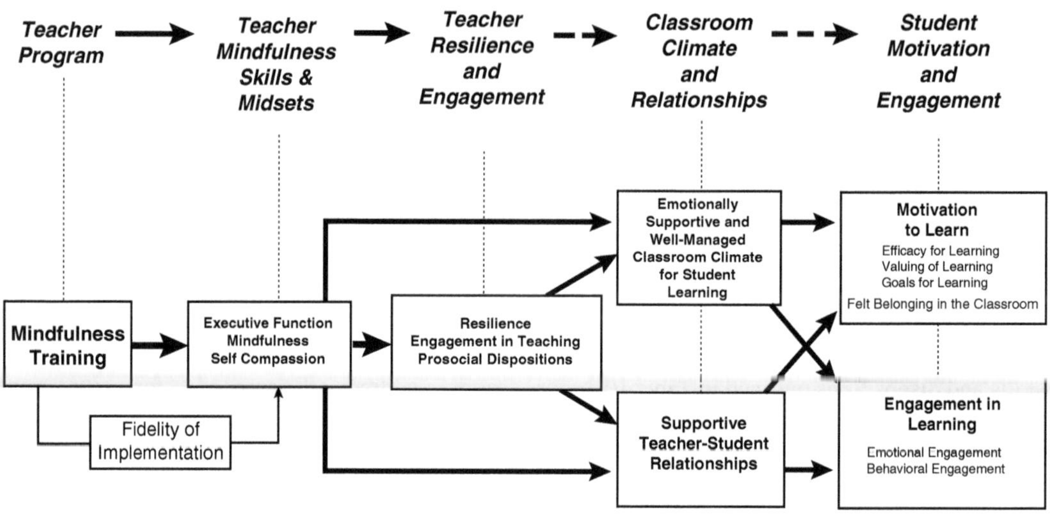

Fig. 10.1 Theory of change: hypothesized effects of mindfulness training on teachers, classrooms, and students

regulation as assessed by third-person measures. Previous research with teachers provides some evidence that MT improves self-reported mindfulness and self-compassion, as well as behavioral measures of sustained attention, working memory, and emotion recognition (Benn, Akiva, Arel, & Roeser, 2012; Flook, Goldberg, Pinger, Bonus, & Davidson, 2013; Frank et al., 2013; Jennings, Snowberg, Coccia, & Greenberg, 2011; Jennings, Frank, Snowberg, Coccia, & Greenberg, 2013; Kemeny et al., 2012; Roeser et al., 2013).

Teacher Resilience, Engagement, and Prosocial Dispositions Research with teachers has also shown that mindfulness practice is associated with reduced stress, improved well-being, and improved efficacy in the classroom (Benn et al., 2012; Flook et al., 2013; Franco, Mañas, Cangas, Moreno, & Gallego, 2010; Jennings et al., 2013; Kemeny et al., 2012; Roeser et al., 2013; Winzelberg & Luskin, 1999). These variables, based on self-report, are consistent with studies suggesting that less stress, more energy and vitality, and greater efficacy is associated with greater work engagement (e.g., Hakanen, Bakker, & Schaufeli, 2006; Tschannen-Moran, Hoy, & Hoy, 1998).

Classroom Climate and Teacher–Student Relationships This stage of our Theory of Change is more conjectural given few published studies have yet examined the effects of teacher mindfulness training on their observed instructional practice and relationships with students. A few small-scale studies exist that provide "existence proofs" that mindfulness training may affect teachers' instructional practice in the areas of emotional support, classroom organization, and relationships with students (Flook et al., 2013; Taylor, Urdan, Cullen, & Roeser, 2014). Future research is needed on the full set of relationships depicted in Fig. 10.1, as well as the student outcomes for which there is no extant evidence as of the writing of this chapter.

Quality of Implementation of MBIs in Education

The Theory of Change in Fig. 10.1 focuses on the putative effects of mindfulness training on teachers, classrooms, and students. The theory begins with an unelaborated consideration of the quality of the implementation of the mindfulness training (see Fig. 10.1). From an educational and applied-developmental perspective on MBIs for teachers, it is clear that high-quality program implementation—what happens within the black box of the intervention—is essential to a program's effectiveness (O'Donnell, 2008). The fact that program implementation quality has received little attention in research on MBIs in education represents an area in need of research. A focus on the implementation quality of MBIs in education, as I endeavor to show in the next section through use of a case study (e.g., Yin, 2014), may hold the key to understanding how (a) how teachers learn mindfulness-based skills and dispositions in such trainings, and (b) how they then transfer mindfulness-based skills and dispositions to the classroom to effect changes such as those hypothesized in the Theory of Change (see Fig. 10.1).

Teaching, Learning, and Transfer in MBIs for Teachers: A Case Study

What is the nature of teaching and learning that goes on in MBIs for classroom teachers, and how can an understanding of teaching and learning in MBIs lead to a broader understanding of the downstream effects these programs on classrooms and students (see Fig. 10.1)? In order to address such questions, my colleagues and I recently conducted a mixed-method case study of the processes of teaching, learning, and transfer within the MBI that mindfulness instructor Margaret Cullen created for public school teachers over a 10-year period (Roeser, Horn-Keller, Stadick, & Urdan, 2012). In terms of her background, Margaret Cullen is a Licensed Marriage and Family Therapist and a Certified MBSR Teacher and was one of the first ten instructors to be certified by the Center for Mindfulness in Worcester, Massachusetts. For 20 years, she has been pioneering mindfulness-based programs in health care, education, business, and academic settings. In 1995, she helped launch the first MBSR program at Kaiser in Oakland, CA; and later collaborated on a revised manual for the entire northern California region. She introduced MBSR to the Cancer Support Community (CSC) in both Santa Monica and Walnut Creek, California where it still thrives, 20 years later. Margaret continues to facilitate support groups, teach mindfulness programs and offer workshops on forgiveness at CSC in Walnut Creek (see Cullen & Pons, 2015).

The goals of the case study were (a) to describe the nature of mindfulness instruction in an MBI for teachers by one expert instructor; (b) to explore how the mindfulness instructor's pedagogical practices might affect teachers' motivation, engagement, and learning of mindfulness skills, and dispositions during the MBI; and (c) to explore how the instructor might support teachers' transfer of the mindfulness skills and dispositions learned in the MBI to the classroom setting. Teacher surveys, interviews, case studies with classroom observations, and detailed analysis of the entire 9-week MBI for teachers, which was captured on HD-video by two cameras and a professional videographer, formed the data sources for the case study (see Roeser, Horn-Keller et al., 2012). To establish that the MBI did in fact assist teachers in developing the mindfulness-based skills and dispositions outlined in Table 10.1 and Fig. 10.1, we analyzed pre-/post-/follow-up data from teacher surveys. Similar to our previous results using randomized control study designs (e.g., Benn et al., 2012; Roeser et al., 2013), results showed that the 13 teachers in the case study reported significant increases in the skills and dispositions of mindfulness and occupational self-compassion from pre-program to post-program to 4-month follow-up (see Fig. 10.2). Thus, the case study was meant to explore how implementation quality, or the processes of teaching, learning, and transfer, were associated with such outcomes for these 13 teachers.

Theoretical Frameworks for Exploring Teaching, Learning, and Transfer in MBIs for Teachers

To explore the nature of teaching, learning, and transfer in the MBI, we drew upon existing constructivist and sociocultural theoretical perspectives on teaching and learning (Rogoff,

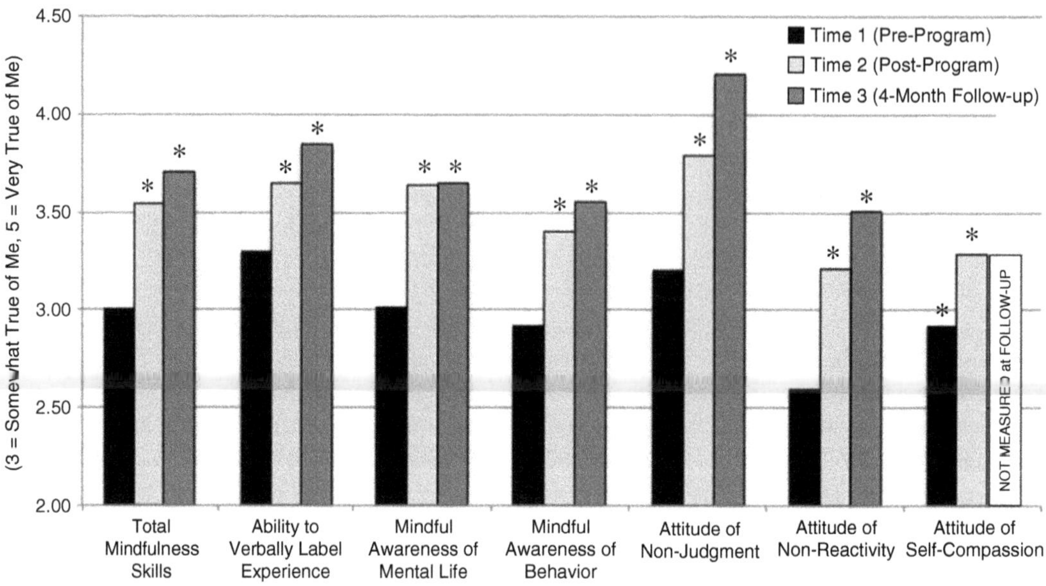

Fig. 10.2 Teacher-reported changes in mindfulness and self-compassion over time: results from an uncontrolled case study of 13 teachers. $N = 13$ public school teachers; *paired t-tests comparing baseline to post-program and follow-up scores $p < .05$

2003; Tharp & Gallimore, 1988). These complementary perspectives posit that teaching and learning inextricably involve social interactional processes—specifically, verbal and non-verbal forms of teaching and modeling by which more-expert others scaffold and guide the development of skills and dispositions among novices (Spindler, 1987; Tharp & Gallimore, 1988). For instance, Lev Vygotsky's (1978) theory of learning emphasized the sociocultural and relational contexts of learning. He posited that novices construct various kinds of knowledge of self, others, and the world through their interactions with more knowledgeable experts who scaffold their development through modeling, verbal teaching, and feedback. Consistent with constructivist and sociocultural theories of teaching and learning, the main hypothesis of the case study was the idea that learning mindfulness skills and dispositions is an "assisted performance"—one that includes both implicit and explicit methods of teaching and modeling that facilitate teacher–participants' learning and transfer of mindfulness skills to the recurrent dilemmas and joys of classroom life (see Fig. 10.1). Although there are numerous kinds of teaching practices and cultural tools that experts use to scaffold learning among novices, for purposes of the case study we focused on four interdependent processes: (1) the nature and variety of teaching activities employed by the instructor; (2) the frequently used vocabulary words of the instructor during group discussions of mindfulness practice; (3) the strategic use of speech and silence by the instructor during guided mindfulness meditations; and (4) the embodied modeling of mindfulness-based skills and dispositions by the instructor.

Nature and Variety of Teaching Activities First, we examined the nature of the activities in the program. It may seem obvious, but the ability of an expert to scaffold the development of a novice's skills and dispositions requires interaction. Interaction refers to activities in which the expert and the novice engage in together, and in which the sharing of information and experience together en route to a learning goal is central (e.g., Dewey, 1902). Did the primary nature and variety of teaching activities in the MBI afford teachers opportunities to interact reciprocally with the instructor around learning the habits of head, heart, and hand associated with mindfulness? To assess this in the

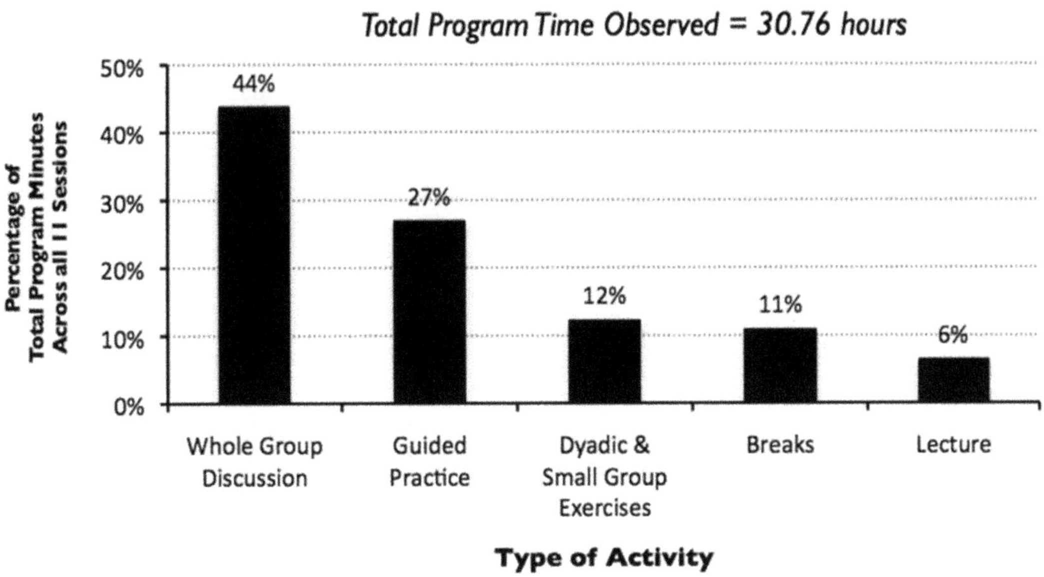

Fig. 10.3 Percentage of total MBI minutes spent in different teaching activities

case study, we coded the approximately 31 h of video of the intervention in terms of the time that was spent in different types of activities. We were particularly interested in seeing how much of the time during the entire intervention was spent in activities that were characterized by experiential forms of learning.

As one can see in Fig. 10.3, the results of the case study revealed that the expert instructor used a variety of pedagogical activities to teach mindfulness skills and dispositions. These activities included guided practice sessions (lying, moving, sitting, and standing mindfulness meditations), whole group discussions of practice, storytelling/poem-reading, lecture, and small group exercises. This variety is characteristic of many MBIs (Cullen, 2011). The most predominant activities in terms of time allotted each week were experiential in nature and included (a) guided group mindfulness practice (e.g., body scan, focused-attention meditation, mindful movement) and (b) whole group discussions of practice. These activities accounted for 71 % of the observed instructional time of the MBI (about 28 h). By contrast, there were only two lectures (total of 2.5 h) in the program (see Fig. 10.3). These findings show that in the most basic sense, this teacher MBI provided a significant amount of opportunities for teachers to learn mindfulness skills and dispositions experientially, and through guided practice with an expert.

In addition, these results implicitly suggest most of teaching activities of this MBI involved joint attention on the part of the instructor and the teachers around the task of learning mindfulness skills and dispositions—the goal (Tharp & Gallimore, 1988). Joint attention is defined as the ability of humans to coordinate attention with a social partner in relation to some object, event, shared experience, or goal. As such, joint attention has been characterized as a "primary cultural guidance device" for teaching and learning new things (e.g., Donald, 2001, p. 201). For instance, joint attention is hypothesized to make possible the acquisition of language and symbolic representation (Tomasello, 1999). More generally, it is hypothesized to be the social process responsible for the development of domain-specific forms of knowledge, and the qualities of awareness and regulation that go along with them. Mindfulness training, for example, inevitably involves the training of attention. Through noting and labeling of attention in the context of joint practice, experts are thought to impart the skills of meta-awareness and the effortful control of attention. Similarly, through shared attention to the ongoing inner vocalization of experience in words, or the continuous affective valencing of experiences as positive, negative or neutral, the skills of meta-cognition and strategic regulation of thinking, and emotional awareness and regulation of emotion, respectively, can be learned. How is this accomplished?

Thompson (2007) describes joint attention as a key process by which a human being learns "the ability to examine one's own thinking *from the perspective of the other* and thereby re-describe one's own cognitive representations of the world" (p. 405). Through joint attention with more expert social others, for instance, novices learn to note and label particular kinds of mental and physical objects and events of significance—often with language. This affords them the possibility of becoming aware of, and naming such objects and events from the perspective of an observer, that is, from a "meta-cognitive" or "witness" perspective. In essence, through interaction, the novice learns to view their experience through the eyes (and words) of the expert.

Because the instructor and the teacher-novices are attending jointly to mindfulness practice as they engage in it together in the MBI, there are ample opportunities for the expert to hear from novices, share information, and offer feedback based on the novices' embodied experiences of trying to learn the skills. Specifically, the instructor can help the novices learn about how to notice and label the qualities of their attention or the presence of thoughts, feelings, or sensations from the perspective of an expert "other." In this way, the teacher-novices learn through social interaction a structure that they then internalize psychologically—the observer-observed structure with regard to their own moment-to-moment experience. This structure affords teachers a means of re-relating to, and re-representing, those aspects of their own mental and physical experience from the vantage point of a "witness" (Engler, 1984). The awareness and psychological distance of this structure, made possible by joint attention and language during mindfulness practice with an expert, serves powerful self-reflective and self-regulatory purposes (Marcovitch, Jacques, Boseovski, & Zelazo, 2008). Specifically, teachers are learning to iteratively reprocess the contents of their experience in ways that allow for the systematic differentiation and integration of higher order forms of domain-specific knowledge schemas and regulatory scripts (e.g., Case, 1992), and more generally, are learning a means of developing their level of consciousness (e.g., Zelazo, 1999).

Several implicit, non-verbal meanings may also be communicated to teachers by the predominance of joint, experiential learning activities in the MBI. These include (a) the implicit value of each teacher as his or her own source of knowledge when learning mindfulness and self-compassion (i.e., self-empowerment), (b) the implicit responsibility of each teacher to determine the quality of his or her learning in the program and at home by participating (i.e., intrinsic motivation to learn), and (c) the implicit importance of being part of a community in which individual teachers can see and hear for themselves that their stress-related struggles and difficulties are not idiosyncratic and personal, but rather shared and professional insofar as other teachers report similar experiences with teaching-related stress (i.e., the normalization of [common] experience). As one teacher noted in her post-program interview:

> *What was most helpful for me was the community, of being in league with your colleagues who are going through something similar or at least know what the heck you're talking about, and being in a space where not only there's some common ground, but there's common experience around how you've tried to cope in the past, and how that coping may not have served you that well. So being more open to other ways to frame the situation and to be more of a problem solver, realizing you are not alone and there is another way.*

Furthermore, via the prolonged nature of learning mindfulness in a community (e.g., 9 weeks, 36 h together), implicit beliefs regarding the relatively fixed versus malleability of one's personal abilities (e.g., attention or emotion regulation), as well as the value of self-compassion and a mastery-goal orientation to learning mindfulness (e.g., Neff, 2003) are likely made salient to the learners. Thus, this kind of experiential, guided professional development activity for teachers may provide an implicit model of motivated learning, norms, and values that teachers can transfer into their own classroom practice with students.

Instructor Vocabulary During Group Discussions of Practice A second core focus of the case study was the mindfulness instructor's use of language during group discussions of mindfulness practice. Language is obviously a primary cultural tool that experts use to scaffold the learning of novices. Vygotsky (1978) hypothesized that novices learn, in part, by internalizing the language of an expert and using that language, in the form of inner private speech, to guide their future action in similar contexts. The basic idea in Vygotsky's theory was that higher order psychological functions and forms of knowledge are derived from social interaction—that these functions and forms first occur between expert and novice as social speech, and then later occur within the novice as private speech and fossilized language or schematized knowledge (e.g., Wertsch, 1991). Based on this idea, we hypothesized that the nature of instructor speech that occurred in group discussions of mindfulness practice, discussions involving question-and-answer and feedback, would be particularly important for teachers' conceptual understanding of mindfulness, as well as their experiential ability to note and label the various psychological constituents of their moment-to-moment experience as they practiced mindful awareness (Tharp & Gallimore, 1988). In sum, we wanted to know, were there identifiable classes of word or "lexicons" that the expert instructor used during group discussions to teach mindfulness?

To examine this question empirically, we transcribed the speech of the instructor during all of the group discussions that occurred across the 11 sessions of the MBI. These discussions constituted about 44 % of the MBI (or about 14 h). We then analyzed the instructor's words by using Wordle software representations and word counts derived from Linguistic Inquiry and Word Count (LIWC—Pennebaker, Francis, & Booth, 2001) software to identify the words she used most frequently. We focused our attention on the instructor's "top 25" most frequently used words in each of the 11 group discussions. Multiple raters thematically grouped these most frequently used words into 12 word families in order to parsimoniously describe their substantive content (see Fig. 10.4). In essence, these emergent word clusters or lexicons revealed substantively what the instructor was offering for internalization to the teachers during group discussions each week for nine consecutive weeks.

Figure 10.4 shows that, in general, the instructor frequently used words reflecting basic program concepts and practices, the conditional nature of examining experience, the nature of knowing what we believe is and what actually is, and mindfulness in relation to sensation-perception, emotion, thought, and insight. This is not surprising, given that the Four Foundations of Mindfulness (mindful awareness of sensation, emotion, thought, and insights into the nature of mind and life) are the underlying thematic basis for the program (see Cullen, 2011). Results showed that the instructor frequently used words that referred to basic mindfulness concepts and practices (concepts and practices in Fig. 10.4), present-centered, mindful awareness in general (awareness), and mindfulness of sensory-perceptual processes (sensation-perception), emotional processes (emotion), and cognitive processes (thought) specifically.

Other lexicons also became apparent. For instance, the instructor's frequently used words about resistance to practice, the nature of epistemological knowing (e.g., what we believe or expect is happening moment to moment versus what *is* actually happening), and reaction and judgment of, versus freedom and responsiveness to, moment to moment experience (automatic reaction as opposed to choiceful responding). One of the more interesting word families that emerged from this analysis was the instructor's frequent use of conditional language during group discussions—language suggestive of curiosity, openness, and ongoing exploration. This word cluster consisted of words such as "may," "might," "kind of," "sort of," and "see if." These words seem to function to encourage the novice towards further inquiry and curiosity with respect to knowing without pressure, coercion, or dogmatism.

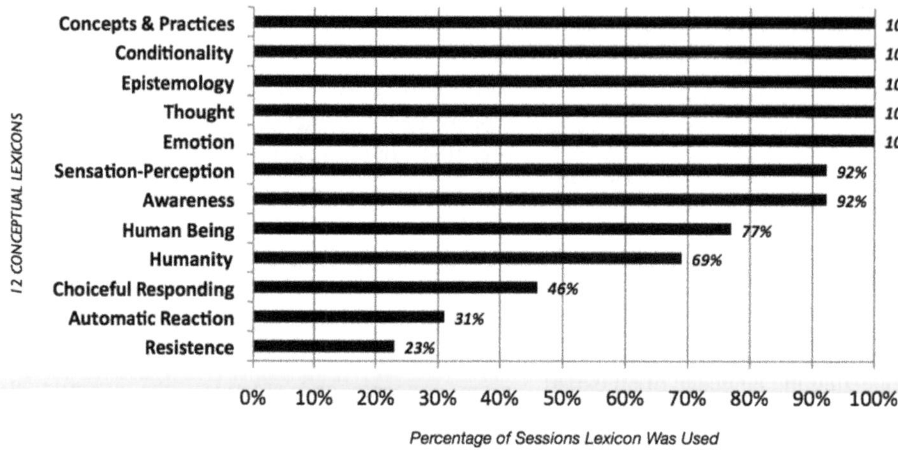

Key for Lexicons and Constituent Words

1. Words Indicative of Key Program Concepts and Practices	[attention, intention, mindfulness, meditation, yoga, compassion, refractory period, relaxation, forgiveness, loving-kindness, practice]
2. **Conditional Language**	[like, may, might, kind of, sort of]
3. Words Indicative of Epistemological Understanding	[really, actually]
4. Words Indicative of Thinking Processes	[think, thinking, thought]
5. Words Indicative of Emotional Processes	[feeling, feel, emotion, angry, anger, interesting, pleasure, want, sadness]
6. Words Indicative of Sensory-Perceptual Processes	[sense, notice, experience, see, find]
7. Words Indicative of Present-Centered Awareness	[time, now, present, moment, change, going, different, towards, back, awareness]
8. Words Indicative of Dimensions of Being Human	[mind, body, brain, heart]
9. Words Indicative of Human Experience	[person, people]
10. Words Indicative of Freedom in Response	[choice, choose, suffering, attachment, freedom]
11. Words Indicative of Reaction and Judgment	[good, bad, positive, negative, neutral, pleasant, unpleasant]
12. Words Indicative of Physical and Psychological Resistance	[resistance, resist]

Fig. 10.4 Percentage of sessions that common lexicons of learning were used by instructor during group discussions across all eleven MBI sessions

In sum, these descriptive results suggest that the mindfulness instructor afforded teacher participants ample opportunities to develop a new vocabulary during these group discussions, a vocabulary reflective of the concepts, practice, and skills and dispositions associated with mindfulness. What is most noteworthy is the frequent and repetitive nature with which the instructor offered these specific lexicons to the teachers for internalization from week to week. This kind of vocabulary provided teachers with a new way of describing their moment-to-moment experience. As one teacher noted in her post-program interview: "*One of the biggest things is that the program has given me is a better language to talk about my emotional life, to recognize patterns in myself and, you know, to have a language for what's happening.*"

Frequency of Instructor Words and Silence During Guided Meditations A third focus of the case study was the mindfulness instructor's use of speech and silence during guided mindfulness meditations. Here, we were interested in a particular type of sociocultural support for learning that Vygotsky called "scaffolding." First, we examined the instructor's scaffolding of learning through the thematic functions of the language utterances she used during guided meditations. To do this, multiple raters transcribed, segmented into utterances, and then thematically coded all the language used by the instructor during the guided meditations across the 11 sessions of the MBI. Figure 10.5 presents the results of this analysis. Given that teachers reported learning the five facets of mindfulness and a disposition of self-compassion from pre- to post-intervention (see Fig. 10.2), we specifically coded utterances in terms of invitations to practice these mindfulness-based skills and dispositions. We also created new codes for other language functions that emerged organically in our analysis. Results are presented in Fig. 10.5.

We found that most of the instructor's speech during guided practices consisted of invitations to practice the five facets of mindfulness described above: acting with awareness, noting and labeling of experience, awareness of mental states, non-judgment of experience, and non-

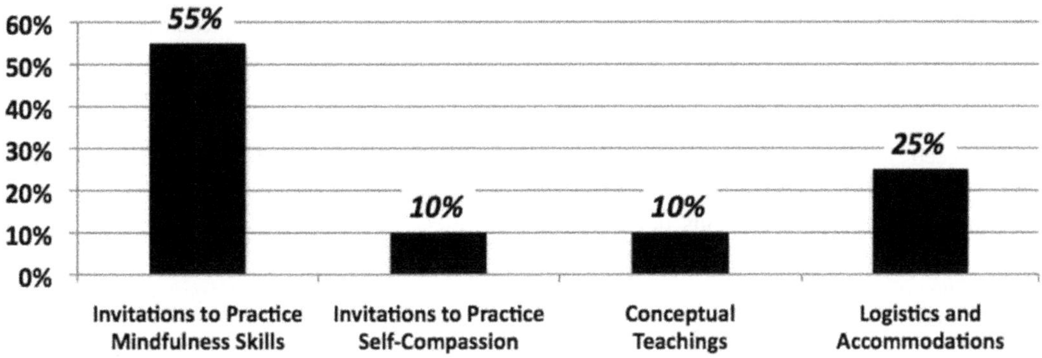

Fig. 10.5 Percentage of instructor's utterances by theme and autonomy-supportiveness during all guided meditation sessions

reactivity to experience. In addition, the instructor also invited the teachers to practice self-compassion—for instance, saying "If the mind wanders from the object of meditation, just note it and gently and kindly escort the attention back to the breath." Over two-thirds of all instructor utterances were invitations to practice these skills and dispositions. Approximately a quarter of the instructor's utterances involved logistics and accommodations to make the practices, especially mindful movement, more accessible to the teachers. For example, during mindful stretching activities, the instructor would offer suggestions for how the exercise could be modified for individuals with specific physical issues. Only about 10 % of all utterances were directive teachings.

Participants noted that these invitations were associated with the development of the skills of mindfulness and self-compassion. In post-program interviews, one teacher noted: "*I think the self-compassion part of this training has been really helpful. Just looking at things differently knowing that you can start over the next day, knowing that you can be there for yourself, that you can really apply forgiveness and kindness to yourself really changes your outlook.*"

These results suggest that this expert instructor offered teachers many opportunities to learn mindfulness skills during guided sessions, and did so using language that positions novices as learners in their own right, rather than positioning them as passive recipients of information from an expert. Theoretically, we hypothesize that the instructor's use of frequent invitations that are autonomy-supportive and inquiry-focused served to cultivate or reinvigorate participating teachers' intrinsic motivation to practice and to learn mindfulness (Deci & Ryan, 2002). As one teacher noted in her interview after the program: "*I think at a personal level, this program has re-awakened my commitment to a regular practice that I hope will bear fruit as time goes on.*"

Another feature of instructor language we investigated during the guided meditation sessions was aimed at examining a second facet of Vygotsky's (1988) concept of scaffolding. On this view, experts scaffold learning among novices by skillfully enacting an *incremental decrease* in their level of guidance and support over time as a novice gains more mastery with a skill. This removal of expert scaffolding over time is hypothesized to allow novices to move from mastery with mentor support, towards independent mastery, and finally towards the internalization and automatization of the acquired skill (Tharp & Gallimore, 1988). Thus, we wondered how an expert instructor might scaffold the development of mindfulness skills during guided meditation practice through the strategic use of speech—conceptualized as a form of external guidance, and silence—conceptualized as an opportunity for novices to engage in self-directed practice. Specifically, we wondered if there was any evidence that the instructor gradually diminished her use of language during these sessions over time and remained silent longer as the teachers gained mastery with the skills of mindfulness.

To assess this, we examined the time signatures of the transcriptions we made of the instructor's speech guided meditation sessions. We simply calculated the amount of time the instructor spoke and guided participants during these sessions, and the amount of time she remained silent. The results showed that, in general, the ratio of instructor speech to silence across all guided practice sessions during the MBI was below 1.00. This means that in general, the instructor spoke less, and was silent more, during these sessions (M=0.81, SD=0.27). We also examined changes in the ratio of talk to silence by the instructor during guided practice activities over the 9 weeks and 11 sessions of the program. As one can see in Fig. 10.6, results showed a linear decline in this ratio from Session 1 to 11 (R^2=.62), suggesting a shift from instructor guidance to silence (and novice self-guidance) over the course of the MBI.

We believe these results are significant for three reasons. First, they suggest a kind of "hand-over" of guidance from the instructor to the teacher-novices over time during the MBI as predicted in Vygotskyian views of skill development (e.g., Tharp & Gallimore, 1988). Second, these results suggest that the instructor was affording the teachers ample opportunities to develop a familiarity and comfort with silence. In fact, "befriending of silence" was rated by teachers in a post-program survey as one of the most important benefits they derived from the MBI. For instance, one secondary teacher, in a post-program interview, described how she transferred this newfound appreciation for silence to her classroom in the form of "wait-time"—allowing students time to think after a question was asked or a response requested:

> *I think the way that this class has affected me personally is that I'm more comfortable with quiet. I don't feel a need to fill the airwaves every five seconds now, which I think is a problem with a lot of teachers. We tend to want to talk a lot because we feel like that's our job. I think this new understanding kind of bled into my classroom where I've started to give a lot more airtime and space, what they call wait-time, to kids. I'm not feeling like I have to rush on to the next thing anymore because I realize that there's something really important about that wait-time and that space.*

One last factor we examined, consistent with Vygotsky's view of skill development, was whether or not the internalization of the instructor's guidance through speech in the form of inner private speech was one process by which teachers transferred the mindfulness skills they learned in the MBI to their classrooms (Vygotsky, 1978). Such "transfer of learning" has been defined as "the influence of prior learning (retained until the present) upon the learning of, or response to, new material" (McGeoch, 1942, p. 394) and "the process that enables us to make previously learned responses in new situations" (Gage & Berliner, 1992, p. 352). There were several instances of transfer mentioned by teachers in their post-program interviews, and these instances provide "existence proofs" of various

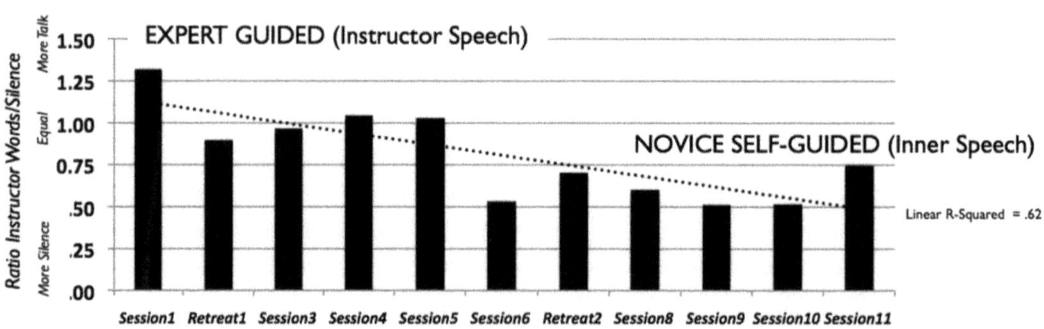

Fig. 10.6 Ratio of instructor speech to silence during guided meditations across all eleven MBI sessions

processes of transfer—imitation, internalization of speech, and use of the expert model as a guide.

For example, in the interview data, one teacher described learning and transferring the disposition of self-compassion: *"I feel like the self-compassion component has been so meaningful to me and so helpful—learning not to beat myself up over this and that, learning to just let go of a lot of things...I hear your voice [instructor voice] through the day reminding me to practice these two."* Another teacher noted in her interview both non-verbal and verbal information that she transferred from the MBI instructor to her classroom:

> *So what I really came away with was this feeling of learning about your non-judgmental style, and that's been such a gift because I judge everything and I'm still judging everything and then I think 'judging, judging' [laughter]. And then* <u>*I hear your voice*</u>*—I just have loved how you diffuse things so easily with your style of 'well, isn't that interesting' or 'let's see about that', or 'what can we do with...' and it's just been really lovely...*

Instructor's Embodiment of Mindfulness Skills and Dispositions Finally, we examined how the mindfulness instructor's embodiment of mindfulness may have been an important, albeit often implicit, form of teaching that occurs in the MBI (Tharp & Gallimore, 1988). The case study results suggest that the expert instructor's embodiment of mindfulness is an important "active ingredient" in an MBI. In a post-program interview, for instance, one female second grade teacher remarked, "The instructor was an amazing role model for how to be a good teacher. She, like, walks the talk." Expertise includes *understanding mindfulness*, so the instructor is able to teach it with clarity. But expertise in this context also includes *embodying mindfulness*. By being mindful, the instructor may implicitly enhance participant motivation (by reflecting a model of participants' own aspirations to be mindful) and participant learning (by modeling the skills and qualities that participants' will be taught during the MBI). By embodying mindfulness, the instructor may also be perceived as authentic and accessible.

To assess all 13 teachers' perceptions of the instructor's embodiment of the skills being taught, we asked them how much they agree with these statements: "The instructor demonstrated good knowledge of the material taught," "The instructor presented the material effectively," "The instructor was a good role for the material we were learning," and "At some point, I developed a faith that I could trust and learn from the instructor." The expert instructor in our case study was evaluated as nearly a "5" on these 5-point items averaged across participants in this and two other trials of the MBI (see Roeser et al., 2002, 2013). We hypothesize that instructor embodiment of mindfulness may "bring the students to the task of learning mindfulness," and also provide teachers with implicit and explicit teachings regarding how to carry themselves and handle stress and interpersonal interactions in their own classrooms.

In sum, results from the case study illustrate some of the ways an expert instructor instructs teachers in the skills and dispositions of mindfulness by embodying mindfulness, using a variety of experiential-oriented teaching activities, and by using language in ways that scaffold mindfulness skill and disposition development. Furthermore, by providing a model of these skills in her own behavior, by offering vocabulary to reappraise moment-to-moment experience, and by affording strategies and the observer-observed structure with regard to conscious awareness, the instructor also supported teachers transfer of these skills to their own classrooms.

Emergent Theory of Teaching, Learning, and Transfer in MBIs for Teachers

Based on these preliminary results of the case study, we have begun to outline a preliminary theory of high quality of implementation of MBIs for teachers. These tentative, generalized propositions are depicted in Fig. 10.7 and briefly summarized here.

First, I propose that the embodied expertise of the mindfulness instructor and the aspiration of the teacher to learn mindfulness are two essential elements in the efficacy of MBIs on teacher outcomes (Cullen, 2011). To date, there exist almost no conceptualizations, assessments, or research on the

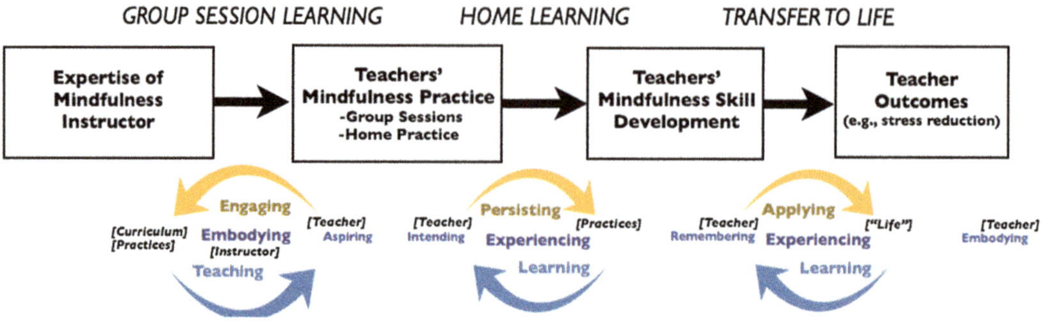

Fig. 10.7 Emerging theory of teaching, learning and transfer in MBIs for teachers

expertise of mindfulness instructors (see Crane et al., 2015 for exception). Based on the results of the case study and the writing of Cullen (2011), I propose that the experiential expertise of the mindfulness instructor in terms of **understanding and embodying mindfulness** in thought, word, and deed during group sessions may be a set of characteristics on which researchers could focus in the future. The instructor's expertise in these regards undergirds everything else they do in the context of implementation MBIs.

Based on the study of teaching, pedagogical expertise might be conceptualized as the practical ability of the mindfulness instructor to "bring the teachers to the task of learning mindfulness" by engaging their aspirations and linking them to what the curriculum and practices have to offer; and to "bring the task of learning mindfulness to the teachers" by teaching them mindfulness skills in emotionally and autonomy-supportive ways and empowering them to realize their intrinsic aspirations (Blumenfeld et al., 1991; Blumenfeld, Mergendoller, & Swarthout, 1987). Finally, the motivation of the instructor may also matters. In the best-case scenario, mindfulness instructors offer such trainings out of an aspiration to assist teachers in assisting themselves in alleviating suffering and realizing happiness. Nonetheless, other motives may be operative that impact on the quality of trainings. These issues involving the person of the mindfulness instructor and their influence on the quality of program implementation merit future research.

The motivation of the teacher in undertaking mindfulness training also undoubtedly matters for their learning of mindfulness skills. But just what are the aspirations of the teachers in attending such trainings? In our own research, we have found that the top four reasons teachers have for voluntarily signing up for an MBI are (1) a desire to lower levels of stress; (2) a desire to become a happier person; (3) a desire to improve one's quality of life; and (4) a desire to relax more. In essence, it appears teachers in our studies self-select into voluntary trainings with classic intrinsic motivations: the desires to alleviate suffering and realize happiness.

The issue of teacher motivation in relation to participating in MBIs in education settings is an important one. Voluntary programs offer an avenue for teachers to self-select given the natural aspirations noted above. Mandated trainings in schools, as part of professional development, may not. More research is needed on these questions, and also on changes in teachers' motivation to (re) engage with mindfulness practice as they go through MBIs (e.g., Grossman & Van Dam, 2011; Shapiro, Carlson, Astin, & Freedman, 2006).

Second, I propose that the expertise and pedagogy of the mindfulness instructor cultivates teachers' aspiration to learn, and thereby their level of engagement and the amount of time they invest in practicing mindfulness during the MBI (by coming to and engaging in group sessions and by doing home practices each day in between sessions). In essence, engaging instruction is hypothesized to cultivate teachers' continuing motivation to learn mindfulness (e.g., Maehr & Braskamp, 1986). I reviewed several dimensions of the pedagogy of one expert mindfulness instructor with the aim of spurring future research on what happens "inside the black box" of MBIs. It seems to me that the rich history of studying teachers, teaching and teacher development has much to offer the field of Contemplative Education in this regard. Studying processes of teaching and learning in mindfulness programs is critical, as I have tried to show, if we are to understand the skills and dispositions taught in such programs might transfer to contexts beyond the training setting.

Third, I propose that teachers' engagement with and practice of mindfulness over time, through personal intention, persistence and learning, and through instructor assistance (in both group sessions and through linguistic guidance on home-practice recordings), gradually lead to teachers' acquisition of mindfulness skills. Research that assesses the development of these skills over time during MBIs, instead of only at the conclusion and follow-up of the program, are needed in the future.

Fourth, I propose that teachers' enhanced mindfulness skills, their intention and remembering to apply those skills, and the visual and verbal scaffolding afforded by the instructor that has been internalized, leads to the gradual transfer of mindfulness skills to life beyond the MBI, for instance, to classrooms. Exploring not only the existence of transfer in terms of observable behavior, but also the means of such transfer (e.g., imitation, private speech, automatized skills) is another important direction for future research. In essence, we are arguing for researchers not just to examine the boxes of teacher, classroom, and student outcomes in the Theory of Change presented in Fig. 10.1, but also the psychosocial proximal processes on the arrows that connect these boxes.

In summary, the results of our case study of one expert mindfulness instructor have eventuated in a provisional theory, depicted in Fig. 10.7. This theory outlines a series of tractable research questions in need of further investigation regarding teaching, learning, and transfer within MBIs generally, and for teachers in particular. In the most basic sense, the hypothesis is that the instructors' embodiment of mindfulness, as well as the forms of teaching they enact during the course of the MBI, provide models for personal comportment and pedagogy that classroom teachers can take back to and enact within their classrooms and lives. In sum, it is for this reason that studying the qualities of mindfulness instructors, as well as their processes of teaching within MBIs, is critically important for understanding the relevance of MBIs in applied educational settings.

Conclusion

The purpose of this chapter was to challenge researchers interested in MBIs in education to look inside the "black box" of these interventions in order to understand how the skills and dispositions of mindfulness are taught and learned. I argued that process studies focused on the implementation of MBIs in education, such as the case study presented here, can help to (a) elucidate the pedagogical practices and uses of language and silence that may characterize highly effective mindfulness instructors as they teach teachers mindfulness-based skills and dispositions; as well as (b) the specific means by which expert mindfulness instructors may scaffold teachers' transfer of these skills and dispositions beyond the training context to settings such as the classroom. I argued that these basic questions regarding teaching, learning, and transfer are at the heart of contemplative education, and are important to address in future research if MBIs are to be successfully scaled, implemented, and sustained in public school settings. Focusing on quality of implementation is one key direction that education-focused researchers might take in order to move the entire fields of Contemplative Science and Contemplative Education forward.

References

Baer, R. A. (2011). Measuring mindfulness. *Contemporary Buddhism, 12*, 241–261.

Baer, R. A., Smith, G. T., Hopkins, J., Krietemeyer, J., & Toney, L. (2006). Using self-report assessment methods to explore facets of mindfulness. *Assessment, 13*, 27–45.

Baer, R. A., Smith, G. T., Lykins, E., Button, D., Krietemeyer, J., Sauer, S., … Williams, J. M. G. (2008). Construct validity of the five facet mindfulness questionnaire in meditating and nonmeditating samples. *Assessment, 15,* 329–342.

Benn, R., Akiva, T., Arel, S., & Roeser, R. W. (2012). Mindfulness training effects for parents and educators of children with special needs. *Developmental Psychology, 48,* 1476–1487.

Birman, B., Desimone, L., Porter, A. C., & Garet, M. (2000). Designing professional development that works. *Educational Leadership, 57,* 28–33.

Bishop, S. R., Lau, M., Shapiro, S., Carlson, L., Anderson, N. D., Carmody, J., … Devins, G. (2004). Mindfulness: A proposed operational definition. *Clinical Psychology: Science and Practice, 11,* 230–241.

Blumenfeld, P. C., Mergendoller, J. R., & Swarthout, D. W. (1987). Task as a heuristic for understanding student learning and motivation. *Journal of Curriculum Studies, 19*(2), 135–148.

Blumenfeld, P. C., Soloway, E., Marx, R. W., Krajcik, J. S., Guzdial, M., & Palincsar, A. (1991). Motivating project-based learning: Sustaining the doing, supporting the learning. *Educational Psychologist, 26*(3–4), 369–398.

Bransford, J. D., Brown, A. L., & Cocking, R. R. (1999). *How people learn: Brain, mind, experience, and school.* Washington, DC: National Academy Press.

Carmody, J., & Baer, R. A. (2008). Relationships between mindfulness practice and levels of mindfulness, medical and psychological symptoms and well-being in a mindfulness-based stress reduction program. *Journal of Behavioral Medicine, 31,* 23–33.

Carmody, J., & Baer, R. A. (2009). How long does a mindfulness-based stress reduction program need to be? A review of class contact hours and effect sizes for psychological distress. *Journal of Clinical Psychology, 65,* 627-638.

Case, R. (1992). *The mind's staircase. Exploring the conceptual underpinnings of children's thought and knowledge.* Hillsdale, NJ: Erlbaum.

Chiesa, A., & Serretti, A. (2009). Mindfulness-based stress reduction for stress management in healthy people: A review and meta-analysis. *Journal of Alternative and Complementary Medicine, 15,* 593–600.

Crane, R. S., Kuyken, W., Williams, J. M. G., Hastings, R. P., Cooper, L., & Fennell, M. J. (2012). Competence in teaching mindfulness-based courses: concepts, development and assessment. *Mindfulness, 3,* 76-84.

Cullen, M. (2011). Mindfulness-based interventions: An emerging phenomenon. *Mindfulness, 2,* 186–193.

Cullen, M., & Pons, G. B. (2015). *The Mindfulness-Based Emotional Balance Workbook: An Eight-Week Program for Improved Emotion Regulation and Resilience.* San Francisco: New Harbinger Publications.

Deci, E. L., & Ryan, R. M. (2002). Self-determination research: Reflections and future directions. In E. L. Deci & R. M. Ryan (Eds.), *Handbook of self-determination theory research* (pp. 431–441). Rochester, NY: University of Rochester Press.

Dewey, J. (1902). *The child and the curriculum.* Chicago, IL: University of Chicago Press.

Donald, M. (2001). *A mind so rare: The evolution of human consciousness.* New York, NY: W. W. Norton.

Eccles, J. S., & Roeser, R. W. (2015). School and community influences on human development. In M. H. Boorstein & M. E. Lamb (Eds.), *Developmental psychology: An advanced textbook* (7th ed.). Hillsdale, NJ: Erlbaum.

Engler, J. (1984). Therapeutic aims in psychotherapy and meditation: Developmental stages in the representation of self. *Journal of Transpersonal Psychology, 16,* 25–61.

Ericsson, K. A., & Charness, N. (1994). Expert performance: Its structure and acquisition. *American Psychologist, 49,* 725.

Flook, L., Goldberg, S. B., Pinger, L., Bonus, K., & Davidson, R. J. (2013). Mindfulness for teachers: A pilot study to assess effects on stress, burnout, and teaching efficacy. *Mind, Brain, and Education, 7,* 182–195.

Franco, C., Mañas, I., Cangas, A. J., Moreno, E., & Gallego, J. (2010). Reducing teachers' psychological distress through a mindfulness training program. *The Spanish Journal of Psychology, 13,* 655–666.

Frank, J. L., Jennings, P. A., & Greenberg, M. T. (2013). Mindfulness-based interventions in school settings: An introduction to the special issue. *Research in Human Development, 10,* 205-210.

Fredrickson, B. L. (2013). Positive emotions broaden and build. *Advances in Experimental Social Psychology, 47,* 1–53.

Fredrickson, B. L., Cohn, M. A., Coffey, K. A., Pek, J., & Finkel, S. M. (2008). Open hearts build lives: Positive emotions, induced through loving-kindness meditation, build consequential personal resources. *Journal of Personality and Social Psychology, 95,* 1045–1062.

Gage, N. L., & Berliner, D. C. (1992). *Educational psychology* (5th ed.). Boston, MA: Houghton Mifflin.

Garet, M., Porter, S., Andrew, C., & Desimone, L. (2001). What makes professional development effective? Results from a national sample of teachers. *American Educational Research Journal, 38*(4), 915–945.

Grossman, P., Niemann, L., Schmidt, S., & Walach, H. (2004). Mindfulness-based stress reduction and health benefits: A meta-analysis. *Journal of Psychosomatic Research, 57,* 35–43.

Grossman, P., & Van Dam, N. T. (2011). Mindfulness, by any other name…: Trials and tribulations of sati in western psychology and science. *Contemporary Buddhism, 12,* 219–239.

Hakanen, J. J., Bakker, A. B., & Schaufeli, W. B. (2006). Burnout and work engagement among teachers. *Journal of School Psychology, 43,* 495–513.

Harrison, J. L. (2014). *Assessing generic and program-specific dose-response relations between engagement in contemplative practices and reductions in teachers' occupational stress and burnout* (Unpublished thesis). Portland State University.

Hofmann, S. G., Grossman, P., & Hinton, D. E. (2011). Loving-kindness and compassion meditation: Potential for psychological interventions. *Clinical Psychology Review, 31*, 1126–1132.

Hölzel, B. K., Lazar, S. W., Gard, T., Schuman-Olivier, Z., Vago, D. R., & Ott, U. (2011). How does mindfulness meditation work? Proposing mechanisms of action from a conceptual and neural perspective. *Perspectives on Psychological Science, 6*, 537–559.

Jennings, P. A., Frank, J. L., Snowberg, K. E., Coccia, M. A., & Greenberg, M. T. (2013). Improving classroom learning environments by Cultivating Awareness and Resilience in Education (CARE): Results of a randomized controlled trial. *School Psychology Quarterly, 28*, 374–390.

Jennings, P. A., Snowberg, K. E., Coccia, M. A., & Greenberg, M. T. (2011). Improving classroom learning environments by cultivating awareness and resilience in education (CARE): Results of two pilot studies. *Journal of Classroom Interaction, 46*, 37–48.

Kabat-Zinn, J. (1994). *Wherever you go, there you are: Mindfulness meditation in everyday life*. New York, NY: Hyperion.

Kabat-Zinn, J. (2011). Some reflections on the origins of MBSR, skillful means, and the trouble with maps. *Contemporary Buddhism, 12*, 281–306.

Kabat-Zinn, J. (2003). Mindfulness-based interventions in context: Past, present, and future. *Clinical Psychology: Science and Practice, 10*, 144–156.

Kemeny, M. E., Foltz, C., Cavanagh, J. F., Cullen, M., Giese-Davis, J., Jennings, P., … Ekman, P. (2012). Contemplative/emotion training reduces negative emotional behavior and promotes prosocial responses. *Emotion, 12*, 338.

Lazarus, R. S., & Folkman, S. (1984). *Stress, appraisal and coping*. New York, NY: Springer.

Lutz, A., Dunne, J. D., & Davidson, R. J. (2007). Meditation and the neuroscience of consciousness. In P. Zelazo, M. Moscovitch, & E. Thompson (Eds.), *Cambridge handbook of consciousness* (pp. 499–555). New York, NY: Cambridge University Press.

Lutz, A., Jha, A. P., Dunne, J. D., & Saron, C. D. (2015). Investigating the phenomenological matrix of mindfulness-related practices from a neurocognitive perspective. *American Psychologist, 70*, 632-658.

Maehr, M. L., & Braskamp, L. A. (1986). *The motivation factor: A theory of personal investment*. Lexington, KY: Lexington Books/DC Heath and Company.

Marcovitch, S., Jacques, S., Boseovski, J. J., & Zelazo, P. D. (2008). Self-reflection and the cognitive control of behavior: Implications for learning. *Mind, Brain, and Education, 2*, 136–141.

McGeoch, J. A. (1942). *The psychology of human learning*. New York, NY: McKay.

Mind and Life Education Research Network (MLERN). (2012). Contemplative practices and mental training: Prospects for American education. *Child Development Perspectives, 6*, 146–153.

Neff, K. D. (2003). The development and validation of a scale to measure self-compassion. *Self and Identity, 2*, 223–250.

O'Donnell, C. L. (2008). Defining, conceptualizing, and measuring fidelity of implementation and its relationship to outcomes in K–12 curriculum intervention research. *Review of Educational Research, 78*, 33–84.

Parker, P. (1998). *The courage to teach. Exploring the inner landscape of a teacher's life*. San Francisco, CA: Jossey-Bass.

Pennebaker, J. W., Francis, M. E., & Booth, R. J. (2001). *Linguistic inquiry and word count: LIWC 2001*. Mahwah, NJ: Erlbaum.

Roeser, R. W. (2014). The emergence of mindfulness-based interventions in educational settings. In T. Urdan & S. Karabenick (Eds.), *Motivational interventions* (pp. 379–419). Edward Elgar, UK: Emerald Group.

Roeser, R. W., Horn-Keller, P., Stadick, M., & Urdan, T. (2012, April). *Teaching, learning and transfer in a mindfulness-based stress reduction program for teachers*. Annual meeting of the American Educational Research Association, Vancouver, BC, Canada.

Roeser, R. W., Marachi, R., & Gelhbach, H. (2002). A goal theory perspective on teachers' professional identities and the contexts of teaching. In C. M. Midgley (Ed.), *Goals, goal structures, and patterns of adaptive learning* (pp. 205–241). Hillsdale, NJ: Erlbaum.

Roeser, R. W., & Peck, S. C. (2009). An education in awareness: Self, motivation, and self-regulated learning in contemplative perspective. *Educational Psychologist, 44*, 119–136.

Roeser, R. W., Schonert-Reichl, K. A., Jha, A., Cullen, M., Wallace, L., Wilensky, R., … Harrison, J. (2013). Mindfulness training and reductions in teacher stress and burnout: Results from two randomized, waitlist-control field trials. *Journal of Educational Psychology, 105*, 787.

Roeser, R. W., Skinner, E., Beers, J., & Jennings, P. A. (2012). Mindfulness training and teachers' professional development: An emerging area of research and practice. *Child Development Perspectives, 6*, 167–173.

Roeser, R. W., & Zelazo, P. D. (2012). Contemplative science, education and child development: Introduction to the special section. *Child Development Perspectives, 6*, 143–145.

Rogoff, B. (2003). *The cultural nature of human development*. New York, NY: Oxford University Press.

Sarason, S. B. (1998). Some features of a flawed educational system. *Daedalus, 127*, 1–12.

Shapiro, S. L., Carlson, L. E., Astin, J. A., & Freedman, B. (2006). Mechanisms of mindfulness. *Journal of Clinical Psychology, 62*, 373–386.

Singer, T., & Lamm, C. (2009). The social neuroscience of empathy. *Annals of the New York Academy of Sciences, 1156*, 81–96.

Skinner, E., & Beers, J. (2015). Mindfulness and teachers' coping in the classroom: A developmental model of teacher stress, coping, and everyday Resilience. In R. W. Roeser & K. Schonert-Reichl (Eds.), *Handbook of mindfulness in education*. New York, NY: Springer.

Spindler, G. D. (1987). *Education and cultural process: Anthropological approaches*. Long Grove, IL: Waveland Press.

Taylor, C. L., Urdan, T. L., Cullen, M. M., & Roeser, R. W. (2014, April). *A qualitative study of the effects of mindfulness training on teachers' professional dispositions and classroom instruction*. Paper presented at the annual meeting of the American Educational Research Association, Philadelphia, PA.

Tharp, R. G., & Gallimore, R. (1988). *Rousing minds to life: Teaching, learning and schooling in social context*. New York, NY: Cambridge University Press.

Thompson, E. (2007). *Mind in life: Biology, phenomenology, and the sciences of mind*. Cambridge, UK: Harvard University Press.

Tomasello, M. (1999). *The cultural origins of human cognition*. Cambridge, MA: Harvard University Press.

Tschannen-Moran, M., Hoy, A. W., & Hoy, W. K. (1998). Teacher efficacy: Its meaning and measure. *Review of Educational Research, 68*, 202–248.

Vago, D. R., & Silbersweig, D. A. (2012). Self-awareness, self-regulation, and self-transcendence (S-ART): A framework for understanding the neurobiological mechanisms of mindfulness. *Frontiers in Human Neuroscience, 6*, 1–30.

Virgili, M. (2013). Mindfulness-based interventions reduce psychological distress in working adults: A meta-analysis of intervention studies. *Mindfulness, 4*, 1–12.

Vygotsky, L. S. (1978). *Mind and society: The development of higher mental processes*. Cambridge, MA: Harvard University Press.

Wallace, B. A. (2007). *Contemplative science: Where Buddhism and neuroscience converge*. New York, NY: Columbia University Press.

Wertsch, J. V. (1991). *Voices of the mind*. Cambridge, MA: Harvard University Press.

Wigfield, A., Eccles, J. S., Schiefele, U., Roeser, R. W., & Kean, P. D. (2006). Development of achievement motivation. In W. Damon & R. M. Lerner (Series Eds.), & N. Eisenberg (Volume Ed.), *Handbook of child psychology. Social, emotional and personality development* (6th ed., Vol. 3, pp. 933–1002). New York, NY: Wiley.

Williams, J. M. G., & Kabat-Zinn, J. (2011). Mindfulness: Diverse perspectives on its meaning, origins, and multiple applications at the intersection of science and dharma. *Contemporary Buddhism: An Interdisciplinary Journal, 12*, 1–18.

Winzelberg, A. J., & Luskin, F. M. (1999). The effect of a meditation training in stress levels in secondary school teachers. *Stress and Health, 15*, 69–77.

Yin, R. K. (2014). *Case study research: Design and methods*. Thousand Oaks, CA: Sage.

Young, S. (2011). *Five ways to know yourself: An introduction to basic mindfulness*. Unpublished manuscript, Burlington, VT.

Young, S. (2015). What is mindfulness?: A contemplative perspective. In R. W. Roeser & K. Schonert-Reichl (Eds.), *Handbook of mindfulness in education*. New York, NY: Springer.

Zelazo, P. D. (1999). Language, levels of consciousness, and the development of intentional action. In P. D. Zelazo et al. (Eds.), *Developing theories of intention: Social understanding and self-control* (pp. 95–117). Hillsdale, NJ: Erlbaum.

Mindfulness Activities and Interventions that Support Special Populations

11

Veronica Smith and Michaela Jelen

Mindfulness Activities and Interventions That Support Special Populations

With tranquil restoration: - feelings too
Of unremembered pleasure: such, perhaps,
As have no slight or trivial influence
On that best portion of a good man's life,
His little, nameless, unremembered, acts
Of kindness and of love. nor less, I trust,
To them I may have owed another gift,
Of aspect more sublime: that blessed mood
In which the burden of the mystery,
In which the heavy and the weary weight
Of all this intelligible world,
Is lightened—that serene and blessed mood
In which the affections gently lead us on, -
Until, the breath of this corporeal frame
And even the motion of our human blood
Almost suspended, we are laid asleep
In body, and become a living soul:
While, with an eye made quiet by the power
Of harmony and the deep power of joy,
We see into the life of things.
Tintern Abbey, William Wordsworth, 1770–1850

Although the subject of Wordsworth's poem, "Tintern Abbey," is memory, it also serves to demonstrate the power of the mind to offer a "tranquil restoration" to the self which, in turn, alters mood and perceptions of the weight of the world, and enhances the ability to see the "life of things" that influence actions of "kindness and of love." These qualities of the mind and their potential benefits have not escaped the attention of professionals in the fields of psychology, general education, and medicine and are beginning to receive attention within the field of special education. Over the past decade, a body of literature has emerged examining the role of mindfulness with children, youth, and adults with special learning needs, and with their teachers and professional caregivers (for selected reviews of this literature see Chapman et al., 2013; Harper, Webb, & Rayner, 2013; Hastings & Manikam, 2013; Hwang & Kearney, 2013, 2014). This work is altering not only the skills and abilities of children with special needs but also the attitudes and beliefs of their teachers and professional caregivers. The aim of this chapter is to examine the practices of engaging in mindfulness with special populations and their teachers. This critical review attempts to take stock and evaluate what is of value of mindfulness with special populations and describe how mindfulness contributes to, in Buddhist philosophy, "the end of suffering," and our evolving acceptance of special needs in contemporary Western contexts.

V. Smith (✉)
Psychological Studies in Education, Department of Educational Psychology, University of Alberta, 6-102 Education North, Edmonton, AB, Canada, T6G 2G5
e-mail: veronica.smith@ualberta.ca

M. Jelen
BC Ministry of Children and Family Development, Victoria, BC, Canada
e-mail: jelenmichaela@gmail.com

K.A. Schonert-Reichl, R.W. Roeser (eds.), *Handbook of Mindfulness in Education*, Mindfulness in Behavioral Health, DOI 10.1007/978-1-4939-3506-2_11

Acceptance of Experience

Mindfulness, as a practice, has been interpreted in educational contexts as a behavioral translation of Buddhist meditation. As such, mindfulness involves behaviors that include observing, describing with no judgment, and focusing awareness in the present moment (Kabat-Zinn, 1990). These behaviors, for special educators, represent a big departure from accepted practices. Our "evidence-base" resides predominantly in behaviorism, where the focus is on changing behavior and providing skills training. In contrast, the major emphasis of mindfulness training is on learning to experience emotions and thoughts skillfully, without evaluation and without the necessity of attempting to change or control the experience.

"Mindfulness is conceptualized as consisting of two facets: present-centered attention and acceptance of experience" (Coffey, Hartman, & Fredrickson, 2010, p. 250). Based on a study examining dispositional and mindfulness factors, Coffey et al. suggested that the ability to identify and differentiate among emotions, and to successfully regulate emotions are important consequences of the activity of mindfulness. Interestingly, when looking at how mindfulness contributes to well-being, they found that the acceptance of one's experience matters more for mental health than does present-centered attention. Acceptance of experience becomes an important notion in the context of special education, especially when we consider the struggle with the practice of *inclusion*. Inclusion of students with developmental disabilities with their same age peers has been on the agenda of special educators for decades (Jorgenson, 1997; Lyon et al., 2001; Shapiro, 1994). Yet, despite the agenda, in practice, there are still difficulties including children in school, as illustrated in the case below.

> *"Why is Bertrand sitting by himself with his iPad instead of interacting with the other students during group time?" I asked. As a special education inclusion consultant, I had a strong interest in encouraging Bertrand's teachers to include him in any activity that might allow him to practice his language and social interaction skills. His Educational Assistant replied, "Oh, he can't sit still during circle-time, he can't keep his hands and feet to himself, so it works out better for everyone if he has computer time on his own." "But he would really benefit from the social participation opportunities offered in the group," I countered. "Well, yes he would, but although he has a placement in this class," she explained, "we really have no idea how to manage his behavior, it is just too stressful everyone. He's not really ready to be included in this class."*

Some of the challenges including Bertrand in activities with his classmates relate to his non-normative behaviors but, beneath this, there is a suggested attitude that children need to be "ready" to be included. To be ready, one needs to behave in the "normative" way, a stance that insists that children adapt to the environment rather than adapt the environment to meet children's needs. This attitude of "readiness" is related to the lack of acceptance, or society's pervasive negative attitude to disability, dubbed "ableist" by Hehir (2007). Biklen (1992), who has written extensively about inclusion, has suggested that the purpose of special education is to "minimize the impact of disability and maximize the opportunities for students with disabilities to participate in schooling and the community" (p. 101). In the United States, the Individuals with Disabilities Education Act (IDEA; 1997, 2004) provides a mandate that requires individualized educational (IEP) teams address how students can gain access to the curriculum and how the school and teachers can meet the needs that arise out of students' disabilities. Yet, despite federally legislated mandates such as IDEA, problems remain in regard to including students in general education classrooms. From a mindfulness perspective, this could stem from a lack of acceptance of experience or a lack of acceptance of disability, itself. Acceptance could shift misguided effort to "cure" disability. Instead, if educators had enhanced ability to identify and differentiate among internal responses to children with disabilities, acceptance may lead to more accurate reflections on the kinds of supports, skills, and opportunities special students need to participate in school as fully as possible. Mindfulness provides an attitude that makes this kind of shift possible.

In the sections below, we review studies that have utilized mindfulness to influence a variety of outcomes. First, we examine mindfulness programs that address educator attitudes and beliefs that enrich well-being and acceptance. Second, we explore programs that address child behaviors or skills that impact upon improved coping in school environments.

Mindfulness Programs for Teachers and Professional Caregivers of Children with Special Needs

Beverly has been a special education teacher for the past 6 years. She used to feel idealistic about what she could accomplish as an educator but lately, she feels inundated by the number of students with special needs. Every year, it seems, more and more children with behavioral and educational needs are being placed in her classroom. This year, she has six of 28 children in her bustling grade 3 class with complex problems that need high levels of support. Robbie and Sean are diagnosed with ADHD and ODD respectfully; they are always getting into arguments and engaging in off task behaviours. It doesn't seem to matter if she lets them sit together or separates them, they always find a way to disrupt the learning of other students. Gemma has a diagnosis of autism spectrum disorder and requires a full time Educational Assistant. Despite not having a designation or Special Education 'code,' Amelia, Ben, and Thomas have learning challenges and it is hard to get them started with their school work. Beverly worries that she might not have the background or the support from the school administration to meet her students' needs. Although she loves her chosen profession, instead of getting easier, teaching seems to be getting harder and she often feels like she is at her wits end. She's really beginning to wonder if she made the correct career choice. Her husband and children have commented that she always seems frazzled and stressed about work rather than the enthusiastic and organized person she was when she first started teaching.

What Are the Issues? Beverly is in trouble. Her troubles are not the children that she has been assigned to teach but how she is coping with the social-emotional pressures of supporting these children on a day-to-day basis. Unfortunately, she is not alone. Many special education teachers like Beverly are at risk of leaving the teaching profession early. Attrition of special educators is on the rise due to a complex set of related circumstances. Billingsley (2003), in a study of the retention and attrition of special education teachers in the United States found that:

> Excessive and prolonged work problems lead to negative affective reactions, such as increased stress, lower job satisfaction, and reduced organizational and professional commitment….[this] clearly weakens the teacher's ability to be effective and therefore reduces their opportunities for the positive intrinsic rewards of teaching. (p. 6)

Mindfulness training may offer a solution; it is hypothesized to reduce biological vulnerability to negative emotional cues (Davidson et al., 2003), and research has demonstrated that those who practice meditation demonstrate activation of the brain that is consistent with improved capability in moderating the intensity of emotional arousal and increasing the experience of positive affect (Linehan et al., 2014). There are a handful of studies that have explored the effect of a mindfulness practice on reducing stress and enhancing well-being and work satisfaction for teachers or professional caregivers who work with high needs populations. These studies are summarized in Table 11.1 and discussed below.

Examples of Programs and Research

Benn et al. (2012) describe the implementation of a 5-week mindfulness program, *SMART-in-Education* (Cullen & Wallace, 2010), that included both special education teachers and parents of children with special needs. *SMART-in-Education*, or *Stress Management and Relaxation Techniques*, is a 36-h program developed to offer the same components of the Mindfulness-based Stress Reduction program (MBSR; Kabat-Zinn, 1990) with additional content that addresses emotion regulation, forgiveness, and kindness, and compassion as it relates to parenting and teaching. In an efficacy trial, teachers and parents who took part in the program reported increased mindfulness in terms of being more present, less judgmental, and more descriptive of their moment-to-moment experiences in contrast to the comparison group. The authors

Table 11.1 Examples of studies examining mindfulness for teachers or professional caregivers of children and youth with special needs

Author(s)	Participants (*N*)	Mindfulness activity	Outcomes targeted	Methodology and findings
Benn, Akiva, Arel, and Roeser (2012)	Special education teachers (23)	*SMART-in-Education* (Cullen & Wallace, 2010)	Mindfulness:	Randomized Waitlist Control
	Parents of children with special needs (20)	– 36 h of didactic and group discussion, mindfulness practices, and homework assignments delivered over nine 2.5 h sessions and 2 full days in a 5 week period	– *Five Facet Mindfulness Questionnaire* (FFMQ; Baer et al., 2006)	In contrast to the comparison group, participants who experienced the program self-reported increased mindfulness in terms of being more present, less judgmental, and more descriptive of their moment-to-moment experiences. Authors determined that these mindfulness competencies mediated reductions in participant's stress and distress with program effects persisting and growing larger in two-month follow-up. Both teachers and parents reported more positive well-being and enhanced relational competence. Teachers reported greater teaching self-efficacy but parents did not report enhancement in parenting efficacy or parent–child interactions
		– Compared with a no treatment control	Well-Being:	
			– *Perceived Stress Scale* (PSS; Cohen et al., 1983)	
			– *State-Trait Anxiety Inventory (S-TAI*; Kendall et al., 1976)	
			– *Centre for Epidemiological Studies Depression (CES-D*; Radloff, 1977)	
			Personal Growth:	
			– *Psychological Well-Being* (three items; Ryff & Keyes, 1995)	
			– *Self-Compassion Scale (SCS*; Neff, 2005)	
			– Positive and Negative affect: (*PANAS*; Watson et al., 1988)	
			– *State Forgiveness Scale* (Brown & Phillips, 2005)	
			– *Interpersonal Reactivity Index (IRI*; Davis, 1983)	
			Vocational Behaviors:	
			– Teaching Self-Efficacy (Midgely et al., 2000)	
			– Parenting Self-efficacy: *Everyday Parenting Scale* (Dunst & Masiello, 2002)	
			– Quality of parent–child interaction: items from the *Parenting Stress Inventory (PSI*) as described by Zaidman-Zait et al. (2010)	

Bethay, Wilson, Schnetzer, Nassar, and Bordieri (2013)	Staff (psychologists, special education teachers and assistants, care staff, nurses, social workers) from a state funded facility that offers 24 h care for individuals with moderate to severe intellectual disabilities	Combined *Acceptance and Commitment Training (ACT; Bond & Hayes,* 2002*) and Applied Behavior Analysis (ABA) (n = 18) contrasted with only ABA (n = 16)*	Psychological distress:	Randomized Control Study
		– *Three 3 h sessions @ 1 week intervals*	– *General Health Questionnaire-12* (Goldberg, 1978) Vocational Behaviors: – *Maslach Burnout Inventory, Human Services (MBI*; Hastings et al., 2004) and *Burnout Believability Scale (BBI*; Bach & Hayes, 2002)	Participants in the ACT + ABA group who reported significant psychological distress at pretest exhibited larger reductions in distress than those who received ABA alone. As well, ACT + ABA participants reported a decrease in the believability of thoughts that are indicative of burnout when compared to the ABA group. The two groups did not differ in the reported frequency of thoughts and feelings that are indicative of burnout consistent with the ACT program model, which emphasizes a reduction in the functional impact of thoughts rather than altering their form or frequency

(continued)

Table 11.1 (continued)

Author(s)	Participants (*N*)	Mindfulness activity	Outcomes targeted	Methodology and findings
Brooker et al. (2013)	Staff employed at residential service homes for adults with disabilities (managers = 22; support staff = 12, total *N* = 34)	*Occupational Mindfulness (OM) Program* (Adapted from *Mindfulness-Based Cognitive Therapy* (*MBCT;* Segal, Williams, & Teasdale, 2002), *MBSR* (Kabat-Zinn, 1990), and Seligman (2002) positive psychology	Mindfulness:	Quasi-experimental pre-post one group design
		2 h sessions × 8 weeks; sessions included focused group work and 40 min homework per 6/7 days	– Five Facet Mindfulness Questionnaire (FFMQ; Baer et al., 2006)	Significant increases in positive affect and the mindfulness facet of observing on the FFMQ. Paradoxically, participants reported enhanced awareness of signs and sources of stress and anxiety, yet positive changes in self-care attitudes and behaviors and interactions with clients and colleagues. More positive attitudes and behavioral changes were reported by support workers than managers. Overall, the program developers concluded that the program yielded a range of benefits to participants and holds significant potential to be transferred to other work settings
			Well-being:	
			– *Perceived Stress Scale* (PSS; Cohen et al., 1983)	
			– *Depression Anxiety Stress Scale—21* (DASS-21; Lovibond & Lovibond, 1995)	
			– PANAS; Watson et al., 1988)	
			– *Satisfaction with Life Scale* (SWL; Diener, 1985)	
			– SCS; Neff (2003)	
			Vocational Behaviors:	
			– *Copenhagen Burnout Inventory* (CBI; Kristensen et al., 2005)	
			– *Minnesota Satisfaction Questionnaire—Short Form* (MSQ-SF; Weiss et al., 1967) for job satisfaction	
			– *Professional Quality of Life Scale* (ProQOL; Stamm, 2009)	
			– *Santa Clara Brief Compassion Scale* (SCBCS; Hwang et al., 2008)	

Jennings, Frank, Snowberg, Coccia, and Greenberg (2013)	Classroom teachers ($n=33$), special education teachers ($n=8$), specialists (e.g., speech and language pathologists) ($n=6$), non-core educators ($n=3$).	*Cultivating Awareness and Resilience in Education (CARE;* Jennings, Snowberg, Coccia, & Greenberg, 2011)	Mindfulness:	Randomized control trial
	Total $N=50$	– 30 h program in day long sessions over 4–6 weeks	– FFMQ; Baer et al. (2006)	Results suggest that CARE had significant positive effects on teachers' general well-being, efficacy, burnout/time pressure, and mindfulness. Teachers who participated in the CARE program described improved ability to "reappraise" stressful situations, a behavior that is associated with emotional regulation. They also reported that improved daily physical symptoms of stress co-occurred with an improved sense of efficacy as a teacher. Like other teachers who participated in mindfulness programs, CARE teachers reported improved observing and non-reacting on the mindfulness measures. Overall, participants reported high levels of satisfaction with the program
		– Intersession coaching and booster session 2 months post program	Well-Being:	
		– Blend of didactic, interactive, and experiential activities	– *PANAS*; Watson et al. (1988)	
		– Emotion skills, mindfulness/stress reduction, and compassion practices	– Emotion Regulation Questionnaire (ERQ: Gross & John, 2003)	
			– CESD-20; Radloff et al., (1977)	
			– Daily Physical Symptoms (DPS; Larson & Kasimatis, 1997)	
			Vocational Behaviors:	
			– Teacher's Sense of Efficacy Questionnaire (TSES; Tsannen-Moran & Woolfolk Hoy, 2001)	
			– MBI; Hastings et al., (2004)	
			– Time Urgency Scale (TUS; Landy et al., 1991)	
			Program Evaluation:	
			– CARE Acceptability	
			Questionnaire (CAQ: Jennings et al., 2013)	

determined that these mindfulness competencies mediated reductions in participants' stress and distress, with program effects persisting and increasing in 2-month follow-up. Additionally, both teachers and parents reported more positive well-being and enhanced relational competence with their children. Importantly, the teachers reported greater teaching self-efficacy and felt better able to gauge how to regulate their response to stressful events. This application of a mindfulness program for special education teachers demonstrated that teachers can develop strategies for stress reduction that generalize to many settings, not only to their classrooms but in other contexts of their life, as well.

Other research has paired teacher training in applied behavioral analysis (ABA), an evidenced-based approach to working with children with special needs (Wong et al., 2014), with a form of mindfulness training called Acceptance and Commitment Therapy (ACT; Bond & Hayes, 2002). The researchers were curious whether ABA training could be enhanced by providing teachers with methods to not only help students with special needs but also to better cope with their personal stress and feelings of burnout related to working with children with additional needs (Bethay et al., 2013). They found that among participants who prior to the program reported significant psychological distress, teachers trained in both ACT and ABA exhibited larger reductions in distress than those who received ABA alone. As well, the ACT + ABA participants reported a decrease in the believability of thoughts related to burnout when compared to the ABA participants. The two groups did not differ significantly in the reported frequency of thoughts and feelings that are indicative of burnout. This finding was consistent with the ACT program model, which emphasizes a reduction in the functional impact of thoughts rather than altering their form or frequency.

Another mindfulness program, developed for staff employed at a residential treatment center for adults with significant disabilities, sought to address staff's response to the range of stressors experienced in the workplace. The program, Occupational Mindfulness (OM; Brooker et al., 2013) combined aspects of Mindfulness-based Cognitive Therapy (Segal et al., 2002), MBSR (Kabat-Zinn, 1990), and Martin Seligman's work in positive psychology. Participants, both support workers and their managers, were provided with structured opportunities for core mindfulness practices and were encouraged to make daily use of a "breathing space" in the workplace and assigned "homework" to establish mindfulness practices in their daily living. At the conclusion of the 8-week program, the researchers found significant increases in positive affect and the mindfulness facet of "observing." Participants reported enhanced awareness of the signs and sources of stress and anxiety which may have been perceived as a negative outcome; however, this awareness was paired with positive changes in self-care attitudes and behaviors and interactions with clients and colleagues. The support workers rated the program positively, a factor that could be related to their attitude and behavior changes. Overall, the program developers concluded that the program yielded a range of benefits to participants and holds significant potential to be transferred to other work settings.

Probably one of the most rigorous studies examining the benefits of mindfulness for teacher educators comes from a recent randomized control trial of the *Cultivating Awareness and Resilience in Education* (*CARE*; Jennings et al., 2011) program (Jennings et al., 2013). While the trial did not exclusively study special educators, they were included in the participant pool. After the 6 week 30-h program, results from teacher self-report measures suggest that CARE had significant positive effects on teachers' general well-being, efficacy, burnout/time pressure, and mindfulness. Teachers who participated in the CARE program described improved ability to "reappraise" stressful situations, a behavior that is associated with emotional regulation. They also reported that daily physical symptoms of stress decreased and co-occurred with an improved sense of efficacy as a teacher. Like other teachers who participated in mindfulness programs, CARE teachers reported improved observing and non-reacting on the mindfulness measures. Overall, participants reported high levels of satisfaction with the program.

What does this research tell us? First, the studies represent an interesting new direction in teacher professional development programs that recognizes that wellness is associated with performance and effectiveness as a teacher. Like our teacher Bev introduced at the beginning of this section, stress and burnout is a serious problem in education today. For special educators, stress is compounded by repeated exposure to challenging behaviors (Koritsas, Iacono, Carling-Jenkins, & Chan, 2010), uncertainty in how to teach some children, and low resources or administrative support to meet student educational needs (Billingsley, 2003). A focus on programs that help teachers reduce stress and bolster well-being, acknowledges the reality of school settings and allows teachers to develop better observational skills of themselves in their circumstances that potentially allows them to respond to student needs more empathically and appropriately, thereby freeing them up to maximize their pedagogical skills with high needs populations.

Mindfulness Programs for Students with Special Needs

James is a 7-year-old boy with attention deficit hyperactivity disorder who attends a rural primary school. He is an affectionate young person who is delayed but progressing well in grade three, except for physical education class. There, he needs a lot of support just to stay in the gym and attend to the teacher. His mother has commented that her son finds the gym over stimulating and he has difficulty focusing in that kind of environment. James is rarely away from school and physical education at his school is scheduled every day.

Jordan is well behaved and sociable in his community, especially when he is in the company of his family. At school, he is able to complete grade level material with particular strengths in math. He finds school a stressful environment and complains to his mother that 'no one likes him' and that his teacher changes the schedule without enough warning. He sometimes refuses to go to school and, even when he is there, he will not participate in activities, saying that he prefers to work alone. His current teacher, Mr. Laughlin, is aware that Jordan is on the autism spectrum and, additionally, sees him as an anxious student who he has referred to the Learning Resource teacher for some social supports.

Lisa is a 14 year-old junior high student who is attends the resource room at her school. Her teacher, Ms. Kirkpatrick, has felt frustrated by Lisa's obsessive-compulsive behaviours and is not sure what to do about them. She says that Lisa becomes angry when she does not provide constant reassurance or when something in the resource room is out of order. Despite regretting her behavior afterward, Lisa often yells and threatens the teacher and the other students, disrupting the learning environment. Lisa has a mild intellectual disability diagnosis and a history of depression, so Ms. Kirkpatrick wants to tread carefully.

What Are the Issues? James, Jordan, and Lisa each have very unique needs. Like many children with mild to moderate disabilities, they find the school environment stressful and unpredictable and are challenged by the work demands at school. It is not uncommon for students with developmental disabilities to respond to the school context with range of maladaptive behaviors: to withdraw, to be noncompliant, and to be aggressive (Allen, 2000). Teachers need to seek ways to reduce student maladaptive behaviors, as they are clearly barriers to benefiting from learning opportunities (Hattie, 2009). Within the special education literature, there are many established treatments for maladaptive behaviors, including functional analysis, antecedent supports, functional communication training, and differential reinforcement, to name a few (Wong et al., 2014). Behavioral treatments have been criticized as, although they are successful in highly controlled context, when fidelity wanes, so too does their effectiveness (Singh et al., 2013). With mindfulness emerging as a promising coping procedure within the typical population, it is not unreasonable to assume that it may be beneficial for individuals with intellectual disabilities and other learning needs (Hwang & Kearney, 2013). Research that has explored the potential of mindfulness to enhance learning outcomes for students with special needs is presented in Table 11.2 and described below.

Table 11.2 Examples of studies examining mindfulness for children, youth, and adults with special needs

Author(s)	Participants (N)	Mindfulness program	Outcomes targeted	Methodology and findings
Adkins, Singh, Winten, McKeegan, and Singh (2010)	Adults with one or more of the following diagnoses ($N=3$):	*Meditation on the Soles of the Feet* (Singh et al., 2011)	<u>Behavior</u>	<u>Multiple baseline across participants</u>
		• Training to shift attention from emotion or trigger prior to behavior	"Maladaptive Behavior"	For all participants the frequency of maladaptive behaviors decreased from the pre-intervention baseline phase to the mindfulness intervention phase and remained low, with mild variability, 9–12 weeks after the intervention
	• Obsessive Compulsive Disorder, Depression, and/or Intellectual Disability	• 1 h, 5 days a week from 2 to 5 weeks; incidental practice encouraged	• Verbal aggression	
		• Support provided by a trained community-based therapist	• Work disruption	
			• Physical aggression	
			• Property destruction	
			• Rectal digging	
			• Urinary Incontinence	
Beauchemin, Hutchins, and Patterson (2008)	Adolescents aged 13–18 years ($N=34$):	Mindfulness Meditation (based on *Wherever you go there you are* (Kabat-Zinn, 1994))	<u>Social Skills, Problem Behaviors, & Academic Performance:</u>	<u>Quasi-experimental Design</u>
	• Learning disabilities	• Teachers trained in 2 h session	– *Social Skills Rating System* (Gresham & Elliot, 1990)	<u>(Pre-post; no-control; no follow-up)</u>
		• Teachers provided students with 5–10 min of mindfulness meditation for several times a day, 5 days per week for 5 weeks	<u>Mental Health:</u>	Teachers rated improved student social skills and academic performance. Students self-reported decreased anxiety following the mindfulness program. No long-term follow-up
			– *State-Trait Anxiety Inventory* (Spielberger et al., 1970)	
Carboni, Roach, and Fredrick (2013)	Children with Attention Deficit Hyperactivity Disorder who were on medication for challenging behaviors ($N=4$)	*MBSR for Children* (Saltzman & Goldin, 2008) and CD of recorded practices from *Building Emotional Intelligence to Cultivate Inner Strength in Children* (Lantieri & Goldin, 2008)	<u>Behavior</u>	<u>Multiple baseline across participants</u>
		• Individual session for 30–45 min per day for 10–20 sessions	– "On task behaviors" in classroom settings ratings based on the *Behavioral Observations of Students in Schools* (BOSS; Shapiro, 2004)	The modest increases of on-task behavior that occurred for all participants during the intervention phase returned close to baseline at 2-week follow-up

Haydicky, Wiener, Badali, Milligan, and Ducharme (2012)	Adolescent males (12–18 years) with Learning Disabilities (LD) ($N = 60$)	*Mindfulness Martial Arts* (MMA; Badali, 2007)	<u>Executive Functioning</u>	<u>Quasi-experimental waitlist control design</u>
	– Subgroups:	• Manualized program; 1.5 h session each week for 20 weeks	– *Behavior Rating Inventory of Executive Functioning; (BRIEF*; Gioa, Isquith, Guy, & Kenworthy, 2000)	In contrast to the waitlist control group, parents reported reductions in externalizing, oppositional behaviors, and conduct problems for their children with LD and ADHD. Parents also reported that their boys with LD + Hyperactive/impulsivity showed improvements in social problems and the executive functioning skill of monitoring. Boys with inattentiveness improved on parent rated social problems. Boys with LD and elevated anxiety self-reported reductions in anxiety
	LD + ADHD (47 %)	• Elements of mindfulness, Cognitive Behavior Therapy, and mixed martial arts	<u>Behavioral Symptoms</u>	
	LD + Hyperactive/impulsive (48 %)		– *Child Behavior Checklist (CBCL*; Achenback & Rescorla, 2001)	
	LD + Anxious/Shy (48 %)		– *Youth Self-Report (YSR*; Achenback, 2001)	
	LD + Inattentive (55 %)			
Idusohan-Mozier, Sawicka, Dendle, and Albany (2013)	Adults with mild to moderate intellectual disabilities and at least one mental health concern (i.e., depression, anxiety, or self-injurious behavior) ($N = 12$)	Program adapted from *Mindfulness-based cognitive behavior therapy* (MBCT; Segal et al., 2002); *Acceptance and Commitment Therapy (ACT*; Hayes et al., 1999; self-compassion (Neff, 2003); and *Meditation on the Soles of Your Feet* (Singh et al., 2003)	<u>Well-being:</u>	<u>Quasi-experimental design (pre- post; no control; 6-week follow up)</u>
		• Adapted for adults with intellectual disabilities	– *The Compassion Scale*; (Neff, 2003)	Improvements in participant's self-reported compassion and kindness for themselves and others, however follow-up scores were closer to baseline. Participant interviews on the HADS revealed that anxiety was reduced at posttest and this difference remained at follow-up. Depression scores were significantly lower at posttest; however, the difference was not maintained at follow-up. Those that completed the program (approximately 80 %), positively rated the experience yet slightly less than half reported that they would continue the practices learned
		• Group ran for 1.5 h for 9 weeks; follow up 6 weeks post intervention	<u>Mental Health:</u>	
		• Caregivers of the adults also attended the sessions and were invited to encourage daily practice	– *Hospital Anxiety and Depression Scale* (HADS; Zigmond & Snaith, 1983)	

(continued)

Table 11.2 (continued)

Author(s)	Participants (*N*)	Mindfulness program	Outcomes targeted	Methodology and findings
Miodrag, Lense, and Dykens (2012)	Adults with Williams Syndrome and Borderline or Mild Intellectual Disability ($N=24$)	*Mindfulness-Based Stress Reduction* (MBSR) (adapted from Kabat-Zinn, 1990)	<u>Biological:</u>	<u>Quasi-experimental (pre-post; no control group; no follow-up)</u>
		• Program conducted during a week-long camp; small-group sessions; 20 min per day for 5 consecutive days	– Physiological measures associated with stress: Salivary cortisol and Salivary Enzyme Alpha-Amylase (sAA) <u>Behavioral Symptoms</u> – Mood Rating Scale (developed by study authors)	As hypothesized, self-reported anxiety and salivary cortisol were associated at the start of each MBSR session. Importantly, both the salivary cortisol and self-reported anxiety were reduced at the end of each session. MBSR did not have a main effect on sAA, which were variable from session to session
Singh et al. (2013)	Adult Smokers with Mild Intellectual Disability ($N=3$)	*Meditation on the Soles of the Feet* (Singh et al., 2011)	<u>Behavior</u>	<u>Changing Criterion Design (12 month maintenance and 3 year follow-up)</u>
		• Phase I: 3 month 10–15 min daily meditation practice; daily monitoring of cigarettes smoked • Phase II: Daily intention to quit smoking; gradual reduction of cigarettes smoked; daily mindful observation of thoughts; meditation of the Soles of the Feet role play 30 min a day for 5 days, guided to use when urge to smoke was strong; 10 days of practice assignments	– Number of cigarettes smoked	All three participants reduced smoking from 13–3[illegible] to 0 cigarettes per day over a period of 77–1[illegible]5 days. Nonsmoking was maintained for all participants after 3 years
Singh et al. (2013)	Adults with Mild Intellectual disability and low frequency but severe aggressive behaviors ($N=34$)	*Meditation on the Soles of the Feet* (*SoF*; Singh et al., 2011)	<u>Behavior</u>	<u>Randomized waitlist control</u>
		• Taught by parents and community support staff for 12-week for 15–30 min per day • SoF program: meditation; focused attention on arousal states; Meditation on the Soles of the Feet practice in simulated incidents	– Physical and verbal aggression	After the SoF intervention, there were observed reductions in both physical and verbal aggression. Fidelity of program implementation, evaluated by certified SoF trainers, was high indicating potential for transfer for SoF to community settings

Singh et al. (2007)	Adults with mild to moderate intellectual disability and comorbid mental health disorder (*N*=3)	Two meditation procedures were taught: *Meditation on the Soles of the Feet* (Singh et al., 2011) and *Recreating-the-scene* (Van Houten & Rolider, 1988)	Behavior	Multiple-baseline across participants
		• Practices were taught, then two practice session per day were supported for 35 weeks	– Physical aggression (e.g., punching, kicking, slapping, or hitting with object)	All three participants reduced aggressive behaviors and maintained reductions at 2-year follow-up. These changes allowed the participants to continue living in their community placements
Singh et al. (2011)	Adolescents (age 14–17) with autism spectrum disorder who had previously been prescribed medication or whose parents had received behavioral training (*N*=3)	*Meditation on the Soles of the Feet* (Singh et al., 2003)	Behavior	Multiple-baseline across participants
		• Taught by participant's mothers for 30-min for 5 consecutive days followed by practice of skills twice a day until behavior was eliminated for 4 consecutive weeks	– Physical aggression towards a sibling or parent (e.g., hitting, kicking or biting)	All three participants reduced aggressive behaviors to near zero incidences and were able to maintain reductions at three-year follow-up. Mothers, who taught the intervention, also reported using *SoF* meditation when they felt stressed
Spek, van Ham, and Nyklicek (2013)	Adults with autism spectrum disorder who were also experiencing symptoms of depression, anxiety and/or rumination (*N*=42)	*Mindfulness-Based Therapy for Autism Spectrum* (MBT-AS) (adapted from *Mindfulness-based cognitive therapy* (MBCT; Segal et al., 2002)	Well-being	Randomized Control Design
		• Small group 2.5 h sessions for 9 weeks with encouragement to practice 40–60 min a day 6 days a week. Guided meditations were provided in audiofiles	– *The Dutch Global Mood Scale* (Denollet, 1993)	Following the mindfulness-based intervention, participants self-reported decreases in anxiety, depression, and rumination with medium to large effects. Further, the intervention group showed an increase in positive affect in contrast to the control group
			Mental Health	
			– *The Symptom Checklist-90-Revised* for anxiety and depression (Derogatis, 1994)	
			– *Rumination-Reflection Questionnaire* (Trapnell & Campbell, 1999)	

(continued)

Table 11.2 (continued)

Author(s)	Participants (*N*)	Mindfulness program	Outcomes targeted	Methodology and findings
Van der Oord, Bogels, and Peijnenburg (2012)	Parents and their children (age 8–12 years) with Attention Deficit Hyperactivity Disorder (ADHD) (*N*=22)	Two programs, Mindful Parenting (MP) and Mindful Child Training (MCT) were developed by the authors based on MBCT (Segal et al., 2002) and MBSR (Kabat-Zinn, 1990) with adaptations for ADHD children (i.e., clear structure, breaks, tangible reinforcement for compliance)	Behavioral Symptoms – Disruptive Behavior Disorder Rating Scale (Pelham et al., 1992)	Quasi experimental waitlist control Parents who participated in the program self-rated reductions of their own ADHD behavior, parenting stress, and overreactivity and improvements in mindfulness awareness
		• Program was conducted in small groups of parents or children (with some joint sessions) for 90 min over 8 weeks	Mindfulness – *Mindfulness Attention and Awareness Scale* (MAAS; Brown & Ryan, 2003) Parenting – *Parenting Stress Index*; De Brock et al., 1992) – *The Parenting Scale* (Arnold et al., 1993) – ADHD Rating Scale (parent); Kooij et al., 2005)	Parents reported child improvements of inattention and hyperactivity/impulsivity. Teacher ratings revealed mild improvements in child inattention; however, no further teacher ratings were found to be statistically significant. Almost 20 % of the participants did not complete the program

van de Weijer-Berjsma, Formsma, de Bruin, and Bogels (2012)	Parents and their children (age 11–15 years) with Attention Deficit Hyperactivity Disorder (ADHD) ($N=10$)	Two programs, *Mindful Parenting* (MP; Bogels et al., 2008; Van der Oord et al., 2012) and *Adolescent Training (AT)*, were developed by the authors. Both programs were inspired by Mindfulness in Schools (Hubbard & Johnson, 2010). To enhance learning, home practice and enhancements were used	Mindfulness	Quasi-experimental design (one group pretest/posttest with follow-up)
		• Parent (with fathers and mothers) and adolescent programs were held concurrently for 8 weekly 90-min sessions	– MAAS (Brown & Ryan, 2003) Behavior Symptoms – *CBCL, YSR, and Teacher Report Form (*Achenback & Rescorla, 2001) – Finders Fatigue Scale (Gradisar et al. 2007) – Subjective Happiness Scale (Lyubomirsky & Lepper, 1999) Executive Functioning – *BRIEF* (Gioa et al., 2000) Computerized Attention Tests – Amsterdam Neuropsychological Tasks (attention, impulsivity, and reaction speed) (De Sonne-ville, 2005) Parenting – *PSI* (De Brock et al., 1992) and PS (Arnold et al., 1993)	No change was found in mindful awareness self-ratings for either adolescents or parents. Adolescents did not report that fatigue or happiness changed as a result of the program. Mixed reports (i.e., parents and /or teacher reports differed) of improvements in attention and reductions in externalizing and internalizing behaviors. Teachers reported that adolescents had better behavior regulation post program, indicating improvements in executive functioning. There were inconsistencies in response to the computerized attention tasks, preventing attribution of changes to the program. Fathers reported reductions in parental stress but mothers did not

(continued)

Table 11.2 (continued)

Author(s)	Participants (*N*)	Mindfulness program	Outcomes targeted	Methodology and findings
Zylowska et al. (2008)	Adolescents ($n=8$) and adults ($n=24$) with ADHD	*Mindfulness Awareness Practices for ADHD* (developed by the authors and informed by Kabat-Zinn, 1990; Segal et al., 2002)	Behavioral Symptoms	Quasi-experimental design (one group, pre-post test)
		• Once per week 2.5 h sessions and daily at home practice for 8 weeks	– ADHD rating scale IV; (DuPaul, 1990) and the SNAP-IV; Swanson, 1995)	Improvements in ADHD symptoms, anxiety, and depressive symptoms were found following the mindfulness-based intervention. Improvements on cognitive tasks that measured attention and cognitive inhibitions were also found
			– Beck Anxiety Depression Indexes; (Beck, Epstein, &Brown, 1992)	
			– Child Depression Inventory; Kovacs, 1992)	
			Cognitive Functioning	
			– The Attention Network Test (ANT; Golden, 1978)	
			– STROOP Task	
			– Trail Making Test (Reitan, 1979)	
			– Digit span on the WISC-3; (Weschler, 1981, 1991)	

Examples of Programs and Research

Of the 14 studies present in Table 11.2, the strongest methodologically are five studies conducted by Nirbhay Singh and his team at the ONE Research Institute in North Carolina (i.e., Adkins et al., 2010; Singh et al., 2007, 2011, 2013). This program of research is commendable for the procedures that were followed to develop the mindfulness practice, *Meditation of the Soles of the Feet (SoF)*, and to test its effectiveness. *SoF* is a practice that is taught to help students recognize the precursors of behaviors or emotions that give rise to maladaptive behavior (e.g., aggression, anger, smoking), to disengage their attention to these precursors, and redeploy their attention to a neutral point in their body, the soles of their feet (Singh et al., 2013). To test the effectiveness of this intervention the research team began by utilizing single-case research designs (SCRD). There is high heterogeneity among the individuals within each of the disability groups. This diversity and the range of abilities and needed interventions makes SCRD a very appropriate research methodology to test program effectiveness. SCRDs are considered the first level of research used to establish the merit of a particular treatment or intervention. SCRD designs provide clear, visual evidence that an independent variable (i.e., such as a mindfulness program) has a replicable effect across a small number of participants (Smith et al., 2007). When there are positive findings, multiple SCRDs can strengthen initial findings by replicating the results across participants with varying needs, abilities, and challenges. Once SCRD studies establish the efficacy of a practice, experimental designs that test the intervention in more controlled ways, such as randomized control trials, are pursued. In the body of work of Nirbhay Singh, we see this carefully planned progression of research. Using a series of SCRD studies he and his team established the effectiveness of the SoF practice to address several maladaptive behaviors in a range of students: anger in an individual with intellectual disability and mental health issues (Singh et al., 2003), aggression in individuals with moderate levels of intellectual disability (Singh et al., 2007), a range of maladaptive behaviors in individuals with and obsessive compulsive disorder or depression (Adkins et al., 2010), aggression in autism (Singh et al., 2011), and smoking cessation in adults with intellectual disability (Singh et al., 2013). These studies helped to refine the adaptations needed to make the *SoF* practice suitable for these populations and establish the efficacy of the procedures. Following these initial studies, the research team moved on to an experimental design that tested the *SoF* practice on aggression in individuals with intellectual disability in a more controlled clinical randomized control trial (Singh et al., 2013). Intervention effects of the SoF practice were observed in decreases in aggression and anger episodes, decreases in maladaptive behaviors, and smoking cessation. Singh et al. (2013) provides an explanation of why the SoF is likely effective: "Given that the mind cannot fully concentrate on two nonhabitual processes simultaneously (Foerde et al., 2006), the *SoF* meditation results in the fading of the anger or emotionally arousing situation. In essence, the individual learns to stop, focus the mind on the body, calm down, be in the present moment, and then make an informed response to the situation, without anger" (p. 164).

Modifications of several mindfulness programs (e.g., MBSR (Kabat-Zinn, 1990), MBCT (Segal et al., 2002), ACT (Bond & Hayes, 2002), and Mindfulness in Schools (Hubbard & Johnson, 2010) to increase the accessibility of the procedures for children and youth with ADHD (Carboni et al., 2013; Van der Oord et al., 2012; van de Weijer-Berjsma et al., 2012; Zylowska et al., 2008), autism (Spek et al., 2013), learning disabilities (Beauchemin et al., 2008; Haydicky et al., 2012; Milligan & Ducharme, 2012), and intellectual disabilities and mental health concerns (Idusohan-Mozier et al., 2013), and Williams Syndrome (Miodrag et al., 2012). Program effects have been mixed but overall positive with reductions in anxiety, depression, and rumination and improvements in social skills, academic performance, executive functioning, well-being, and on task behavior. One study (Miodrag et al., 2012) found that salivary cortisol was associated with reductions in self-reported anxiety at the end of each mindfulness session but cautioned that, "We do not know how this would translate into longterm stable effects" (p. 143).

What does this research tell us? This growing body of research, the majority of which has been published in the last 5 years, indicates a belief that people with disabilities can and do benefit from programs that are more "psychological" in nature, as long as adaptations are made to increase accessibility (Idusohan-Mozier et al., 2013). As such, the effects of the application of mindfulness have been observed in the seemingly disparate conditions of ASD, intellectual disabilities, ADHD, mental health concerns, and other developmental issues. Positive outcomes have been seen through behavioral changes, decreased anxiety, better focus and attention at school, and improvements in well-being and attitudes toward school. However, these positive findings need to be considered with caution. Many of the studies described above include small samples or use weak designs (i.e., pre-post test with no comparison group). In addition, with the exception of the unique *SoF* meditation (i.e., Adkins et al., 2010; Singh et al., 2007, 2011, 2013), no research addresses the issue of which components of the mindfulness program influence the changes observed or were perceived by the participants as the most meaningful. Few studies explore long-term impact of the program (with the exception of Singh et al., 2013) and whether the students are able to maintain the mindfulness practices without adult supports. Knowledge of whether and for whom supports are needed may add to future successful applications of mindfulness programs and approaches with special populations

Conclusions and Future Directions

The research on mindfulness programs that have been offered to special education teachers and professional caregivers is promising. Effects of the programs include reductions in stress and "burnout," more effective "reappraisal" of situations and high acceptance of the programs by teachers. Programs that contribute to teacher wellness are likely to have far reaching consequences, especially in regard to student outcomes. There is a well-established relationship between teacher attitudes toward their teaching and their effectiveness as teachers (Osher et al., 2007) and teacher quality is highly associated with student outcomes (e.g., Allen, Pianta, Gregory, Mikami, & Lun, 2011; Hamre & Pianta, 2005). Whether or not enhanced mindfulness practices influence teacher attitudes of acceptance toward students with disabilities is suggested but the exact mechanisms of how mindfulness can contribute to shifts in interactions with these students requires further exploration. Several researchers caution that it is likely that short duration programs may not be sufficient to establish a mindfulness "practice" that will sustain enhanced coping and response to stressful workplace settings. Other supports within the workplace or school setting may need to be established in order to support teacher practices in this regard. Clearly more research is needed in this area.

For children with special needs, mindfulness appears to have positive outcomes, especially in regard to decreased anxiety, improved on task behavior, and decreased depression and rumination. This review reveals that mindfulness is a promising approach for delivering needed supports for students with special needs. Given the complexities involved with the development and evaluation of such programs, it is not surprising that empirical support for them is still quite limited. While there are promising effects for some targeted developmental issues, more work is needed to specify who will benefit from mindfulness programs and how the positive effects can endure and translate to other settings. In order for mindfulness to be adopted by students, schools, and other agencies, future research must continue to demonstrate efficacy, effectiveness, and social validity across large diverse samples of individuals and contexts.

References

Adkins, A. D., Singh, A. N., Winten, A. S. W., McKeegan, G. F., & Singh, J. (2010). Using a mindfulness-based procedure in the community: Translating research to practice. *Journal of Family Studies, 19*, 175–183.

Allen, D. (2000). Recent research on physical aggression in persons with intellectual disability: An overview. *Journal of Intellectual and Developmental Disability, 25*, 41–57.

Allen, J. P., Pianta, R. C., Gregory, A., Mikami, A. Y., & Lun, J. (2011). An interaction-based approach to enhancing secondary school instruction and student achievement. *Science, 333*, 1034–1037.

Beauchemin, J., Hutchins, T. L., & Patterson, F. (2008). Mindfulness meditation may lessen anxiety, promote social skills, and improve academic performance among adolescents with learning disabilities. *Complementary Health Practice Review, 31*(1), 34–45.

Benn, R., Akiva, T., Arel, S., & Roeser, R. W. (2012). Mindfulness training effects for parents and educators of children with special needs. *Developmental Psychology, 48*, 1476–1487.

Bethay, J. S., Wilson, K. G., Schnetzer, L. W., Nassar, S. L., & Bordieri, M. J. (2013). A controlled pilot evaluation of acceptance and commitment training for intellectual disability staff. *Mindfulness, 4*, 113–121.

Biklen, D. (1992). *Schooling without labels: Parents, educators, and inclusive education*. Philadelphia, PA: Temple University Press.

Billingsley, B. S. (2003). *Special education teacher retention and attrition: A critical analysis of the literature* (COPSSE Document No. RS-2E). Gainsville, FL: University of Florida, Center on Personnel Studies in Education.

Bond, F. W., & Hayes, S. C. (2002). ACT at work. In F. W. Bond & W. Dryden (Eds.), *Handbook of brief cognitive behavior therapy* (pp. 117–139). New York, NY: Wiley.

Brooker, J., Julian, J., Webber, L., Chan, J., Shawyer, F., & Meadows, G. (2013). Evaluation of an occupational mindfulness program for staff employed in the disability sector in Australia. *Mindfulness, 4*, 122–136.

Carboni, J. A., Roach, A. T., & Fredrick, L. D. (2013). Impact of mindfulness training on the behavior of elementary students with attention deficit/hyperactivity disorder. *Research in Human Development, 10*(3), 234–251.

Chapman, M., Hare, D. J., Caton, S., Donalds, D., McInnis, E., & Mitchell, D. (2013). The use of mindfulness with people with intellectual disabilities: A systematic review and narrative analysis. *Mindfulness, 4*, 179–189.

Coffey, K. A., Hartman, M., & Fredrickson, B. L. (2010). Deconstructing mindfulness and constructing mental health: Understanding mindfulness and its mechanisms of action. *Mindfulness, 1*, 235–253.

Cullen, M., & Wallace, L. (2010). *Stress management and relaxation techniques in education (SMART) training manual*. Unpublished manual, Impact Foundation, Aurora, CO.

Harper, S. K., Webb, T. L., & Rayner, K. (2013). The effectiveness of mindfulness-based interventions for supporting people with intellectual disabilities: A narrative review. *Behavior Modification, 37*(3), 431–453.

Hastings, R. P., & Manikam, R. (2013). Mindfulness and acceptance in developmental disabilities: Introduction to the special issue. *Mindfulness, 4*, 85–88.

Hattie, J. (2009). *Visible learning: A synthesis of over 800 meta-analyses relating to achievement*. New York, NY: Routledge.

Haydicky, J., Wiener, J., Badali, P., Milligan, K., & Ducharme, J. M. (2012). Evaluation of a mindfulness-based intervention for adolescents with learning disabilities and co-occurring ADHD and anxiety. *Mindfulness, 3*, 151–164.

Hehir, T. (2007). Confronting ableism. *Educational Leadership, 64*, 8–14.

Hwang, Y., & Kearney, P. (2013). A systematic review of mindfulness intervention for individuals with developmental disabilities: Long-term practice and long lasting effects. *Research in Developmental Disabilities, 34*, 314–326.

Hwang, Y., & Kearney, P. (2014). Mindfulness and mutual care for individuals with developmental disabilities: A systemic literature review. *Journal of Child and Family Studies, 23*, 497–509.

Idusohan-Mozier, H., Sawicka, A., Dendle, J., & Albany, M. (2013). Mindfulness-based cognitive therapy for adults with intellectual disabilities: An evaluation of the effectiveness of mindfulness in reducing symptoms of depression and anxiety. *Journal of Intellectual Disability Research, 59*(2), 93–104.

Jennings, P. A., Frank, J. L., Snowberg, K. E., Coccia, M. A., & Greenberg, M. T. (2013). Improving classroom learning environments by cultivating awareness and resilience in education (CARE): Results of a randomized controlled trial. *School Psychology Quarterly, 28*(4), 374–390.

Jennings, P. A., Snowberg, K. E., Coccia, M. A., & Greenberg, M. T. (2011). Improving classroom learning environments by cultivating awareness and resilience in education (CARE): Results of two pilot studies. *Journal of Classroom Interaction, 46*, 37–48.

Jorgenson, C. (1997). *Restructuring high schools for all students: Taking inclusion to the next level*. Baltimore, MD: Paul Brooks.

Kabat-Zinn, J. (1990). *Full catastrophe living: Using the wisdom of your body and mind to face stress, pain and illness*. New York, NY: Delacorte.

Koritsas, S., Iacono, T., Carling-Jenkins, R., & Chan, J. (2010). *Exposure to challenging behaviour and support worker/house supervisor well-being*. Melbourne, Victoria, Australia: The Centre for Developmental Disability Health Victoria.

Lyon, G. R., Fletcher, J. M., Shaywitz, S. E., Shaywitz, B. A., Torgenson, J. K., Wood, F. B., … Olson, R. K. (2001). Rethinking learning disabilities. In C. E. Finn, A. J. Rotherman, & C. R. Hokanson (Eds.), *Rethinking special education for a new century* (pp. 259–287).

Washington, DC: Thomas B. Fordham Foundation and Progressive Policy Institute.
Miodrag, N., Lense, M. D., & Dykens, E. M. (2012). A pilot study of a mindfulness intervention for individuals with Williams syndrome: Physiological outcomes. *Mindfulness, 4*, 137–147.
Segal, Z. V., Williams, J. M. G., & Teasdale, J. D. (2002). *Mindfulness-based cognitive therapy for depression: A new approach to preventing relapse*. New York, NY: Guilford.
Shapiro, J. P. (1994). *No pity: People with disabilities forging a new civil rights movement*. New York, NY: Random House.
Singh, N. N., Lancioni, G. E., ManiKam, R., Winton, A. S. W., Singh, A. N. A., Singh, J., & Singh, A. D. A. (2011). A mindfulness-based strategy for self-management of aggressive behavior in adolescents with autism. *Research in Autism Spectrum Disorders, 5*, 1153–1158.
Singh, N. N., Lancioni, G. E., Winton, A. S. W., Adkins, A. D., Singh, J., & Singh, A. N. (2007). Mindfulness training assists individuals with moderate mental retardation to maintain their community placements. *Behavior Modification, 31*(6), 800–814.
Singh, N. N., Lancioni, G. E., Karazsia, B. T., Winton, A.S., Meyers, R. E., Singh, A. N., Singh, A. D., & Singh, J. (2013). Mindfulness-based treatment for individuals with mild intellectual disability. *Mindfulness, 4*, 158–167.
Smith, T., Scahill, L., Dawson, G., Guthrie, D., Lord, C., Odom, S., … Wagner, A. (2007). Designing research studies on psychosocial interventions in autism. *Journal of Autism and Developmental Disorders 37*, 354–366.
Spek, A. A., van Ham, N., & Nyklicek, I. (2013). Mindfulness-based therapy in adults with an autism spectrum disorder: A randomized control trial. *Research in Developmental Disabilities, 34*, 246–253.
van de Weijer-Berjsma, E., Formsma, A. R., de Bruin, E. I., & Bogels, S. M. (2012). The effectiveness of mindfulness training on behavioral problems and attentional functioning in adolescents with ADHD. *Journal of Child and Family Studies, 21*, 775–787.
Van der Oord, S., Bogels, S. M., & Peijnenburg, D. (2012). The effectiveness of mindfulness training for children with ADHD and mindful parenting for their parents. *Journal of Child and Family Studies, 21*(1), 139–147.
Wong, C., Odom, S. L., Hume, K., Cox, A. W., Fettig, A., Kucharczyk, S., … Schultz, T. R. (2014). *Evidence-based practices for children, youth, and young adults with autism spectrum disorders*. Chapel Hill: The University of North Carolina, Frank Porter Graham Child Development Institute, Autism Evidence-Based Practice Review Group.
Zylowska, L., Ackerman, D. L., Yang, M. H., Futrell, J. L., Horton, N. L., Hale, T. S., … Smalley, S. L. (2008). Mindfulness meditation training in adults and adolescents with ADHD: A feasibility study. *Journal of Attention Disorders, 11*(6), 737–746.

Preparing Teacher Candidates for the Present: Investigating the Value of Mindfulness-Training in Teacher Education

12

Geoffrey B. Soloway

Introduction

Teaching is stressful. Diverse student abilities and exceptionalities, challenging classroom behavior, coupled with standardized testing and curricular expectations contribute to a demanding context for K-12 teachers (Hansen & Sullivan, 2003; Kyriacou, 2001). However, levels of teacher stress is not solely based on circumstances happening to teachers, distress is meditated by the complex interaction between teachers' disposition, values, skills, and coping mechanisms (Mearns & Cain, 2003; Montgomery & Rupp, 2005). Teacher distress negatively impacts the whole system of education, especially classroom culture and student learning (Jennings & Greenberg, 2009). How can Teacher Education respond to the problem of teacher stress and burnout while simultaneously preparing new professionals for excellence in teaching? This chapter investigates mindfulness and mindfulness-based training as a relevant model in Teacher Education for developing resilient and effective teachers.

Teacher Education has traditionally focused on three main areas: content knowledge, pedagogical skills, and development of disposition (Cochran-Smith, 2001; Darling-Hammond et al., 2005; Fullen & Hargreaves, 1992; Grant, 2008). While all three are widely seen as integral components of Teacher Education, development of disposition remains elusive. The field of Teacher Education, it seems, is still in the process of developing models of effective teacher disposition and in cultivating strategies for applying these models in practice. Generally speaking, disposition has been defined in terms of the trends or habits of mind that repeatedly affect teachers' actions and judgments within variable contexts (Borko, Liston, & Whitcomb, 2007; Johnson & Reiman, 2007; Katz & Rath, 1985). Disposition is a matter of how we, as teachers, adapt to a constantly changing set of opportunities and challenges; how we, as individuals, function within a dynamic system of interpersonal exchange. This understanding is in line with the definition articulated by The National Council for Accreditation of Teacher Education (NCATE, 2006) who identifies disposition as consisting of the professional attitudes, values, and beliefs that are active in supporting student development and when interacting with the school community at large. Needless to say, disposition is a multidimensional construct, with many different meanings in the field of Teacher Education (Johnson & Reiman, 2007; Koeppen & Davison-Jenkins, 2007; Murray, 2007).

The importance of cultivating "the person" for "the profession" is not a new area of focus in

G.B. Soloway (✉)
Mindwell, Bowen Island, BC, Canada
e-mail: Geoff@mindwellcanada.com

K.A. Schonert-Reichl, R.W. Roeser (eds.), *Handbook of Mindfulness in Education*, Mindfulness in Behavioral Health, DOI 10.1007/978-1-4939-3506-2_12

Teacher Education. Over the past 20 years, the published work of teacher educators such as Parker Palmer's (1998) "The Courage to Teach," Jack Miller's (1994) "The Contemplative Practitioner," and Noddings's (1992) "The Challenge to Care in Schools" have highlighted the importance of addressing the inner lives of teachers. Collectively, their research has elucidated various properties of effective teaching (e.g., integrity, presence, and caring). More recent research in the field has elucidated further characteristics of effective teacher disposition that include reflectivity, honesty, and empathy (Evans & Nicholson, 2003; Ryan & Alcock, 2002), as well as holding high expectations for students, and being lifelong learners (Major & Brock, 2003; NBPTS, 2002). Even though disposition is theoretically regarded as a central aspect in Teacher Education, we have witnessed little integration of formalized training programs that explicitly focus on developing disposition in Teacher Education.

In this chapter I present a summary of study completed as a doctoral dissertation that explores the added value of a dispositional development program in Teacher Education. The program implemented is called Mindfulness-Based Wellness Education (MBWE). The primary purpose of the study was to gain insight into the experiences of teacher candidates going through an experiential course focused on developing a mindful disposition. In the following sections, I provide a rationale for choosing mindfulness and a brief background on the implementation of mindfulness-based training in other professional preparation programs. I then introduce MBWE, the training used in this study, provide an overview of the methodology used in the study, and present five themes as the results of the study with a discussion on the relevance to Teacher Education.

Mindfulness

Mindfulness is a cognitive-social-emotional ability that can be learned and developed. Mindfulness is an intentional way of being, calling us back into the present moment experience of our lives in contrast to running on our automatic patterns of reactivity. In a moment of mindfulness, we have heightened awareness of our body, emotions, thoughts, and surroundings, which allows us to gain a clearer understanding of our unfolding experience. Often, our behavior is triggered automatically as we react immediately to an initial emotion and/or thought. Mindfulness provides perspective for us to see more clearly and know our automatic reactions, empowering us with the ability to respond more appropriately. Mindfulness practice nurtures self-compassion and helps us in coming to know and relate to the internal dialogue we all have. The practice of mindfulness and learning to relate to our thoughts and emotions is central to mental, social, emotional, and physical health.

Mindfulness is primarily concerned with attentiveness: a waking up to the here and now of the moment. Meditation, a central formal practice in the cultivation of mindfulness, is like a dress rehearsal, tuning our brains for staying present. The guidelines of mindfulness meditation practice are simple—be present. Yet, we quickly come to realize this practice is not easy. Undertaking the practice of mindfulness includes heightening sensitivity to the busyness of our own thought patterns, and to the specific ways in which we automatically react to our unfolding experience. Within this context, the challenge is to continually bring ourselves back into present moment awareness while embodying both patience and acceptance towards our own busy minds. Non-judgment is therefore a key element in allowing us to take note of our reactions to events as they occur without being consumed by thoughts or emotions. The practice of mindfulness heightens awareness of the activity in our minds rather than seeking to change or control the contents of our minds. The opposite of controlling is allowing or letting be, which facilitates an up close and personal experience of life just as it is. Although we are coming into more direct experience with our feelings, thoughts, and bodily sensations, there is also a greater sense of spaciousness to our experience. This spaciousness offers an important perspective as to the nature of our thoughts, unpleasant bodily sensations, or debilitating emotions coloring our experience. Practicing mindfulness is scaffolding for learning how to stay with, and process, the full experience of our lives; mindful awareness cultivates a disposition that seeks to liberate the mind from its own reactive or automatic set of behavioral responses. This tendency toward inner freedom extends beyond a seated posture into ways of being and relationships with ourselves, others, and the world.

Mindfulness-Based Training for Human Service Professionals

In addition to the clinical studies investigating the health benefits of mindfulness training, there is growing interest in the integration of mindfulness-based training for human service professionals. Specifically, there is interest in professional preparation programs such as counseling (Schure, Christopher, & Christopher, 2008; Shapiro, Brown, & Biegel, 2007), nursing (Cohen-Katz et al., 2005), social work (Ying, 2009), dentistry (Lovas, Lovas, & Lovas, 2008), and medicine (Saunders et al., 2007; Shapiro, Astin, Bishop, & Cordova, 2005). Complementing the stress reduction benefits, those studies reveal the professional value of mindfulness training, such as the development of presence in the practitioner. Within such studies, the ability to attend fully to and connect with the client is what Siegel (2007) refers to as attunement, which is essential in the process of developing a therapeutic relationship. The patient's healing is thus directly responsive to the cultivation of therapists' disposition of mindfulness.

Such findings are certainly relevant to the teaching profession, if for no other reason, because teachers' effectiveness is so clearly dependent upon their ability to connect and develop healthy relationships with their students (Hamre & Pianta, 2001; Jennings & Greenberg, 2009; Zins, Weissberg, Wang, & Walberg, 2004). Many Teacher Education programs highlight the importance of classroom climate and teacher-student relationships, often covering a descriptive analysis and approach to these topics. However, few programs provide specific opportunities for developing the competencies that create healthy teacher-student relationships (LeBlanc & Gallavan, 2009; Riley, 2011; Schwartz, 2008). Drawing on existing literature, we can expect mindfulness to enhance teacher presence and in turn positive teacher-student relationships. The current study seeks to uncover additional benefits of mindfulness training in Teacher Education. The next section introduces, MBWE, the program used in this study.

Mindfulness-Based Wellness Education

MBWE was first offered in Teacher Education at the Ontario Institute for Studies in Education of the University of Toronto (OISE/UT) in 2006. The program was developed by Dr. Corey Mackenzie, Dr. Patricia Poulin, and myself in response to the growing problem of teacher stress and burnout as a method for cultivating resiliency in future teachers. MBWE blended the popular Mindfulness-Based Stress Reduction (MBSR) program with a model of wellness promotion (Soloway, 2005; Soloway, Poulin, & Mackenzie, 2010). This 9-week program was run in the context of an elective course entitled "Stress and Burnout: Teacher and Student Applications."

MBWE uses a "wellness wheel" (Fig. 12.1) to explore mindfulness through various dimensions of one's experience. During each week of the course, different dimension of wellness are explored. Each week, teacher candidates are invited to maintain a daily formal mindfulness practice, such as mindful sitting or yoga, and more informal practices that address bringing mindfulness to activities such as listening, speaking, socializing, or engaging with nature. Teacher candidates are also asked to choose a practice that supports the dimension of wellness they are focusing on that week, such as healthy eating or spending quality time with friends and family. For example, during the first week of the course, teacher candidates explore their physical wellness through physical exercise and through

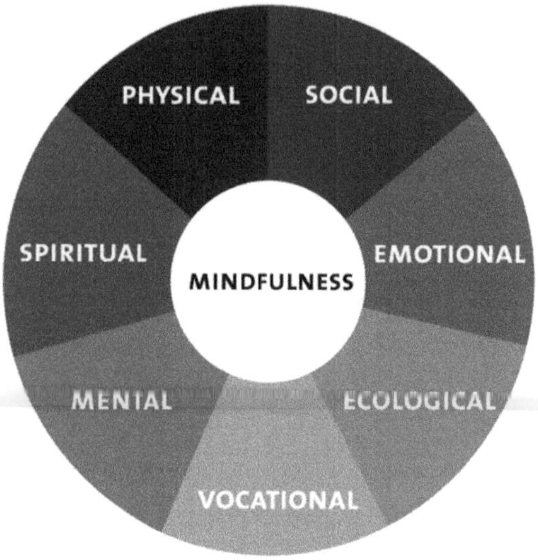

Fig. 12.1 Wellness wheel

mindfulness practices such as mindful eating and the body scan.

Teacher candidates are given a CD with mindfulness practices that are each 20 min long, a wellness workbook, and a course reader at the beginning of the course. Teacher candidates are encouraged to work up to maintaining a 20-min formal mindfulness practice three times a week, and completing a shorter mindfulness practice on other days in order to maintain a regular daily practice. The overall trajectory of the MBWE curriculum begins with a primary focus on personal development and gradually builds into a more integrated consideration of one's professional capacities as a teacher.

In the first 2 years of offering the MBWE course, two studies with teacher candidates enrolled in MBWE demonstrated that active participants exhibited significantly greater increases in mindfulness, life satisfaction, and teaching self-efficacy when compared to a control group (Poulin, 2009; Poulin, Mackenzie, Soloway, & Karaoylas, 2008). In addition to the positive statistical results, teacher candidates also shared their feedback that provoked further investigation. The following quotation from one teacher candidate, for example, elaborates in her own words how they experienced the MBWE program:

> I honestly think that the MBWE program should be a requirement for every teacher candidate at OISE/UT because there are so many things that I learned about how to deal with the challenges in the classroom that I never learned from the other classes. It was all about developing myself as a teacher, as a person first, and then teaching second. That is so important because it really affects how you teach and it effects the classroom environment.

These types of responses to MBWE inspired me to further identify the broader personal and professional benefits teacher candidates were experiencing.

Methodology: Action Research Design

Being in the unique position as instructor of the "Stress and Burnout" class at OISE/UT, I used this opportunity as the context for my doctoral dissertation. The primary research question was intended to uncover the benefits teacher candidates were experiencing by participating in MBWE as part of Teacher Education, which is presented in this chapter. The secondary research question was focused on learning about teacher candidates' experiences in order to improve the program. To answer these questions, I employed an action research design over three consecutive semesters. MBWE runs as a one-semester course. Using an action research design, I applied a grounded theory approach in creating my research questions, in choosing participants, in directing the inquiry, and when interpreting the data. Over three consecutive semesters, I interviewed a total of 23 teacher candidates who took the MBWE program. I chose to interview participants at the completion of the academic school year hoping to gain information on the impact of the course over teacher candidates' entire year (i.e., including the second practicum experience). Further, teacher candidates filled out mid-course and end-of-course feedback forms (anonymously) about the program. Feedback from teacher candidates' experiences in the first round of data collection was used to inform the teaching of the subsequent MBWE program sessions and, in turn, change the later experiences of teacher candidates taking the program (Fig. 12.2).

Teacher candidates self-selected to enroll in the Stress and Burnout class. The description of the course that teacher candidates had access to prior to selecting the course did not include any mention of mindfulness practice. By signing up for Stress and Burnout, teacher candidates identified themselves as being interested in the topic of stress, and/or looking for strategies in reducing their stress and stress of their future students. The sample in this study consisted of teacher candidates who participated in the Stress and Burnout class (MBWE program) during three consecutive semesters. I chose a diverse sample to interview. Criteria of diversity were based on the teaching level of teacher candidates (primary/junior, junior/intermediate, intermediate/senior), gender, ethnicity, and age.

I conducted interviews with participants that lasted between one and one-and-a-half hours. Interviews were semi-structured to allow for new themes and questions to emerge while ensuring coverage of a specific topic (Punch, 2009). Interviews were analyzed using multilevels of coding in following a grounded theory approach: (1) open coding, (2) theoretical coding, and (3) selective coding (Charmaz, 2006). At each level of coding, a new set of themes emerged. The first rounds of coding were done inductively and the final stages were done deductively—focusing on particular points of complexity and interest (Glaser, 1978).

Findings

This study demonstrated five central themes from data: (1) Reflective Practice, (2) Teacher Identity, (3) Social and Emotional Competence and Well-being on Practicum, (4) Learning to Fail—Learning to Teach, and (5) Engagement in Teacher Education. In what follows, I will briefly outline essential features of each main theme.

Reflective Practice

The practice of reflection is regarded as an important aspect of teacher education (Grimmet & Erickson, 1988; Loughran, 2006; LaBoskey, 1994). Yet, despite its popularity within the realm of theory, best practices and processes for cultivating a reflective practitioner remain unclear (Hatton & Smith, 1995; Korthagen, 2004; Zeichner, 2009). Reflection can be understood as a dialectical process whereby one suspends immediate judgments and preconceptions to

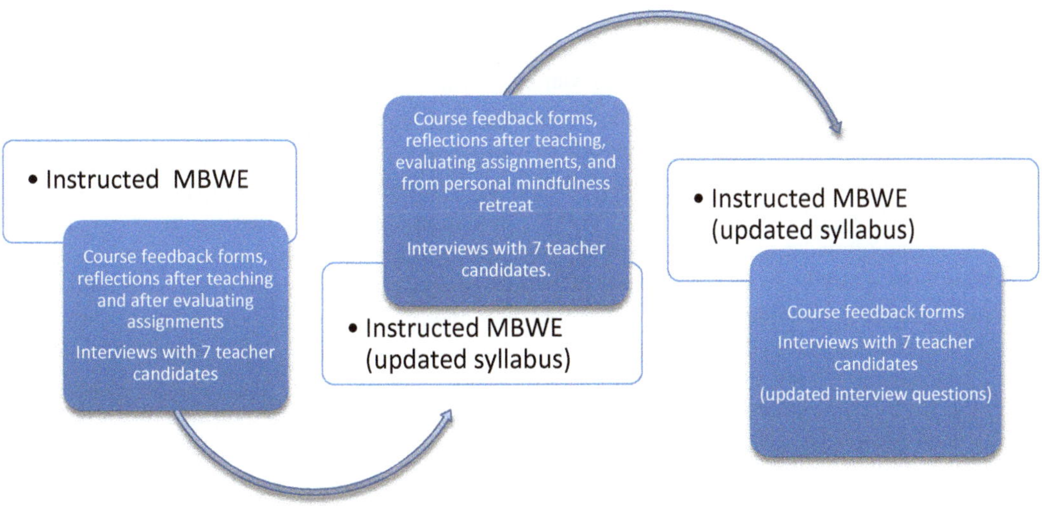

Fig. 12.2 Iterative process of teaching and researching mindfulness-based wellness education

allow for a more careful consideration of one's actions and decisions (Dewey, 1933). This emphasis on reflection *within action* was popularized in the 1980s by Donald Schön (1983, 1987) in his seminal works on professional practice: "The Reflective Practitioner" and "Educating the Reflective Practitioner." In those texts, Schon distinguished between *reflection-on-action* and *reflection-in-action*. Reflection-on-action looks back on what occurred in practice in order to improve on future endeavors. By contrast, reflection-in-action implies awareness and modification while in the very midst of the practice itself. Schön (1983) argued that reflection-in-action offers us a much needed alternative for adaptive problem solving. Rather than relying on technical knowledge from fixed sources (i.e., solving problems based on existing theory), reflection-in-action relies on the identification and assimilation of feedback while in the midst of practice. Here, reflection shapes the unfolding of action.

Reflection-in-action refers to the process of heightening awareness while in the midst of the action itself, as opposed to thinking back about the practice after it occurs. Mindfulness practice involves modifying one's awareness on a continual moment-by-moment basis. Whereas most reflection in Teacher Education is conducted as reflection-on-action, the practice of mindfulness meditation contributes to the skills of reflection-in-action. For example, in a simple sitting meditation, one learns to recognize the speed and frequency with which our thoughts begin to wander. The practice thus involves becoming aware of how the mind has wandered, taking note where the mind has gone, and then returning oneself to the chosen focus. Again, this exercise serves as a key insight and reminder about the nature of the mind and how quickly we can lose track of its intended focus and intention. Developing mindfulness is thus the practice of maintaining awareness of the continuing unfolding of moments.

The novel experience of learning mindfulness is a practice of reflection-in-action: a learning process in regulating attention to stay present from moment-to-moment. Below, a teacher candidate described her experience of reflection-in-action:

> The biggest thing that mindfulness helped me with was my reflection. Not just reflecting after a class, it was a conscious reflection while I was actually doing things. I would find that I was able to stop in certain places of a lesson, and actually right at that moment, make a conscious decision to reflect—I was more aware of what was going on, instead of waiting till the end when everything was finished…throughout my life I always thought that I was a pretty reflective person, but than came to realize that I would wait much too long, and I would miss a lot of opportunity to make better right at that time.

Learning how to drop back into the present is the first step of reflection-in-action because it provides the necessary perspective from which to reflect. Often, teachers are simply caught up in the busyness of teaching in the classroom setting, and thus neglect their own moment-to-moment awareness of how the class is unfolding. Below, a teacher candidate describes the application of reflection-in-action in her class:

> By staying in the moment I was also able to adapt on the spot and change the lesson to meet the needs of the students and go with the flow of how the lesson was moving along. I was also able to ask good follow up questions to the students and provide good answers on the spot.

Training in mindfulness supported teacher candidates in cultivating the skills and abilities to revisit present moment awareness during key moments in the classroom, enabling them to choose a best course of next action.

The skills learned from reflection-on-action do not necessarily translate into skills for reflection-in-action. Providing authentic opportunities for teacher candidates to practice reflection-in-action only occur during practice teaching opportunities in Teacher Education, and those experiences are typically filled with high levels of stress and anxiety which makes bringing awareness in the moment of teaching very challenging. Highlighting the value of mindfulness training in the development of reflective practitioners is an important finding for Teacher Education. Whereas a pedagogy of reflection in

Teacher Education remains ambiguous, the pairing of mindfulness practice and reflection offers new strategies for promoting insight into developing reflective practitioners.

Teacher Identity

Developing teacher identity is a common learning objective in Teacher Education (Danielewicz, 2001; Kosnick & Beck, 2009; Rodgers & Scott, 2008). Though teacher identity has been conceptualized in various ways, the literature frequently defines identity in Teacher Education using both personal and professional dimensions (Beijaard, Meijer, & Verloop, 2004; Stenberg, 2010). Usually considered under the rubric of personal identity are the various attitudes, beliefs, and values that inform one's pedagogical practice. It is generally accepted that varying degrees of self-awareness in this respect will inevitably contribute to the decisions and interactions that are made in the classroom (Connelly & Clandinin, 1999; Korthagen, 2004). By comparison, professional identity refers more specifically to teachers' perceptions of their own roles as a teacher. This includes all matters of authority and responsibilities, philosophy of teaching, and teaching practice that are all heavily influenced by continued experience in the classroom and self-concept (Tillema, 2000; Warin, Maddock, Pell, & Hargreaves, 2006). Considered together, teacher identity encompasses the changing perceptions teachers hold for themselves outside of the classroom, in the classroom, and in the wider school community.

Participating in MBWE includes engaging in mindfulness practices and completing weekly reflections on various dimensions of wellness that contribute to teacher candidates self-knowledge. In turn, teacher candidates gain insight into more deeply held personal values and beliefs. Korthagen (2004) highlights the importance of creating opportunities for clarifying values and beliefs as an integral part to personal and professional identity development. Samantha, a teacher candidate, described her personal engagement in MBWE:

> And that's why I want to make it a lifestyle and not just a thing to do... I took this [MBWE] on as something that I needed rather than something I would put into a classroom. It was something I wanted to teach myself and then live the teaching.

Florence, another teacher candidate, came into Teacher Education after already having trained and worked as a nurse. Being a health care professional, she was already introduced to the stresses of working in the field. Florence had no background with mindfulness or yoga prior to beginning MBWE. By the completion of the course, Florence became an advocate for mindfulness training as part of professional preparation. Florence described her experience of grappling with deep issues—not simply working at a superficial level—an essential part of core change:

> Equity and social justice was our major focus in school. I think other courses in Teacher Education did a good job making us aware of the injustices and yes there was a big focus on change and what you can do to change, but I don't think a lot of people are necessarily strong enough to do that and I didn't find any other course focused on building that strength. Strength to deal with situations. The idea of strength—you have to know who you are and know your identity and know how to deal with situations that will be very uncomfortable for you.... Exploring the many aspects of myself through the course opened my eyes to a lot of challenges I had with my own values and beliefs and my own identity. I thought I was strong and knew what I wanted, what I valued, and what I could contribute into a classroom. Digging into myself, I realized there were major gaps that I needed to work on.

Clarifying values and beliefs in one's life is an ongoing process in human development. This theme highlights the intensive process of grappling with personal values and beliefs that is facilitated when engaging mindfully with one's life. Whereas other courses in Teacher Education call awareness to issues of social justice and serve to heighten awareness of biases as they may relate to being in the classroom and teaching,

MBWE directs focus within teacher candidates' personal lives to see how they are enacting their values and beliefs and to help them recognize the disconnect between their actions and values.

In addition to supporting personal dimensions of identity development, MBWE also encouraged teacher candidates to contemplate their identity in the classroom. Teaching identity includes how one believes he or she is being perceived, and how one perceives oneself in the classroom and in the profession. For example, MBWE focuses on mindful teaching, which is discussed and practiced as ways of staying present in the classroom amidst all the busyness. Tania, a teacher candidate, spoke about how she wants to be seen in the classroom:

> MBWE is the course that pops up in my brain whenever I am thinking about planning a lesson, or just how I want to approach my role as a teacher. I want to be that kind, patient and welcoming teacher, and this class [MBWE] helped me to start cultivating that.

The quote below from Deborah, a teacher candidate, distinguishes between the idea of mindful teaching and the skills necessary for enacting mindful teaching that are practiced in MBWE:

> The course taught a lot about the kind of teacher I want to be. It taught me a lot about how I wanted to set up my classroom, how I want to be seen…I think the strengths of this program is that it says, yes you might want to be a mindful teacher but do you know how to be a mindful teacher, you want to be a thoughtful teacher but do you know how to be a thoughtful teacher.

This theme makes an important link to teaching practice, as teacher candidates found the MBWE program valuable in developing their professional identity. MBWE provides opportunity for teacher candidates to move beyond fanciful wishes of whom they would like to be in the classroom and to learn the skills for enacting mindfulness in the classroom. Teacher candidates developing their personal and professional identity is part of the process of adult development, and plays a significant role in how teacher candidates see themselves in the classroom as well as experience themselves in the classroom. Teaching plays a critical role in the development of healthy children and adolescents, and thus it seems only natural that we apply high standards of consideration to the development of their educators.

Social and Emotional Competence and Well-Being on Practicum

Over the past decade, research on social and emotional learning continues to demonstrate the importance to healthy child and adolescent development as well as academic outcomes (Greenberg et al., 2003; Zins et al., 2004). Jennings and Greenberg (2009) reconceived social and emotional competence (SEC) within the sphere of teacher development. Accordingly, teacher SEC and well-being are characterized using the existing framework of social and emotional learning, including five central competencies: self-awareness, social awareness, responsible decision-making, self-management, and relationship management (Jennings & Greenberg, 2009; Zins et al., 2004). Jennings and Greenberg's (2009) model of "the pro-social classroom" explains the effects of teacher SEC and well-being in connection to improving the teacher-student relationship, improving classroom management, and enabling social and emotional learning for students. Hong (2010) similarly argues that emotional intelligence is one key aspect of teacher identity that contributes to the long-term sustainability of teachers. In the following quotation, Hong (2010) articulates the gap between Teacher Education and the emotional realities of teaching:

> This lack of systematic efforts to provide pre-service teachers with a realistic understanding of teachers' emotional experiences and developmental stages raises one of the most important issues in teacher education programs. Bridging the gap between theory and practice is critical in this situation, because the gap between the educational theories pre-service teachers learn in college and the demanding reality in-service teachers learn in the classroom and in the broader school context can make them feel lost. (p. 1540)

Offering mindfulness-based learning in Teacher Education is an opportunity to begin bridging the gap between theory and realities of teaching. Beginner's mind is a principle introduced in MBWE reminding teacher candidates to notice their automatic social or emotional patterns of behavior in the classroom. In contrast to getting stuck in our typical perceptions, constructs, and labels, beginner's mind invites us to see each moment unfolding with fresh eyes (Kabat-Zinn, 1990). Shunryu Suzuki (2003), in his book "Zen Mind, Beginner's Mind," says, "In the beginner's mind there are many possibilities, but in the expert's there are few (p. 21)." Fresh eyes in a classroom are more open to seeing without existing judgment. A teacher's practice of beginner's mind can be applied in multiple ways in teaching and learning. Below, Tom, a teacher candidate discusses the benefits of integrating this principle into his teaching practice on practicum:

Daily I try to keep in mind two of the foundations of mindfulness practice, beginner's mind and letting go. I keep reminding myself that "no moment is the same as any other." As a teacher it is important for me to start every day with "fresh eyes" rather than seeing the reflection of my own thoughts about the students and my co-workers. By neglecting preconceived notions, I am giving every student the chance to grow.

Beginner's mind is a principle that brought teacher candidates "back into the present" in the classroom, opening up new spaces of social and emotional awareness within themselves and for developing connection with students.

Teacher social and emotional competence and well-being are relatively new constructs within Teacher Education; however, their value has long been implicitly understood in relation to teacher–student relationship and classroom management. Teacher candidates shared that MBWE cultivated skills and competencies that could be accessed while teaching on practicum. Teacher candidates reported that taking time to slow down and practice mindful teaching contributed to positive interactions with their students, which in turn diminished classroom management issues and enhanced their overall teaching experience. Infusing mindfulness-based practices in Teacher Education provided teacher candidates the opportunity to develop the daily competencies required to be successful in the classroom.

Learning to Fail: Learning to Teach

The paradigm of constructivism constitutes both a theory of knowledge and a theory of education. Constructivism describes knowledge as being actively constructed by the individual and his or her assimilation of new experiences with the past (Richardson, 2003). A constructivist approach shifts the focus of teaching from the teacher to the student. Whereas the teacher-centered approach has traditionally favored passive transmission of information within a lecture-style format, the constructivist model challenges teachers to find more innovative scenarios centered on the students' experience of learning. A problem in Teacher Education is that constructivist learning theory is often taught using a teacher-centered approach. Mindfulness is often taught from a constructivist approach where the learner gains knowledge through their direct experience with the practice. For example, a primary step in learning mindfulness is becoming more aware of when we are no longer present. This theme highlights the experience of teacher candidates constructing new insight into teaching when given the opportunity to "fail" learning mindfulness.

In going through the MBWE program, many teacher candidates spoke about their experience of learning mindfulness. Indeed, learning to practice mindfulness is not easy. Especially for new practitioners, the task of "quieting the mind" represents a new and uncomfortable set of problems. Chief amongst these is the demand for a renewed relationship to failure. In typical learning situations, the experience of failure falls under the category of "final results." In the MBWE program, teacher candidates were taught to become mindful of their experience of failure as it occurred specifically *within* practice. For example, one of the common misperceptions about mindfulness practice is that the practitioner is trying to "blank" one's mind. As a result, when thoughts enter the mind or when one gets lost in one's preoccupations, the new practitioner will often see themselves as having failed. In mindfulness practice however, one comes to accept that the mind will continually wander away from the chosen point of focus. The challenge is to realize that the mind has wandered and to bring it back to the chosen focus without condemning oneself for not having achieved unwavering attention. In other words, it is the process of "failing" that enables learning, a circular pattern that happens over and over again in mindfulness practice.

In MBWE, what is important is how teacher candidates relate to their failures. Embodying the attitude of acceptance, patience, and non-judgment towards themselves positively influenced their teaching practice. Next, Rosa described her experience learning and grappling with mindfulness practice:

> Attempting and sometimes feeling like I failed at mindfulness practice, gave me insight to a different perspective on learning, and the experiences of feeling inadequate when immediate understanding does not always occur. I feel like this experience helped me to better understand students who might not 'get it' the first time around, and the importance of being patient with them and the pace at which they are learning.

The process of failing is a humbling process and provides insight into the process of learning. We often fail many times, especially when undertaking the practice of learning something new. Providing teacher candidates with the experience of failure and learning to relate constructively to this experience plays a formative role in teacher candidates' resiliency and vision of teaching. The following quotation from a teacher candidate describes her relationship of learning mindfulness to her emerging vision of teaching.

> As a student in MBWE, having never meditated nor done much yoga in the past, the subject matter in this course was almost entirely new to me. Through the experience of learning something entirely new, I gained great insight regarding the actual process of learning. Most importantly, I feel that the practice of having an open heart, being non-judgmental and a beginner's mind is crucial for learning. In learning anything new, not just mindfulness practice, keeping an open mind helps to better internalize and engage in the material, while being non-judgmental about the self-learning process and the subject matter, makes for fewer obstacles towards the goal of new knowledge and skill acquisition. Knowing this, I hope to teach these ideas to my future students, so that they may be more open to the process of learning science and biology.

Mindfulness training can be understood as a pedagogical strategy in Teacher Education to create genuine opportunity for teacher candidates to grapple with learning a new challenging skill. Teacher candidates also gained insight into the emotional dimension of failure and learned how to navigate challenging emotions and related thoughts. Developing a more direct relationship with the emotional landscape of failure enabled teacher candidates to stay present in their experience, to be resilient in their process of learning, and to develop a more empathetic response to their students' learning process. Learning to fail is an important experience for teacher candidates when learning to teach.

Engagement in Teacher Education

Within the literature, student engagement is broadly distinguished into three categories: behavioral, emotional, and cognitive (Finn, 1993; Klem & Connell, 2004; Marks, 2000; Reeve, Jang, Carrell, Jeon, & Barch, 2004). Klem and Connell (2004) explain each of these components:

> Behavioural engagement includes time students spent on their work, intensity of concentration and effort, tendency to stay on task and propensity to initiate action when given the opportunity. Emotional components of engagement include heightened levels of positive emotion during the completion of an activity, demonstrated by enthusiasm, optimism, curiosity and interest. Cognitive components of engagement include students' understanding of why they are doing what they're doing and its importance. (p. 262)

Kuh et al. (2007) assert that these various dimensions of engagement are inextricably linked to certain structural or institutional factors that dictate schedules, curriculum, opportunity for collaboration with peers, resources, and the overall support that is offered within the student experience. It is significant that these factors are seen not only to affect the students' involvement in the course—i.e., the nuts and bolts of their being in the classroom—but more importantly, their active engagement with course content and materials both inside and out of class. This theme articulates the value of mindfulness for teacher candidate Engagement in Teacher Education.

Mindfulness practice supported teacher candidates in staying emotionally engaged in their Teacher Education program. More specifically, the process of paying attention heightened awareness of negative ruminations that teacher candidates get caught up during their experience in Teacher Education. Rumination refers to having persistent thoughts occurring; over-analyzing that becomes worrying or brooding. Rumination contributes to stress and in turn mental health issues, which are increasing in incidence within higher education (Cairns, Massfeller, & Deeth, 2010; Guthman, 2010). One common rumination that negatively impacted teacher candidates' engagement was a critique of their Teacher Education experience. Many teacher candidates criticize their training as being too theoretical and not practical enough as illustrated by Deborah below:

> Especially in January when I started this class (MBWE) there was an extreme type of negativity going on in all the classrooms and I had it as well. There was a lot of frustration regarding what we were getting out of this education. Like you did practicum and that was so much to take in at once. I was saying I don't know why I am here because I didn't feel I was getting the lesson planning training or things like that. A lot of the classroom discussion was around what we wanted to get out of the program and there was a lot of tension in classes and a lot of negativity... I just tried to commit to being present and let go of the frustration. In terms of sitting and listening to a lecture, instead of thinking about other things.

Further, many teacher candidates drifted toward potential job prospects at the halfway mark of the program as school districts started their hiring process. Challenging emotions and wandering thoughts often disengage learners cognitively, emotionally, and behaviorally. Heightening self-awareness and coping skills supported teacher candidates in learning to let go of unhelpful ruminations that disengage them from their learning and help them reinvest in their learning process.

For many, bringing awareness to their ruminating tendencies is an important step in helping teacher candidates let go of them and return to a place of presence. The quotation below by Rosa, a teacher candidate, describes her experience of mindfulness supporting their engagement through this process:

> MBWE also enhanced my experience of other courses I have been taking in Teacher Education. Reflecting on my school experience, I largely had a mentality in which I just wanted school to be over ... something resonated with me from mindfulness practice and as a result I have applied awareness to my schooling. Because of mindfulness practices I have learned to be aware of my present education experience and enjoy the process of my schooling.

In addition to the content of the MBWE being relevant to professional preparation, mindfulness supports students in their process of learning in all courses; mindfulness can be understood as an enabling factor for engagement in higher education.

Teacher candidates also spoke about the prevalence of group work in their courses and consequently, of the need to develop positive working relationships with their peers. MBWE was seen to support teacher candidates in reducing relational stresses that accompany working in a group of diverse voices and opinions. More specifically, teacher candidates talked about the practice of acceptance and non-judgment with others during activities in other classes. In the following quotation, Florence talks about regulating her own behavior when interacting in her other classes.

> In the class where we talk about very controversial issues, acceptance played a bit part. In the past when listening to someone I would jump on something when I didn't agree with it, and I learned to listen and not judge immediately. As well, not to judge them afterwards based on a opinion that they had. Before, I would judge a person based on a thought.

Engaging in mindfulness practice, teacher candidates were supported in their personal and collegial relationships, and encouraged with regards to their participation in other courses. Overall, teacher candidates felt their experience in MBWE enabled them to cognitively, behaviorally, and emotionally engage in their teacher education program.

Future Directions

This chapter provides an overview of a qualitative action research dissertation conducted over two years in Teacher Education. Since the study of mindfulness training in Teacher Education is a relatively new area of research, a grounded theory approach was used to unearth new areas for further study. The five main themes found in this study, Reflection-in-action, Teacher Identity, Social and Emotional Competence and Well-Being on Practicum, Learning to Fail—Learning to Teach, and Engagement in Teacher Education, are not meant to be generalized to all teacher candidates going through mindfulness training programs, or even the MBWE program. These themes are considered to be central foci for future research topics in the relatively new study of Mindfulness in Education. Continuing to investigate these themes qualitatively and quantitatively will enhance clarity in the relationships between mindfulness training, teacher education, and educational impact. Considering mindfulness is still a relatively new concept and practice in the field of education, continued research translating the purpose and value of mindfulness into recognizable constructs and priorities of Teacher Education is necessary.

This study investigated an elective course on mindful well-being focusing primarily on personal development, with a secondary focus of professional application. Another approach would be to look at a mindfulness-based program for teachers that is solely focused on professional development, for example, preparing teachers to teach mindfulness in their future classrooms. Another model for preparing teacher candidates is through mindful teacher education. Mindful teacher education would include teacher educators going through their own training in mindfulness, and learning to infuse mindfulness into their other teacher education classes. Comparing teacher candidates experiences in all three models may offer insight into the type of mindfulness-based training that are most effective and feasible in Teacher Education.

Curiously, teacher educators have years of experience in the K-12 classroom yet very little training in teaching adults. One underlying assumption in Teacher Education maintains that experience teaching in the K-12 classroom is sufficient for preparing teacher candidates. This assumption can be problematic for two reasons. First, teacher educators typically have experience teaching children and adolescents whereas teacher candidates are adult learners. Second, developing adult disposition is not an area many K-12 teachers would be knowledgeable in or have experience facilitating, and yet dispositional development is a core element of Teacher Education. Developing disposition in professional preparation raises concerns because it blends the lines between personal and professional. Faculties of Education, for example, typically focus on content knowledge and professional practice, not the inner life of the student. Personal development is regarded theoretically as a critical element in Teacher Education however not as closely followed in practice. Teacher Education would benefit from specialists, i.e., mindfulness-based educators, who can co-facilitate mindfulness-based training with teacher candidates, as well as teacher educators undergoing training in mindfulness.

Conclusion

When we think back to the most influential teachers we have had in our lives, are they the ones who had the greatest knowledge in their field or the ones with engaging lesson plans? More often it is the presence of a teacher that ignites student interest and then able to utilize knowledge and pedagogical strategies to further learning in the classroom. This exploratory study found that mindfulness training in the context of Teacher Education provided practical learning opportunities for teacher candidates to develop the skills, knowledge, and dispositional goals of Teacher Education. The real world of teaching transcends fixed and clearly defined ways of being in the classroom because no two students are the same. Teacher education is not trying to create a mold of an expert teacher, but rather lead new teachers on a path with the skills and awareness to continue to develop as a person and as a professional. Whereas teacher education is most often based on preparing teacher candidates for the future, mindfulness training is a key new insight for preparing teachers for the present—the place where all the complexities of teaching and living unfold.

References

Beijaard, D., Meijer, P., & Verloop, N. (2004). Reconsidering research on teachers' professional identity. *Teaching and Teacher Education, 20*(2), 107–129.

Borko, H., Liston, D., & Whitcomb, J. (2007). Apples and fishes: The debate over dispositions in teacher education. *Journal of Teacher Education, 58*(5), 359–364.

Cairns, S. H., Massfeller, H. F., Deeth, S. C. (2010). Why do postsecondary students seek counselling? *Canadian Journal of Counselling, 44*(1), 34–50.

Charmaz, K. (2006). *Constructing grounded theory*. London, UK: Sage.

Cochran-Smith, M. (2001). The outcomes question in teacher education. *Teaching and Teacher Education, 17*, 527–546.

Cohen-Katz, J., Wiley, S., Capuano, T., Baker, D. M., Deitrick, L., & Shapiro, S. (2005). The effects of mindfulness-based stress reduction on nurse stress and burnout: A qualitative and quantitative study, part III. *Holistic Nursing Practice, 19*(2), 78–86.

Connelly, M., & Clandinin, D. J. (1999). *Shaping a professional identity*. London, Ontario, Canada: The Althouse Press.

Danielewicz, J. (2001). *Teaching selves: Identity, pedagogy and teacher education*. Albany, NY: State University of New York Press.

Darling-Hammond, L., Banks, J., Zumwalt, K., Gomez, L., Sherin, M. G., Griesdorn, J., & Finn, L. E. (2005). Educational goals and purposes: Developing a curricular vision for teaching. In L. Darling-Hammond & J. Bransford (Eds.), *Preparing teachers for a changing world* (pp. 169–190). San Francisco, CA: Jossey-Bass.

Dewey, J. (1933). *How we think*. Boston, MA: D.C. Heath.

Evans, J., & Nicholson, K. (2003). Building a community of learners: Manhattan College Elementary Education Program. *Teacher Education Quarterly, 30*(1), 137–150.

Finn, J. D. (1993). *School engagement and students at risk*. Washington, DC: National Center for Education Statistics.

Fullen, M., & Hargreaves, A. (1992). *Teacher development and educational change*. Bristol, PA: The Falmer Press.

Glaser, B. G. (1978). *Theoretical sensitivity*. Mill Valley, CA: The Sociology Press.

Grant, C. A. (2008). Teacher capacity. In M. Cochran-Smith, S. Feiman-Nemser, D. J. McIntyre, & K. E. Demers (Eds.), *Handbook of research on teacher education* (pp. 128–133). New York, NY: Routledge.

Greenberg, M. T., Weissberg, R. P., O'Brien, M. U., Zins, J. E., Fredericks, L., Resnik, H., & Elias, M. J. (2003). Enhancing school-based prevention and youth development through coordinated social, emotional, and academic learning. *American Psychologist, 58*(7), 466–474.

Grimmet, P., & Erickson, G. L. (1988). *Reflection in teacher education*. New York, NY: Teachers College Press.

Guthman, J. (2010). College students exhibiting more severe mental illness. Retrieved February 26, 2011, available at: http://www.apa.org/news/press/releases/2010/08/students-mental-illness.aspx.

Hamre, B., & Pianta, R. C. (2001). Early teacher-child relationships and trajectory of school outcomes through eighth grade. *Child Development, 72*, 625–638.

Hansen, J., & Sullivan, B. (2003). Assessment of workplace stress: Occupational stress its consequences, and common causes of teacher stress. North Carolina: Information Analysis.

Hatton, N., & Smith, D. (1995). Reflection in teacher education: Towards definition and implementation. *Teaching and Teacher Education, 11*(1), 33–49.

Hong, J. I. (2010). Pre-service and beginning teachers' professional identity and its relation to dropping out of the profession. *Teaching and Teacher Education, 26*, 1530–1543.

Jennings, P. A., & Greenberg, M. T. (2009). The prosocial classroom: Teacher social and emotional competence in relation to student and classroom outcomes. *Review of Educational Research, 79*(1), 491–525.

Johnson, L. E., & Reiman, A. J. (2007). Beginning teacher disposition: Examining the moral/ethical domain. *Teaching and Teacher Education, 23*(5), 676–687.

Kabat-Zinn, J. (1990). *Full catastrophe living: Using the wisdom of your body and mind to face stress, pain and illness*. New York, NY: Dell.

Katz, L. G., & Rath, J. D. (1985). Dispositions as goals for teacher education. *Teaching and Teacher Education, 1*(4), 301–307.

Klem, A. M., & Connell, J. P. (2004). Relationships matter: Linking teacher support to student engagement and achievement. *The Journal of School Health, 74*(7), 262–273.

Koeppen, K. E., & Davison-Jenkins, J. (2007). *Teacher dispositions: Envisioning their role in education*. Lanham, MD: Rowman & Littlefield Education.

Korthagen, F. (2004). In search of the essence of a good teacher: Towards a more holistic approach in teacher education. *Teaching and Teacher Education, 20*, 77–97.

Kosnick, C., & Beck, C. (2009). *Priorities of teacher education*. New York, NY: Routledge.

Kuh, G. D., Kinzie, J. Buckley, J. A., Bridges, B. K., & Hayek, J. C. (2007). *Piecing together the student success puzzle: Research, propositions and recommendations*. ASHE higher education report (Vol. 32, No. 5). San Francisco, CA: Jossey-Bass.

Kyriacou, C. (2001). Teacher stress. *Educational Review, 53*(1), 27–35.

LaBoskey, V. K. (1994). *Development of reflective practice*. New York, NY: Teachers College Press.

LeBlanc, P. R., & Gallavan, N. P. (2009). *Affective teacher education*. Lanham, MD: Rowman & Littlefield Education.

Loughran, J. (2006). *Developing a pedagogy of teacher education*. New York, NY: Routledge.

Lovas, J. G., Lovas, D. A., & Lovas, P. M. (2008). Mindfulness and professionalism in dentistry. *Journal of Dental Education, 72*(9), 997 1009.

Major, E. M., & Brock, C. H. (2003). Fostering positive dispositions toward diversity: Dialogical explorations of a moral dilemma. *Teacher Education Quarterly, 30*(4), 7–26.

Marks, H. M. (2000). Student engagement in instructional activity: Patterns in elementary, middle and high school years. *American Education Research Journal, 37*(1), 153–184.

Mearns, J., & Cain, J. E. (2003). Relationships between teachers' occupational stress and their burnout and distress: Roles of coping and negative mood regulation expectancies. *Anxiety, Stress, & Coping: An International Journal, 16*(1), 71–82.

Miller, J. P. (1994). *The contemplative practitioner*. Toronto, Ontario, Canada: OISE Press.

Montgomery, C., & Rupp, A. A. (2005). A meta-analysis for exploring the diverse causes and effects of stress in teachers. *Canadian Journal of Education, 28*, 458–486.

Murray, F. B. (2007). Disposition: A superfluous construct in teacher education. *Journal of Teacher Education, 58*(5), 381–387.

National Board for Professional Teaching Standards (NBPTS). (2002). *What teachers should know and be able to do*. Arlington, VA: National Board for Professional Teaching Standards.

National Council for Accreditation of Teacher Education (NCATE). (2006). *Professional standards for the accreditation of schools, colleges, and departments of education: 2006 edition* (2006th ed.). Washington, DC: National Council for Accreditation of Teacher Education.

Noddings, N. (1992). *The challenge to care in schools: An alternative approach to education*. New York, NY: Teachers College Press.

Palmer, P. J. (1998). *The courage to teach: Exploring the inner landscape of a teacher's life*. San Francisco, CA: Jossey-Bass.

Poulin, P. A. (2009). *Mindfulness-based wellness education: A longitudinal evaluation with students in initial teacher education* (Ph.D. dissertation, OISE/UT).

Poulin, P. A., Mackenzie, C. S., Soloway, G., & Karaoylas, E. C. (2008). Mindfulness training as an evidenced-based approach to reducing stress and promoting well-being among human services professionals. *International Journal of Health Promotion and Education, 46*, 72–80.

Punch, K. F. (2009). *Introduction to research methods in education*. Thousand Oaks, CA: Sage.

Reeve, J., Jang, H., Carrell, D., Jeon, S., & Barch, J. (2004). Enhancing student's engagement by increasing teacher autonomy support. *Motivation and Emotion, 28*(2), 147–169.

Richardson, V. (2003). Constructivist pedagogy. *Teachers College Record, 105*(9), 1623–1640.

Riley, P. (2011). *Attachment theory and the teacher-student relationship*. New York, NY: Routledge.

Rodgers, C. R., & Scott, K. H. (2008). The development of the personal self and professional identity in learning to teach. In M. Cochran-Smith, S. Feiman-Nemser, D. J. McIntyre, & K. E. Demers (Eds.), *Handbook of research on teacher education* (pp. 732–755). New York, NY: Routledge.

Ryan, P. M., & Alcock, M. A. (2002). Personal and interpersonal attributes in selecting teachers. *Action in Teacher Education, 24*(1), 58–67.

Saunders, P. A., Tractenberg, R. E., Chaterji, R., Amri, H., Harazduk, N., Gordon, J. S., … Haramati, A. (2007). Promoting self-awareness and reflection through an experiential mind-body skills course for first year medical students. *Medical Teacher, 29*(8), 778–784.

Schön, D. A. (1983). *The reflective practitioner: How professionals think in action*. New York, NY: Basic Books.

Schön, D. A. (1987). *Educating the reflective practitioner: Toward a new design for teaching and learning in the professions*. San Francisco, CA: Jossey-Bass.

Schure, M. B., Christopher, J., & Christopher, S. (2008). Mind–body medicine and the art of self-care: Teaching mindfulness to counseling students through yoga, meditation, and qigong. *Journal of Counseling and Development, 86*, 47–56.

Schwartz, M. (2008). Teacher preparation for character development. In L. Nucci & D. Narvaez (Eds.), *Handbook of moral and character education* (pp. 583–600). Hillsdale, NJ: Erlbaum.

Shapiro, S. L., Astin, J. A., Bishop, S. R., & Cordova, M. (2005). Mindfulness-based stress reduction for health care professionals: Results from a randomized trial. *International Journal of Stress Management, 12*(2), 164–176.

Shapiro, S. L., Brown, K. W., & Biegel, G. M. (2007). Teaching self-care to caregivers: Effects of mindfulness-based stress reduction on the mental health of therapists in training. *Training and Education in Professional Psychology, 1*(2), 105–115.

Siegel, D. (2007). *The mindful brain*. New York, NY: W.W. Norton.

Soloway, G. B. (2005). *Mindfulness-based wellness education*. Unpublished masters research paper, OISE of the University of Toronto, Ontario.

Soloway, G. B., Poulin, A., & Mackenzie, C. S. (2010). Preparing new teachers for the full catastrophe of the

21st century classroom: Integrating mindfulness training into initial teacher education. In A. Cohan & A. Honigsfeld (Eds.), *Breaking the mold of pre-service and in-service teacher education*. Lanham, MD: Rowman & Littlefield Education.

Stenberg, K. (2010). Identity work as a tool for promoting the professional development of student teachers. *Reflective Practice, 11*(3), 331–346.

Suzuki, S. (2003). *Zen mind, beginner's mind*. New York, NY: Weatherhill.

Tillema, H. H. (2000). Belief change towards self-directed learning in student teachers: Immersion in practice or reflection in action. *Teaching and Teacher Education, 16*, 575–591.

Warin, J., Maddock, M., Pell, A., & Hargreaves, L. (2006). Resolving identity dissonance through reflective and reflexive practice in teaching. *Reflective Practice, 7*(2), 233–245.

Ying, Y. W. (2009). Contribution of self-compassion to competence and mental health in social work students. *Journal of Social Work Education, 45*(2), 309–323.

Zeichner, K. M. (2009). *Teacher education and the struggle for social justice*. New York, NY: Routledge.

Zins, J. E., Weissberg, R. P., Wang, M. C., & Walberg, H. J. (2004). *Building academic success on social and emotional learning: What does the research say?* New York, NY: Teachers College Press.

Embodied Presence: Contemplative Teacher Education

13

Richard C. Brown, Genét Simone, and Lee Worley

I'm slowly becoming more willing to be seen—more relaxed, with more mindfullness, hoping to take less cover behind the self-created teacher cocoon. This kind of transparency paradoxically fills me with great anxiety about not-knowing what is going to happen. Yet I feel more alive—constantly being mindful of the shifting situations in the class, making choices in split-second moments to remain open rather than closed... (TKL'09)

This student's story exemplifies the transformative process that graduate students experience during their studies in the Contemplative Education program at Naropa University, located in Boulder, Colorado. It is one of many reflections collected since the program's inception in 2000, describing an "inner shift" that occurs when students engage in a variety of contemplative practices during two summer intensives, and carefully-sequenced online courses that extend through 2 years. These students, classroom teachers for the ages of early childhood through adulthood, go through a metamorphosis that changes them from the inside-out—from being facilitators of knowledge and skills to being teachers who are able to "read" situations and respond with a synchronized body and mind. As in the story above, this synchronization of body and mind occurs organically in the moment; it is not forced or planned. However, for that organic unfolding to occur on a regular basis, and in the midst of a teacher's often hectic life, a solid foundation of skills must be learned and practiced.

The concept of a synchronized body and mind in teaching is often overlooked in teacher education and professional development in the USA, especially with current federal, state, and local emphasis on rigorous academic standards aimed at preparing a generation of citizens capable of competing in a world economy. Indeed, ever since the landmark report "A Nation at Risk" (1984), and the more recent Obama Administration's "Race to the Top" funding initiative,[1] the federal and state emphasis on "high standards" has directly impacted pedagogy and curriculum in all major subject areas to the detriment of more creative, social, emotional,

[1] A 2009 initiative by the Obama Administration, the American Recovery and Reinvestment Act, included a program called "Race to the Top." This initiative offered competitive grants to schools in the USA that could prove they were providing innovative curriculum, closing "the achievement gap," attracting and retaining highly-qualified administrators and teachers, and raising test scores. Since 2009, the U.S. Department of Education has offered additional "phases" of funding for these, and other, initiatives.

R.C. Brown (✉) • L. Worley
Naropa University, Boulder, CO, USA
e-mail: rbrown@naropa.edu; lworley@naropa.edu

G. Simone
Woodring College of Education, Western Washington University, Bellingham, VA, USA
e-mail: Genet.Simone@wwu.edu

K.A. Schonert-Reichl, R.W. Roeser (eds.), *Handbook of Mindfulness in Education*, Mindfulness in Behavioral Health, DOI 10.1007/978-1-4939-3506-2_13

and intrapersonal skills. More importantly, it has redefined standards for teacher education and professional development by equating effective teaching with adoption of the Common Core Standards and higher student test scores on a variety of state-driven assessments. The results of these initiatives, unfortunately, place teachers in the predicament of having to "teach to the test" or risk being removed from their posts when scores are less than desirable. These outcomes are being vigorously debated in a variety of states with some, like Texas and Virginia, opting out of federal funding altogether in order to avoid the punitive measures of noncompliance.[2]

Although adoption of the Common Core Standards, or better scores on state-driven assessments, are not inherently detrimental to children's learning, they do overlook a critical feature of teachers' success with their students' learning: the teacher's self-awareness—a mindful awareness of what is occurring, not just from a detached self-other perspective, but also from the perspective of the teacher's own mind, heart, and senses. There is a symbiotic relationship between good teachers and their students, which is dependent upon the teacher's inner and outer intelligence.

What we offer in the Contemplative Education Department at Naropa University provides the foundation from which the path of a teacher's evolution into fuller inner and outer development is paved, and we find that THAT is what leads to better student learning. We call the primary feature of the teacher's inner and outer development *embodied presence.*

In this chapter, we emphasize the somatic or physical dimensions of embodied presence, highlighting a uniquely potent dimension of our program's approach. We discuss the emotional and conceptual aspects as well, but more as context for bodily presence. We provide a definition of embodied presence, and how it directly relates to the practice of mindful awareness that is being explored in this series. We offer examples from students' writings and faculty observations, and provide sample exercises used in our program that aim to help students understand in a visceral way what it means to become more embodied and more present. The results of such inner work can be quite surprising, satisfying, and far-reaching. One student wrote in her journal:

> Over time, and with practice, I have begun to build a connection to my experience by paying attention to my sensations, thoughts and feelings to root me in my presence. I am beginning to shift my perspective, from a primary concern about how I am seen to feeling the moment and moving from there. I have become much more flexible in teaching …, and that flexibility is reflected in a freshness in my being after the class is done: I feel replenished, rather than depleted. (CT'10)

What Embodied Presence Is *Not*

Before elaborating on what we mean by embodied presence, we would like to first explain what it is *not*. Embodied presence is not a teaching "disposition" as is framed by the National Council for Accreditation of Teacher Education (NCATE), a primary organization that identifies and enforces standards expected in most teacher training institutions in the United States.[3] As explained in Standard 1: *Candidate Knowledge, Skills, and Professional Dispositions,* Professional Dispositions are

> attitudes, values, and beliefs demonstrated through both verbal and non-verbal behaviors as educators interact with students, families, colleagues, and communities. These positive behaviors support student learning and development. NCATE expects institutions to assess professional dispositions based on observable behaviors in educational settings.[4]

[2]Office of the Governor Rick Perry. (2010, January 13). Gov. Perry: Texas Knows Best How to Educate Our Students: *Texas will not apply for Federal Race to the Top Funding.* Retrieved June 25, 2014: http://governor.state.tx.us/news/press-release/14146/); and Richmond Times-Dispatch (2013, October 10). Virginia News: Va. not pursuing $45 million Race to the Top grant. Retrieved June 25, 2014: http://www.timesdispatch.com/news/state-regional/va-not-pursuing-million-race-to-the-top-grant/article_9128279c-a917-5346-a402-f8afade4a475.html

[3]With the July 1, 2013 de facto consolidation of NCATE and TEAC into CAEP as the new accrediting body for educator preparation, please visit http://caepnet.org for general information (TEAC=Teacher Education Accreditation Council; CAEP=Council for the Accreditation of Educator Preparation).

[4]NCATE Mission Statement: www.ncate.org

According to these national standards, "dispositions" have a rather solid quality that is observable, measurable, and capable of being assessed. What we are providing in our contemplative education program—embodied presence—does not negate that focus. We agree that teachers should be observed handling situations with honesty, consistency, and a positive, problem-solving demeanor that supports the learning needs of every student.

However, these national standards do not address the importance of training teachers in establishing the underlying foundation that will help them, in authentically personal and professional ways, negotiate the tricky territory of daily events as they unfold in a classroom. To uphold the belief that all children can learn requires teachers to be fully present to the plethora of multifacted situations that arise each day, with mind and body synchronized—in short, having an embodied presence. Training in the development of embodied presence means working with the under-current of energy that subsequently affects professional dispositions in an authentic way. Our education starts where our teachers are, mentally and emotionally, and with regard to their body. We provide them with opportunities to learn directly about the aspects of their "being" that inform their teaching and interactions with others. Faculty members in our program also participate in this learning process, supporting students in the Master's program in their growth toward embodied presence from the inside-out. In this way, the flowering of teachers' "dispositions" is not an add-on to previous curriculum and methods found in teacher training programs, but rather a process of infusion where one's entire being is transformed, and then emerges with honesty, sincerity, and an open heart. Working from this pedagogy of embodied presence, one student remarked,

> I have been using my breath as a focal point in my instruction … [and] my instruction is more vivid, because I am experiencing it within my body simultaneously. At the very least, including myself in the instruction makes me feel calm, allowing me to connect authentically with my experience and provide creative sequences for my students. (EB'09)

Here, we see an example of the symbiotic relationship between the development of embodied presence and one person's teaching practice; the former informs the latter, thereby strengthening the overall delivery of instruction.

Second, *embodied presence* is not "acting." Teaching is often compared to putting on a performance or acting for an audience. As such, teacher educators uphold the belief that teachers should receive training in acting so they can put on a great performance to keep students engaged with their learning. As Finkel (2000) noted:

> …we always hear that a teacher is like an actor, and a good class is like a theatrical performance. Most of us do remember fondly those brilliant teachers/actors we may have had. …we left their classes inspired, moved. But did we learn anything? (p. 1)

Although we can agree that there is an element of theatrical performance in teaching, rather than equating the two, we need to understand this relationship in a more holistic, contemplative context. Embodied presence is quite different from professional acting training. An excerpt from a student versed in performing makes this distinction clear:

> I remember beginning presence work with an expectation that 'acting' would be easy for me, but I quickly discovered I possessed an underdeveloped ability to be present and unattached to the spontaneity of each moment. I found myself preparing and over-thinking, and allowing that to determine my actions. I was very tightly attached to making sure I appeared to be 'doing the right thing' and 'moving and speaking with grace.' I was so concerned with how I appeared that I couldn't connect with the experience of presence at all. (CT'10)

This sentiment is summed up by Worley (2001), who writes, "Before we can act genuinely, we need to discover how to be genuine" (p. 4). It is from this perspective that we have drawn our ideas of teaching presence to teachers. We use a more communally based theater model where the separation between performers and audience is not so rigid. Moving this analogy to a classroom, rather than creating a sensational show for a passive audience, the teacher models a quality of unconditional openness. Here, the mind and body of the teacher, and the minds and bodies of the students, meet in the space between. This *receptive presence*[5] while initiated and cultivated in the body and speech of the teacher includes more of the whole situation—the students, time of day, spatial arrangement of the room, current events, and so on. In this way, the teacher's "performance" can be considered more "shamanistic" in its approach because it draws on the collective wisdom and intelligence of the audience/class to evoke the spirit of learning. In Palmer's (1998) words, it is able to call forth "the community of truth,"

> where we are held together not only by our personal powers of thought and feeling, but also by the power of 'the grace of great things' … the subjects around which the circle of seekers [is] gathered—not the disciplines that study these subjects, not the texts that talk about them, not the theories that explain them, but the things themselves. (pp. 106–107)

This all-encompassing approach invites into a situation all of its aspects in an organically unfolding manner. To be a teacher in this realm means providing not only the opportunity to use everything at one's disposal, but also having an awareness of what is actually there in the first place, and knowing how to use it.

In our culture, we often interpret "actor" or "acting" as being somewhat artificial, where the actor (or teacher in this case) follows a script and pauses in all the right places. Having presence does not deny the value of direct instruction, but goes beyond those limitations; the teacher steps out from behind the metaphorical desk onto the "stage," and becomes fully engaged around the classroom. Everyone and everything is included in this grand ensemble of learning. The teacher is an anchor whose presence in body, voice, and mind empowers the students, themselves, to become fully immersed in the learning process. Having such presence, an embodied teacher brings together the students' collaborative energies in a circle of mutual discovery, where the outcomes may surprise both teacher and students and lead to an excitement for life and learning.

We need to be clear, however, that developing an embodied presence is not an exercise of simply learning a few techniques that are haphazardly applied in the classroom; development at such a deep level requires time and a special context in which embodied presence may be cultivated. Frameworks for self-understanding must be provided on a regular basis through a variety of intellectual, artistic, and physical modes. There needs to be plenty of space for examination of the inner self and support from a caring community of like-minded practitioners. These features, and more, are found within the larger framework of Contemplative Education.

Contemplative Education at Naropa University

> *The basic idea was an institute that would create an interface, a dialogue, between Buddhism and the intellectual culture of the West, as well as with other spiritual traditions. … [Chögyam Trungpa] talked about creating sparks by juxtaposing different traditions. The idea was that if you look at things from different perspectives, you can get to their essence.* (in Midal, 2005, pp. 143–144)

Naropa—rather than being a Buddhist school—was envisioned by its founder[6] as being "Buddhist-inspired." It is non-sectarian in its investigation of contemplative principles and practices from many of the world's wisdom traditions. Graduates are provided knowledge and skills "to meet the world as it is and to change it for the better."[7]

The pedagogical approach at Naropa is the contemplation, or mindfully aware investigation,

[5] This term, "receptive presence" was coined by Lee Worley, and is used throughout her work and writings.

[6] Chögyam Trungpa Rinpoche (1939–1987) was the 11th descendent in the line of Trungpa tulkus, important teachers of the Kagyü lineage of Tibetan Buddhism. After fleeing Tibet in 1959 when the Chinese Communist Party took control, Chögyam Trungpa Rinpoche established a number of learning centers in the West, one of which was Naropa University (est. 1974) in Boulder, Colorado.

[7] Naropa University Mission Statement.

of one's thoughts, emotions, and actions in such a way as to experience them without creating additional overlays that distort their essence. Contemplation leads to experiences where the separation between a subject, and the object being observed is softened.

Emphasis on "nowness" always plays a large role in contemplative education training. The living moment becomes the basis for reflecting on the past or planning for the future. In their coursework at Naropa, students are inspired and encouraged to bring their whole beings to bear on the subject being studied in the moment at hand, and to stay abreast of the waves of moments as they flow forward. Learning in this way has the tendency to provide students with a more relaxed and accepting perspective about their world—one in which they, and others, can be regarded as "basically good."

The idea that human beings are inherently good and sane, and basically intelligent, is fundamental to the concept of contemplative education and is at the root of Naropa University's vision. Chögyam Trungpa coached his early students to appreciate that sanity is more basic to human beings than insanity and that the world is a workable place. Becoming brave about getting to know ourselves, we discover that we are basically good—that our very nature is sane and clear. Seeing this with some certainty in ourselves, we also become aware of how our thoughts and emotions can distort how we perceive the world. With this new awareness of how our minds operate, and the ability to keep a clearer perspective, the world appears more welcoming. We have a place in its evolutionary processes.

Contemplative Education and the Teacher's Inner Life

Contemplative teacher education begins with disciplines that develop the inner life of the teacher, by which we mean the constellation including one's physical manifestation, sense perceptions, intellect, and emotions. This "inner landscape" (Palmer, 1998) grows and develops throughout one's life, influences one's actions, and provides guideposts for determining a life purpose. When we ask ourselves the metaphysical question, "Who am I?" we are seeking to locate and understand our inner life—our "authentic self" (Kessler, 1991; Senge, Scharmer, Jaworski, & Flowers, 2004, p. 221).

For a teacher, this sense of self, or inner life, tends to become overrun with beliefs about the teacher's expected role as disciplinarian, curriculum expert, and ethical role model. Although those particular traits are certainly needed for effective teaching, they fall short of reaching the full realm of the teacher's inner life, where the energy and potential for masterful teaching resides. Of course, not paying attention to that inner life can still result in a teacher who can negotiate the complicated, ever-changing, and highly charged territory of the classroom, but we believe that neglecting to support the teacher's inner life ultimately manifests a feeling of disconnection between the teacher's heart and the students' needs and aspirations (Gatto, 1992; Liston, 2000; Tomkins, 1996). Palmer (1998) calls this "living a divided life," where the identity and the integrity of the teacher are not symbiotically attuned. Such misalignment can lead to misunderstandings and missed opportunities for authentic learning and personal growth—those meaningful "teachable moments" that teachers hope to experience. One student in our program commented:

> I have hidden behind this teacher mask for so long that I'm not sure I know how to function without it… I think I am finally starting to feel the discomfort and disconnect of living a divided life. I am coming to see and understand the many ways I deceive myself. I think all this inner exploration we've been doing over the last year and a half has revealed the extent of my delusions. As difficult as this revelation is to bear, I feel that it is a sign of progress on the path. (AC'09)

The disconnect of wearing a "mask" is quite palpable for this teacher, and although those feelings may go unnoticed by others, they create enough discomfort inside the teacher to genuinely impact instruction.

Anyone attuned to teaching can admit that the profession is certainly not exempt from stressful experiences and feelings.

> Faced with a system that tends to ignore their emotional and developmental needs, teachers are tossed around year after year by a multitude of energy-sapping demands; indeed, the list of things for which teachers are responsible grows longer with every shift in the social and political tides … Since schools are not typically designed to actively and intentionally support the teachers' quest for meaning, teachers who once felt a passion for their craft begin to "burn out," and may end up leaving the profession altogether. (Farber, 1984, 1991; Friedman, 1991; Little & Turk, 1985, in Simone, 2009, pp. 28–29)

For those who stay in the teaching profession, it is clear that their health and overall well-being needs to be taken into account. Organizations like *The Center for Courage & Renewal* have been instrumental in providing renewal for teachers through seasonal retreats, and others, like the Garrison Institute—aimed at nurturing the minds, bodies, and spirits of teacher—are appearing.

In our teacher education program, we are continually engaged in contemplating these questions: What *is* the teacher's inner life, and how can it be cultivated and nurtured? Which practices or exercises lay the most dependable foundation for that cultivation? How can developing an embodied presence enhance student learning in school? After using contemplative approaches with teachers for over two decades, we know that such an undertaking requires a great deal of patience, perseverance, and trust between teacher educators and their students (who are teachers themselves).

How, then, do people cultivate this inner self in order to reach a stage where they can experience an embodied presence? We have learned that the keys to inner growth and realization are the practices of *mindfulness* and *awareness* or—more accurately—*mindful awareness*. Mindful awareness is the basis for a set of skills that can be developed in a relatively short period of time, but which take a lifetime of honing.

Mindful Awareness and the Body

> *The faculty of voluntarily bringing back a wandering attention, over and over again, is the very root of judgment, character, and will. No one is compos sui [master of himself] if he have it not. An education which should improve this faculty would be the education 'par excellence.'* (James, 1984, p. 424)

In Naropa University's Contemplative Education graduate program, activating the inner life begins through unbiased, compassionate investigation using methods based on mindful awareness. The mindfulness dimension involves the seemingly simple act of bringing a focused, yet open, attention to one's experiences, and repeating that mental shift as much as possible throughout the day. Doing this cultivates one's ability to think more clearly and act more deliberately because more information—both subtle and overt—is allowed to arise and be nonjudgmentally considered before moving ahead.

Awareness is understood as holding a spacious, extended quality of mind within which mindfulness can continually reoccur. It could be said that mindfulness is a tool for aligning and stabilizing mind and body while awareness is the integration of oneself within the larger environment. Chögyam Trungpa (1998) elegantly describes the union of the two methods of mindfulness and awareness:

> Right mindfulness does not simply mean being aware; it is like creating a work of art. If you are drinking a cup of tea with right mindfulness, you are aware of the whole environment as well as the cup of tea. You can therefore trust what you are doing; you are not threatened by anything. You have room to dance in the space, and this makes it a creative situation. The space is open to you. (p. 99)

In other words, there is awareness of the space in conjunction with attention on a particular object or person. Being located in the "whole environment" in this way, tends to produce a level of confidence in one's direct experience. With this understanding in mind, the sequence of teacher training in Naropa University's Contemplative Education program starts with practices in mindful awareness that are focused on sensory experiences, emotions, thoughts, and the dimensions and dynamics of space. One student wrote in her journal:

> What Presence allows for is a deep grounding within the physical form of the body in space. [Then, speaking about the concept of fear] What

> does fear *feel* like? I feel it in my shaking belly, in a quickening of my heart rate, in tears that come to my eyes. As I breathe into and through the physical sensations they eventually dissolve. (AB'09)

In the past decade, many research studies have been conducted that provide scientific evidence supporting the development of mindful awareness practices on a person's body and mind, and overall health and well-being. The strong effects of mindful awareness on the health of the body suggests that a more fully embodied mindful awareness may have even greater benefits, as Daniel Siegel (2007) has begun to explore:

> In mindful awareness we are often focusing on aspects of our bodily function ... If in mindfulness practice our mind is filled with word-based left-sided chatter at that moment, we could propose that there is a fundamental neural competition between right (body-sense) and left (word-thoughts) for the limited resources of attentional focus at that moment. Shifting within mindful awareness to a focus on the body may involve a functional shift away from linguistic conceptual facts toward the nonverbal imagery and somatic sensations of the right hemisphere. (p. 47)

In our program we are discovering that when mindful awareness is developed in many domains, particularly in the body, teachers have a broad base of presence upon which to draw in order to nourish themselves and to support a more enlivened classroom learning culture. "While teaching we might even forget we even have bodies. But just as in meditation, when our physical bodies are upright, receptive, and present, we are more able to directly contact our inner resources and be more responsive to our students" (Brown, 2011, pp. 77–78).

Embodied Presence

Teachers who have learned mindful awareness practices in our summer program have found them beneficial to their work with children and adults in a variety of learning environments. Students report being able to work more effectively in difficult situations that previously caused a great deal of stress; they seem to have a larger perspective, which enables them to be more patient, resourceful, and confident with decisions. Through essays and journals, students have provided a variety of reflections that include premises about their contemplative education, such as:

1. Intellectual understanding deepens when it is linked to body awareness.
2. With embodied presence, the teacher's thoughts and actions become clearer and more genuine, leading to increased confidence when relating to students and the subject matter.
3. Challenging and unpredictable classroom situations can be met with more flexibility and adaptability by teachers; they are able to more calmly meet difficult situations in a relaxed, yet authoritative manner.
4. Embodied presence practices enliven a sense of curiosity, improvisation, and playfulness in teachers when responding to teachable moments.
5. Embodied presence expands teachers' awareness so that it embraces the entire learning environment. As such, more careful attention is given to the arrangement of the room, use of time, grouping of students, and coordination of the lessons.

These aspects of expanded awareness also invite broader participation from unexpected quarters of the learning environment as teacher and students find new and refreshing ways to be together. All of these effects are evidence, at least from our students' experience, of an increased stable teaching presence and an increased capacity for mixing effective pedagogy with in-the-moment responsiveness.

Using Presence Exercises in Educating Teachers

During two summer programs, and also online in their classes, teachers in our program engage in mindfulness meditation and other practices such as mindful eating, speaking, and walking. The intention of these practices is to thoroughly integrate mindful awareness in their emotional, perceptual, and intellectual lives. Among the most integrative of all these practices are the ones that focus on the cultivation of authentic communication, which occurs through movements in body and speech. Many teacher educators tend to overlook this dimension, but it is a critically important to the conveyance of knowledge and the receptivity of the teacher. Often, it is the messengers, not the messages, that impact students the most. "We teach who we are," writes Palmer (1998):

> Every class comes down to this: my students and I, face to face [are] engaged in an ancient and exacting exchange called education. The techniques I have mastered do not disappear, but neither do they suffice ... Only one resource is at my immediate command: my identity, my selfhood, my sense of 'I' who teaches—without which I have no sense of the 'Thou' who learns. (p. 10)

And who is the "I" who teaches? It is the one who speaks clearly, listens attentively, and stands or moves with intention and grace. Although conventionally speech is thought to mean the talking aspect of body/mind, speech also includes how a teacher stands or sits—the messages that come from body language, as well as the skills of listening and of responding appropriately to the messages coming from students. One student, noticing the subtlety of how her presence was contributing to disconnection with her students, wrote:

> When I give my students directions, I notice that I speak quickly. I can hear my words blending together and feel my eyes rolling into my head. I speak on the exhale of my breath as if I am sighing in boredom. When I ask if there are any questions I speak in a tone that would make any student hesitate to raise their hand. (EB'10)

There are many embodied presence practices we use to bring students in our MA program to a level of development that expands their awareness of the thoughts and emotions residing within; we have chosen three to share: *Lying Down to Standing Up*, *Presenting Yourself*, and *Embodied Reading and Listening*. Below, for each practice, we provide the underlying premise, followed by the sequence of steps used (i.e., method), and finally some potential results of each exercise.

Lying Down to Standing Up Exercise

Premise The body has intelligence that is often ignored in ordinary life. This creates for the student/teacher a nonconceptual arena, an opportunity for exploring the dilemma: What should I do, to do this right?

Method Teachers create a 20-min improvisational movement "performance" that starts from a lying down position on the floor and ends in a standing position. They should not use any familiar vocabulary of movement, such as yoga asanas, calisthenics, or dance forms, but instead allow the body to dictate its preferences for moving. All class members do these solo performances simultaneously. There is also an explicit instruction that this is not a performance for others, but for each person alone. Teachers are told that the ratio of time spent on the floor to standing up is theirs to decide. Once they have moved from lying on the floor, however, they should not return to that posture.

Result Having called this 20-min piece a performance raises several levels of anxiety. Some teachers feel they are not performers and, thus, do not know what to do. Others make large, "artistic" movements and do not fulfill the request to let the body lead the movement by following its own desires. Still others are stumped by what the teacher wants and look about helplessly, hoping to get a clue from what the others are doing.

In discussion afterwards, this exercise offers teachers a lot of information about themselves, personally, as well as about being a student. Some of the learning is quite uncomfortable. Generally, however, after more practice, this exercise can be enjoyable once the performer relaxes and permits the body to lead. Knowing from the beginning that one is moving from lying down to standing means that awareness of each moment can be the focus. No energy is demanded for making big choices about where one is headed. Used over time, this basic form can be refined in many ways, such as doing the exercise with the eyes closed, or engaging in a "moving duet" with a partner. There are always surprises, no matter how many times the exercise is repeated. We find that, beyond the boredom of repetition are unimagined well-springs of new inspiration.

Presenting Yourself[8]

Premise The body/mind through awareness can utilize the energy of the audience (or class) to cocreate the moment of meeting. This is particularly helpful for teachers, who tend to experience their energy only dispersing throughout the day and not being replenished at a mutual rate.

Method A space is arranged as a "stage" with an offstage area on either side and space for the audience (i.e., class) in front. All students sit in the audience, and regard the empty stage. They do not speak or physically respond to any aspect of the performances about to occur. They simply witness the performances of classmates. The purpose of the exercise is experiencing how being seen feels in the body when they are "onstage" with the audience or class silently looking at them.

To start, one student comes to edge of the performance space and prepares to make an entrance. It starts with an initial gesture, such as a bow to the stage area, a moment of stillness, or a stretch. The person then enters the stage and stops somewhere onstage. The person stands, mindfully aware, without making any gesture or speech. The student is simply seen by the audience for a moment. The student then exits the stage on either side (not in front), and another student voluntarily rises to repeat the sequence until all of the students have presented themselves.

Result Students may discover their discomfort with being seen and the anxiety that causes different manifestations to arise, such as feelings of *fight or flight*, the need to apologize, or to hide and consequently abandon awareness. For some, a pleasure in being seen arises. Subsequent repetitions can include adding a gesture that arises spontaneously in response to the experience of being seen.

Ultimately Presenting Yourself assists students to trust the moment, to feel the audience for inspiration, and to remain present and aware of the whole. When this occurs, the audience and the performer can "meet in the space between," each side bringing its intelligence to that middle and sparking the learning of the moment—a learning that is often as surprising to the performer/teacher as it is to the audience/students.

Embodied Reading and Listening

Premise Teachers, by training, usually pay attention to content alone and miss the sensory and emotional undertones that enrich the meaning of what is being said. This exercise involves mindful awareness of sound and body during speaking and listening. It integrates conceptual understanding with internal sense perceptions and attunes teachers to their students' communication on both a sensory and content level. It fosters synchronized, authentic, and heart-felt speech and listening.

Method At the beginning level of this practice,[9] pairs of teachers are asked to select a poem or a children's story and to take turns reading it to each other. The readers are instructed to read very slowly in order to enunciate clearly and appreciate the words that they are sharing. Reading slowly also allows readers to hear the sound of

[8] This more advanced exercise, sometimes called the "Stage," supports and furthers the development of presence. Before tackling the challenge of being publicly "seen" students should become familiar with mindful awareness in a more private, individual way, and also in small groups.

[9] More advanced levels involve teachers reading from a text that they would normally read to their own students.

their own voice and actually feel the vibrations of sound in the body.

The listener sits close by and does not look at the reader, focusing only on the sounds and meaning of what is being read. In both roles, listener and reader are asked to lower the locus of offering and receiving to the area of the heart. Shifting communication from the head to the heart further engages the body as an instrument of speaking and listening.

Results The reader and listener may notice and integrate several dimensions: The conceptual content that is being read, sense perceptions (particularly sound), the feeling tones in the voice, and inner responses to those dimensions. This last dimension might be experienced as a tinge of quivering fear from the reader or a feeling of warmth and tenderness in the chest of the listener. Essential to this practice is allowing whatever feelings that arise to coexist without judgment with the other dimensions of the exercise.

Preliminary to the embodied reading and listening exercise, teachers clarify the sense of hearing through other exercises involving mindfully listening to the sounds of a stream or of traffic, wind in the leaves, or children playing on a playground. As with all mindful awareness practices, when one notices the mind commenting on the sounds, one gently and nonjudgmentally lets go of thoughts that arise, and returns to listening to the sounds themselves. One student commented:

> I find that when I'm able to stay with my breath during meditation, I'm able to hear the sound around me - birds chirping, kettle boiling, car engines in the distance, my neighbour's baby crying … But when my thoughts get the better of me, all I can hear is my own voice—and the sounds all around me disappear. My mind chatter separates me from my surroundings … When there is silence in me, there is greater connectedness with the world around me and the world seems much more alive. (KTL'09)

This teacher uses the memory of the Embodied Reading and Listening activity she experienced in the summer program to change the way she speaks to her own class:

> When I catch my "auto-pilot" voice in class, I remember how I felt reading aloud last summer at Naropa. I remember feeling comforted as I let the sounds slowly form on my lips. It was as if I was massaging myself into relaxation. As those memories arise, my tone softens and the speed of my voice slows down. I pause and breathe as I find accurate words to describe the task for my students. I am soothed in the process and able to reconnect with them. (EB'10)

Another teacher articulates how embodied reading has improved and enlivened his classroom instruction:

> I read from Fredrick Douglass's autobiography, and my students were enthralled. I took my time and read carefully and clearly and, even though the language was old fashioned and a bit advanced for 8th graders, they picked up on the ideas he was speaking about with no problem. This was a wonderful way to give a first-hand account and a personal voice to such a major issue (slavery) in American History. (AC09)

Through these and other exercises, our students begin to trust the intrinsic intelligence of their bodies and senses. Although understanding and examining the functions of the thinking mind is essential to learning, it is a fundamental skill in contemplative education to be able to distinguish among thinking, perceiving, and feeling. When those separate capacities are clearer in the teacher's experience, they function better independently and in greater harmony with each other.

Embodied Teaching through "Bridge Practices"

It is a big step from practicing embodied presence in a safe university environment to skillfully integrating presence during the busyness of a typical school day. To help with that transition, we encourage our students to engage in "bridge practices" which are practices that help integrate mindfulness into daily activities. One example of a bridge practice is walking meditation, which is normally done during long sessions of mindful awareness meditation. It involves mindfully attending to the sensations in the soles of one's feet and the swing of the legs as one walks, usually slowly, around the meditation area. During walking meditation, there are many subtle distractions, so students learn to reestablish mindful awareness while in motion; in this way, walking meditation is a method for bridging mindful awareness with the world. We encourage our students to use an adapted form of walking meditation when walking from their car to the classroom or when walking down a hallway between classes. When using this adapted walking meditation in school, teachers walk at their normal pace, but still practice awareness as they go. To prepare for walking meditation as a bridge practice in schools, during our summer program, we practice walking meditation using different speeds and in a variety of environments.

Another bridge practice is standing meditation. Here, the focus of mindfulness is on feeling the direct contact of one's feet with the floor while standing and, at the same time, opening one's awareness to the surrounding space of the room. The key to this practice, as in all mindfulness practices, is allowing one's direct experience (in this case the sense of touch) to function without being obscured by conceptual commentary. That is, when thoughts arise during standing meditation, one gently lets them go and returns to the sensory experience of one's feet on the floor. Teachers are encouraged to use standing meditation for brief periods, such as while monitoring tests or supervising student discussion groups. Teachers report feeling a stronger connection with their bodies, a sense of being "grounded" on the earth, and they see it as an opportunity to return to the present moment. One student, fairly new to the teaching profession, shared this story:

> There I was, standing in front of a classroom of fidgety third-graders, who were really not that interested in what I was teaching. My mind was racing, and then it went blank. It was apparent to everyone that I was losing control, and fast! Then, I remembered the standing meditation, so I just flashed on that and felt my feet on the floor. I felt the floor holding me up solidly and surely; I took a deep breath, and then—suddenly, without any thought at all, I knew what to do. I redirected the lesson, and the children got right back into their learning. (JS'08)

Contemplative Academics

Fundamentally, contemplative education is "weaving academic study and the practices of mindfulness and awareness" (Midal, 2005, p. 146). In order to thoroughly transform their own students' learning, teachers in our program must themselves integrate contemplative practice into their academic learning experiences. Over the years, the Naropa Contemplative Education program has not only taught contemplative practices, but also infused all the academic endeavors with contemplative dimensions. Thus, in our program, all traditionally academic activities, such as reading, writing, discussion, exams, and studying, have contemplative dimensions associated with them; those aspects of education are further enhanced with ongoing exercises in embodied presence. It is beyond the scope of this chapter to explore all the ways in which embodied presence is integrated into academics in our program, so we will focus on just one: the Master's Project.

Master's Projects are developed over the course of the final two online semesters and provide the means for students to explore more deeply and multidimensionally any topic of their choice that resonates with their lives as teachers. Students' examinations and analyses of Master's Project topics can be deeply personal explorations of their own teaching practice or more widely applicable research studies with children in school. Experiencing and then describing experiences via the Master's Project, students in our program develop an approach to their academic work that is precise, sensory, and experiential, and becomes a living model for them to integrate contemplative intelligence into their academic work.

At the end of their projects, students present their work to faculty, peers, and (sometimes) family members and are assessed not only on the content of their study in terms of its thoughtfulness, depth, and organization, but also their embodied presence as they deliver information to their audience. After each presentation, in addition to a critique of the content, faculty members provide feedback about each student's presence, as observed through the aesthetics of room arrangement, the student's clarity of voice, his or her pacing of the presentation, and authenticity when responding to participants' questions. Students report that this approach to the presentation actually provides further insights for them into the meaning of the project itself. In this way, the presentation becomes yet another venue for practicing embodied awareness and learning something new from that experience. Furthermore, their practice of embodied presence during the presentation fosters an unexpectedly profound connection with the audience.

Conclusion

Teachers become contemplatives with the aspiration that their approach to teaching students will have depth and meaning, and genuinely reflect who they are. The fruition of our program, contemplative teaching, can be said to be the embodied presence of the teacher fully engaging with students in academic pursuits in the broadest sense of that term. Teachers communicate their presence and begin to transform their learning community from the inside-out. Doing so cultivates improvisational, intuitive teaching—embracing teachable moments and letting go of the "agenda" if it is not working.

No two teachers in our program take their Naropa education into their classrooms in the same way. It is at the core of our approach to provide the space and opportunity—indeed the encouragement—for each teacher to let the heart and mind find its unique manifestation in each particular learning environment. This recent graduate, a primary-school teacher, recalled a poignant moment of inner-awareness-to-outer-manifestation as she was seated on the floor one day with her young students clustered around:

> I felt slow and steady, and my whole body was aware of the energy in the classroom space. I noticed the children's bottoms moving and their hands busy in their laps as they sat there before me. I slowly changed my position from sitting cross-legged to sitting on my knees. The children asked if they could sit like me. This took a few minutes, but soon they found stillness in this new position. From this transition, one of the students asked about the paint jars on the corner shelf that I had forgotten about. Right then, on the spot, I came up with an activity to paint our letter of the week. This was not at all what I had planned to do. Before painting [our letter], we all sat there gently tickling our faces with our favorite brushes. I appreciated the simplicity [of the moment]—a light buzzing radiated through my body. As we painted the letter D, the children were very quiet and seemed to enjoy this new approach to learning. (JH'10)

References

Brown, R. (2011). The mindful teacher as the foundation of contemplative pedagogy. In J. Simmer-Brown & F. Grace (Eds.), *Meditation and the classroom: Contemplative pedagogy for religious studies* (pp. 75–83). Albany: State University of New York Press.

Farber, B. (1984). Teacher burnout: Assumptions, myths, and issues. *Teachers College Record, 86*(2), 321–338.

Farber, B. (1991). *Crisis in education: Stress and burnout in the American teacher*. San Francisco, CA: Jossey-Bass.

Finkel, D. (2000). *Teaching with your mouth shut*. Portsmouth, NH: Boynton/Cook.

Friedman, I. A. (1991). High- and low-burnout schools: School culture aspects of teacher burnout. *The Journal of Educational Research, 84*, 325–333.

Gatto, J. T. (1992). *Dumbing us down: The hidden curriculum of compulsory schooling*. Philadelphia, PA: New Society.

James, W. (1984). *Psychology: Briefer course*. Cambridge, MA: Harvard University Press.

Kessler, R. (1991). The teaching presence. *Holistic Education Review, 4*(4), 4–15.

Liston, D. (2000). Love and despair in teaching. *Educational Theory, 50*(1), 81–102.

Little, M. D., & Turk, D. C. (1985). Sources of stress and dissatisfaction in experienced high school teachers. *The Journal of Educational Research, 78*, 178–185.

Midal, F. (2005). *Recalling Chögyam Trungpa*. Boston, MA: Shambhala.

National Commission on Excellence in Education. (1984). *A nation at risk: The full account*. Portland, OR: USA Research Inc.

Palmer, P. (1998). *The courage to teach: Exploring the inner landscape of a teacher's life*. San Francisco, CA: Jossey-Bass.

Senge, P., Scharmer, C. O., Jaworski, J., & Flowers, B. S. (2004). *Presence: An exploration of profound change in people, organizations, and society*. New York, NY: Doubleday.

Siegel, D. J. (2007). *The mindful brain*. New York, NY: W.W. Norton.

Simone, G. (2009). *Professional development as a process of renewal: Case studies of the courage to teach program*. Saarbrücken, Germany: VDM Verlag Dr. Müller Aktiengesellschaft.

Tomkins, J. (1996). *A life in school: What the teacher learned*. Reading, MA: Perseus Books.

Trungpa, C. (1998). *The myth of freedom and the way of meditation*. Boston, MA: Shambhala.

Worley, L. (2001). *Coming from nothing: The sacred art of acting*. Boulder, CO: Turquoise Dragon Press.

On Attentive Love in Education: The Case of Courage to Teach

14

Daniel P. Liston

Introduction

About 10 years ago, I found myself in a fairly deep, dark, and anxious funk; I was disheartened and depressed (see Liston, 2000, 2002). I had been an elementary and middle school teacher in both large urban and small town settings, attended graduate school to examine the problems and promises of public education, contributed to the inquiry on schooling and teaching, and had become a recognized scholar in my field. But, it wasn't working. My scholarship sat on the shelves in libraries; my university students faced the same damn obstacles I had encountered as a teacher; and the university's intellectual and professional arena around teacher development seemed dry, arid, and uninspiring. Many of our teaching candidates headed off to their classrooms passionate andprepared (in the progressive tradition[1]), and yet new and veteran teachers would walk into my Masters' classes discouraged and depleted. More and more it seemed that experienced and practicing teachers in Colorado's Front Range came to the university looking for intellectual, professional, and emotional sustenance in the teacher education curriculum—but they didn't seem to be receiving the nourishment they sought. I went searching for ways to address their distress and my discomfort.

I sensed that there was something ill-conceived about the way we were approaching the headaches and heartaches of teaching and teacher education. We seemed to be fooling ourselves that we had in our hands (or on the horizon) surefire curricular, instructional, or institutional solutions. We seemed impelled to go forward with (really) only a glimmer of an understanding of ourselves and those who we aspired to teach. And, we seemed to have embraced conceptions of teaching, learning, and reason that left the realm of affect and emotion in ourselves, and in

[1] Many teacher candidates are prepared within a progressive, rather than traditional, orientation and this preparation factors into the headaches and heartaches of beginning classroom teachers. Those prepared within the progressive child-oriented approach usually find themselves employed in fairly traditional and skill-focused schools. The relationship between schools of education and K-12 public schools has a long and complicated history. See for example Labaree (2004), Clifford und Guthrie (1988) and Zeichner (2009).

D.P. Liston (✉)
University of Colorado at Boulder,
Boulder, CO, USA
e-mail: Dan.Liston@colorado.edu

K.A. Schonert-Reichl, R.W. Roeser (eds.), *Handbook of Mindfulness in Education*,
Mindfulness in Behavioral Health, DOI 10.1007/978-1-4939-3506-2_14

our students, behind. I knew that I had become a teacher and a scholar as much for the desires of my heart as the inclinations of my head, but somehow, the heart had been left behind.

So, I explored the work of philosophers, sociologists, educational researchers, and literary scholars who were examining the forgotten terrain of emotion. I began to develop a framework that underscored the role of emotion, and awareness of the affective dimension of our personhood and relationships, in teaching and learning. I discovered Parker Palmer's *The Courage to Teach* in which he recognizes the potentially depleting work of a profession that requires working with one's head, heart, and soul to engage and transform young lives. Over time, I became a facilitator of Courage to Teach/Lead professional development retreats.[2] I also began to pursue a more contemplative and mindful approach to my professional and personal challenges. I read and engaged with the work of Thomas Keating and his practice of "centering prayer" (see Keating, 1996a, 1996b, 1998, 1999), as well as others writing in a more contemplative vein.

One of the outcomes of this scholarly and experiential exploration was a growing appreciation and understanding of *love* as an essential affective/emotional dimension of teaching and learning. As a result of my own personal experience, contemplative forays, and examination of the scholarly literature on reason and emotion, I came to understand the centrality and complexity of love in teaching and learning (see Liston, 2000, 2002, 2004, 2008, 2012). In fact, it is now difficult for me to conceive of teaching without this complex notion of love. It is a multifaceted concept, one that includes a romantic love of learning (the lure of learning in teaching), an attentive love toward self and others (especially students and colleagues), and an enlarged love with transcendent capacities to deal with the emotional heartache and appreciate the beauty of teaching and learning.

In teaching, we inevitably confront obstacles to expressing this lure of learning and attending to students. Schools tend not to encourage or support these loving engagements. At times, the obstacles can lead to frustration, discouragement, and even despair. In this essay, I explore the thesis that love and attention to inner, other, and outer realms are central to teaching and learning, and that many teachers who have the potential to be excellent teachers leave teaching because of the institutional obstacles that contort and distort their loves and their ability to grow them. There is a great deal of pain and suffering in those departures. In the first part of the essay, I focus on Keating's contemplative approach and note the role of love. Next, I sketch the basic outlines of attentive love utilizing the insights of three philosophers: Iris Murdoch, Simone Weil, and Sara Ruddick.

The Courage professional development and renewal program of Parker Palmer, that uses his text and is delivered in the form of retreats, recognizes these dynamics of love slighted and lost, helps teachers live with the accompanying grief, and provides the tools and pathways of understanding to handle the inevitable tensions that come with teaching.[3] Thus, in the second part of this essay I focus on the interaction of love and attention within the Courage to Teach work as one example that aims to attend to the inner life of the teacher and the cultivation of these twin qualities, as the "work before the work" in educational reform and renewal. Here, I identify and elaborate several contemplative elements, grounded in attentive love, that are present in Courage renewal work. In particular, I highlight aspects of facilitator modeling, the Courage circle of trust framework (see http://www.couragerenewal.org/approach/), and the Courage practice of clearness committees. Through these elements, participants in Courage retreats come to grapple, and more capably deal with, the professional issues that bedevil them. Attentive love,

[2] http://www.couragerenewal.org/programs/facilitator-prep

[3] The Center for Courage and Renewal (formerly the Center for Courage to Teach) is the organization that developed around the efforts to address Palmer's insights into and experiences with teachers. In the section on Courage work, I will describe this effort more completely and focus on the Courage work with teachers rather than the work with other serving professions.

especially its contemplative features, plays a key role here. Retreat participants come to know themselves better and discern the troubling and engaging features of their professional terrain, and they come to do so as a community of loving-kindness that supports one another and reaffirms that teachers are "not alone."

Contemplation and Love

What is love, and how is it related to attention and teaching? To begin to explore these questions, I begin with Thomas Keating's (1996a, 1996b) approach to the contemplative journey. Keating posits the contemplative journey is, at its core, "an exercise of letting go of the false self" (p. 20). In a trilogy of texts, he plumbs the depths of a particularly Christian approach to meditation (Keating, 1996a, 1996b, 1998). The journey Keating delineates is a nuanced, demanding, and attentive process. Keating's efforts to portray the central tenets of centering prayer are extensive and substantive. Here, I utilize Keating's (1996a) pointed elaboration of centering prayer, which is best conveyed and understood as a discipline that is

> ... designed to withdraw our attention from the ordinary flow of our thoughts. We tend to identify ourselves with that flow. But there is a deeper part of ourselves. This prayer opens our awareness to the spiritual level of our being. This level might be compared to a great river on which our memories, images, feelings, inner experiences, and the awareness of outward things are resting. Many people are so identified with the ordinary flow of their thoughts and feelings that they are not aware of the source from which these mental objects are emerging. Like boats or debris floating along the surface of a river, our thoughts and feelings must be resting on something. They are resting on the inner stream of consciousness, which is our participation in God's being. That level is not immediately evident to ordinary consciousness. Since we are not in immediate contact with that level, we have to do something to develop our awareness of it. It is the level of our being that makes us most human. The values that we find there are more delightful than the values that float along the surface of the psyche. We need to refresh ourselves at this deep level every day. Just as we need exercise, food, rest, and sleep, so also we need moments of interior silence because they bring the deepest kind of refreshment." (pp. 34–35)

Keating further describes the methods of centering prayer as well as the extraneous noise and distinct kinds of thoughts, which frequently accompany this meditative process (pp. 109–115).

Central to this meditative practice is a particular quality of attentiveness: It is an attentiveness to and a process of letting go of the false self, and a resulting understanding of the true Self—or "no self" (1999, p. 44). It usually entails an individual sitting (or walking) in silence—employing a sacred word to attune and reorient the individual to the meditative method. For Keating, centering prayer is a process that results in seeing much of our own, and the world's, engagements as shining, usually thin (but sometimes quite thick) chimera (i.e., the false self) that tend to lure us away from what really matters (true Self). Throughout his written work, Keating underscores the continual and ongoing nature of this contemplative process and contrasts it with a putative achievement of "mindfulness bliss."[4] Keating maintains that centering prayer allows us to tap into the inner stream of consciousness, "the level of our being that makes us most human," where we find the values that matter most. Others who practice the meditative and contemplative arts have tapped into this inner stream and uncovered a wealth of understanding.

Love is a central theme in Thich Nhat Hanh's approach to mindfulness. In *Teachings on Love*, Hanh (1998) comments extensively on the variety of ways in which love constitutes part of this "inner stream." Hanh writes:

> Mindfulness is the energy that allows us to look deeply at our body, feelings, perceptions, mental formations, and consciousness and see clearly what our real needs are, so we will not drown in the sea of suffering. Eventually love fills our mind and our will, and all our actions from that time on manifest love. (p. 15)

[4] This is a point worth underscoring. Sometimes, the putative and received notion of "meditation" or "mindfulness" is one that construes contemplation as an approach that magically dissolves daily tensions and dilemmas and delivers the practitioner transcendent bliss. Keating emphasizes throughout his works that centering prayer will not deliver an unending state of bliss, but instead enables individuals to see themselves, others, and the world more clearly. This discerning function of centering prayer coincides with the attentive love I elaborate later.

Hanh claims that the practice of mindfulness taps into the significance of love. He writes about the importance of self love, love between individuals, the role of love in understanding others, deep listening, and loving speech. His love meditations encourage an awareness that knowing oneself is "the first practice of love" and that through looking deeply and attending fully to another person's pain, the doors of love and understanding can be opened (see Hanh, 1998, Chaps. 3 and 4). Hanh joins the company of many others in recognizing this connection between mindfulness and love. Thomas Keating, Joanna Macy (1991), Henry Nouwen (1996), and Thomas Merton (2004) have also elaborated the multiple connections between contemplation and love. These authors (and others) provide rich tools for exploring the conceptual terrain of loving, teaching, and living.

Within the last decade contemplative and mindful practices have gained a small and notable foothold in segments of US culture. For some individuals, contemplative and meditative practices provide rich pathways through which to explore and dwell in life's pains, paradoxes, beauty, and intrigues. Unfortunately for some teachers and a segment of the larger public, these meditative explorations appear thoroughly spiritual, more or less religious, and seem to utilize concepts that do not seem to be appropriate for educational contexts.[5] In short, some shy away from mindfulness practices due to religious connotations, whereas others do not see the "payoff" in exploring professional concerns.[6] It seems to me that within the academic and university settings, scholarly acceptance of and inquiry into mindfulness practices, although now growing in some disciplinary sectors (see Zajonc, this volume), has been limited and approached with some skepticism. And, scholarly investigations of emotion and reason have been, and continue to be, relatively sparse, and discussions of love nearly absent.[7]

Explorations of Love in Teaching: Conceptual and Experiential

A decade ago I realized that something new was needed for teachers and educational scholars to help explore this important terrain of emotion and reason. Personally and professionally, I have pursued two distinct routes: (1) conceptual and phenomenological understandings of teaching's emotional and intellectual struggles, and (2) an experiential exploration of teachers' frustrations, delights, and heartaches in the daily course of teaching in schools. The first route was more intellectually focused while the second route was more experientially engaged. As part of the second path, I participated in, and later became a facilitator of, Courage to Teach/Lead retreats.[8]

As a scholar, I sought out and developed further elaborations of teaching's emotional terrain as well as the distinct kinds of love present in teachers' lives (e.g., Liston & Garrison, 2004). In order to accomplish this intellectual task, I turned to the realms and discipline I knew best: teachers' narrative accounts and philosophical analysis. I attempted to discern the ways reason and emotion intermingled and elaborated three distinct *teaching loves*: the lure of learning in teaching, attentive love toward students, and an enlarged love to deal with teachers' despair. This elaboration of teaching's loves enabled me to develop a set of concepts that could integrate teachers'

[5] See Rachel Kessler's *Soul of Education* as well as more popular press items: San Francisco parents… https://www.facebook.com/pages/SF-Parents-Against-TM-in-Public-Schools/201123776750702; and Olesen, http://educationcurrent.wordpress.com/

[6] This observation is based on my experience working with teachers and administrators in Colorado's Front Range.

[7] During the last 10 years, greater attention has been paid to emotions in many academic fields. David Brooks' *The Social Animal* (2011) is a helpful introduction to the psychological research on emotion. The Stanford online encyclopedia provides a help overview of recent developments in the philosophy of emotion. See http://plato.stanford.edu/entries/emotion/

[8] In our Colorado Courage organization, we have worked with teachers and educational leaders, clergy and lay religious leaders, foundations' staff, and others in the serving professions. Here, as I noted earlier, I focus on the work with teachers and educational leaders.

experiences with my growing understanding of both the contemplative and scholarly terrains.

Experientially, I pursued a further understanding of teachings' loves and heartaches through Courage to Teach/Lead retreats, first as a participant and then as a facilitator. Over time, I became aware of the ways in which Courage professional development attempts to address the three various teaching loves. Here, I will focus on the ways in which Courage retreats attune participants to features of what I have called "attentive love." In the Courage setting, attentive love acts as a bridge concept and set of experiences and practices, connecting teachers to a more contemplative orientation. Courage retreats are, for some participants, an introduction to and initial engagement with a contemplative orientation via practices that encourage attentive love.[9]

Attentive Love in Teaching and Facilitating[10]

In attempting to understand the role of attentive love in educational practice I turned to three western philosophers—individuals who had addressed the western split dividing reason and emotion—philosopher and mystic Simone Weil; novelist and philosopher Iris Murdoch; and mother, feminist, and philosopher Sara Ruddick. In the last century, these three philosophers developed and articulated conceptual elements of attentive love.

In various writings, Weil (1951, 1963, 1981, 1998) elaborates the qualities of *attention* and the role it plays in developing a spiritually and deistically oriented attentive love. For Weil, attentive love serves as a sort of antidote to the force, power, and gravity that pervade our material lives (Springsted, 1986). Based in part upon Weil's elaboration, Murdoch and Ruddick articulate their conceptions. In Murdoch's (1971) first substantial philosophical text, *The Sovereignty of Good*, she transforms Weil's deistic understandings of attentiveness into a non-deistic but nevertheless spiritual view of love, beauty, and the Good. Sara Ruddick, a philosopher and mother, explores the commingling of reason and emotion in one of life's most precious and difficult endeavors, that of being a parent. In *Maternal Thinking*, she takes Weil's and Murdoch's spiritually aligned conceptions of attentive love and elaborates a more secular view (Ruddick, 1995). In the next section, I will highlight elements of attentive love with minor references to both teaching and Courage facilitation. In the subsequent section, I explore more fully these elements within Courage retreats.

Elements of Attentive Love

As a way of connecting individuals with each other and within themselves, attentive love entails the following: (1) the presumption that good exists within each individual (e.g., shared humanity and goodness); (2) the attempt to discern and see others (colleagues and students) more clearly and justly (mindfully, with great respect and ethical awareness, as well as attention to others); and (3) the understanding that in order to see more clearly we need to reduce the noise of our selves (emotional self-awareness and regulation, and a less self-centric/more altruistic perspective).

Attentive love in teaching is frequently a struggle and a sacrifice. It is a struggle and a sacrifice to see beyond our egoistic selves so as to see students more clearly with empathy, noninstrumental understanding, and compassion. But, it is not only struggle. Attentive love provides a healing place from which to attend to others and ourselves. It is a stance that provides a place of relief and restoration—a boat mooring of sorts.[11] In Courage retreats facilitators attempt to attend lovingly to the participants.

[9] I should underscore that the presentation and analysis of Courage retreats is one I have developed and is neither necessarily shared by the Center for Courage and Renewal nor by all facilitators. I have shared this text with other facilitators and many acknowledge features of attentive love in the Courage retreat settings. Here, I am advancing my own views.

[10] Elsewhere I have elaborated this notion of attentive love in relation to critical pedagogy and reverence in teaching. See Liston (2008, 2012).

[11] Susan Kaplan helped to clarify this point in her reading of the manuscript.

Presumption of Goodness

It is not unusual for any of us to overlook the actual and potential "good" that exists within others. And, it is not unusual for teachers to mistakenly perceive the struggles and qualities of their students. As teachers we frequently see the world and students through our own anxieties and fears. When teaching is construed (for us or by us) as controlling and directing others, discerning this good is not a priority or a need. When teaching is defined solely as drilling and skilling kids to achieve higher standardized test scores, we do not honor students. But, when teaching is viewed as a way to help others take part in the challenges and pleasures of understanding our political, cultural, and natural worlds, and become more capable in transforming these worlds, then we frequently need to affirm and understand (as much as we can) our students' goodness. In Courage to Teach retreats, a central goal is to reengage the teachers' sense of wonder about learning, teaching, and themselves. Part of that engagement with wonder depends on an affirmation of good within themselves and their students.

It is an act of faith and a persistently reinforced belief that we seek to understand, to reach out beyond ourselves for "that which is good." It is a desire that may not always be consciously present and certainly conflicts with other desires and needs. But, it is a yearning that defines, in part, what it means to be human. It is a desire that Simone Weil captures quite well. She writes, "At the center of the human heart, is the longing for an absolute good, a longing which is always there and never [adequately] appeased by any object in this world" (Weil quoted in Bell, 1998, p. 71).

A yearning for transcendence, a longing for something greater than ourselves is what Weil uncovers in her exploration of love. For her, we long to reach beyond ourselves, to see and to participate in something larger than ourselves. Another element in our students' and colleagues' goodness is the expectation that, in this world, they will be treated decently. Weil writes:

> At the bottom of the heart of every human being, from earliest infancy until the tomb, there is something that goes on indomitably expecting, in the teeth of all experience of crimes committed, suffered, and witnessed, that good and not evil will be done to him. It is this above all that is sacred in every human being. (Weil quoted in Bell, 1998, p. 71)

Weil maintains that each and every human being is sacred. When teaching, we connect students with material that has, among other purposes, the potential to take them beyond themselves, to attend to the world and themselves more clearly, and to act in ways that are decent and loving. In teaching, we can attend lovingly to the good in our students so that they, in turn, can develop their search for the good. In facilitating we attend lovingly to the good and underlying sense of wholeness in our teachers and educational leaders and when that occurs these teachers and leaders can develop their own inner journey and search for the good.

Discerning Things Clearly and Justly

Sara Ruddick (1995) writes in her book *Maternal Thinking* that attentive love "implies and rewards a faith that… to the loving eye the lovable will be revealed… Attentive love, or loving attention, represents a kind of knowing that takes truthfulness as its aim but makes truth serve lovingly the person known" (1989, pp. 119–120). In teaching, this requires that we look with loving, clear-sighted attention to our students to connect them with the educational tasks at hand. Attentive love in teaching readies students for an engagement with the worlds around them through the curriculum. In elementary settings when students are young and skills undeveloped, in high school when students have become numb to learning, or at most any educational level when beginning a new topic of study, we, as teachers, need to prepare students for the tasks, challenges, and pleasures of learning. Attentive love enables teachers to see the student more clearly and identify what preparation and/or further connections should occur. In Courage facilitating, we utilize "circles of trust," "third things" (frequently, pieces of poetry), and "clearness committees" to dig more deeply into our selves, allow others to be "heard into speech," and enable a grand diversity of views to be voiced.

So what are the qualities of this attentiveness? Iris Murdoch (1971) claims that we attend throughout the moments of our days. We look at our students and observe their mannerisms, frustrations, interests, anxieties, dress, and fascinations. We hear their concerns. Murdoch writes:

> In particular situations 'reality' as that which is revealed to the patient eye of love is an idea entirely comprehensible to the ordinary person. The task of attention goes on all the time and at apparently empty and everyday moments we are "looking," making those little peering efforts of imagination which have such important cumulative results (1971, pp. 40 and 43).

Teachers are constantly observing and noting students' characteristics and features. Attentive teachers can speak volumes about their students. In order to see and speak those volumes, these teachers have to suspend temporarily their own expectations, bracket their agendas, and set aside their concerns so as to apprehend the student's reality on his or her own terms. This is not an easy task; it requires effort, discipline, and—at times—sacrifice. In facilitation, I have found that this attention to participants follows a similar path. In order to see retreat participants more clearly, I have to suspend my expectations and framings in an attempt to see the participant more clearly. Murdoch reminds us that attending lovingly to others is a complicated endeavor:

> Human beings are far more complicated and enigmatic and ambiguous than languages or mathematical concepts, and selfishness operates in a much more devious and frenzied manner in our relations with them.... Our attachments tend to be selfish and strong, and the transformation of our loves from selfishness to unselfishness is sometimes hard even to conceive of.... The love which brings the right answer is an exercise of justice and realism and really looking. The difficulty is to keep the attention fixed upon the real situation and to prevent it from returning surreptitiously to the self with consolations of self-pity, resentment, fantasy, and despair.... It is a task to come to see the world as it is. (1971, p. 91)

When engaged in intellectual and pedagogical pursuits, our selfish desires can obstruct our understandings. We can impose our meanings on historical reconstructions or, because of our frustrations of the moment, fail to grasp a mathematical algorithm. Our egos can get in the way. In our pedagogical interactions, we may be much more prone to see obscurely. It is difficult to see our students unencumbered by the noise of our teacher egos. Our own conceptions, anxieties, satisfactions, and dreams can get in the way. There is in teachers, as humans, the inclination to see the world as they want to see it, not to view it with attentiveness and loving kindness. It is a struggle to see others and the world with loving, clear-sighted attention. It is an effort to reduce the noise of our egoistic selves. Courage retreats attempt to enable teachers and educational leaders to attend to themselves, students, and colleagues with loving, clear-sighted attention. The retreat process, especially the clearness committee, facilitates this clarity of vision. Intuitively many teachers and leaders approach students in this fashion but have lost (or never fully practiced) this orientation to themselves and colleagues.

Reducing the Noise of the Self

It is an effort to attend to students. The struggle is not that attentive love requires attending to each and every student in all of our class sessions. Rather it is a task to suspend our own expectations, bracket our own agendas, and set aside our concerns so as to see the matter at hand from our students' point of view. The degree of difficulty varies. With some students, we are able to see fairly clearly the obstacles and issues at hand, and we can facilitate their learning. With others, it may take a few days of trying on different interpretations, distinct framings, so as to see the student before us with clear-sighted attention. And yet with others, we have to examine not only their situation but ourselves; we have to look at what in us is getting in the way of seeing them more clearly. Lisa Delpit, the accomplished literacy scholar, writes about this quality of attention as a form of listening, as a way of attending to others when differences become obstacles. She writes that when this occurs we need:

> a very special kind of listening, listening that requires not only open eyes and ears, but open hearts and minds. We do not really see through our eyes or hear through our ears, but through our beliefs. To put our beliefs on hold is to cease to

> exist as ourselves for a moment—and that is not easy. It is painful as well, because it means turning yourself inside out, giving up your own sense of who you are, and being willing to see yourself in the unflattering light of another's angry gaze. It is not easy, but it is the only way to learn what it might feel like to be someone else and the only way to start the dialogue. (1998, p. 297)

How do we put our beliefs on hold to attend to the other before us? How do we reduce the noise of our egos? Sara Ruddick and Iris Murdoch lay out some rudimentary features: we talk with others; we attempt to see the good in the situation or student; and we refocus our attention on an object which is a source of contemplation and energy.

There are times when in order to see the student or situation more clearly we have to refocus our gaze, look away in an effort to gain some distance and detachment from the current scene. Murdoch talks of prayer and reorientation as two options. Not all of us are spiritually oriented. However, I think we have within us the power to redirect our gaze on something of value. In this vein, Murdoch writes: "Whatsoever things are true, whatsoever things are honest, whatsoever things are just, whatsoever things are pure, whatsoever things are lovely, whatsoever things of good report; if there be any virtue, and if there be any praise, think on these things." (1971, p. 56)

Conversations with others, refocusing on the good within the situation or student, and a reorientation of our gaze allows us a degree of detachment from the noise of ourselves. None are, for sure, guaranteed methods. Nevertheless, all seem to provide a measure of redirection, detachment, and reengagement. Within the larger contemplative community, there are a great number and variety of mindfulness practices that facilitate this redirection and place of detachment, with meditation, centering prayer, tai chi, and yoga among them.[12] In what follows I will detail features of the Courage retreat principles and structure that encourage these aspects of attentive love and, as such, introduce teachers to the meditative arts and mindfulness.

[12] See http://www.contemplativemind.org/practices/tree.html

Courage Retreats and Attentive Love

Many teachers engage in attentive love with their students; it is a form of care and support that frequently develops quite naturally. However, school structures and cultures all too often obstruct this loving disposition. Courage to Teach retreats support an engagement with attentive love and remind teachers that it is possible to care in this fashion not only for students and colleagues, but also to attend lovingly to themselves (see Palmer, Jackson, Jackson, & Sluyter, 2001; Palmer, 2004). In this section, I elaborate how certain features of the Courage Retreat encourage the development of attentive love in educators.

Attentive love is practiced in Courage retreats in a number of distinct ways. It is modeled by facilitators in their personal dispositions and interactions, as well as in providing a supportive, inviting, and safe place for participants to explore their professional heartaches and joys. Attentive love is also present in the circle of trust format—in the norms ("Touchstones") that guide this group and individual reflective process.[13] It is also embedded within the "clearness committee"—a time of intense personal reflection and community support for the self-identified "focus" person.[14] In what remains, I describe further the ways in which facilitator modeling, the circle of trust norms and practices, and the clearness committees encourage attentive love. However before I discuss those three domains, it will be helpful to briefly describe the elements and structure of a Courage retreat.

Courage Retreats

Although the length and duration of Courage retreats vary from a 2-h local introduction, a half- or whole-day "sampler," all the way to a two-night getaway located within a retreat setting, the basic elements of Courage retreats are fairly stable and established. Generally, a retreat experi-

[13] See Appendix 1 for a delineation of commonly used "Touchstones".

[14] See http://www.couragerenewal.org/clearnesscommittee/ for Parker Palmer's description of the Clearness Committee process.

ence includes one or more circle of trust[15] sessions (90–120 min long). Each session incorporates time for individual reflection as well as small group (dyads or triads) interactions. In the circle, skilled facilitators create a quiet and purposeful space in which the noise within and around us can subside, enabling each participant to hear his or her own inner voice. Participants explore the intersection of their personal and professional lives, making use of their own stories, as well as insights from poets, storytellers, memoirs, and a range of wisdom traditions. It is a process which affirms the integrity of the retreat participants with an understanding that each participant is capable of articulating his or her own voice—in community with others.

In a circle of trust, the group (10–25 individuals) sits in a circle with a centerpiece that serves as a visual focal point and has as a central substantive focus—a poem, a brief text, or a musical piece. "Touchstones" (group norms) guide the interactional process. The poems or "third things" (the third element in addition to the participants and the facilitator) tend to highlight tensions and perspectives on life's inner journey. It is common that the circle begin with a moment of silence, followed by a facilitator's introduction to and reading of the text, and then a segment of time is devoted to participants' responses and connections to the text—their distinct, heartfelt, and personal ruminations. It's important to note that the interactional format of the circle is not a conversation between or among participants but instead a "sharing into the circle." It is important to add that individuals share if they are so moved. Following the circle sharing, a time for solitary reflection and journaling is offered, and this is frequently followed by small group interactions focused on the fruits of the individual reflective process. Within the small groups individuals are encouraged to take the time to allow each person to talk, followed by questions and conversation on the personal issues raised and significant themes covered. Sometimes, the entire retreat group is reconvened after the small group interactions.

[15] See http://www.couragerenewal.org/approach/

In addition to the circle format, retreats may also offer opportunities to form clearness committees. In a clearness committee, one person who wishes to share a particularly pressing issue, one that occurs at the intersection of soul and role, invites others to join him or her in an exploration of that issue. In a clearness committee, the members first listen to the focus person's description of the problem and then are invited to pose "open and honest" questions. Generally, this process encourages a deep reflection on the part of both the focus person and the members of the committee. It requires discipline and discernment to identify powerful open and honest questions—questions that are neither curiosity nor agenda driven, and ones that will encourage the focus person's inner dialogue. Moreover, the questions are not expected to solve the dilemma for the focus person but rather to facilitate a deeper understanding of the issue and its inner dimensions.

Courage retreats are not limited to circle and clearness committee formats, but these two components form the backbone of many extended (1–3 days) retreat experiences. Along with facilitator modeling, these two programmatic structures are modalities through which aspects of attentive love are conveyed.

Facilitator Modeling

In my professional life, Courage facilitation has been a gift. Although I am inclined to look upon children as sacred beings and am open to seeing them more clearly and justly, adults have always presented a challenge to me. I am less likely to attend with care and attention to an adult's entangled features and dispositions, to discern who they are, to view them attentively and lovingly. Participating in and facilitating Courage retreats has changed (some of) that. Facilitators attempt to support and embody the values that define the retreat space and honor each participant's "inner source of truth"—their sacred nature.[16] One overarching goal and cornerstone of the circle process is the creation of a trusting community. Without a

[16] See Appendices 1 "Touchstones" (http://www.couragerenewal.org/touchstones/) and 2 "Key Principles of Formation" (http://www.couragerenewal.org/approach/).

trusting environment, it is difficult to engage in the courage work or the practice of attentive love.

Facilitators work to create a retreat space that is inviting and safe. The ways in which this is accomplished vary widely among facilitators but frequently include a retreat location of natural beauty; the creation of a meeting space that is pleasant to behold through the use of centerpieces and other design elements; the initial gift of a personal welcome card and chocolate; and the facilitator's willingness to show up as a whole person acknowledging strengths and frailties. All of these elements, when offered with integrity and clear intention, contribute to the creation of a retreat space that is inviting, safe, and contained. This safe space is enhanced further when facilitators are able to communicate their individual sense of vulnerability as well as the need for participants to approach their own individual vulnerabilities as well as those of others. When this vulnerable terrain is voiced by facilitators, it seems to contribute strongly to a sense of retreat trust and participants' willingness to attend lovingly to themselves and others. I'll explain further.

Vivian Gussin Paley (1986) is fond of noting that when we attend to young children (preschool and early elementary students) we notice that their concerns revolve around three fs: friendship, fantasy, and fairness. A good education, in Paley's estimation, honors those early childhood dispositions. Over time, in my work as a facilitator, I have noticed that adults can be welcomed warmly and honestly by acknowledging our strengths and vulnerabilities—our own age-appropriate three fs. At some point, I came to embrace the realization that we adults tend to make mistakes or "fuck up."[17] On good days we learn to *f orgive* ourselves and those around us, as well as embrace a *f aith* in ourselves and others that enables us to reengage. These have become my adult, developmentally appropriate, three fs. The Courage work, with its emphasis on personal formation, supports these three fs. Central to the Courage notion of "formation" are a set of "key principles of formation."[18] One of the principles is that:

> At the heart of formation is the understanding that there is a "hidden wholeness" at work in the natural world, in our lives, in our work—a hidden wholeness that often takes the form of paradox. Working with paradox helps us to see how things that are seemingly opposites, when more clearly understood, actually complement and co-create each other. You cannot know light without darkness, silence without speech, solitude without community. Understanding and exploring paradox is central to the pedagogy underlying this approach to inner work (see Appendix 2)

The paradox inherent in the notion that positive personal growth comes from serious personal challenges and mistakes, along with the notion that we have within us a "hidden wholeness" to deal with these paradoxes, has supported my adult-oriented three fs and informed my attentive love toward self and others. We are most vulnerable when we are facing our frailties and weaknesses. The three fs, in conjunction with the recognition of a hidden wholeness, allow facilitators to face and embrace these small truths.

With this framing I, as a facilitator, am more inclined: to see the good within my adult participants; to attempt to view participants more clearly and justly; and to quiet the noise within me. Without an understanding of paradox and our hidden wholeness, as well as a forgiveness toward and faith in my own and others' inevitable fuck-ups, I might have a tendency to run roughshod over others. When we, as facilitators, live and inhabit these realizations, we model for others a stance worth inhabiting, one that attends lovingly to others.

Circle of Trust

A circle of trust is guided by several touchstones, and here I will highlight two of them. However before I do, it is important to convey the key assumptions that guide facilitators in their creation of a circle of trust—or as Palmer calls it—the

[17] I apologize to any reader who might be offended by such language. In my Irish Catholic, working class cultural heritage it is a term used, perhaps, too freely. Here, I use it to acquire my first "f" and to capture and evoke the associations and frustrations that attend our inevitable minor and more serious mistakes and misjudgments.

[18] See Appendix 2.

formation space.[19] Earlier I noted that facilitators work to create a retreat space that is inviting and safe. They also attempt to design settings that are engaging and challenging. In the Courage repertoire, six paradoxes guide the creation of circles of trust and the retreat space. Here are some of the paradoxes that a facilitator of formation must know how to cultivate if the space is to bear good fruit:

1. The space must be open and yet bounded.
2. The space must be hospitable yet "charged."
3. The space must invite the voice of the individual and yet hold it in creative tension with the voice of the group.
4. The space must honor personal stories and yet expand them with archetypal stories of tradition.
5. The space must support solitude and yet surround it with the resources of community.
6. The space must invite and encourage speech yet invite and encourage silence as well (Palmer, n.d.).

In Courage work, these paradoxes guide the individual's formation process. In order for participants to discern their inner truths, to enter into a contemplative space, and to attend to themselves and others lovingly, the tensions must be inhabited. In the circle of trust aspects of these tensions are highlighted by the touchstones.

Two touchstones that guide the circle process and encourage an attentive orientation include: "When the going gets rough, turn to wonder" and "Trust and learn from the silence." Certainly other touchstones provide boundaries and norms for the circle and encourage attentive loving, but these two touchstones seem especially to encourage participants to be more mindful and loving.

"When the Going Gets Rough, Turn to Wonder" When my professional or personal life becomes entangled and gnarly, I frequently get hijacked by the entanglements. When I become hijacked, I don't search for the good in others or attempt to see them clearly. The "turn to wonder" touchstone reminds participants that when reading and responding to a piece of personally provocative poetry or hearing another person's tale that triggers a potent remembrance, the turn to wonder may help gain a bit of detachment and lead toward further discernment.

As a participant in or a facilitator of a circle of trust, I continually remind myself that rough times need not produce tough and hardened lives. The circle's poetry and other third things frequently invite participants into the frustrations of life's outer and inner journeys. The turn to wonder touchstone requests that we not get caught in those frustrations. Instead, we are invited to a more cognitively and affectively flexible stance.

"Trust and Learn from the Silence" In Courage retreats, we try to befriend silence. Today's aural world is filled with all sorts of noise. This noise resonates in the external world and reverberates within each individual's inner life. The admonition to trust and learn from the silence sets the stage for inner reflection, and it is also a critical element in the circle's life. Palmer (2004) writes that:

> …silence is a vital ingredient in a circle of trust, reminding us again of how countercultural these practices really are … Our culture is so fearful of the silence of death that it worships nonstop noise—perhaps as a secular sign of "eternal life!" In the midst of all that noise, small silences can help us become more comfortable with the Great Silence toward which we are all headed. Small silences bring us "little deaths," which, to our surprise, turn out to be deeply fulfilling. For example, as we settle into silence where our posturing and pushing must cease, we may experience a temporary death of the ego, of that separate sense of self we spend so much time cultivating. But this "little death," instead of frightening us, makes us feel more at peace and at home. (pp. 159–161)

Accepting silence into the warp and woof of the circle slows down the tempo of the retreat and beckons each individual to dwell in a newly found space.

I recall one retreat series in which a younger teacher used her iPod and earplugs during times of silent reflection. I understood that for some individuals music can become background noise and set the stage for reflection, but I also thought that dwelling in silence was something that might be useful for this individual. I chose not to say

[19] Thanks to Estrus Tucker and Susan Kaplan for suggesting the inclusion of these formation principles.

anything or intervene. During our second or third retreat, she forgot her iPod at home and so was left without musical resources during times of silence. At one point during the music-less experience, she looked up at me and commented that this newfound silence was an experience she had not had before—one that altered significantly her retreat experience. This time she ventured into silence, and she had a distinctly different experience. I had the sense that this time she was on an inner journey. Palmer (2004) comments that

> … silence brings not only little deaths but also little births—small awakenings to beauty, to vitality, to hope, to life. In silence we may start to intuit that birth and death have much in common. We come from the Great Silence without fear into this world of noise. Perhaps we can return without fear as well, crossing back over knowing that the Great Silence is our first and final home. (p. 161)

Befriending silence in retreat can open doors to a loving attentiveness. I can quiet the noise of self and others so that greater clarity is within reach.

Clearness Committee

The clearness committee is a discernment process[20] and requires committee members to formulate open and honest questions to a set of issues or dilemmas posed by the focus person. Frequently, the focus person will come to the committee with a dilemma that entails a conflict between his or her "role and soul." Such conflicts usually entail a significant crossroad between external role-based expectations and internal soul-driven desires. The conflict may be an unresolved sense of loss or grief—a personal or professional loss that affects their daily living and work life; or it may entail an experience of conflicting inner desires and distinct professional paths—do I follow up this new job opportunity which will allow me to develop new capacities (that I may or may not have), or do I stick with what I know to be tried and true. In a clearness committee, a group of 4–6 individuals gather to support the inner reflection, the inner journey, of a focus person. For the duration of time (2 h generally), committee members are prohibited from:

> …trying to advise, fix, save, or set this person straight. For two hours, they are allowed to speak to the focus person only by asking honest, open questions—questions that have no hidden agenda, questions that are not advice in disguise, questions that are not intended to lead in a certain direction—only questions that can help the focus person remove the blocks to inner truth and discover inner wisdom. (Palmer, 1998, p. 141)

Learning to ask open and honest questions is a demanding and discerning process. It requires that we attempt to attend lovingly to another individual's story and dilemma and pose questions that encourage an inner dialogue for the focus person. Participants learn the distinctions among questions that attempt to fix the person's problem; give advice in question guise; or frame the issue with a particular set of assumptions. In the retreat experience, the committee members gain practice and experience at discerning which questions represent open and honest responses. Facilitators use a variety of simulations along with conceptual elaborations to distinguish those questions that are most helpful. Some of the guidelines for open and honest questions include posing:

- Questions that the questioner could not possibly anticipate the answer to
- Questions that assist the focus person to explore his or her concerns rather than satisfy the committee member's curiosity
- Questions that go to the person as well as the problem—questions about feelings as well as facts
- Simple and direct questions[21]

In order to formulate such questions, the committee member inevitably engages in a process of discerning which questions are more about his or her own curiosity, his or her need for fixing, or his or her framing of the person's conundrum. In order to formulate powerful questions, the committee members need to attend to their own motivations for, engagements with, and interests in the questions they raise. Frequently, members are advised that "If you

[20] http://www.couragerenewal.org/parker/writings/clearness-committee

[21] Adapted from a Courage Handout entitled "Open Questions" (n.d.).

aren't sure about the question, be quiet, wait, and if it keeps surfacing, ask it."[22] This process of discernment requires that the committee members attempt to see clearly and identify the good within the focus person. In order to accomplish that feat, they need to quiet the noise of their own entanglements with the issues. These are features and acts of attentive love.

Conclusion

Courage retreats provide teachers and educational leaders many gifts. In today's educational world, these gifts are sorely needed. Although standards and assessments are critical pieces of the schooling picture, they are not the only critical elements. Since the passage of, and the creation of the infrastructure for "No Child Left Behind" (NCLB), commentators have been highlighting the missing elements. Many teachers and scholars argue capably that the NCLB vision of schooling grossly simplifies and frequently misdirects the complex process of schooling, teaching, and learning (see Ravitch, 2010; Smoot, 2010). Within this conversation scholars and teachers point to the need to return to rich curricula and passionate and caring teaching. Courage retreats provide at least two missing critical gifts. Courage reawakens and affirms in teachers a sense of attentive love toward students, colleagues, and most especially themselves.[23] It allows teachers to recall what once may have been an intuitive response within the classroom and provides a set of norms and practices that support this loving attentiveness toward self and others. Courage retreats also introduce teachers and leaders to a more silence-filled and contemplative stance to teaching's and life's dilemmas. As noted earlier, mindfulness practices frequently tap into the significance of love. Courage retreats represent another significant pathway to love, one that may lead participants to a more mindful and contemplative space. Courage work is certainly an affirmation of and engagement with attentive love; in many ways, it is best described as courageous love.[24]

Appendix 1: Touchstones (http://www.couragerenewal.org/touchstones/)

- *Be present as fully as possible.* Be here with your doubts, fears, and failings as well as your convictions, joys, and successes, your listening as well as your speaking.
- *What is offered in the circle is by invitation, not demand.* This is not a "share or die" event! During this retreat, do whatever your soul calls for, and know that you do it with our support. Your soul knows your needs better than we do.
- *Speak your truth in ways that respect other people's truth.* Our views of reality may differ, but speaking one's truth in a circle of trust does not mean interpreting, correcting, or debating what others say. Speak from your center to the center of the circle, using "I" statements, trusting people to do their own sifting and winnowing.
- *No fixing, saving, advising, or correcting each other.* This is one of the hardest guidelines for those of us in the "helping professions." But it

[22] Ibid.

[23] In many ways, this attentive love toward self can lead to an enlarged love—especially when the situation is critical and the need is great. When a teacher despairs, the attentive love toward himself/herself and, particular, others can be expanded to an enlarged love toward their life situations and their immediate and expanding contexts. Enlarged love is, in many ways, attentive love practiced with a larger, more generalized scope and addressing a significant and demanding need. See Liston (2000).

[24] I am deeply indebted to the Courage organization, Parker Palmer, Marcy Jackson, Rick Jackson, Cindy Johnson, Terry Chadsey, and many others for their creation of a powerfully supportive community and the elaboration of a set of principles and practices to engage in and live by. When I was introduced to the Courage community, I immediately felt, but could not articulate, a powerful sense of care, love, and attention. These folks model this stuff day in and day out. I also want to thank Susan Kaplan, Vern Rempel, Michele Seipp, Estrus Tucker, and Paul Michalec for reading earlier drafts of this essay. Their critical and supportive comments improved the text.

is vital to welcoming the soul, to making space for the inner teacher.

- *Learn to respond to others with honest, open questions* instead of counsel, corrections, etc. With such questions, we help "hear each other into deeper speech."
- *When the going gets rough, turn to wonder.* If you feel judgmental, or defensive, ask yourself, "I wonder what brought her to this belief?" "I wonder what he's feeling right now?" "I wonder what my reaction teaches me about myself?" Set aside judgment to listen to others—and to yourself—more deeply.
- *Attend to your own inner teacher.* We learn from others, of course. But as we explore poems, stories, questions, and silence in a circle of trust, we have a special opportunity to learn from within. So pay close attention to your own reactions and responses, to your most important teacher.
- *Trust and learn from the silence.* Silence is a gift in our noisy world, and a way of knowing in itself. Treat silence as a member of the group. After someone has spoken, take time to reflect without immediately filling the space with words.
- *Observe deep confidentiality.* Nothing said in a circle of trust will ever be repeated to other people.
- *Know that it's possible* to leave the circle with whatever it was that you needed when you arrived, and that the seeds planted here can keep growing in the days ahead.

Appendix 2: Key Principles of Formation

1. *Everyone has an inner teacher.*

   Every person has access to an inner source of truth, named in various wisdom traditions as identity, true self, heart, spirit, or soul. The inner teacher is a source of guidance and strength that helps us find our way through life's complexities and challenges. Circles of Trust give people a chance to listen to this source, learn from it and discover its imperatives for their work and their lives.

2. *Inner work requires solitude and community.*

   In Circles of Trust, we make space for the solitude that allows us to learn from within, while supporting that solitude with the resources of community. Participants take an inner journey in community where we learn how to evoke and challenge each other without being judgmental, directive, or invasive.

3. *Inner work must be invitational.*

   Circles of Trust are never "share or die" events, but times and places where people have the freedom within a purposeful process to learn and grow in their own way, on their own schedule and at their own level of need. From start to finish, this approach invites participation rather than insisting upon it because the inner teacher speaks by choice, not on command.

4. *Our lives move in cycles like the seasons.*

   By using metaphors drawn from the seasons to frame our exploration of the inner life, we create a hospitable space that allows people of diverse backgrounds and perspectives to engage in a respectful dialogue. These metaphors represent cycles of life—such as the alternation of darkness and light, death, and new life—shared by everyone in a secular, pluralistic society regardless of philosophical, religious, or spiritual differences.

5. *An appreciation of paradox enriches our lives and helps us hold greater complexity.*

   The journey we take in a Circle of Trust teaches us to approach the many polarities that come with being human as "both–ands" rather than "either–ors," holding them in ways that open us to new insights and possibilities. We listen to the inner teacher and to the voices in the circle, letting our own insights and the wisdom that can emerge in conversation check and balance each other. We trust both our intellects and the knowledge that comes through our bodies, intuitions, and emotions.

6. *We live with greater integrity when we see ourselves whole.*

   Integrity means integrating all that we are into our sense of self, embracing our shadows and limitations as well as our light and our gifts. As we deepen the congruence between our inner and outer lives, we show up more fully in the key relationships and events of our lives, increasing our capacity to be authentic and courageous in life and work.

7. *A "hidden wholeness" underlies our lives.*

   Whatever brokenness we experience in ourselves and in the world, a "hidden wholeness" can be found just beneath the surface. The capacity to stand and act with integrity in the tragic gap between what is and what could be or should be—resisting both the corrosive cynicism that comes from seeing only what is broken and the irrelevant idealism that comes from seeing only what is not—has been key to every life-giving movement and is among the fruits of the Circle of Trust approach.

References

Bell, R. (1998). *Simone Weil: The way of justice as compassion*. New York, NY: Rowman and Littlefield.

Brooks, D. (2011). *The social animal*. New York, NY: Random House.

Clifford, G., & Guthrie, J. (1988). *Ed School: A brief for professional education*. Chicago, IL: University of Chicago Press.

Delpit, L. (1988). The silenced dialogue: Power and pedagogy in education other people's children. *Harvard Educational Review, 58*(3), 280–298.

Hanh, T. N. (1998). *Teachings on love*. Berkeley, CA: Parallax Press.

Keating, T. (1996a). *Open mind, open heart*. New York, NY: Continuum.

Keating, T. (1996b). *Crisis of faith, crisis of love*. New York, NY: Continuum.

Keating, T. (1998). *Invitation to love*. New York, NY: Continuum.

Keating, T. (1999). *The human condition*. New York, NY: Paulist Press.

Kessler, R. (2000). The soul of education: Helping students find connection, compassion and character as school. Washington, DC: Association for Supervision and Curriculum Development.

Labaree, D. (2004). *The trouble with Ed schools*. New Haven, CT: Yale University Press.

Liston, D. P. (2000). Love and despair in teaching. *Educational Theory, 50*(1), 81–102.

Liston, D. P. (2002). Despair and Love in Teaching. In S. M. Intrator (Ed.), *Stories of the courage to teach*. San Francisco, CA: Jossey-Bass.

Liston, D. P. (2004). The lure of learning in teaching. *Teachers College Record, 106*(3), 459–486.

Liston, D. P. (2008). Critical pedagogy and attentive love. *Studies in Philosophy and Education, 27*(5), 387–392.

Liston, D. P. (2012). Reverence and love in teaching. In A. G. Rud & J. Garrison (Eds.), *Reverence and teaching*. New York, NY: Palgrave Macmillan.

Liston, D. P., & Garrison, J. (Eds.). (2004). *Teaching, learning, and loving*. New York, NY: Routledge/Falmer.

Macy, J. (1991). *World as lover; world as self*. Berkeley, CA: Parallax Press.

Merton, T. (2004). *The inner experience*. New York, NY: HarperCollins.

Murdoch, I. (1971). *The sovereignty of good*. New York, NY: Routledge.

Nouwen, H. J. (1996). *The inner voice of love*. New York, NY: Doubleday.

Olesen, T. (2014, July 21). *Mindfulness is religion in schools*. Retrieved from http://educationcurrent.wordpress.com/

Paley, V. G. (1986). On listening to what children say. *Harvard Educational Review, 56*(2), 122–132.

Palmer, P. (1998). *The courage to teach*. San Francisco, CA: Jossey-Bass.

Palmer, P. (2004). *A hidden wholeness*. San Francisco, CA: Jossey-Bass.

Palmer, P. (n.d.). The art and craft of formation. Center for Courage and Renewal, Seattle, Washington.

Palmer, P., Jackson, M., Jackson, R., & Sluyter, D. (2001). The courage to teach: A program for teacher renewal. In L. Lantieri (Ed.), *Schools with spirit*. Boston, MA: Beacon.

Ravitch, D. (2010). *The death and life of the great american school system: How testing and choice are undermining education*. New York, NY: Basic Books.

Ruddick, S. (1995). *Maternal thinking*. Boston, MA: Beacon.

San Francisco parents against TM in public schools. Messages posted to https://www.facebook.com/pages/SF-Parents-Against-TM-in-Public-Schools/201123776750702

Smoot, B. (2010). *Conversations with great teachers*. Bloomington: Indiana University Press.

Springsted, E. (1986). *Simone weil and the suffering of love*. Cambridge, MA: Cowley.

Weil, S. (1951). *Waiting for god*. New York, NY: G.P. Putnam's Sons.

Weil, S. (1963). *Gravity and grace*. London, UK: Routledge and Kegan Paul.

Weil, S. (1981). *The Illiad or the poem of force* (M. McCarthy, Trans.). Wallingford, PA: Pendle Hill Pamphlet #91.

Weil, S. (1998). Simone Weil. In E. Springsted (Ed.). Maryknoll, NY: Orbis Books.

Zeichner, K. (2009). *Teacher education and the struggle for justice*. New York, NY: Routledge.

Mindfulness and Organizational Change

15

Rona Wilensky

Introduction

Can the introduction and addition of mindfulness practices to organizational change initiatives accelerate individual and institutional transformation? In principle, this is a testable hypothesis. Before anyone sets out to do so, however, it is important to first explore the reasoning that might underlie this idea. This chapter will address why and how mindfulness practices could have a positive, measurable impact on individual and organizational change within a school, or for that matter, any work setting.

To move from the abstractions of "mindfulness practices" and "individual and organizational transformation," I explore this question in the context of one particular set of mindfulness meditation practices and of two specific change processes that were developed apart from each other but which bear striking and important resemblances. The mindfulness meditation practices that are considered here are rooted in the Shambhala lineage but can be found across a wide range of mindfulness traditions, including those which are strictly secular (e.g., Kabat-Zinn, 2013; Kornfield, 1993). The organizational change strategies I consider are the Immunity to Change model developed by Robert Kegan and Lisa Laskow Lahey of Harvard University (Kegan & Lahey, 2001, 2009) and the Constructivist Listening school change strategy developed by Julian Weissglass of the University of California, Santa Barbara (Weissglass, 1998) and adopted by the now disbanded National Coalition of Equity in Education, which Weissglass founded.

"Section I: A Set of Mindfulness Practices" summarizes the mindfulness practices I will be referencing as well as the cognitive and emotional competencies that they support, many of which are well established in the research literature. "Section II: The Immunity to Change Model" presents the Immunity to Change model and highlights the specific ways the competencies described in "Section I: A Set of Mindfulness Practices" can support, augment, and accelerate the change mechanisms of the model. "Section III: Constructivist Listening" follows the same strategy for the Constructivist Listening school change model albeit in a more concise fashion. "Section IV: Bringing Mindfulness and Organizational Change Together" considers the common features of these models that lend themselves to complementarity with mindfulness practices, and looks at how mindfulness practices might be introduced into these or similar models. The final section discusses some qualitative pilots that could explore the opening hypothesis as well as deepen the causal connection I am proposing.

R. Wilensky (✉)
PassageWorks Institute, Boulder, CO, USA
e-mail: Rona.Wilensky@gmail.com

K.A. Schonert-Reichl, R.W. Roeser (eds.), *Handbook of Mindfulness in Education*,
Mindfulness in Behavioral Health, DOI 10.1007/978-1-4939-3506-2_15

It is important to emphasize that nothing in this paper is meant to suggest that mindfulness practices be used on their own or instead of these change models to achieve the same outcomes. Rather the assumption is that these two models are successful and robust on their own terms. The premise of this chapter is that the effectiveness of both (or of similar models) could be *enhanced* through the incorporation of mindfulness practices into their implementation.

Section I: A Set of Mindfulness Practices

The meditation practice being considered in this discussion goes by a variety of names—*shamatha, shinay, calm abiding, one pointedness, concentration,* and *mindfulness-awareness*. The core process involves the experience of placing and returning attention to a particular object of meditation in order to stabilize the mind. The foundational practice is placing attention on the breath as the object of mindfulness, becoming aware of when the attention has wandered from the breath, and returning the attention to the breath. Over time and during intense practice sessions such as those found in retreat settings, practitioners often find greater and greater stability of the attention on the breath; in other words, infrequent, or at times nonexistent, wandering of the attention. Newer practitioners, such as might be encountered in a school or organizational change process, are more likely to repeatedly experience wandering of the mind along with continual opportunities to return it *gently* to focusing on the breath. The benefits proposed here for including mindfulness practices in change initiatives are not dependent on participants achieving the absence of mind wandering that advanced practitioners obtain. Rather it is rooted primarily in the capacities strengthened by becoming aware of mental and physical distractions and responding to their vagaries with gentleness.

The three crucial elements of this practice and its benefits are described below, along with two additional practices—contemplation and compassionate abiding. Some, but by no means all, of the outcomes listed here have been verified by Western experimental science. The list as a whole is primarily based on the first person experiences of generations of meditators, documented in both classical texts and the writings of contemporary Western practitioners. It also reflects my experience over 11 years of regular practice during which I have personally experienced all of these outcomes. I would add that this list is not exhaustive; it is tailored to those benefits and outcomes that have a bearing on the issue of the relationship between mindfulness practices and personal and organizational change.

The first element of mindfulness-awareness meditation is sitting in an upright but relaxed posture (either on a chair or on a cushion) paying attention to the sensations of breathing in the body. This aspect of the technique

- Enhances the ability to focus and pay attention (Seppala, 2014). This increased attentional capacity can be applied elsewhere in life (e.g., listening, looking, or working attentively)
- Is relaxing and stress reducing in and of itself, as the mind synchronizes with the body and the parasympathetic nervous system is activated (Mindfulnet.org, 2014)
- Is training in noticing physical sensations associated with the breath and posture, which enhances the capacity to take advantage of the information processing done by the entire nervous system, not just the prefrontal cortex. As a result of this practice, over time practitioners are more apt to notice "what their gut" is telling them, or when their body is engaging in habitual somatic responses to stress (Kabat-Zinn, 2013)
- Provides an experience of simply being, not doing. This allows practitioners to become familiar with what "being" is and their reaction to it. It also provides an opportunity for the arising of emotions that have been kept at bay through busyness, e.g., sadness/grief, anger/rage, anxiety/fear (Chodron, 2007)

The second element of mindfulness meditation is based on the phenomenon that eventually, without conscious intention, the practitioner becomes aware that the attention has wandered from the breath. The minds of ordinary practitioners will always wander and awareness will always notice. The instruction at this point is to note what point of focus the mind has wandered to and then gently return the focus to the breath, to notice the distraction and let it go, to neither repress the distraction nor indulge in it. This aspect of the technique

- Is part of enhancing the capacity of the mind to pay attention by repeatedly bringing attention back to its object
- Enhances the already present but often underdeveloped capacity to be aware of what the mind is doing and to see the workings of the mind—thoughts and emotions—as "objects" of this awareness. This contrasts to being inside of thoughts and emotions. With the cultivation of greater self-awareness, practitioners "have" thoughts and emotions instead of thoughts and emotions "having" them (Kegan & Lahey, 2009)
- Allows practitioners to become familiar with ongoing internal narratives that often "have" them. When habitual thoughts are identified "on the cushion" as repetitive story lines, they are more easily recognized as such when "off the cushion"
- Familiarizes practitioners with this nonconceptual awareness capacity which everyone innately has. According to meditation masters, this awareness faculty, which Gaylon Ferguson (Ferguson, 2010) calls "natural wakefulness," is capable of perceiving internal and external reality with greater clarity than everyday mind because it functions apart from the filters of habitual self-talk
- Allows practitioners to experience themselves as neither fixed nor solid. They see and experience thoughts and emotions as *just* thoughts and emotions that arise and, so long as these are not continually stoked by perseverating, subside. This reduces attachment to these "objects" and makes it easier for minds to change. In this experience, practitioners also experience a "self" that is not the same as habitual thoughts and emotions, suggesting that it is safe to change one's mind and even change one's perceived identity

The third element of mindfulness meditation is a combination of *not judging* the contents of the thoughts or emotions that arise and returning the mind *gently* to the breath. This aspect of the technique

- Allows for the development of kindness, acceptance, and humor toward habitual thoughts and emotions—toward the habitual self. "There it is, again. And again. And again"
- Sets a pattern that can be transferred to any change process by replacing aggression toward what has been (and continues to show up) with gentleness and even amusement
- Provides practice in being nonjudgmental that can be extended toward others. "If this is going on in me, what is everyone else going through?"

The Shambhala tradition talks about the importance of cultivating both "fearlessness" and "gentleness" in mindfulness meditation—having the courage to see what is really going on inside (and outside) of the practitioner and being gentle toward ourselves and others both for what is and for the process of becoming something else (Chodron, 1997). These qualities are cultivated through the meditation practice described above and through the additional technique of a *contemplation practice* (Mipham, 2004). Contemplation practice allows individuals to intentionally cultivate qualities such as openheartedness, kindness, compassion, curiosity, forgiveness, and gratitude toward self and others through the intentional contemplation of these ideas. In this practice, phrases describing these ideas become the object of meditation. Contemplation practice is usually undertaken subsequent to the (at least partial) stabilization of the mind through the foundational breath awareness practice.

Finally, a *compassionate abiding practice* (Chodron, 2007) encourages individuals to fully feel the bodily sensations of their emotions while dropping the thoughts that usually go with them.

Rather than simply acknowledging emotional experience and returning to the breath, in this modality practitioners stay with the arising, duration, and subsiding of the physical sensations of strong emotions. Such a practice should not be done by those with a history of trauma or serious emotional/mental disorders without therapeutic support, and even then it is contraindicated for some disorders. For everyone else, this practice allows individuals to

- Experience the transitory nature of emotion (the feeling will subside by itself when not restoked by thoughts or self-talk)
- Discover that these feelings, even if painful, are not lethal
- Learn that these emotions can be tolerated without having to relieve them by acting in response to them

In short, compassionate abiding practice teaches practitioners to learn to stay with their feelings and to develop compassion for both the self who is experiencing them and the history that generated them. Traditional teachings (Chodron, 2007; Mipham, 2004) say that learning to abide with these feelings in all their intensity will not only lessen their power, but will ultimately lead to less frequent occurrence and possible cessation. From the point of view of Western science, this is still an open question.

Section II: The Immunity to Change Model

In their work on what they call Immunity to Change, Kegan and Lahey (2001, 2009) take up the question of why people in organizations do not change their behavior when they have compelling reasons as well as a genuine commitment to do so. The model can apply to all forms of behavior, including personal wellness habits and family-based interactions, but the primary focus of Kegan and Lahey's research and consulting work is on changing behavior in the workplace, including schools (Wagner, Kegan, Lahey, & Lemons, 2005). In particular, the model is concerned with the resistance of well-meaning people to making changes that they, their coworkers, and/or their bosses have identified as beneficial to the individual and to the organization.

The core insight that underlies the Immunity to Change theory and the interventions that accompany it is that individuals who don't make changes that seem to be in their best interest usually have competing, but unconscious, commitments to their current (dysfunctional) behaviors based on unexamined but deeply held ideas about what is in their best interest. In other words, there are good reasons for their failure to change, but these reasons are usually hidden from the view of everyone, including the individual in question.

In turn, these hidden/competing commitments rest on what Kegan and Lahey (2001, 2009) call "big assumptions" about the world, about the individual, and most importantly about what is necessary for the individual to be safe in the world. These big assumptions are rooted in past experiences, some stemming from as far back as childhood and others from earlier periods in adulthood. Whatever their origin, the big assumptions lead to unconscious commitments to behaviors that are no longer in the individual's best interest and are associated with painful, at times traumatic, experiences which negatively affected the individual's sense of psychological and/or physical safety. The commitments and behaviors that stem from these big assumptions manage the intense anxiety associated with those earlier experiences by making sure the individual is never in a similar situation again. With an origin in deeply personal, highly vulnerable, and usually painful situations, it is not surprising that individuals keep these commitments and assumptions from the view not only of others, but also of themselves; high levels of anxiety and vulnerability are not consistent with how adults are expected to behave, especially in the workplace.

These hidden big assumptions and competing commitments, nevertheless, have a powerful influence on day-to-day public (and private) life. In the first place, they constitute a mind-set through which the individual sees the surrounding world. Moreover, because "big assumptions are held as fact, they actually inform what people see, leading them to systematically (but unconsciously) attend to certain data and to avoid or ignore other data" (Kegan & Lahey, 2001). In other words, big assumptions create blind spots—about ourselves, about others, and about the world.

In the second place, these forces internally tug at individuals, pulling them in directions that are often directly contrary to where they say they want to go. This leads to a sense of personal frustration and failure on the part of those wanting to make changes in their behavior, to disappointment from others who would also like to see these changes, and to the general perception that adults are not capable of change. This latter notion, when widely accepted, leads easily to the popular idea in education reform that if you really want to change the system, you need to replace those currently employed and start all over again.

Although every individual's big assumptions are rooted in their own particular history and manifest in personally distinctive ways, the longitudinal research of Kegan and Lahey (2009) has identified three successive stages in adult development that account for many of the experiences of normative adults—the socialized mind, the self-authoring mind, and the self-transforming mind. According to Kegan and Lahey, "these three adult meaning systems make sense of the world, and operate within it, in profoundly different ways" (2009). In addition, "each successive level … is formally higher than the preceding one because it can perform the mental functions of the prior level as well as additional functions… [with] the implication … that a higher level of mental complexity outperforms a lower level" (2009). Significantly, from the point of view of the relationship between this model and mindfulness meditation, movement from one stage to the next is accompanied by an increased capacity to look "at" one's mental functioning rather than to be captive to looking "through" one's current mind-set. I return to this point below.

The interventions designed by Kegan and Lahey (2001, 2009) to bring to light the competing commitments and big assumptions that thwart change also support individuals in shifting from a lower level of mental complexity to the next higher one. This process not only allows the particular desired changes to take place, but also simultaneously enhances the overall effectiveness and capacity of the individual as he/she moves to a higher level of mental functioning. For a complete description of these levels of mental functioning and detailed guidance on why and how to do this work, readers should consult *Immunity to Change* (2009) as well as Kegan's earlier work, *In Over Our Heads* (1998). Here I provide a distillation of their change process in order to identify those elements that could be enhanced by the mindfulness practices described in "Section I: A Set of Mindfulness Practices".

The heart of the Immunity to Change work is the creation of a personal "immunity map" that surfaces competing commitments and their underlying big assumptions in four columns. A sample map, reproduced from their book, is provided in Table 15.1 (Kegan & Lahey, 2009).

The first column, entitled Commitment, identifies the important new behavior that the individual would like to undertake. Ideally this new behavior represents the "one big thing" that if the person did differently would make a significant difference in their individual performance and their interactions with others. In identifying this one big thing, individuals are strongly encouraged to formally seek the feedback of their colleagues (and even of their family members) to make sure they are working on something that will actually make a difference in their lives.

The second column, entitled Doing/Not Doing Instead, takes honest stock of the habitual behaviors that are contrary to the Commitment. For example, with a Commitment in column one to "better focus on a few critical things" then examples in the Doing/Not Doing Instead column include such current behaviors as "letting new opportunities distract me; accepting more tasks and sacrificing non-work related things; not balancing time commitments between the urgent and the important; and not asking people to help."

The third column entitled "Hidden Competing Commitments" begins the process of surfacing the thoughts and feelings that account for the

Table 15.1 A sample four column map

Commitment"	Doing/not doing instead	Hidden competing commitments	Big assumptions
To better focus on a few critical things	I let new opportunities distract me, adding to my list of things to do	(I fear missing a good opportunity) I'm committed to being independent and capable of anything	If I'm dependent on others and unable to do many things well, I lose my self-respect
	I accept more tasks and sacrifice non-work-related things	(I fear letting my team down; if I put myself first, I feel guilty and selfish) I'm committed to being selfless	If I put myself first, I'll become what I dislike in others—superficial and trivial
	I don't consistently balance time commitment to urgent and important rankings	(I dislike leaving boxes unchecked—it's harder to drop something than just do it) I'm committed to always finding a way to get it done	If I don't find a way to get things done, I'll stop being valuable
	I don't ask people to help me"	(I fear that I can't count on people) I'm committed to not needing anyone	If I need anyone, I will be hurt by them

habitual behaviors in column 2 that undermine accomplishing the goal in column 1. Kegan and Lahey recommend getting at these hidden/competing commitments by first posing the question "if you imagine doing the opposite of the undermining behavior (of column 2) do you detect in yourself any discomfort, worry, or vague fear?" (2001) and second by "transforming that passive fear into a statement that reflects an active commitment to preventing certain outcomes" (2001). See column 3 in Table 15.1 for details on how these statements get formulated. From these hidden/competing commitments, the final step is the identification of the big assumptions that underlie them. The instruction is to "create the beginning of a sentence by inverting the competing commitment and then fill in the blank" (2001).

Just as this hypothetical individual immunity map shows the powerful reasons why he/she didn't focus on a few critical things, so too do all immunity maps reveal the ways in which important new behaviors threaten the current foundations of an individual's very identity. The critical question in the Immunity to Change process is whether the big assumptions at the root of the map are true. Testing those assumptions is the centerpiece of the next phase of the change process.

Once the immunity map has been constructed and honed so that its assumptions are testable, the map's author is encouraged to take the following steps (Kegan & Lahey, 2009):

- Pay attention to when and where the big assumptions are activated in life and when they are inaccurate.
- Create a biography of the big assumptions to learn when they got started, what their history is, and whether they are still valid.
- Test the big assumptions by intentionally behaving counter to how they would have you act, see what happens, and reflect on the results.

Finally, the author of the map is instructed to resurvey the people consulted on the chosen Commitment of column 1 to find out what, if any, progress they have seen, and what effect any changes in behavior have had on them.

This work can be done by individuals pursuing their own professional goals, but in order to provide the greatest support for the process (and for progress) Kegan and Lahey (2009) strongly recommend that individual change work be done within a team context and that individual goals be aligned with change goals associated with the collective work of that group. This requires that people share their immunity maps with each other and give each other permission to name the reappearance of old behaviors and competing commitments. This external scaffolding provides tremendous support as people tackle what has been unconscious and habitual.

Given this brief overview of a complex undertaking, how might the introduction of mindfulness practices enhance success and help overcome obstacles? Answering this question requires the identification of points of vulnerability within the model as well as ways that mindfulness connects to overall psychological functioning.

The practices described in "Section I: A Set of Mindfulness Practices" enhance the Immunity to Change model in two primary ways: first, by strengthening the capacity of the mind to be aware of itself and of behavior, and second, by enhancing the capacity of individuals to tolerate emotional discomfort and, in particular, anxiety.

The development of the immunity map is usually done with the assistance of someone trained to facilitate the inner exploration that generates the information in the map. Immediately following the "aha" that the map provides, the individual is asked to begin the work of (1) noticing how the hidden commitments and big assumptions operate in day-to-day life, and (2) replacing old behaviors with new behaviors. Both of these steps require awareness—first, the capacity of the mind to see itself acting in accordance with hidden commitments or big assumptions, and second, the capacity of the mind to see itself being, as it were, "off task"—engaging in habitual behaviors rather than the new ones. The awareness capacity required in this change work is the identical capacity that is strengthened by breath awareness practice—noticing and not being attached to the content of thoughts, and noticing when the mind is thinking rather than paying attention to the breath.

A few quotes from *Immunity to Change* (Kegan & Lahey, 2009) highlight the importance of this increased self-awareness:

> If I'm (engaging in the old behavior) it's because I don't realize it. (p. 193)

> When things get busy, I go on auto pilot and fall back into my old patterns. (p. 196)

> I'm trying to change, but ...keeping it at the top of my mind is always difficult to do. (p. 196)

Despite the tremendous insight that immunity maps provide into the origins of resistance to change and in spite of the incredible support that is provided by having teammates aware of each others' immunity maps and having permission to call each other out on lapses, the challenge of making change also involves the challenge of increased self-awareness. Ultimately, each individual is the only one who is with his/her personal thoughts, emotions, and behaviors all the time. Without a robust capacity for self-awareness and self-reflection, it will be difficult for individuals to catch themselves enacting old habits and to engage in enough repetitions of replacement behaviors to truly uproot those habits. Teachers in particular, whose day-to-day work is more isolated than many professionals, have an especially high need for practices which strengthen their capacity to be aware of what they are thinking, feeling, and doing in the moment. Mindfulness meditation provides just such a mental fitness regime to continually raise the baseline level of self-awareness.

The second challenge of the Immunity to Change work is that it tampers with the psychological system that each individual has unconsciously designed to manage the sources of their greatest anxieties. In dismantling their old anxiety management systems, participants in the Immunity to Change process are opening themselves to the challenging feelings they have been avoiding, to the fact that it is "gut wrenching (to) look at (one)self in a self-reflective way" (Kegan & Lahey, 2009), and to the truism that in the early stages of change, new behaviors are distinctly uncomfortable. Without alternative anxiety management systems, without a tolerance for emotional discomfort, without a sense of kindness toward oneself, and without the experience that not all emotions reflect the truth of a current situation but often harken back to the past, many individuals are likely to abandon change efforts instead of experiencing these discomforts.

The mindfulness and compassionate abiding practices described in "Section I: A Set of Mindfulness Practices" offer individuals antidotes to these obstacles. In the first place, mindfulness practice activates the parasympathetic nervous system (Mindfulnet.org, 2014) and provides an alternative anxiety management system to engaging in the habitual behaviors flowing from hidden commitments and big assumptions.

Mindfulness practice also cultivates kindness toward oneself and one's perceived failings by reinforcing the importance of gentleness when bringing the ever-errant mind back to the breath. Each sitting session provides countless opportunities to notice oneself fail at holding attention to the breath, to bring oneself back to the task with compassion, and to take advantage of the fact that each new breath is a fresh opportunity to try again. In turn, compassionate abiding practice provides experience with both the impermanence and harmlessness of the physical sensations of intense emotions. Both practices give the individual opportunities to reflect on whether the events and thoughts that trigger the uncomfortable feelings of anxiety, fear, or stress are genuine threats or simply relics of the past.

A regular mindfulness practice also builds in a daily period of self-reflection. Although the purpose of a daily practice is not to revisit what has happened elsewhere but rather to experience what is happening in the present moment, inevitably recent thoughts, emotions, and actions resurface in the quiet of that time. The practitioner may not have caught him or herself in the midst of habitual behaviors with enough time to change direction, but even noticing them later strengthens self-awareness and is a reminder of one's commitments. The most important "move" at such moments is not to berate oneself for having failed to make the changes one is committed to, but to have compassion for the strength of the hidden commitments that lead one astray, to summon the courage to continue on the path toward change, and to celebrate the awareness of the misstep. This is identical to the process of trying to place the mind on the breath, noticing that it has wandered and gently returning it—over and over again. Realizing exactly how difficult mindfulness is, let alone one's own change process, can generate greater kindness toward others who are also grappling with the power of habitual behaviors.

Finally, it is important to remember that, in addition to facilitating change in particular behaviors, Kegan and Lahey (2009) are facilitating movement upward in the stages of adult development they have identified. Sitting practice can be of use in this more abstract task as well. It can assist individuals who are plateaued at the stage of "socialized mind" where "(they) are shaped by the definitions and expectations of (their) personal environment" (Kegan & Lahey, 2009). Practitioners in this stage of development have the opportunity in their sitting practice to experience a sense of self that exists apart from their connection to their affiliative groups. This can support letting go of an identity defined by being a member of a group and moving on to the next stage of self-authoring where "(the) self coheres by its alignment with its own belief system/ideology/personal code: by its ability to self direct, take stands, set limits and create and regulate its boundaries on behalf of its own voice" (2009). Sitting practice for individuals at this second plateau of adult development provides the opportunity to experience a sense of self that is distinct from the substance of their self-authoring—the wants, needs, goals, and desires which in a meditative process are identified as thoughts rather than the totality of identity. This in turn facilitates the transition to the self-transforming mind which can "step back from and reflect on the limits of (its) own ideology or personal authority; see that any one system of self-organization is in some way partial or incomplete; be friendlier toward contradiction and opposites (and) seek to hold on to multiple systems rather than projecting all but one onto the others" (2009). This self-transforming mind may in fact be the "don't know mind" that is cultivated in all mindfulness traditions (Suzuki, 1999).

In these particular ways, mindfulness practice has the potential to support growth in the mental complexity of adult minds. As Kegan and Lahey note, such development and neuro-plasticity was not even assumed possible as recently as 30 or so years ago (2009).

Section III: Constructivist Listening

Julian Weissglass' model of change (Weissglass, 1998) was developed to explicitly deal with supporting changes in the behaviors of educators in the face of overwhelming evidence that in schooling, the more things change the more they remain the same. Weissglass argues that the reason for the well-documented failure of most educational change efforts is that they have attended more to curricular, economic, and political policies than to the psychological and social needs of the people who needed to do the actual changing. His starting premise is that any effort at institutional change in schooling (or elsewhere) must give equal priority to addressing and supporting changes in individual thinking and behavior.

Reading the works of Kegan and Lahey (2009) on one hand and Weissglass (1998) on the other, it is possible to discern a common view that the absence and/or failure of individual change efforts is rooted in the cognitive, emotional, and behavioral consequences of past trauma. Where Kegan and Lahey (2009) highlight competing commitments and big assumptions that stem from these painful experiences, Weissglass (1998) gives primacy to the historical and ongoing suppression of emotional release[1] from those same experiences, especially ones associated with early childhood. In his view, the suppression of emotional release, which he identifies as a manifestation of cultural disapprobation toward the expression of emotions, blocks healthy growth and change through the generation of dysfunctional behaviors and an inability to think clearly. For Weissglass, change in individual attitudes, behaviors, and thinking only becomes possible when individuals are provided with safe opportunities for the release of these previously suppressed emotions (1998).

While this theory and intervention could support change in any area, Weissglass is an educational reformer, and his interest is in the way teachers teach and behave with their students—in particular how they teach and behave with students who are culturally or educationally different from themselves. He has, therefore, focused his work on supporting teachers' emotional release from those particular distressful experiences of childhood that relate to learning, schooling, and to all forms of individual and social difference. In Weissglass' model (1998), the lack of release from these particular wounds is what keeps teachers unconsciously attached to their habitual behaviors and attitudes toward teaching methods, toward ideas about how students learn and what constitutes intelligence, as well as in their attitudes toward colleagues, leaders, and the diversity of students that they encounter. The ongoing distress is seen as "a primary source of unintelligent and uncaring behavior" (1998). In turn, its emotional release contributes not only to recovery from these effects, but also to the increased capacity to evaluate experience, think more clearly, and be more effectively professionally (1998).

The core intervention of Weissglass' model (1998) is to provide individuals with structured opportunities to be listened to attentively as they recall early memories of learning, schooling, and social difference. As these stories emerge, they are often accompanied by emotional release in the form of crying, trembling, or other physical expression. It is this release that heals the speaker. Weissglass calls this particular form of attentive listening "Constructivist Listening" and distinguishes it from other such forms through its focus on being of benefit primarily to the speaker (1998).

Constructivist Listening requires only the communication of interest, caring, and acceptance. The listener does not need to always understand the speaker's stream of thought. The listener's job is simply to hold the space to "enable the talker to express his or her feelings, to construct personal understandings, and to use his or her intelligence to respond creatively to situations rather than rely on habits or old coping strategies" (Weissglass, 1998). The outcome for the speaker is the "construct(ion) of new meanings, (the) reevaluation of why they are who they are, why they teach the way the teach, and why they relate to children and colleagues the way they do" (1998). The cathartic release allows the speaker to "exercise freedom to choose new ways to respond to the world" (1998). Strikingly, this outcome mirrors that desired by Kegan and Lahey (2009).

[1]The forms of emotional release that Weissglass names include: crying, tantruming, trembling, laughing, yawning, excessive talking, and perspiration (1998).

The primary structure of intervention in Weissglass' model (1998) is found in the dyad in which the two participants alternate in the speaking and listening roles, taking equal amounts of time. A further intervention is found in support groups in which each person has an equal amount of time to be a speaker while the other members act as listeners. In each setting, confidentiality is maintained, with the additional proviso that the listener(s) may not bring up what they have heard even to the speaker, although the speaker can choose to reengage the topic with any listener.

The structures that support emotional release and cognitive reframing are complemented in National Coalition of Equity in Education trainings with multiple opportunities to learn new information and new perspectives on teaching, learning, and valuing difference. The processes that support healing from the past are what allow individuals to be available to these new learnings and to truly hear the perspectives of students and colleagues who are different from themselves. Together the healing and learning lay the groundwork for teachers to act differently in the classroom and in their lives, to work with each other to create new policies and practices to support the learning of all students, and to become allies to individuals from socially marginalized groups.

Constructivist Listening is not only used to excavate and release the past, it is also a form of ongoing support as individuals move forward in their lives with commitments to new behaviors in their teaching practice and within their school communities. Ongoing dyadic or support group relationships can be used to assist individuals in constructing cognitive meaning from new experiences, processing feelings that arise in the course of the school day, or thinking aloud about what actions to take in complex situations (Weissglass, 1998). Here, then, is another similarity to the Immunity to Change model (Kegan & Lahey, 2009) insofar as both acknowledge the long-recognized limitations of increased self-understanding in transforming behavior. In response, each model has devised a distinctive social structure to provide ongoing support. In the Immunity to Change model, this takes the form of allowing colleagues to remind one of the contents of the immunity map; in the Constructivist Listening model, ongoing social support takes the form of accessing dyadic interchanges with a trusted ally.[2] But in this commonality of social support also resides a common point of potential breakdown. Accessing support requires accessing individuals who may not be available when needed. This lack of availability can be temporary—the support person is not present at the moment of need or is too distracted to provide it—or it can result from bigger challenges—career changes, relocations, illnesses, or even death.

A regular mindfulness practice, which includes both breath awareness practices as well as practices for dealing with emotional distress, offers the Constructivist Listening model the same immediate benefit that it offers the Immunity to Change model—its supports are always available because they are internal to the practitioner.[3] Beyond that significant structural benefit, mindfulness practice potentially offers substantive assistance to the processes of cognitive, emotional, and behavioral transformation in three ways. First, a regular practice offers the possibility of altering practitioners' attachment to their historical identities and opinions by acquainting them with a more open capacity for awareness independent of those identities and opinions. If this is so, meditation would facilitate greater openness to new ways of being and doing in the world. Second, it is known that meditation increases practitioners' ongoing self-awareness (Seppala, 2014). This capacity could allow individuals engaged in change processes to more

[2] A variation of this ongoing dyadic support is found in the Focusing model of Eugene Gendlin (Gendlin, 1988). Developed to support personal change, its distinguishing characteristic is its encouragement of attention to somatic clues as an indication of the need for curiosity about and processing of experience and feelings. David Rome (2014) explores this potential in his book, *Your Body Knows the Answer: Using Your Felt Sense to Solve Problems, Effect Change and Liberate Creativity.*

[3] The internal supports provided by mindfulness are also beneficial to individuals who are engaged in therapeutic processes, whose "aha" moments are not enough to translate into daily behavior change.

quickly catch themselves in thoughts, emotions, or behaviors that are the habitual residue of the past. Third, and of particular importance to the Constructivist Listening model in which emotional release from painful experiences is the central strategy, mindfulness practices provide practitioners with immediately accessible tools for self-care, self-compassion, and self-management which could be accessed when intense emotions are triggered (Seppala, 2014).

Mindfulness could also increase the skillfulness of listening within dyads and support groups when these are available by increasing the attention paid to the speaker (Seppala, 2014). By increasing the mental focus of practitioners, mindfulness could enhance the work of being the attentive listener in the Constructivist Listening process. Comfortable with the silence of meditation and the process of "learning to stay," practitioners could more easily refrain from interrupting the monologue of the speaker. Engaging in contemplative practices that focus on developing compassion, kindness, and openheartedness could further enhance the listener's capacity to hold an inviting container for the speaker's processing. Finally, the stress reduction outcomes of mindfulness practices (Seppala, 2014) could be a crucial balm to the overload that school staff faces when they are trying to change themselves and their organizations even as they must keep schools running smoothly for students.

Section IV: Bringing Mindfulness and Organizational Change Together

Mindfulness practices offer the potential to complement these two models of change because of the particular characteristics these models have in common, and it follows that such practices could equally support other change processes that share some or all of these features. I identify four commonalities and then consider why these particular characteristics invite mindfulness practices as additional scaffolding.

The first common characteristic of these two models is that each sees change in individual behavior as essential to change in organizations. They share a common understanding that change requires more than transformations in structures and policies, or in organizational systems and rules. Although these organizational transformations are critically important supports to allow people to work in new ways, they alone will not lead to new outcomes, such as increased student learning (broadly defined) in the case of schools, or increased productivity in the case of businesses. Kegan, Lahey, and Weissglass share a common belief that institutional changes must be matched by changes in the ways that individuals within organizations function on their own and interact with colleagues and clients.

Importantly, these theorist/practitioners go beyond the conviction that individuals and their behaviors must be engaged and committed to the proposed changes in order to accomplish hoped-for outcomes. More significantly, they share the view that people must actually change *who* they are as well as *what* they do. In the Immunity to Change model, participants are supported in moving to a new stage of adult development. In the Constructivist Listening model, participants are encouraged to heal from past wounds and cast off dysfunctional identities that developed out of emotional suppression.

The second commonality is that these change processes are designed to take place *within* an organizational community. Individual employees do not go off to workshops and then return to their work settings to implement what they have learned. Nor do they listen to a presentation, take it in, and do with it as they will. Instead, individuals within the same organization are asked to work together on the simultaneous transformation of themselves and their organization. Not only are these collaborative processes, but they are also ones that drop deeply beneath the familiar conventions of group problem solving. They ask people to uncover and share their vulnerabilities. Gone is the conventional pose that everyone has their act together.

The third commonality is that each process not only begins collaboratively, but is also sustained collaboratively through intentional external support systems comprised of colleagues who are given roles in assisting each other in sticking with their best intentions. Both models recognize the power of relationships to sustain individual initiative and effort.

The fourth and final commonality of these two change processes is that they focus on the transformation of both thoughts *and* feelings. In each process, individuals are engaged in interventions that demand the reexamination of their ideas about themselves and about the world. They are also asked to look at, experience, and transform how they feel about themselves and the world. Significantly, participants are asked to integrate the cognitive and the emotional—to see and respond to themselves and to the world with their minds and their hearts. In short, they are asked to become more whole.

Mindfulness complements these approaches for many reasons that I have already touched on and will summarize here. This list represents my extrapolation from the research and the classical traditions of what mindfulness has to offer the processes of personal and organizational change. Most are possibilities that are not only not validated in the research, but are not yet even being explored:

- Mindfulness could support individual transformation through the development of a new relationship to personal experience and by looking at, instead of through, thoughts and emotions.
- Mindfulness practices could loosen attachment to habitual thoughts and feelings.
- Mindfulness could develop the capacity to stay with and work through emotional discomfort.
- Mindfulness could cultivate the courage to look at personal demons and own them with kindness as an integral aspect of self.
- Mindfulness could cultivate the capacity to move beyond shame and embarrassment, making it more possible to share one's inner life with others.
- Mindfulness cultivates kindness and compassion (Seppala, 2014), qualities that could make it safe to work with others in deep and personal ways.
- Mindfulness reduces stress and anxiety (Seppala, 2014) which are intrinsic to transformational change. The potential of mindfulness to mitigate these obstacles to deep change is significant.
- Mindfulness could cultivate the self-awareness that allows those involved in holistic change processes to monitor their own progress when they are not engaged in the powerful social support structures that each of the change processes discussed here includes to enhance the likelihood of success.

The alignment in goals, content, and processes between mindfulness practices and these two change models are the basis for this chapter's central hypothesis: adding instruction in mindfulness to the repertoire of interventions and structures used in these or similar models of transformational change and supporting the adoption of a regular personal mindfulness practice by participants would enhance the simultaneous transformation of individuals and organizations. Conversely, participating in these kinds of change processes might simultaneously enhance the power of a mindfulness practice for personal transformation through the excavation and awareness of the specific history and content of habitual patterns. This would echo the powerful synergy often experienced by individuals who participate in both mindfulness practices and psychotherapy Didonna (2009).

How then to introduce mindfulness practices into these models? The short answer is: in the same way that all the other elements of the models are introduced and reinforced. The first step is to explain what mindfulness is and why it matters to the work at hand. This would then be followed by instruction and modeling conducted by trained individuals. Next, comes the inclusion of mindfulness practices within the retreats, workshops, meetings, and coaching sessions that support the other key elements of the model. There should also be reminders about why regular outside practice is beneficial, just as there might be reminders about the practice of other elements of the model. Individual mindfulness instruction can also be made available to address questions that inevitably arise in the early stages of practice. This would be similar to offering individual coaching sessions for other model elements. Finally, it is important that those who facilitate the core change process have themselves incorporated mindfulness into their lives, in the same way that they have lived and benefited from the other model elements.

The viability of such experiments would in part depend on whether there are (or should be) quantitative outcome measures of the impact of these models on their participants. For my purposes, it is sufficient to suggest some preliminary action research that would yield suggestive results. First, I would encourage senior trainers in these or similar organizational change processes to learn and practice mindfulness for themselves as a self-experiment. First person subjective experience of mindfulness by those with the highest levels of expertise in these models would inevitably yield direct and powerful insight into the complementarity I propose. If the outcome of such a first person "experiment" suggested promising possibilities, these individuals might choose to add simple, short, breath, and body awareness practices into some of their trainings—using videos or voice recordings of mindfulness teachers if necessary—and notice whether such practices impact the dynamics of the training sessions themselves. If the effects of this second "experiment" were promising, the next step would be to expand this component and specifically encourage ongoing mindfulness practice to participants. Comparing feedback and outcomes from the sessions that include mindfulness to others that did not, as well as to their past experience of feedback and outcomes from the core program, would influence what, if any, next steps should be taken.

We have a long history of failed efforts to change organizations and the individuals within them, and each of us has our own long history of failed efforts to change our own daily behaviors and states of mind. Clearly, this is hard work. The models of Kegan and Lahey and of Weissglass are notable for their emphasis on the simultaneity of organizational and individual change and for their holistic approach to engaging the cognitive and affective realms of individual members of organizations. What these models of change, and others like them, do is powerful, important, and when it works, truly transformational. The goal of adding the suite of mindfulness practices described in this chapter is to support this work with the hope that mindfulness practices would increase efficacy as well as the proportion of participants who are able to thoroughly apply these strategies to the enhancement of their own lives and that of their organizations.

References

Chodron, P. (1997). *When things fall apart: Heart advice for difficult times*. Boston, MA: Shambhala.

Chodron, P. (2007). *Practicing peace in times of war*. Boston, MA: Shambhala.

Didonna, F. (Ed.). (2009). *Clinical handbook of mindfulness*. New York, NY: Springer.

Ferguson, G. (2010). *Natural wakefulness: Discovering the wisdom we were born with*. Boston, MA: Shambhala.

Gendlin, E. (1988). *Focusing-oriented psycho-therapy: A manual of the experiential method*. New York, NY: Guilford.

Kabat-Zinn, J. (2013). *Full catastrophe living: Using the wisdom of your body and mind to face stress*. New York, NY: Bantam.

Kegan, R. (1998). *In over our heads: The mental demands of modern life*. Cambridge, MA: Harvard.

Kegan, R., & Lahey, L. (2001). The real reason people won't change. *Harvard Business Review, 79*(10), 85–92. Reprint RO110E.

Kegan, R., & Lahey, L. (2009). *Immunity to change: How to overcome it and unlock the potential in yourself and your organization*. Cambridge, MA: Harvard.

Kornfield, J. (1993). *A path with heart: A guide through the perils and promises of spiritual life*. New York, NY: Bantam.

Mindfulnet.org. (2014). *The neuroscience of mindfulness*. Retrieved from http://www.mindfulnet.org/page25.htm

Mipham, S. (2004). *Turning the mind into an ally*. Boston, MA: Shambhala.

Rome, D. (2014). *Your body knows the answer: Using your felt sense to solve problems, effect change and liberate creativity*. Boston, MA: Shambhala.

Seppala, E. (2014). *20-scientific-reasons-to-start--meditating-today*. Retrieved from http://www.emmaseppala.com/

Suzuki, S. (1999). *Zen mind, beginner's mind*. Boston, MA: Weatherill.

Wagner, T., Kegan, R., Lahey, L., & Lemons, R. W. (2005). *Change leadership: A practical guide to transforming our schools*. San Francisco, CA: Jossey-Bass.

Weissglass, J. (1998). *Ripples of hope: Building relationships for educational change*. Santa Barbara, CA: University of California Center for Educational Change in Mathematics and Science.

Mindful School Leadership: Guidance from Eastern Philosophy on Organizing Schools for Student Success

16

Gordon S. Gates and Barbara Gilbert

Current educational reform focuses on three school improvement strategies: measuring student achievement on standardized tests and performance benchmarks, implementing instructional interventions for struggling learners, and sanctioning schools that fail to make desired improvements (McDonnell, 2012). Proponents of these policies contend that through instituting various control tactics involved in simplifying, standardizing, and assessing educational outcomes (Foster, 2004), educators will be better positioned to meet the needs of minority and low socioeconomic status students, the underserved students most at risk of dropping out (Schoen & Fusarelli, 2008). Researchers find limited support for this argument as studies show gains in achievement for some student demographic groups but not others and the observed effects tend to be small (Chiang, 2009; Dee, Jacobs, Hoxby, & Ladd, 2010; Lee, 2006). Critics of such policies attribute some of difficulty in making progress to school leaders who vacillate between implementing thoughtful, comprehensive changes that strengthen teaching and acting quickly and reactively to avoid sanctions (de Wolf & Janssens, 2007; Mintrop & Sunderman, 2009).

Recently, scholars in the field of organizational studies have noted that the increase in student achievement desired by legislators and reformers (Balfanz, Herzog, & MacIver, 2007), such as that expressed in the 2001 US federal government's legislation on no child being left to fail or drop out of school (Chiang, 2009), emerges from a different set of principles than those present within the top-down, sanctions-driven approach (Borko, Wolf, Simone, & Uchiyama, 2003). Organizations found to consistently achieve their desired goals without major failures—labeled as high reliability organizations (HROs)—operate through iterative and sustained processes of learning enabled by collective mindfulness (Weick & Roberts, 1993; Weick & Sutcliffe, 2006). Examples of organizations that exhibit high reliability include nuclear powered submarines, chemical plants, air traffic control centers, and firefighting command systems. Weick posits, "The key difference between HROs and other organizations is the sensitivity or mindfulness with which people in most HROs react to even very weak signals that some kind of change or danger is approaching" (Coutu, 2003, p. 86). What is most noteworthy about HROs is the presence of mindfulness needed for handling problems, although what they are applauded for

G.S. Gates (✉)
Washington State University, Pullman, WA, USA
e-mail: gates@wsu.edu

B. Gilbert
Harvard University, Cambridge, MA, USA
e-mail: barbara_gilbert@gse.harvard.edu

K.A. Schonert-Reichl, R.W. Roeser (eds.), *Handbook of Mindfulness in Education*,
Mindfulness in Behavioral Health, DOI 10.1007/978-1-4939-3506-2_16

is their consistency in securing required outcomes (Levinthal & Rerup, 2006; Weick & Sutcliffe, 2007).

Several scholars suggest the strategies identified in HRO research provide direction for how schools might address low student performance, the achievement gap, and a host of other challenges in public education (Eck, 2011; Hoy, Gage, & Tarter, 2006). Stringfield (1996) for instance, suggested that adopting HRO principles would mean

> administrators would need to clarify goals; create and clarify standard operation procedures regarding curriculum, instruction, and the handling of various students and task management issues; greatly increase goal-directed staff development; further open access to rule-making; improve two-way staff evaluation procedures and practices; be clearer and more flexible in dealing with situations in which special needs of children must be met….; replace teachers' isolation with more collegial working relationships; and finally, a school would need to allocate funds not just to procure new equipment, but to maintain existing equipment. (p. 5)

Bellamy, Crawford, Marshall, and Coulter (2005) also endorse turning to HROs, though reservedly. They reviewed literature to propose HROs to provide a metaphor for fail-safe schools and recommend limited adoption of HRO tenets given what they contend are significant structural and decision-making differences between HROs and schools, such as teacher autonomy, lack of standardization, and decentralization in schools. Educational literature that discusses HRO scholarship, therefore, takes an array of positions to guide school leadership toward improvement (i.e., high reliability) in student outcomes.

Perhaps unsurprisingly, mindfulness also evidences contrasting treatment in the educational literature that seeks to determine the appropriateness of HRO theory for accomplishing the goals of school reform. Stringfield, Reynolds, and Schaffer (2008) in their study on the implementation of HRO strategies in 12 Welsh secondary schools make no mention of mindfulness. Bellamy et al. (2005), on the other hand, unequivocally propose the notion of "*mindfulness*, for constant vigilance that recognizes that problems can occur at any time. A useful mindset that supports this vigilance is an assumption that every program, curriculum, instructional strategy, and teacher is fallible" (italics in original, p. 401). Yet, Bellamy et al.'s analysis is less focused on understanding mindfulness than discussing issues that pertain to mindlessness. Their premise mirrors that of HRO literature specifically and Western psychology generally where mindfulness and mindlessness are interpreted as opposites (Bishop et al., 2004; Langer, 1989; Weick & Sutcliffe, 2006).

Mindlessness is defined by Carson and Langer (2006) as a rigid mindset in which one "is oblivious to context or perspective" (p. 30). Cast in highly negative terms, researchers speak, among other concerns, of the "deleterious effects of mindless information processing" (Langer & Piper, 1987, p. 280) as contributing to catastrophic failure (Fiol & O'Connor, 2003; Weick, Sutcliffe, & Obstfeld, 1999). Hoy (2003) too adopts this stance in making his case about the relevance of mindful practice for school leadership. He discusses the various ways educators experience mindlessness to the detriment of school operations. We agree that there is value in exposing "some of the basic causes of mindlessness that influence our daily behavior—repetition, premature cognitive commitment, an emphasis on outcomes, and context confusion" (p. 95). Yet, the focus on mindlessness to represent and explain mindfulness denotes an important conceptual shift. We contend further analysis is warranted to better identify and present the potential of *mindfulness* in organizing for high reliability in general and in particular for educator practice concerned with improving student learning or what we propose calling "mindful school leadership."

In this chapter, we turn to Buddhist philosophy for analysis of the potential benefits of mindfulness for educational reform (Bishop et al., 2004; Rosch, 2008; Weick & Putnam, 2006). Our discussion begins by reviewing literature that draws on writings translated or presented to convey various traditions in Buddhism to an

American or Western audience. Following our examination of teachings concerned with mindfulness from this tradition, we offer a brief synopsis of HRO research to integrate and propose ways to reframe or enhance understanding of mindfulness as applicable to organizational work. While we include references to educational literature and the principalship in both of the prior sections, it is in the third that we focus our attention on connecting and pushing the relevance of our argument for researchers and practitioners of leadership in schools. With the chapter's purpose and outline stated, we proceed to our discussion on the psychology of awareness offered within Eastern teachings.

Mindfulness in Buddhist Philosophy

Stephen Batchelor (1997), in *Buddhism Without Beliefs*, clarifies a common misunderstanding held by many in the West that defines and dismisses Buddhism as a faith tradition. Batchelor shares the path of the Four Noble Truths, which are foundational tenets for Buddhism, to argue:

> There is nothing particularly religious or spiritual about this path. It encompasses everything we do. It is an authentic way of being in the world. It begins with how we understand the kind of reality we inhabit and the kind of beings we are that inhabit such a reality. Such a vision underpins the values that inform our ideas, the choices we make, the words we utter, the deeds we perform, the work we do. It provides the ethical ground for mindful and focused awareness, which in turn further deepens our understanding of the kind of reality we inhabit and the kind of beings we are that inhabit such a reality. (pp. 10–11)

John Dewey traveled China and Japan from 1919 to 1921 and reached an understanding similar to Batchelor's. Dewey's writings were heavily influenced by Buddhist philosophers in whom "he found reinforcement for his lifelong effort to understand human experience" (Jacobson, 1988, p. 5). The perspective of the above scholars grounds and reinforces our examination as reasonable and appropriate for informing educational leadership theory and practice.

Buddhism's Four Noble Truths embrace two propositions that (a) as a result of self-centeredness, individuals suffer from existential dissatisfaction and (b) there is a cure for this unhappiness. The intent of Buddhist mindfulness training is to help practitioners dismantle habituated, egocentric behaviors and "patterns that prevent us from knowing what we are" (McLeod, 2002, p. 30). Zen Buddhism, for example, suggests that the path to mindfulness may be best understood through the cultivation of beginners' mind. Other Buddhist traditions use different language, but they agree that "The mind of the beginner is empty, free of the habits of the expert, ready to accept, to doubt, and open to all the possibilities. It is the kind of mind which can see things as they are" (Suzuki & Dixon, 1970, pp. 13–14). Accordingly, Buddhism proffers a holistic philosophy and practice that helps to conscientiously develop a nonjudgmental awareness of body, feelings, and the mind. Below, we propose five principles of mindfulness that are relevant to school leadership that both complement and challenge understandings of mindfulness offered in HRO literature. These include: attention to the present, receptivity to experience, proclivity to question, cultivation of compassion, and respond with wisdom.

Attention to the Present Although a belief in self provides some measure of stability in an impermanent world, Buddhist teachers are clear: Our notion of self frequently sets up conditions for egocentricity and feeds a psychological need to control (Chodron, 2012; Loori, 2008; Nairn, 1999). A tenet of Buddhism is that individuals, made uncomfortable by the fact "that all life is transient, constantly appearing and disappearing, constantly changing" (Katagiri, 2008, p. 4), tend to develop and hold to a belief in the existence of an independent and unchanging self across a linear progression of time (Batchelor, 2000; Gyatso, 1998). In holding to "a wish to make life—which is basically fluid—into something certain and fixed" (Chodron, 2001, p. 10), human behavior, thoughts, and feelings evidence what is described as attachment. Rather than operating from what is, human perception and interaction is often negatively influenced by normative values and beliefs—including notions of what should and should not be, as well as what is and is not desired. Weick and Putnam (2006) share that it is attachment which "encourages people to reject or ignore concepts associated with negative and neutral feelings (e.g., uncertainty, absorption) and to develop misperceptions of themselves, their work, and their context" (p. 281). The applicability of this tenet becomes clear with recognition that in schools today there is much interpreted as deficient including the lack of parent support, poorly prepared students, congested and over-regulated curriculum, insufficient funding, to name just a few of the challenges. Educational accountability has been shown to exacerbate such perception and further confound the ability of educators to institute meaningful change to address the needs of failing students (Anagnostopoulos & Rutledge, 2007; Mintrop & Sunderman, 2009).

Buddhism, however, presents more than the diagnosis but advances a comprehensive approach to handling the problem of attachment. Mindfulness training is forwarded as the tool, or collection of methods more accurately, which are concerned with learning to observe when and how attachment arises. The various forms and practices of meditation are key to developing necessary mental skills. In meditating, no matter the type or technique, individuals strengthen their capacity to recognize what they are adding to or subtracting from the present moment. Mindfulness meditation is a discipline for learning about how to be present or give attention to whatever arises in the here and now.

Kabat-Zinn (1994) identifies meditation as a process of non-doing in which one is focused on being rather than busily doing. Non-doing is a particularly difficult concept for Westerners to understand or appreciate, as social value is given to progress that tends to be equated with action directed at the achievement of goals. Some Eastern philosophers suggest that the almost exclusive focus on doing that is prevalent in the West is not only a primary source of dissatisfaction, stress, and defensiveness but limits perception of what is possible and of consequence to living fully (Carroll, 2004). Through a process of identifying and removing what is added to or subtracted from the present in terms of goals, expectations, desires, etc., mindfulness meditation is hypothesized to cultivate an attitude of openness, acceptance, and curiosity to what occurs moment-to-moment without trying to fix it or wanting to get rid of it (Nanda, 2009). Hanh (2008) shares this teaching on the primacy of being to promise "We only have one moment to live, and that is the present moment. If we come back to the present moment, we'll be in contact with innumerable wonders in and around us" (p. 65). Katagiri (2008) further clarifies,

> What you can see is right now, a moment, the present time. But this present is not just the present; it's connected with the whole universe. This is how you can see the universe. If you see this universe, you realize that you are part of a dynamic reality that is constantly changing according to the conditions of every moment. (p. 230)

Buddhist philosophy in this way connects being present to the primacy of experience.

Receptivity to Experience A second principle of mindfulness that is relevant to education is the intent of meditative practice for developing the capacity to "observe things as they are, and to let everything go as it goes" (Suzuki & Dixon, 1970, p. 33). The various techniques of meditation build concentration needed for staying focused on the present rather than the mental wandering that frequently arises when things are not going as desired. In schools, for example, few if any changes to operations occur without some hitch or resistance, which can become extreme in some situations, from those who are comfortable with or benefit from previous arrangements (Enomoto & Conely, 2008; Starr, 2011). Keeping focused and on message when dealing with micropolitics of faculty interaction is critical (Maxcy & Nguyen, 2006). Meeting with upset parents is no less difficult and as the task falls to principals, there is "motivation to learn how to 'cool out' dissatisfied parents, to deal with their discontent in ways that prevent further escalation and if possible enhance parental satisfaction" (Lortie, 2009,

p. 174). Mindfulness meditation tends to employ simple supports such as a focus on the breath, coming in and going out in its natural rhythm to develop the mental skills, which can be useful in such situations.

According to Buddhism, there is nothing but right now and that which is right now is a process: changing, happening, coming, and going, which can be observed in each cycle of respiration. Suzuki discusses the development of calm that follows observing the breath. He states that it is analogous to "a general housecleaning of your mind" (p. 110) and is an important first step in helping one find balance in body, feelings, and the mind. More importantly, he explains that when mediation is practiced over time, the various constraints coloring one's perceptions become known. The nature of awareness that is possible from this discipline translates into all aspects of an individual's life both personal and professional. Because meditative practice develops concentration with no other purpose than to be, meditation readies the mind for being receptive to experience.

The metaphors of a pool of water or mirror are used in various Buddhist traditions to speak to this quality of receptiveness and the characteristics of the mind that are associated with it (Rosenberg, 1998; Sunim, 1999). When a pond is stirred, its water becomes cloudy and its surface less reflective. The mental equanimity and concentration that are nurtured by meditation are likened to the process of the sediment in the water settling. The practice of meditation is described in this way as playing an important role to perceiving and appreciating experience. With mindfulness, experience provides access or an approach to knowledge that is without bias of prior conceptualization of phenomena (e.g., schema), including the limitations that arise from language or labels, as well as feelings based on prior experience and socialization. For example, Nh'ãat (2006) shares that misconceptions occur when one "use[s] words to point to something—an object or concept—but they may or may not correspond to the 'truth' of that thing, which can only be known through a direct perception of its reality" (p. 28). Buddhist teachings on mindfulness advance a radical epistemology: the phenomenological world can be experienced, but not completely or accurately represented. Engaging in mindfulness meditation encourages and enhances the capacity to experience phenomena as constantly emerging and in process.

Proclivity to Question A third principle relevant to education found in Buddhist traditions is the postulate of an inherent problem with attempts to solidify knowledge and establish control over phenomena given the vastness and fluidity of the universe. Eastern philosophers have been intensely interested in understanding epistemological problems associated with knowledge because phenomena are interconnected and constantly changing.

Several ideas repeated by Buddhist teachers further define the problem. First, there is the tendency of the mind to begin each moment of experience by "making the smallest distinction" (Loori, 2008, p. 106). This systematically translates life into a litany of dualistic thinking that constrains understanding to sets of fixed categories such as love–hate, winners–losers, acceptance–rejection. This process of differentiation, or "relative mind," is particularly problematic because it filters one's perceptions, guards one against others, and limits one's ability to interact freely with the world. Relative mind creates negative emotional responses in an attempt to reduce vulnerability and in an effort to establish certainty, solidify the self, and control others or conditions. Through meditation, individuals come to an awareness of this tendency of relative mind and learn to quiet its operation. The task during mindfulness meditation is to recognize such thoughts, feelings, or sensations and to return to the breath or what are termed as objects of support. Examples of other supports in meditating include the sound of a bell or voice when using a guided meditation or the placement of feet in a walking meditation.

When individuals have developed sufficient skill in regaining equanimity and possessing concentration, insight into the nature of relative mind and its attachment may arise (Rosenberg, 1998;

Sunim, 1999). A mindful individual peels back the layers of mental preconceptions and emotional responses that obscure the ability to remain open and engaged in the world as it is moment-to-moment. As such, life becomes "more about holding questions than finding answers" (Chodron, 2001, p. 10). Batchelor (2000) explains that through meditation, individuals "learn how to suspend the habit of reaching for a word or phrase with which to fill the emptiness opened by the question. The meditator seeks not a solution to this question but a living, ongoing response" (p. 45). Questions, according to this philosophy, rather than answers mark the door to understanding and action.

Helsing (2007) provides a recent analysis of educational research that promotes questioning as fundamental to effective teaching given the pervasiveness of uncertainty in its practice. Copeland (2003) for similar reasons makes this argument for effective instructional leadership. Researchers find expert practitioners use inquiry to inform and develop their professional practice. Asking questions is the heart of the inquiry model presented in the literature for both effective teaching and schools.

Cultivation of Compassion A fourth principle of mindfulness that is relevant to education concerns the cultivation of compassion. Meditation and self-reflection are processes through which one develops understanding of one's responsibilities "as an individual living with other individuals [with the capacity to] see who you are and how you are without illusion, judgment or resistance of any kind" (Gunaratana, 2002, p. 14). Insight arises out of questioning the nature of reality and one's relationship with the world. A key component of this, Gunaratana explains, is how the mechanics of selfishness are revealed as "meditation changes your character by a process of sensitization, by making you deeply aware of your own thoughts and deeds" (p. 16). People are born and die, relationships begin and end, and possessions come and go. Meditation cultivates compassion for self and for others through attention to feelings that arise from shared experiences, and the recognition that each of us is not much different in our desires, hopes, fears, etc. From these insights, motivation grows for being mindful, avoiding causing harm to others, and acting to serve humanity. Together the three qualities provide the backbone for skillful and compassionate action (Chodron, 2012; Loori, 2008; Rosenberg, 1998).

Few write as powerfully about the development and exercise of compassion as a professional skill for educators than Parker Palm (2007) in *The Courage to Teach*. Feminist scholarship in educational leadership contends that compassion is also a key proficiency or trait that contributes to leader effectiveness (Christman & McClellan, 2008). More than a few proponents of Buddhism endorse such claim (Batchelor, 1997; Carroll, 2004; Gyatso & van den Muyzenberg, 2009). Thus, the description and definition of compassion found in Buddhism can be seen as promising for informing educator practice.

Compassion plays a prominent role in Buddhism. The stance advanced in Buddhist philosophy, however, has little to do with behaving in ways that conform to normative ideals of acting charitably. Compassion in Buddhism is described as maintaining an intention or state of mind that Gyatso (1998) regards as "nonviolent, nonharming, and nonaggressive. It is a mental attitude based on the wish for others to be free of their suffering and is associated with a sense of commitment, responsibility, and respect towards the other" (p. 114). Sitting in meditation provides repeated opportunities in handling negative thoughts, unpleasant feelings, and difficult sensations that lead to development of compassion. Social interactions or encounters that give rise to these same kinds of emotional and psychological reactions will occur, yet given the increase in skillfulness from meditative practice, an individual is better able to respond compassionately. Certain Buddhist teachers posit that "When our identification with mind and body is loosened and to some degree seen for what it is, we become more open to the concerns of others, even when we don't agree with them, even when we have to oppose them" (e.g., Beck, 1997, p. 113). This is how "you claim your courage, your kindness, your strength…This is a way of extending warmth and acceptance to whatever is going on for you right now" (Chodron, 2012, p. 41).

Respond with Wisdom Buddhist teachings explain mindfulness as enhancing an individual's capacity to respond wisely to any situation that arises and is the fifth principle we wish to discuss. A powerful exposé on such teaching is found in *Fragrant Palm Leaves* by Thich Nhat Hanh (1998). In sharing excepts from his journals written when he was a young man studying in New England and then living back in Vietnam during the war, Hanh gives personal examples that reveal how he became an advocate for both peace and engaged Buddhism. Reflecting on his experience, he wrote "I knew early on that finding truth is not the same as finding happiness. You aspire to see the truth, but once you have seen it, you cannot avoid suffering" (p. 89). His narrative, however, soundly rejects negative reactions that are judgmental about the events large and small that happened during the war. He extends this analysis to assessments that arise for interactions or events that people consider as positive. Once he has made these points, Hanh shares the teaching on which he ponders: "Truth cannot be borrowed. It can only be experienced directly…[in] the reality of the present moment" (p. 89). Hanh's journal poignantly conveys mindfulness as being "present in the real stream of time and looking directly at life itself" (Katagiri, 2008, p. 11), no matter what is there.

Buddhism proposes the principal weakness arising from thought and emotion surfaces "When we're not aware of our feelings, we're driven by them, pushed around…we react automatically" (Rosenberg, 1998, p. 74). Leithwood and Beatty (2009), Lortie (2009), and Hoy (2003) describe the press of many and hurried decisions, conflict, and high stakes in the work of school administrators that reveal the potential significance of how mindfulness enables individuals to respond with wisdom. Since mindfulness is awareness without added attachment or prior conception, choice becomes possible. Goldstein (2008) exposes this idea when he states that "Awareness gives us the option of *choosing wisely*; we can choose which patterns should be developed and cultivated, and which should be abandoned" (italics in original, p. 25). A psychology of empowerment, in which volitional choice is an ever-present possibility, underlies Eastern mindfulness. Teachings on meditation delineate processes for using engagement with and reflection on tendencies to succumb and react, to distinguish and stimulate our capacity to create and respond. The promise of being fully present is that it renders both access and discernment for choosing a wise response. Rosenberg (1998) explains that in being mindful one "feel[s] more alive than ever, more focused and intelligent, though your intelligence isn't based on knowledge acquired over time....it is much more trustworthy in terms of what it sees and the actions that come out of that seeing" (p. 133).

Organizing for Reliability and Mindfulness

The five principles described above can serve to enrich the discussion on mindfulness in HROs generally, and in educational institutions in particular. Mindfulness in the HRO literature explicitly draws on Ellen Langer's (1989) definition, which parallels and contrasts in critical ways with Eastern mindfulness (see Roeser, 2014; Rosch, 2008; Weick & Putnam, 2006). Studies by Langer and associates examine the effects of holding a flexible mindset, creating and refining categories of understanding, being open to new ways of knowing, and cultivating multiple perspectives. Brown and Langer (1990) explain "Mindfulness theory encourages us to take a second look at the way our perceptual processes structure experience, in order to discover that they are more malleable and susceptible to individual control than may be apparent at first glance" (p. 312). According to this view, a mindful individual is guided by existing rules and routines rather than mindlessly governed by preconceptions or past distinctions. As such, mindfulness is "understood as the process of drawing novel distinctions" in a way that "keeps us situated in the present" (Langer & Moldoveanu, 2000, pp. 1–2).

Weick and colleagues define mindfulness "as a rich awareness of discriminatory detail generated by organizational processes" (Weick & Sutcliffe, 2006, p. 516). They find mindfulness in HROs is supported by a preoccupation with failure, reluctance to simplify interpretations, sensitivity to operations, commitment to resilience, and deference to expertise. Since these five cognitive processes have been well described in literature (Eck, 2011; Weick & Sutcliffe, 2007), we offer an abbreviated account of the processes in order to connect and explain the relevance of the five principles identified in our previous discussion of Eastern mindfulness. Table 16.1 below presents the comparisons that we wish to draw between these two bodies of literature and which we explain in greater detail in the narrative that follows.

Preoccupation with Failure HROs purposely create and sustain a belief that failures provide valuable signals that "a static world is based on preconceived notions of how the world is" (Carson & Langer, 2006, pp. 35–36) has been compromised and requires attention. People in HROs are mindful of the lessons learned from "near-miss events" and carefully attend to "what *could have* happened, and *why* it didn't happen" (Kaplan, 2002, p. 337). As such, individuals working within HROs candidly acknowledge failure and near failure when they occur so that the organization is better able to refocus on current conditions and detect "possible weakness in other portions of the system" (Weick & Sutcliffe, 2001, p. 56). In contrast to other organizations, management of HROs purposefully avoid the negative connotation of "error" and the tendency towards useless recriminations when errors are made. Indeed, the literature offers many cases of individuals who self-reported mistakes and were rewarded for doing so.

Table 16.1 Comparison of Western and Eastern mindfulness

HRO processes	Buddhist principles
Preoccupation with failure	Attention to the present
Sensitivity to operations	Receptivity to experience
Reluctance to simplify	Proclivity for questions
Commitment to resilience	Cultivation of compassion
Deference to expertise	Respond with wisdom

Western and Eastern mindfulness are thus similarly interested in nonjudgmental attention to what is happening moment-to-moment (e.g., Kabat-Zinn, 1994). In both cases, mindfulness is seen to direct attention and guide inquiry on what is actually occurring moment-to-moment. Although HROs encourage a preoccupation with failure, Eastern philosophy rejects the binary of success and failure, and instead, brings to the foreground the notion of nonjudgmental attention. Both strategies endeavor to create the conditions—a baseline if you will—for seeing as much information as possible. Yet, Fiol and O'Connor (2003) are critical of the emphasis on failure in HRO literature, and contend that it is not the search for failure alone that is important for mindfulness and improved decision-making. They claim that a focus on failure without success "may completely eliminate any sense of control [and] is likely to drive a firm into the ground as quickly as a singular focus on success" (p. 64).

Wears and Nemeth (2007) also critically examine the diagnostic difficulty that attends hindsight bias that arises with too narrow a focus on failure. They recommend attention be given to constraints or a work ecology approach that is holistic. The skill and outlook delineated in nonjudgmental attention to the present found within Buddhist notions of mindfulness speak to both sets of concerns. Although Eastern philosophy tends to dismiss the relevance and possibility of control, it is keenly interested in developing and strengthening the quality of choicefulness by individuals in the presence of the so-called failures or successes alike.

Too many educators, students, and even parents feel their ability and choice are threatened or diminished through standardized achievement assessments that label, compare, and bestow rewards and sanctions for performance (Barrett, 2009; Finnigan & Gross, 2007; Lyons &

Algozzine, 2006; Thompson, Warren, & Carter, 2004). Blame has been given too large a role in too many schools. There is preoccupation with failure in education, but it frequently may be of the wrong kind. Blame signals the misplacement of attention to past behavior and future consequences. Philosophers of Eastern mindfulness speak of learning from the past and preparing for the future; however, they also warn of treating both with caution since they are imagined. We propose the processes involved in preparing, taking, and reporting student performance outcomes will look and feel different (e.g., less fault finding, decrease in worrying, and more collaborative opportunity seeking in professional learning communities or in parent involvement to support student learning) when attention to the present is part of classroom and school-wide practices.

Sensitivity to Operations The preferred methodology in HROs for achieving high stakes outcomes involves a commitment to ongoing inquiry and flexible problem-solving. Mindfulness in HRO theory involves continuous updating that requires individuals to remain sensitive to changing operational needs and conditions (Weick & Sutcliffe, 2001). Updating processes feed into learning and subsequent training, which are key elements in HROs for avoiding errors given the "inherent difficulty of handling information in ill-structured or constantly changing situations" (Swuste, 2008, p. 442). Continuous observation, testing, and modification support development of habitualized actions, preconceptions, and labels (Ford & Backoff, 1988) that strengthen the ability to manage change. As key attributes of routinization, these organizing tools facilitate problem solving that is helpful as complexity increases.

Western mindfulness as such is focused on sense-making for the purpose of doing (e.g., learning, routinizing, solving problems), while Buddhist practice is experiential for the purpose of being (e.g., noticing) (Nairn, 1999; Sunim, 1999). HROs concentrate on conceptual understanding of phenomena (e.g., creating routines, making measurements, decision-making). In contrast, Eastern practice sets out a process of ongoing deconstruction of understanding. The problem for mindfulness through sensitivity to operations involves the way routines, standard procedures, and the other like operational features function as confirming evidence for establishing expectations (Weick & Sutcliffe, 2007). Learning routines, technological advancements, and enhanced coordination reduce perceived uncertainty and increase felt control, as well as shift attention to operational norms and protocol compliance (Woods, 2005). Sensitivity to operations in this way leads to preference of categorically based knowing from perceptually based knowing (Weick, 2006). With an emphasis on being receptive to experience, Eastern mindfulness provides a healthy antidote to reliance

> on our routines when we least need them. When work's surprises require us to adapt and innovate, we can find ourselves instead reaching for familiar habits, making us ineffective...Adapting to surprises and chaos need not be a monumental task but a simple shift from holding on to letting go, from maintaining a point of view to not having one at all, from trying to solve a problem to listening for solutions. (Carroll, 2004, p. 195)

One of the major problems to reforming schools pertains to the nay saying by those who claim, for example, to have tried particular changes before to no effect (Anagnostopoulos & Rutledge, 2007; Enomoto & Conely, 2008; Hoy, 2003). Such educators know too well their practice. Rather than leveraging uncertainty and ambiguity—that are an inherent part of teaching and learning (Helsing, 2007)—to engage in inquiry, their sensitivity to operations is used in some instances to protect known procedures and minimal expectations for those who have traditionally been underserved by schools (Shields, 2004). The principle of receptivity to experience as such identifies a valuable tool aligned with literature on building capacity for school improvement (Copeland, 2003).

Reluctance to Simplify Interpretation People in HROs resist the urge to simplify or streamline processes, and instead, focus on developing a complex understanding of their work. The commitment to complexity is important because they believe they cannot afford failures (LaPorte & Consolini, 1991). Although complete failure is rare in HROs, individuals are well aware of the need to be cognizant of organizational "expectations, of the limited horizon of these expectations and of the need for ongoing corrections" (Czarniawska, 2005, p. 271). Expectations come in many forms including those present in goals, role differentiation, standard procedures, strategic plans, etc. Expectations are shortcuts, abbreviations, or generalizations for describing, explaining, and influencing behavior. There is utility in such abstraction, including conservation of resources and advancement of predictability, thus the actions that maintain complexity related to reluctance in simplifying have come under criticism as incurring significant costs that are unnecessary in many situations or contexts (LaPorte, 1996; Vogus & Welbourne, 2003).

The operationalization of Eastern mindfulness and its affect on organizational outcomes have yet to receive the same scrutiny that cognitive processes of organizing for high-reliability outcomes have. Mindfulness as expressed in the proclivity for questions, neither leads, requires, nor maintains complex structures or organizational procedures. Eastern mindfulness, rather, appears to support "conceptual slack" (Weick & Sutcliffe, 2001), in which members embrace "a willingness to question what is happening, rather than feign understanding, and greater usage of respectful interaction to accelerate and enrich the exchange of information" (pp. 70–71). Thus, we see enactment of this principle as particularly relevant for research, theory, and practice concerned with furthering the kind of inquiry and decision-making needed for distributed leadership to be effective (Leithwood & Mascall, 2008; York-Barr & Duke, 2004).

Commitment to Resilience The notion of resilience in the organizational literature on HROs refers to the possibility of lapses in reliability regardless of preparation and planning. Commitment to resilience captures the ongoing effort to recognize and cope with errors and limit their negative consequences (Blatt, Christianson, Sutcliffe, & Rosenthal, 2006). Procedures are adopted in HROs that reflect or anticipate mistakes will occur. Frequent updates on monitored inputs and scheduled changes in tools or training provide ongoing surveillance to adjust to changes before they disrupt or violate parameters (Fiol & O'Connor, 2003; Van Dyck, Frese, Baer, & Sonnentag, 2005; Vogus & Welbourne, 2003). Redundancy in systems names another tactic with backups or recoveries in order to provide fail-safe operations (Parnes et al., 2007).

Sagan (2004) examines a number of ways redundancies in organizations backfire to threaten reliability. Social shirking and overcompensation are particularly relevant. Stated simply, social shirking occurs as people in an organization are aware of the duplication in their efforts and therefore assume that someone else will correct some noted issue. Inaction should not be viewed as necessarily calculated or negligent, but evidence of confusion. Disorder can be seen where something is everyone's responsibility, but no one steps up to take care of problems given the pressures of their other duties for which they are directly responsible. With overcompensation, pressure arises as improvements in one area provide opportunities for action in another area that increase exposure to risk. In both threats to reliability, pressure is increased in the organization from various sources that influence mindfulness.

The cultivation of compassion presented in Eastern teachings on mindfulness speaks to these issues in ways that literature on HROs does not. Carroll (2004) translates the applicability of compassion at work to the problems that arise in our jobs, viewing them not as tiresome obstacles or demoralizing fights, but important experiences. He notes: "If we take a moment to slow down and open up to our work circumstances, we will discover that work is continually inviting us to help, not hide; to listen openly, not close up; to connect, not detach" (pp. 6–7). For educators, the practice of mindfulness meditation provides the skills to notice feelings (e.g., being rushed to move to teaching the next concept, defending a decision made on student discipline, or ignoring visiting a classroom because there is not a problem) and we contend to strengthen reflective practice of practitioners as called for by Dewey and Schon among others (Rodgers, 2002). Indeed, compassion for self and others encourages skillful, responsive behavior rather than reactive and limited action, which create added problems or perpetuate blame given hindsight bias when failure results (Wears & Nemeth, 2007). Literature on teacher and administrator stress (Hawk & Martin, 2011; Metzger, 2003) speaks to compassion as a mechanism for coping with limited resources and high demands found in schools.

Deference to Expertise Mindfulness in the organizational literature also emphasizes deference to expertise. In organizations that operate in rapidly changing and potentially dangerous environments, complexity is built into the system to allow the full participation of every individual. Attention, as well as the ability to hold knowledge and roles loosely, is found to be critical. HROs as such tend to operate as tightly coupled systems, in which many of the subsystems "are interdependent, with little or no slack between them" (Bierly, Gallagher, & Spender, 2008, p. 393). A potential negative consequence of the pronounced interdependence arises when one organizational component fails, which can result in catastrophic, systemic losses. HROs meet this challenge by forming informal networks of knowledgeable people who can "quickly self-organize into ad hoc networks to provide expert problem solving. These networks have no formal status and dissolve as soon as a crisis is over" (Weick & Sutcliffe, 2001, p. 71). Fenema (2005) posits that within these informal networks, the complicated and fluid relationships that exist guide the majority of organizational decisions; and it is their willingness to value flexibility over rank that enhances organizational resilience.

Our interpretation of Eastern mindfulness compliments findings related to this cognitive process of "deference to expertise." Trust surfaces in both approaches as significant. Further, in HROs, when trouble happens, decision-making migrates, frequently downward, to the level where expertise resides. HROs thus recognize the importance of empowerment for people to make choices that will be positive and for the greater good. The discipline of meditation described in Eastern philosophy also operates to empower, but facilitates such action through steadying and focusing the quality of attention.

The nature of autonomy in schools has been assessed as a key obstacle to organizing schools for high reliability (Bellamy et al., 2005). Yet, to forfeit the full meaning of reliability in student achievement or other student learning outcomes allows schools to operate in ways that permit as acceptable the failure of some students. Although we hold serious reservations about accountability policies given major weaknesses identified by Foster (2004), Lortie (2009), Mintrop and Sunderman (2009), and others we contend some of the noted problems could be mitigated though adoption of mindful practice. Weick and Sutcliffe's (2006) unequivocal assertion of mindfulness' value or relevance for any organization is particularly salient to our position. Mindfulness, as a kind of nonjudgmental awareness and attention, is critical to all organizations they claim, as "Attention is scarce when it is undisciplined and obstacles interfere with clear comprehension, but attention is more plentiful and sufficient when it becomes more stable and vivid" (p. 521). Literature on HROs exposes the relevance of shifting decisions to those with expertise—in addition to avoiding blame, learning for problem solving, creating redundancies, etc.—while Eastern mindfulness provides a robust vehicle to developing equanimity and concentration of attention necessary to respond with wisdom. Practitioners of educational leadership need wisdom in guiding schools to the kinds of improvement that can help make learning more than a probability for many students, but a possibility for all.

Implications for Mindful School Leadership

Our purpose in examining mindfulness in Eastern philosophy, and comparing it to uses of mindfulness in organizational literature, was to draw attention to some of the broader implications of an integrative psychology of mindfulness for educational administration. The principles of attention to the present, receptivity to experience, proclivity for questions, cultivation of compassion, and respond with wisdom that we identified within literature on Buddhism were shown to complement, modify, or challenge Western psychology's view of mindfulness in the organizational literature on HROs, and its more cognitive and action-oriented formulations of mindfulness. Eastern mindfulness forwards insight on a number of questions or issues raised in HRO research about the processes of preoccupation with failure, sensitivity to operations, reluctance to simplify interpretations, commitment to resilience, and deference to expertise that hold promise for strengthening theory about how to secure consistently high organizational performance for desired outcomes.

Our analysis of Eastern philosophy and HRO research highlighted what we appreciate as the applicability and potential of mindfulness by school personnel, with emphasis on those involved in leadership. Since our analysis focused largely on Eastern mindfulness, we will reference our comments in this section to this material, with limited consideration to five cognitive processes in HROs as these have been discussed elsewhere as applicable to education (e.g., Hoy et al., 2006). We will also incorporate literature from educational leadership as needed to substantiate or connect our ideas to the field, but we are purposefully brief. Our aim is to lay out the broad picture since what we propose marks a beginning. Hoy, Gage, and Tarter (2006) perhaps best stated the problem and direction of inquiry we encourage as they argued the conceptualization and measure of mindfulness in "schools is in its early stage…Qualitative case studied, for example, would be helpful in demonstrating specific examples of mindful and mindless behavior" (p. 252).

To begin, Eastern philosophy advises, if we are to take mindfulness seriously, that the practice of meditation must come to the foreground. Kabat-Zinn's (2003) work on mindfulness-based stress reduction has led the way in removing some of the mysticism and objections to the relevance of these practices in secular settings like schools. Yet, Dane (2011) shared that while meditation has gained attention in many fields, its treatment remains limited in management. In educational leadership the situation appears not much better, even though school administrators report conflict and ambiguity as significant sources of stress, particularly when dealing with demands made by stakeholders such as parents or legislators (Hawk & Martin, 2011; Metzger, 2003).

There are many forms of mindful practice that can be incorporated into educational settings as evidenced by the other chapters in this handbook. Indeed, meditation can be done in the context of any daily activity (Hanh, 1991). We propose that researchers begin with examination of how and with what kinds of tasks, issues, and people administrators and teacher leaders intentionally adopt a mindful stance. Recent autoethnographic studies by McDonald and Gates (2015) and Fabian (2015) explore the work experiences of a superintendent and central office administrator who were practicing mindfulness meditation and applying their developing skills to their work in schools. Using first-person descriptions, their examples illustrate the value of mindfulness for school administrators in coping with uncertainty and high demands, listening to others, and responding with purpose. We invite others to employ this and additional methods as well as to other areas of professional responsibility to create a vibrant line of inquiry. For example, Horng, Klasik, and Loeb (2010) recently distinguished six areas of principal work, all of which could be sites for the introduction of mindful practice: administration (e.g., supervising students, addressing discipline problems, following and fulfilling various policies, scheduling events, etc.), organization management (e.g., working with budgets, managing noncertified staff, attending to facilities, etc.), daily instruction (e.g., coaching and evaluating teachers, teaching students, etc.), instructional programs (e.g., evaluating curriculum, using assessment data, planning teacher professional development, etc.), internal relations (e.g., attending meetings, communicating with parents, working with students, etc.), and external relations (e..g, fundraising, communicating with the central office, and interacting with local organizations, etc.). We share this list to explicitly declare that we view mindfulness as relevant for each, and to begin a discussion of how such practice might specifically be incorporated into the work of school administrators in the service of improving reliability in student outcomes. Yet, we desire to award particular attention to two specific areas of professional responsibility since both are noted in literature on the principalship as critical or promising.

First, research on instructional leadership of principals generally includes the notion of building the leadership capacity of teachers (York-Barr & Duke, 2004). Heck, Marcoulides, and Lang (1991) reported principals who employ collaborative decision-making and flexible rule structures as associated with higher-reliability in student outcomes. Leithwood and Mascall (2008) recently replicated these findings. Researchers attribute differences in teaching between teachers in effective and less effective schools to principals' supervision and collaboration, yet the large percentage of unexplained variance in these models suggests further study is needed (Luyten, Visscher, & Witziers, 2005). Drawing on HRO literature, we suspect mindfulness may hold part of the elusive answer to uncovering how principals and teachers work together on instructional issues that bolster resilience for student outcomes (see also Roeser, Skinner, Beers, & Jennings 2012). Helsing's (2007) review of teacher's work supports such contention as she argues

> Teaching is inherently uncertain because it is centered on human relationships and involves predicting, interpreting, and assessing others' thoughts, emotions, and behavior. Furthermore, the lack of a knowledge base or technical culture in the field results in little consensus about the goals or methods of good teaching. (p. 35)

The second area we believe mindfulness can make a significant impact on educational leadership and administration pertains to the cultivation of compassion. Scholarship on school administration has long noted the presences of values, both implicit and explicit, in the choices made about schooling children and exposes the deference, difficulties, and dilemmas experienced by school leaders given social privilege and cultural reproduction. The normative and ideological nature of educator practice is described in literature on social justice (Shields, 2004), distribution of leadership (Leithwood & Mascall, 2008; Wahlstrom & Seashore Louis, 2008), school politics (Flessa, 2009), and educational accountability (Daly, 2009; Normore, 2004). Yet it is McClain, Ylimaki, and Ford's (2010) examination of compassion that articulates how a wisdom-centered leadership advanced in Eastern philosophy provides meaningful analysis and guidance with regard to the problems that confront school leaders everyday. These authors note how much of the prior literature is "written extensively about the social justice and human responsiveness of authentic democratic education... focuses on characteristics of effective decisions rather than ongoing ways of cultivating wisdom and compassion in democratic leadership" (pp. 346–347). We lend our voice to theirs in noting the significance of efforts to explore compassion as a key component, trait, characteristic, or quality of school leadership. How is it that those involved in leadership come to believe, see, and act to create a vision for education that each moment with each child, in or out of school, is precious?

In conclusion, those interested in applying or organizing schools using the principles and processes from research on high reliability can find support and direction within the chapter for framing further inquiry and investigation. Our position as such is aligned with studies by Stringfield et al. (2008) and Hoy et al. (2006) as well as treatises by Eck (2011) that advocate adoption of HRO processes to schools. Proponents of Eastern mindfulness, however, would state that the advancement of conceptual understanding misses what is most meaningful within their philosophy. And it is this assertion that we argue makes our discussion relevant and valued for school leadership concerned with educational reform. Eastern wisdom points to mindfulness as a simple but not easy task of being fully present. Researchers, reformers, and even practitioners may debate the appropriateness of policy concerned with high reliability, contest definitions, and present contradictory findings from studies in their recommendations for organizing and leading schools toward improved outcomes. The applicability of HRO literature for changing educational organizations, however, stems less from its concern for reliability and more from what it offers educators for becoming mindful in carrying out their day-to-day work with students and parents, as well as with their fellow teachers and administrators. Through presenting our complementary framework of HRO processes and Buddhist principles we hope to support and encourage professional practice informed by and directed towards being, present, and mindful.

References

Anagnostopoulos, D., & Rutledge, S. (2007). Making sense of school sanctioning policies in urban high schools. *Teachers College Record, 109*(5), 1261–1302.

Balfanz, R., Herzog, L., & MacIver, D. (2007). Preventing student disengagement and keeping students on the graduation track in high-poverty middle-grades schools: Early identification and effective interventions. *Educational Psychologist, 42*(4), 223–236.

Barrett, B. (2009). No Child Left Behind and the assault on teachers' professional practices and identities. *Teaching and Teacher Education, 25*, 1018–1025.

Batchelor, S. (1997). *Buddhism without beliefs: A contemporary guide to awakening*. New York, NY: Riverhead Books.

Batchelor, S. (2000). *Verses from the center: A Buddhist vision of the sublime*. New York, NY: Riverhead Books.

Beck, C. J. (1997). *Everyday Zen: Love and work*. London, England: Thorsons.

Bellamy, G. T., Crawford, L., Marshall, L. H., & Coulter, G. A. (2005). The fail-safe schools challenge: Leadership possibilities from high reliability organizations. *Educational Administration Quarterly, 41*(3), 383–412.

Bierly, P. E., Gallagher, S., & Spender, J. C. (2008). Innovation and learning in high-reliability organizations: A case study of United States and Russian nuclear attack submarines, 1970-2000. *IEEE Transactions on Engineering Management, 55*(3), 393–408.

Bishop, S., Lau, M., Shapiro, S., Carlson, L., Anderson, N., Carmody, J., & Devins, G. (2004). Mindfulness: A proposed operational definition. *Clinical Psychology: Science and Practice, 11*(3), 230–241.

Blatt, R., Christianson, M. K., Sutcliffe, K. M., & Rosenthal, M. M. (2006). A sensemaking lens on reliability. *Journal of Organizational Behavior, 27*(2006), 897–917.

Borko, H., Wolf, S. A., Simone, G., & Uchiyama, K. P. (2003). Schools in transition: Reform efforts and school capacity in Washington state. *Educational Evaluation and Policy Analysis, 25*(2), 171–201.

Brown, J., & Langer, E. (1990). Mindfulness and intelligence: A comparison. *Educational Psychologist, 25*(3 & 4), 305–335.

Carroll, M. (2004). *Awake at work*. Boston, MA: Shambhala.

Carson, S. H., & Langer, E. J. (2006). Mindfulness and self-acceptance. *Journal of Rational-Emotive & Cognitive-Behavior Therapy, 24*(1), 29–43.

Chiang, H. (2009). How accountability pressure on failing schools affect student achievement. *Journal of Public Economics, 93*, 1045–1057.

Chodron, T. (2001). *Buddhism for beginners*. Ithaca, NY: Snow Lion.

Chodron, T. (2012). *Living beautifully with uncertainty and change*. Boston, MA: Shambhala.

Christman, D., & McClellan, R. (2008). "Living on barbed wire": Resilient women administrators in educational leadership programs. *Educational Administration Quarterly, 44*(1), 3–29.

Copeland, M. (2003). Leadership of inquiry: Building and sustaining capacity for school improvement. *Educational Evaluation and Policy Analysis, 25*(4), 375–395.

Coutu, D. L. (2003). Sense and reliability: A conversation with celebrated psychologist Karl E. Weick. *Harvard Business Review, 6*(4), 84–90.

Czarniawska, B. (2005). Karl Weick, concepts, style and reflection. *The Editorial Board of the Sociological Review, 53*(1), 267–278.

Daly, A. (2009). Rigid response in an age of accountability: The potential of leadership and trust. *Educational Administration Quarterly, 45*(2), 168–216.

Dane, E. (2011). Paying attention to mindfulness and its effects on task performance in the workplace. *Journal of Management, 37*(4), 997–1018.

de Wolf, I. F., & Janssens, F. J. G. (2007). Effects and side effects of inspections and accountability in education: An overview of empirical studies. *Oxford Review of Education, 33*(3), 319–396.

Dee, T., Jacobs, B., Hoxby, C., & Ladd, H. (2010). The impact of No Child Left Behind on students, teachers, and schools. *Brookings papers on economic activity* (pp. 149–207). Brookings Institute Press.

Eck, J. (2011). Best in the world: High performance with high reliability. In J. Eck, S. Stringfield, D. Reynolds, E. Schaffer, & G. Bellamy (Eds.), *Noteworthy perspectives: High reliability organizations in education* (pp. 36–44). Denver, CO: McREL.

Enomoto, E., & Conely, S. (2008). Changing of the guard: How different school leaders change organizational routines. *Journal of School Leadership, 18*(3), 278–301.

Fabian, J. (2015). Moving forward by sitting still: An autoethnographic study of mindfulness. In G. Gates

(Ed.), *Mindfulness for educational practice* (pp. 39–58). Charlotte, NC: Information Age.

Fenema, P. (2005). Collaborative elasticity and breakdowns in high reliability organizations: Contributions from distributed cognition and collective mind theory. *Cognition, Technology & Work, 7*(2), 134–140.

Finnigan, K., & Gross, B. (2007). Do accountability policy sanctions influence teacher motivation? Lessons from Chicago's low-performing schools. *American Educational Research Journal, 44*(3), 594–629.

Fiol, C. M., & O'Connor, E. J. (2003). Waking up! Mindfulness in the face of bandwagons. *Academy of Management Review, 28*(1), 54–70.

Flessa, J. (2009). Educational micropolitics and distributed leadership. *Peabody Journal of Education, 84*, 331–349.

Ford, J. D., & Backoff, R. W. (1988). Organizational change in and out of dualities and paradox. In R. E. Quinn & K. S. Cameron (Eds.), *Paradox and transformation: Toward a theory of change in organization and management* (pp. 81–121). Cambridge, MA: Ballinger.

Foster, W. (2004). The decline of the local: A challenge to educational leadership. *Educational Administration Quarterly, 40*(2), 176–191.

Goldstein, J. (2008). A heart full of peace. In M. McLeod (Ed.), *The best Buddhist writing 2008* (pp. 19–27). Boston, MA: Shambhala.

Gunaratana, B. H. (2002). *Mindfulness in plain English*. Boston, MA: Wisdom.

Gyatso, T. (1998). *The art of happiness: A handbook for living (with H. C. Cutler)*. New York, NY: Riverhead Books.

Gyatso, T., & van den Muyzenberg, L. (2009). *The leader's way: The art of making the right decisions in our careers, our companies, and the world at large*. New York, NY: Broadway Books.

Hanh, T. (1991). In A. Kotler (Ed.), *Peace is every step: The path of mindfulness in everyday life*. New York, NY: Bantam Books.

Hanh, T. (1998). *Fragrant palm leaves: Journals 1962-1966*. New York, NY: Riverhead Books.

Hanh, T. (2008). Nothing to do, nowhere to go: Practices based on the teachings of Master Linji. In M. McLeod (Ed.), *The best Buddhist writing 2008* (pp. 54–68). Boston, MA: Shambhala.

Hawk, N., & Martin, B. (2011). Understanding and reducing stress in the superintendency. *Educational Management Administration & Leadership, 39*(3), 364–390.

Heck, R., Marcoulides, G., & Lang, P. (1991). Principal instructional leadership and school achievement: The application of discriminant techniques. *School Effectiveness and School Improvement*, 2(1), 115–135.

Helsing, D. (2007). Regarding uncertainty in teachers and teaching. *Teaching and Teacher Education, 23*, 1317–1333.

Horng, E., Klasik, D., & Loeb, S. (2010). Principal's time use and school effectiveness. *American Journal of Education, 116*(4), 491–523.

Hoy, W. (2003). An analysis of enabling and mindful school structures: Some theoretical, research and practical considerations. *Journal of Educational Administration, 41*(1), 87–108.

Hoy, W., Gage, C., & Tarter, C. (2006). School mindfulness and faculty trust: Necessary conditions for each other? *Educational Administration Quarterly, 42*(2), 236–255.

Jacobson, N. P. (1988). *The heart of Buddhist philosophy*. Carbondale, IL: Southern Illinois University Press.

Kabat-Zinn, J. (1994). *Wherever you go there you are: Mindfulness meditation in everyday life*. New York, NY: Hyperion Press.

Kabat-Zinn, J. (2003). Mindfulness-based interventions in context: past, present, and future. *Clinical Psychology: Science and Practice, 10*(2), 144–156.

Kaplan, H. (2002). Event reporting, mindfulness and the high reliability organization: Is the glass half empty? *Vox Sanguinis, 83*(Suppl. 1), 337–339.

Katagiri, D. (2008). *Each moment is the universe*. Boston, MA: Shambhala.

Langer, E. J. (1989). *Mindfulness*. Cambridge, MA: Da Capo Press.

Langer, E. J., & Moldoveanu, M. (2000). The construct of mindfulness. *Journal of Social Issues, 56*(1), 1–9.

Langer, E. J., & Piper, A. I. (1987). The prevention of mindlessness. *Journal of Personality and Social Psychology, 53*, 280–287.

LaPorte, T. R. (1996). HROs: Unlikely, demanding and at risk. *Journal of Contingencies and Crisis Management, 4*(2), 60–71.

LaPorte, T. R., & Consolini, P. M. (1991). Working in practice but not in theory: Theoretical challenges of "high-reliability organizations". *Journal of Public Administration Research and Theory: J-PART, 1*(1), 19–48.

Lee, J. (2006). *Tracking achievement gaps and assessing the impact of NCLB on the gaps: An in-depth look into national and state reading and math outcome trends*. Cambridge, MA: The Civil Rights Project at Harvard University.

Leithwood, K., & Beatty, B. (2009). Leadership for emotionally hot climates. *International Studies in Educational Administration, 37*(1), 91–103.

Leithwood, K., & Mascall, B. (2008). Collective leadership effects on student achievement. *Educational Administration Quarterly, 44*(4), 529–561.

Levinthal, D., & Rerup, C. (2006). Crossing an apparent chasm: Bridging mindful and less-mindful perspectives on organizational learning. *Organization Science, 17*(4), 502–513.

Loori, J. D. (2008). The great way. In M. McLeod (Ed.), *The best Buddhist writing 2008* (pp. 104–111). Boston, MA: Shambhala.

Lortie, D. (2009). *School principal: Managing in public*. Chicago, IL: University of Chicago Press.

Luyten, H., Visscher, A., & Witziers, B. (2005). School effectiveness research: From a review of the criticism to recommendations for further development. *School Effectiveness and School Improvement, 16*(3), 249–279.

Lyons, J., & Algozzine, B. (2006). Perceptions of the impact of accountability on the role of principals. *Education Policy Analysis Archives, 14*(16), 1–16.

Maxcy, B., & Nguyen, T. (2006). The politics of distributing leadership: Reconsidering leadership distribution in two Texas elementary schools. *Educational Policy, 20*(1), 163–196.

McClain, L., Ylimaki, R., & Ford, M. (2010). Wisdom and compassion in democratic leadership: Perceptions of the Bodhisattva ideal. *Journal of School Leadership, 20*, 323–351.

McDonald, T., & Gates, G. (2015). Mindfulness in educational leadership: Coping with stress and improving professional practice in the superintendency. In G. Gates (Ed.), *Mindfulness for educational practice* (pp. 59–80). Charlotte, NC: Information Age.

McDonnell, L. (2012). Educational accountability and policy feedback. *Educational Policy, 27*(2), 170–189.

McLeod, K. (2002). *Wake up to your life: Discovering the Buddhist path of attention*. New York, NY: HarperCollins.

Metzger, C. (2003). Self/inner development of educational administrators: A national study of urban school district superintendents and college deans. *Urban Education, 38*(6), 655–687.

Mintrop, H., & Sunderman, G. L. (2009). Predictable failure of federal sanctions-driven accountability for school improvement—And why we may retain it anyway. *Educational Researcher, 38*(5), 353–364.

Nairn, R. (1999). *Diamond mind: A psychology of meditation*. Boston, MA: Shambhala.

Nanda, J. (2009). Mindfulness: A lived experience of existential-phenomenological themes. *Existential Analysis, 20*(1), 147–162.

Nh'ãat, H. (2006). *Understanding our mind*. Berkeley, CA: Parallax Press.

Normore, A. H. (2004). The edge of chaos: School administrators and accountability. *Journal of Educational Administration, 42*(1), 55–77.

Palmer, P. (2007). *The courage to teach* (2nd ed.). San Francisco, CA: Jossey-Bass.

Parnes, B., Fernald, D., Quintela, J., Araya-Guerra, R., Westfall, J., Harris, D., & Pace, W. (2007). Stopping the error cascade. *Quality and Safety in Health Care, 16*, 12–16.

Rodgers, C. (2002). Defining reflection: Another look at John Dewey and reflective thinking. *Teachers College Record, 104*(4), 842–866.

Roeser, R. W. (2014). The emergence of mindfulness-based interventions in educational settings. In S. Karabenick & T. Urdan (Eds.), *Advances in motivation and achievement* (Interventions, Vol. 18). New York, NY: Emerald.

Roeser, R. W., Skinner, E., Beers, J., & Jennings, P. A. (2012). Mindfulness training and teachers' professional development: An emerging area of research and practice. *Child Development Perspectives, 6*, 167–173.

Rosch, E. (2008). More than mindfulness: When you have a tiger by the tail, let it eat you. *Psychological Inquiry, 18*(4), 258–264.

Rosenberg, L. (1998). *Breath by breath*. Boston, MA: Shambhala.

Sagan, S. (2004). The problem of redundancy problem: Why more nuclear security forces may produce less nuclear security. *Risk Analysis, 24*(4), 935–946.

Schoen, L., & Fusarelli, L. D. (2008). Innovation, NCLB, and the fear factor: The challenge of leading 21st-century schools in an era of accountability. *Educational Policy, 22*(1), 181–203.

Shields, C. (2004). Dialogic leadership for social justice: Overcoming pathologies of silence. *Educational Administration Quarterly, 40*(1), 109–132.

Starr, K. (2011). Principals and the politics of resistance to change. Educational Management Administration & Leadership, 39(6), 646–660.

Stringfield, S. (1996). Attempts to enhance students' learning: A search for valid programs and reliable, systemic implementation supports. In R. Blum & J. Arter (Eds.), *A handbook for student performance assessment in an era of restructuring* (pp. 2–6). Arlington, VA: Association for Supervision and Curriculum Development.

Stringfield, S., Reynolds, D., & Schaffer, E. (2008). Improving secondary students' academic achievement through a focus on reliability: 4- and 9-year findings from the High Reliability Schools project. *School Effectiveness and School Improvement, 19*(4), 409–428.

Sunim, H. (Ed.). (1999). *Only don't know*. Boston, MA: Shambhala.

Suzuki, S., & Dixon, T. (1970). *Zen mind, beginner's mind* (1st ed.). New York, NY: Walker/Weatherhill.

Swuste, P. (2008). "You will only see it, if you understand it" or occupational risk prevention from a management perspective. *Human Factors and Ergonomics in Manufacturing, 18*, 438–453.

Thompson, G., Warren, S., & Carter, L. (2004). It's not my fault: Predicting high school teachers who blame parents and students for students' low achievement. *The High School Journal, 87*(3), 5–14.

Van Dyck, C., Frese, M., Baer, M., & Sonnentag, S. (2005). Organizational error management culture and its impact on performance: A two-study replication. *Journal of Applied Psychology, 90*(6), 1228–1240.

Vogus, T., & Welbourne, T. (2003). Structuring for high reliability: HR practices and mindful processes in reliability-seeking organizations. *Journal of Organizational Behavior, 24*(7), 877–903.

Wahlstrom, K., & Seashore Louis, K. (2008). How teachers experience principal leadership: The roles of professional community, trust, efficacy, and shared responsibility. *Educational Administration Quarterly, 44*, 458–495.

Wears, R. L., & Nemeth, C. P. (2007). Replacing hindsight with insight: Toward better understanding of diagnostic failures. *Annals of Emergent Medicine, 49*(2), 206–209.

Weick, K. (2006). Faith, evidence, and action: Better guesses in an unknowable world. *Organization Studies, 27*(11), 1723 –1736.

Weick, K. E., & Putnam, T. (2006). Organizing for mindfulness: Eastern wisdom and Western knowledge. *Journal of Management Inquiry, 16*(3), 275.

Weick, K. E., & Roberts, K. H. (1993). Collective mind in organizations: Heedful interrelating on flight decks. *Administrative Science Quarterly, 38*(3), 357–381.

Weick, K. E., & Sutcliffe, K. M. (2001). *Managing the unexpected: Assuring high performance in an age of complexity* (1st ed.). San Francisco, CA: Jossey-Bass.

Weick, K. E., & Sutcliffe, K. M. (2006). Mindfulness and the quality of organizational attention. *Organization Science, 17*(4), 514–524.

Weick, K. E., & Sutcliffe, K. M. (2007). *Managing the unexpected: Resilient performance in an age of uncertainty* (2nd ed.). San Francisco, CA: Jossey-Bass.

Weick, K. E., Sutcliffe, K. M., & Obstfeld, D. (1999). Organizing for high reliability: Processes of collective mindfulness. *Research in Organizational Behavior, 21*, 81–123.

Woods, D. (2005). Creating foresight: Lessons for enhancing resilience from Columbia. In W. Starbuck & M. Farjoun (Eds.), *Organization at the limit: Lessons from the Colombia disaster* (pp. 289–308). Malden, MA: Blackwell.

York-Barr, J., & Duke, K. (2004). What do we know about teacher leadership? Findings from two decades of scholarship. *Review of Educational Research, 74*(3), 255–316.

Part III

Mindfulness in Education: Science and Applications with Students

Mindfulness Matters in the Classroom: The Effects of Mindfulness Training on Brain Development and Behavior in Children and Adolescents

17

Kristen E. Lyons and Jennifer DeLange

Introduction

A growing body of research suggests that even short-term mindfulness training may lead to changes in brain functioning and neuroanatomy. For example, mindfulness training has been found to improve the brain's ability to selectively focus attention (Jha, Krompinger, & Baime, 2007; Napoli, Krech, & Holley, 2005) and to increase the functional connectivity between brain regions (Kilpatrick et al., 2011), improving the brain's ability to efficiently process information. There is also evidence that mindfulness training physically reshapes the brain, both by increasing the density of brain in regions responsible for learning and memory (Hölzel, et al., 2010) and by strengthening the physical connections to brain regions involved in self-control (Tang et al., 2010). This research (which has primarily been conducted with adults) has led to a growing interest in bringing mindfulness training into school settings (e.g., Shapiro et al., 2015; Zelazo & Lyons, 2012), in order to improve academic achievement.

K.E. Lyons (✉) • J. DeLange
Metropolitan State University of Denver, Denver, CO, USA
e-mail: klyons7@msudenver.edu; jdelang1@msudenver.edu

The aim of this chapter is to provide an overview of the effects of mindfulness training in children and adolescents from a cognitive neuroscience perspective. There are good reasons, we believe, to suspect that integrating mindfulness exercises into classrooms may improve self-regulation, thereby increasing student's ability to learn and succeed academically. The chapter is divided into five sections: First, we review what mindfulness practice is, and how it can be implemented in classrooms at all ability and grade levels. Second, we explain the theoretical basis for why mindfulness practice should facilitate academic achievement from a cognitive neuroscience perspective. Third, we review specific research findings from developmental psychology and cognitive neuroscience on the effects of mindfulness training, and discuss directions for future research. Finally, we discuss practical guidelines for teachers and administrators who wish to integrate mindfulness practice into their schools and classrooms.

What is Mindfulness and How Is It Practiced?

Mindfulness is a contemplative practice that originated in the Buddhist tradition. It was popularized in the West and secularized by John Kabat-Zinn who developed the Mindfulness-Based Stress

K.A. Schonert-Reichl, R.W. Roeser (eds.), *Handbook of Mindfulness in Education*, Mindfulness in Behavioral Health, DOI 10.1007/978-1-4939-3506-2_17

Reduction (MBSR) program in 1979 as a way to help patients manage chronic illnesses, pain, and other medical conditions (Kabat-Zinn, 2003). This program and its derivatives (such as Mindfulness-Based Cognitive Therapy; Segal, Teasdale, & Williams, 2004) are now widely used with a variety of populations ranging from cancer patients (e.g., Ledesma & Kumano, 2009) and individuals suffering from mental health disorders (e.g., Goldin & Gross, 2010) to prisoners (e.g., Shonin, Van Gordon, Slade, & Griffiths, 2013), medical students (e.g., de Vibe et al., 2013), returning soldiers (e.g., Rees, 2011), and individuals dealing with normal day-to-day stress (e.g., Chiesa & Serretti, 2009).

In secular contexts, mindfulness is defined as paying attention, on purpose, to the present moment, with an attitude of kindness and nonreactivity (Kabat-Zinn, 2003). Conceptualized in this way, mindfulness training is not a specific regimen of actions or behaviors but rather is a general approach that one can take to a variety of life events. Therefore, one can practice mindfulness in a wide range of settings, ranging from a formal sitting or walking meditation to daily activities such as sharing a meal with a friend, to even mundane activities such as completing one's daily chores. Participating in a formal mindfulness training program, such as MBSR, is thought to facilitate individuals' ability to bring mindfulness to their daily life activities at home and at work or school.

The standard MBSR program consists of weekly group meetings supplemented by daily home practice (Kabat-Zinn, 2003). The program includes a variety of activities to practice different aspects of being mindful, though a few core exercises are repeatedly practiced throughout the course. One core practice is a meditation on one's breath. In this activity, individuals sit or lie down quietly while focusing their attention on their breath, focusing exclusively on each in-breath and each out-breath. If they notice that their attention has wandered (e.g., to thoughts about the future or the past), then their task is to gently bring their attention back to the present moment without judgment or reactivity. Another core practice in the program is the body scan, in which participants lie down quietly and successively attend to each part of their body, from the tip of their toes to the top of their heads, and simply notice how each part of their body feels without judging or reacting. If the mind wanders (as it will inevitably do), participants' task is to gently bring one's focus back to the body. Trained instructors or audio recordings guide participants through these meditations, which typically last between 15 min and 1 h.

Clearly, these kinds of activities are beyond the capabilities of most children, and even many adolescents. Therefore, educators and clinical practitioners have worked to adapt the core elements of mindfulness training to be more developmentally appropriate for use with children and adolescents. These adaptations typically include decreasing the duration of the practice, making the exercises less abstract (often by introducing physical props), and utilizing more movement-based activities (see Zelazo & Lyons, 2012). For example, to help preschoolers focus on their breath, teachers can have students place stuffed animals on their bellies and "rock them to sleep" with their breathing (e.g., Hawn Foundation, 2011; Kaiser-Greenland, 2010). To practice the body scan, teachers can have students stand and use a real or imaginary hula-hoop to successively "scan" the different parts of their bodies (e.g., Johnson, Forston, Gunnar, & Zelazo, 2011).

When teaching mindfulness to older children and adolescents, training activities should become gradually more abstract with increasing grade levels to correspond with age-related increases in children's ability to think abstractly and metacognitively reflect on their thinking (Flavell, Miller, & Miller, 1985). For example, young adolescents may practice mindful awareness of thoughts by imagining that they are standing high on a hill looking down at a train, with each train car carrying one of their thoughts—with their task being to simply notice each thought as it passes by without adding emotional responses or cognitive judgments (Broderick, 2013). Older adolescents may be given even less scaffolding, for example, practicing mindfulness of emotions by being told to ride the waves of their emotions like a surfer riding a wave (Broderick, 2013).

In addition to these more formal activities, students can practice brief moments of mindfulness throughout the school day. For example, a teacher might ring a bell which prompts students to pause and take five mindful breaths (e.g., at the start of a new activity or when the students return from recess). Students can also pick an activity, such as writing their name or opening a door, and practice bringing full mindful awareness to this routine activity every day for a week. Teachers can also integrate mindfulness into regular school activities, such as by asking high school students to notice with all of their senses what they are observing in chemistry class or to mindfully notice their emotions as they read a poem (see other chapters in this volume for details).

Thus, there is increasing evidence that students of all grade and ability levels can practice mindfulness if educators implement it in developmentally appropriate ways based on the cognitive and emotional maturity level of their students. To facilitate this, there are now several commercially available programs and curricula for teaching mindfulness to students from preschoolers to high school students, including *MindUp* (Hawn Foundation, 2011), *Inner Kids* (Kaiser-Greenland, 2010), *Stressed Teens* (Biegel, 2010), and *Learning to Breathe* (Broderick, 2013). Most of these programs include books or lesson plans, as well as teacher training programs to help prepare teachers to lead their students through the practices.

Why Should Students Practice Mindfulness?

The widespread popularity of the MBSR program can be attributed to its significant impacts on health and well-being. Short-term mindfulness training (lasting from a few days to a few weeks) has been found to reduce stress (e.g., Shapiro, Astin, Bishop, & Cordova, 2005), alleviate mental health symptoms (Hofmann, Sawyer, Witt, & Oh, 2010; Teasdale et al., 2000), and increase subjective well-being (Carmody & Baer, 2008). Training has also been found to improve overall physical health (Grossman, Niemann, Schmidt, & Walach, 2004) and boost immune functioning (Davidson et al., 2003). Most relevant for educators, there is also strong evidence that mindfulness training in healthy nonclinical populations improves self-regulation (Chiesa, Calati, & Serretti, 2011; Shapiro et al., 2015; Zelazo & Lyons, 2012), with associated changes observed in brain structure (Hölzel et al., 2011; Tang et al., 2010) and brain function (e.g., Goldin & Gross, 2010; Kozasa et al., 2012).

Self-regulation involves a variety of automatic and consciously controlled processes that are critical for success in school and in life. Self-regulation includes both executive function (i.e., the ability to selectively focus and sustain attention, inhibit inappropriate responses, flexibly shift in response to changing task demands, and maintain and manipulate information in working memory; Zelazo, Carlson, & Kesek, 2008) and emotion-regulation (i.e., the ability to control how one experiences and expresses emotions; Gross, 1998). A number of studies have demonstrated that childhood self-regulation is a robust predictor of success in school (Blair & Diamond, 2008; Ursache, Blair, & Raver, 2012), and longitudinal studies have found that childhood self-regulation predicts physical health, addiction status, income, and criminal activity in adulthood, even after controlling for IQ and the family of origin's socioeconomic status (Moffitt et al., 2011). Thus, interventions that improve self-regulation are likely to have immediate as well as cascading benefits for students.

Mindfulness training is an ideal intervention for improving self-regulation because it targets both "top down" aspects of self-regulation (i.e., conscious control over one's attention, actions, and emotions) and simultaneously dampens "bottom up" reactivity (i.e., automatic responses such as anger or fear or value judgments) that interfere with students' ability to pay attention and learn (Zelazo & Lyons, 2012). This may be particularly helpful in classroom settings, where teachers are expected to promote the development of large numbers of students who may vary in the areas of self-regulation in which they need improvement.

A second reason that educators should consider implementing mindfulness training in schools is that the robust effects of training that have been found in adults are likely to be even more robust if training is implemented during childhood or adolescence. This is because the brain is more plastic (i.e., more likely to be affected by environmental inputs) in earlier developmental periods (Huttenlocher, 2009). By introducing mindfulness practices to their students when the neural networks supporting cognitive control and emotion-regulation are still developing (Giedd et al., 1999), teachers can literally help shape the development of these regions in their students' brains. These changes are likely to have profound impacts on students' ability to succeed in school by increasing students' ability to consciously control their attention, keep in mind and manipulate information, inhibit inappropriate responses, and by reducing the influence of negative emotional responses that impede school achievement (Roeser & Peck, 2009).

In short, mindfulness training has the potential to train students' brains so that they are better equipped to learn. Given the rather minimal costs in terms of time and money of implementing mindfulness training and the potential for cascading benefits, it is easy to justify the infusion of mindfulness training into schools.

The Impact of Mindfulness Training on Self-Control Behavior and the Brain

Over the last 15 years, there has been a surge of research investigating the effects of mindfulness training in healthy adults (e.g., Chiesa et al., 2011; Tang et al., 2007). This research has provided evidence that mindfulness training may lead to improvements in at least two aspects of self-regulation that are of critical importance for success in school and success in life, namely executive function (EF) and emotion-regulation (Grossman et al., 2004; Tang & Posner, 2009). More recently, research has begun to investigate whether such training effects are also observed in children and adolescents. This research is much more preliminary (Burke, 2010; Shapiro et al., 2015; Zelazo & Lyons, 2012) although there are promising reasons to suspect that mindfulness training may be an effective way to improve self-control in both typically and atypically developing youth.

Effects of Mindfulness Training on Executive Function

Effects on Attention The capacity to selectively focus and sustain attention is fundamental to learning. The first step in encoding material is attending to it: If students cannot ignore irrelevant distractions (e.g., noise from their classmates or text messages from friends) to maintain their focus on their class work or homework, information simply cannot be encoded into long-term memory (Cowan, 1988). Students who are better able to focus and sustain their attention will also likely do better on exams, when they must ignore distractions to focus on the task at hand.

Research consistently shows that mindfulness training improves adults' performance on tests of selective attention (Chiesa et al., 2011; Jha, Stanley, Kiyonaga, Wong, & Gelfand, 2010; Tang & Posner, 2009). Recently, investigators have begun to explore whether mindfulness training in youth leads to similar improvements; preliminary findings suggest that this may be the case. For example, Johnson et al. (2011) found that 5 weeks of mindfulness training improved preschoolers' performance on the Flanker Task, a measure of selective attention; in contrast, no changes were observed from pre- to post-test in an active control (literacy training) group. Similar effects have been observed in elementary school students: Napoli et al. (2005) found that mindfulness-based training implemented in school over the course of several months led to greater improvements on teacher-ratings of student attention and students' performance on behavioral tests of selective attention relative to a control group of children who did not complete training. Among adolescents, there is preliminary evidence to suggest that mindfulness training administered in a clinical setting reduces parent-reported attention problems among early adolescents (e.g., Semple, Lee, Rosa, & Miller, 2010).

To date, no studies have investigated the effects of mindfulness training on children's or adolescents' brain structure or functioning (an important direction for future research). However, it seems reasonable to speculate that similar mechanisms of change that have been observed in adults are also likely to be observed in children. Thus, one might extrapolate that the observed improvements on behavioral measures of selective attention in children are likely to be supported by increases in functional brain activity in the anterior cingulate, a region of the brain implicated in conflict monitoring and resolution (e.g., Hölzel et al., 2007). Behavioral changes may also be accompanied by structural changes in the density of neural connections to this region, as has been observed in adults (Tang et al., 2010; Tang, Lu, Fan, Yang, & Posner, 2012). Future research is needed to investigate whether these effects of mindfulness training that have been observed in adults extend to children's and adolescents' brain function and structure.

Effects on Working Memory Working memory is the ability to keep in mind and manipulate information (Baddeley, 1992). The classic (now perhaps outdated) example of working memory is attempting to keep in mind a phone number before being able to write it down. Research indicates that working memory is a more robust predictor of school achievement than IQ (Alloway & Alloway, 2010), perhaps because the need for reliance on working memory in school is so pervasive. According to information processing theory, working memory serves as a gateway into long-term memory: If information is attended to, then it will pass into working memory, but what happens while the information is in working memory determines whether the information will be transferred to long-term memory or be forgotten (Baddeley, 1992; Baddeley & Hitch, 1974; Shiffrin & Schneider, 1977). Working memory also influences how well students can solve a variety of academic problems (e.g., Passolunghi & Siegel 2004; Swanson & Sachse-Lee, 2001). For example, when solving a word problem on a math assignment, students must rely on working memory to read and make sense of the prompt to figure out what question is being asked of them, identify the relevant information, and compute the appropriate algorithm. At a more mundane level, students must rely on working memory to keep in mind directions so as to be able to complete assignments and follow classroom guidelines. Failing to do so can lead to failure to adequately complete assignments and poorer quality relationships with teachers, which are associated with poorer school achievement (Hamre & Pianta, 2006).

As with attention, research with adults has shown that mindfulness training improves performance on measures of working memory (e.g., Jha et al., 2010; Mrazek, Franklin, Phillips, Baird, & Schooler, 2013). There is also some initial evidence from developmental studies that mindfulness training administered in schools improves working memory. For example, one study found that parents reported improvement in their children's working memory after mindfulness training in elementary school students who initially scored low in EF (Flook et al., 2010). To date, there is not good documentation that mindfulness training improves performance on behavioral tests of working memory in children, but there is ample evidence that working memory can be improved via computerized training regimens in both children and adults, and that such training leads to increases in functional brain activity in regions supporting working memory, including prefrontal and somatosensory regions (see Klingberg, 2010 for a review). It remains to be seen whether similar effects will be observed as a result of mindfulness training in children.

Effects on Inhibitory Control Inhibitory control is the ability to stop oneself from making an inappropriate response (Munakata et al., 2011). The ability to prevent oneself from acting in ways that one should not develop dramatically over the course of childhood and adolescence (Zelazo & Carlson, 2012), anecdotally illustrated by children's difficulty with games such as *Simon Says* or *Red Light Green Light*. In school settings, inhibitory control is important for helping students to stay on task (e.g., preventing oneself from chatting with a friend when one is supposed to be concentrating on a math assignment), follow classroom rules (e.g., not blurting out the answer, but instead raising one's hand), and maintain positive social relationships with other students and the teacher (e.g., by not hitting or saying mean things when one gets upset) (Best, Miller, & Naglieri, 2011; Fitzpatrick, McKinnon, Blair, & Willoughby, 2014). Inhibitory control is also important in testing situations, in which one must inhibit giving wrong answers that may come to mind quickly but are in fact incorrect.

Inhibitory control has not been a traditional target of mindfulness training in research with adults. However, a number of studies with children and adolescents have documented that mindfulness training reduces behavioral problems stemming from poor inhibitory control in children and adolescents with behavioral problems (Van de Weijer-Bergsma, Formsma, de Bruin, & Bögels, 2012; Van der Oord, Bögels, & Peijnenburg 2012; Zylowska et al., 2008). There is also preliminary evidence that training teachers in mindfulness leads to reductions in typically developing preschoolers' problem behaviors, such as hitting, biting, screaming, and destroying physical property (Singh, Lancioni, Winton, Karazsia, & Singh, 2013), perhaps due to improvements in inhibitory control. Among typically developing adolescents, trait levels of mindfulness, assessed using self-report questionnaires, correlate with scores on tests of inhibitory control (Oberle, Schonert-Reichl, Lawlor, & Thomson, 2012). Thus, it seems reasonable to suspect that training in mindfulness may lead to improvements in inhibitory control in children and adolescents. Given the lack of research on the effects of mindfulness training on inhibitory control in adults, it is difficult to speculate about specific ways that training may cause changes in functional brain activity during inhibitory control tasks. However, one might hypothesize that behavioral changes in this ability are likely to be supported by more efficient functioning in the neural network documented to support inhibitory control, namely the frontal and parietal cortices (Rubia et al., 2001).

Effects of Mindfulness Training on Emotion-Regulation

Emotion-regulation is a multifaceted process that involves both the experience of emotions (e.g., the extent to which one is able to prevent oneself from becoming overwhelmed by feelings of sadness or anger) and the expression of emotions (e.g., the extent to which one is able to control when and how emotional responses are displayed; Gross, 2002). Emotions are a powerful force, influencing how well other psychological functions operate with the potential to facilitate, as well as impede, cognitive function (Cole, Martin, & Dennis, 2004). Similar neural networks support emotion-regulation and cognitive control (Etkin, Egner, & Kalisch, 2011), including regions implicated in self-awareness and self-correction, such as the anterior cingulate and medial prefrontal cortices. In other words, cognitive and affective functions are yoked together the brain. Hence, emotional and cognitive processes have considerable influence over one another.

Because of the integration between emotional and cognitive processes, adept emotion-regulation is fundamental to school success. Individual differences in emotion-regulation have been found to predict adaptive social functioning in preschoolers (Rubin, Coplan, Fox, & Calkins, 1995); school readiness and academic competence in early childhood (Ursache et al., 2012); academic success and productivity in the classroom; and standardized early literacy and math achievement scores (Graziano, Reavis, Keane, & Calkins, 2007). Findings by Graziano et al. (2007) also suggest that children who have difficulty regulating their emotions have trouble learning in the classroom and are less productive and accurate when completing assignments. Hence, interventions that improve children's ability to regulate their emotions have the potential to impart a number of benefits that directly contribute to academic success.

Research suggests that mindfulness practice in children and adolescents is associated with increased emotional well-being and decreased emotional distress (e.g., Biegel, Brown, Shapiro, & Schubert, 2009; Kuyken et al., 2013; Semple et al., 2010). Youth trained in mindfulness have been found to report lower levels of psychological distress and increased self-esteem (Tan & Martin, 2012). They have also been found to report lower levels of conflict, anxiety, and stress (Sibinga et al., 2013), as well as a reduced tendency to develop suicidal ideation or thoughts of self-harm (classic examples of emotional dysregulation; Britton et al., 2014).

Even when reporting sadness, adults who have been trained in mindfulness show distinct neural responses. Specifically, they are more likely to activate regions of the brain associated with body sensations and less likely to activate regions of the brain associated with emotional reactivity (Farb et al., 2010). The tendency to recruit regions associated with body sensations during sadness is associated with reduced symptoms of depression. Hence, mindfulness training may facilitate individuals' ability to maintain emotional equilibrium, even in the face of negative emotions or life events. How such issues play out in children and adolescents remains unknown at this point.

Regulation of negative emotion through mindful practices has been shown to increase activity in areas of the brain associated with conscious control of behaviors (regions of the prefrontal cortex) and decrease activity in areas associated with automatic emotional reactions (namely, the amygdala) (Modinos, Ormel, & Aleman, 2010). Research indicates that there is an inverse correlation between activities in the two brain regions, suggesting that increased activity in the prefrontal cortex serves to downregulate activation in the amygdala. Ochsner, Bunge, Gross, and Gabrieli (2002) have also found that mindfulness may moderate activity in the neural networks that are used in the cognitive control of negative emotion. Taken together, these findings support the notion that mindfulness practice modulates brain activity in multiple emotion processing systems, contributing to an overall improved ability to control how and when emotions are experienced and expressed.

Directions for Future Research

Research on the effects of mindfulness training for youth is still very preliminary (Burke, 2010; Greenberg & Harris, 2012; Shapiro et al., 2015; Zelazo & Lyons, 2012). A number of studies have demonstrated the feasibility of conducting mindfulness training with youth of all ages (see Shapiro et al., 2015 for a review), as well as the feasibility of implementing such training among typically and atypically developing youth (Burke, 2010; Zoogman, Goldberg, Hoyt, & Miller, 2015). In recent years, studies have begun to investigate whether such training has demonstrable effects on cognitive and affective regulation in children and adolescents (Shapiro et al., 2015; Zoogman et al., 2015) with most studies finding that there are significant improvements in children and adolescents as a result of training (Zoogman et al., 2015). Nevertheless, there are clear gaps in the literature and a number of open questions concerning the efficacy of mindfulness training for children and adolescents.

Much of the extant literature on the effects of mindfulness training (in adults and children) has serious methodological limitations (Davidson, 2010; Greenberg & Harris, 2012). One primary concern is the lack of adequate control groups. According to a recent meta analysis, of 20 published studies investigating the effects of mindfulness training for youth, only about half included an active control group (Zoogman et al., 2015). Many studies have simply used a pre-/post-test design with no control group, or compared outcomes in the trained group to a passive "wait-list" control group.

To determine if mindfulness training improves neurocognitive functioning in children and adolescents, it is necessary to compare outcomes between those who participate in mindfulness training and those who participate an active control training condition matched in terms of superficial characteristics (e.g., receiving special instruction in small groups, receiving daily home practice activities). The challenge for researchers is to select a training program that controls for these elements and does not inadvertently tap into any of the core elements of mindfulness training thought to drive change (i.e., practicing paying attention with purpose and nonreactivity). Designing a study with an appropriate control group can be challenging, as many "control" training programs may indirectly train these capacities (e.g., taking a health class may cause participants to attend more to their physical activity and notice the food they are eating; participating in a book-reading class may lead to practice in metacognitive reflection). Nonetheless, more rigorous comparisons to active control groups (e.g., a relaxation training condition) will be required for research in this area to advance beyond its current preliminary state.

A second important direction for future research concerns the kinds of outcome measures that are included. To date, many studies in this area have relied on self-, parent-, or teacher-reports. This can raise issues of validity and reliability, as individuals performing the assessment are likely to be informed of the child's training status, and therefore may be biased in their observations or reports. Studies therefore should also include behavioral outcome measures (such as standardized or computerized tests) to assess whether objective changes have occurred.

Third, few (if any) studies with children and adolescents have examined whether there are developmental differences in the efficacy of training. This type of design presents challenges, as the training activities and assessments that are developmentally appropriate for one age group may not be developmentally appropriate for use with another age group. Overcoming this challenge is important for both theory and practice, as it will inform us as to the ages at which mindfulness training is most impactful and when teachers should begin implementing mindfulness training with their students.

Fourth, future research should investigate the moderators of training efficacy. Training is unlikely to be equally effective for all individuals; thus, it is important to determine who is most likely to benefit from training. For example, there is some preliminary evidence that those who are initially poorer in terms of self-control tend to benefit more from training (Flook et al., 2005; Zoogman et al., 2015). Future research with children and adolescents should investigate the extent to which preexisting individual differences in cognitive or emotional maturity predict change as a result of trainings.

In a similar vein, not all training is likely to be equally effective. Varying the duration, frequency, and instructor of training may impact training efficacy for children and adolescents. For example, correlational research indicates that in training studies, some participants practice more regularly than others, and those that do show more improvements at post-testing (e.g., Huppert & Johnson, 2010). Although it is tempting to attribute the relatively greater improvement as resulting from the increased frequency of practice, it is possible that a third variable may drive this relationship (e.g., that individuals who practiced more frequently faced overall higher levels of stress and that higher levels of stress predict greater change as a result of mindfulness training). To determine whether training frequency influences training efficacy, carefully controlled research needs to test this experimentally. Likewise, experimental studies are needed to determine the ideal duration of training (e.g., in terms of weeks) and length of individual training activities. Such information will be instrumental in guiding teachers' decisions about when and how to implement mindfulness training in schools. Of course, these dimensions are likely to differ between children of different grade and ability levels, posing an additional question for future research.

Another aspect of training that is important to investigate is the characteristics of the trainer and the degree of teacher training required for training to be effective. Many people have argued that it is necessary for teachers to have their own mindfulness practice in order to teach mindfulness to others (e.g., Burke, 2010); however, the degree of teacher training that is necessary to impart change in students has yet to be determined experimentally. If mindfulness training is to be scaled up from small intervention studies to a mainstream educational practice, it is likely not feasible to require all teachers to have a deep mindfulness meditation practice of their own. Future studies should examine what degree of training is necessary for teachers to be able to effectively train their students.

In addition, while teachers are likely to be the primary source of training, an open question concerns the role of parents in supporting mindfulness practice in youth. Many studies have documented that targeting parents is an effective way to improve outcomes in children (e.g., Golan & Crow, 2004; Koutakis, Stattin, & Kerr, 2008). Investigating whether mindfulness interventions that include parents as well as children are more effective than those targeting children alone is an important question that ought to be addressed experimentally.

Finally, future research with children and adolescents should investigate the mechanisms of change by which mindfulness practice causes changes in the brain and behavior. In particular, it is important to identify how the *active ingredients* of mindfulness training (e.g., sustained attention, nonreactivity) impact different aspects of self-control (e.g., selective attention, working memory, emotion-regulation). This line of research would be invaluable to teachers to help them determine how best to help students with needs for improvement. It would also help researchers to better understand how self-control develops, and why there are such dramatic individual differences in this ability.

How Should Educators Implement Mindfulness Training?

The most important principle for teachers to keep in mind when implementing mindfulness training is: *use it or lose it*. The brain is literally shaped by experience; neural connections that are used more frequently become strengthened while neural connections that are used infrequently fade away (e.g., Neville & Bavelier, 1998; Rosenzweig & Bennett, 1996). In this way, the brain adapts to environmental demands, becoming more efficient and preparing the developing human to thrive in the environment in which he or she will live.

One of the basic principles of learning is that spaced practice is superior to an equal amount of condensed practice (Cepeda, Pashler, Vul, Wixted, & Rohrer, 2006). In other words, it is better to practice something in short spurts spread out over a longer period of time than to "cram" the same amount of practice into a short period of time. Thus, teachers should institute short mindfulness practices throughout the school day rather than scheduling one extended period of formal practice each day.

In addition to implementing more formal mindfulness training activities, teachers should also infuse mindful inquiry into otherwise standard lessons (e.g., asking students to focus on their sensory experiences during chemistry class, prompting students to attend to their breathing during physical education, or asking students to reflect on their thoughts during a social studies or literature lesson). Doing so is likely to be beneficial for several reasons. First, students are better able to retain new information if it is integrated into an existing schema (Brewer & Nakamura, 1984). By capitalizing on their students' preexisting knowledge (e.g., about chemistry or literature), teachers can help students to better retain the basic principles of mindful awareness, weaving this new knowledge into their students' existing mental frameworks. Second, by practicing mindfulness in a variety of contexts, students have the opportunity to draw connections between how mindfulness is practiced in different settings, thereby processing elements of the practice at a deeper level (Craik & Tulving, 1975). In addition, decontextualization of mindfulness practice is likely to lead to better transfer, enabling students to see that mindfulness can be brought to a wide variety of problems and settings to help students better focus and manage their emotional responses (Perkins & Salomon, 1989).

Of course, before implementing mindfulness training in their classrooms, teachers should complete appropriate training. Adequate training is necessary to ensure that training is likely to be effective. Training is also important because, while the risks of mindfulness training are minimal, teachers should be cautioned that promoting mindful awareness may lead some students to become aware of negative emotions which were previously not a focus of their conscious attention (e.g., Broderick, 2013). Knowing how to best manage these kinds of responses is critical, if mindfulness training is to be implemented in schools.

Conclusions

Over the last decade, there has been a surge of interest in bringing mindfulness training to children and youth. Though the field of developmental contemplative science that studies mindfulness training in children and youth is still in its infancy in many ways (Roeser & Zelazo, 2012), it holds much promise. By integrating mindfulness practice into the school day, teachers can promote self-control, emotional well-being, and academic achievement in their students, with potential benefits extending from the early life into adulthood.

References

Alloway, T. P., & Alloway, R. G. (2010). Investigating the predictive roles of working memory and IQ in academic attainment. *Journal of Experimental Child Psychology, 106*, 20–29. doi:10.1016/j.jecp.2009.11.003.

Baddeley, A. (1992). Working memory. *Science, 255*, 556–559.

Baddeley, A. D., & Hitch, G. (1974). Working memory. *Psychology of Learning and Motivation, 8*, 47–89.

Best, J. R., Miller, P. H., & Naglieri, J. A. (2011). Relations between executive function and academic achievement from ages 5 to 17 in a large, representative national sample. *Learning and Individual Differences, 21*, 327–336. doi:10.1016/j.lindif.2011.01.007.

Biegel, G. (2010). *The stress reduction workbook for teens: Mindfulness skills to help you deal with stress.* Oakland, CA: New Harbinger Publications.

Biegel, G. M., Brown, K. W., Shapiro, S. L., & Schubert, C. M. (2009). Mindfulness-based stress reduction for the treatment of adolescent psychiatric outpatients: A randomized clinical trial. *Journal of Consulting and Clinical Psychology, 77*, 855–866. doi:10.1037/a0016241.

Blair, C., & Diamond, A. (2008). Biological processes in prevention and intervention: The promotion of self-regulation as a means of preventing school failure. *Development and Psychopathology, 20*, 899–911. http://dx.doi.org/10.1017/S0954579408000436.

Brewer, W. F., & Nakamura, G. V. (1984). The nature and functions of schemas. In R. S. Wyer Jr. & T. K. Srull (Eds.), *Handbook of social cognition* (pp. 119–160). Hillsdale, NJ: Erlbaum.

Britton, W. B., Lepp, N. E., Niles, H. F., Rocha, T., Fisher, N. E., & Gold, J. S. (2014). A randomized controlled pilot trial of classroom-based mindfulness meditation compared to an active control condition in sixth-grade children. *Journal of School Psychology, 52*, 263–278. doi:10.1016/j.jsp.2014.03.002.

Broderick, P. C. (2013). *Learning to breathe: A mindfulness curriculum for adolescents to cultivate emotion regulation, attention, and performance*. Oakland, CA: New Harbinger Publications.

Burke, C. A. (2010). Mindfulness-based approaches with children and adolescents: A preliminary review of current research in an emergent field. *Journal of Child and Family Studies, 19*, 133–144. doi:10.1007/s10826-009-9282-x.

Carmody, J., & Baer, R. A. (2008). Relationships between mindfulness practice and levels of mindfulness, medical and psychological symptoms and well-being in a mindfulness-based stress reduction program. *Journal of Behavioral Medicine, 31*, 23–33. doi:10.1007/s10865-007-9130-7.

Cepeda, N. J., Pashler, H., Vul, E., Wixted, J. T., & Rohrer, D. (2006). Distributed practice in verbal recall tasks: A review and quantitative synthesis. *Psychological Bulletin, 132*, 354–380. doi:10.1037/0033-2909.132.3.354.

Chiesa, A., Calati, R., & Serretti, A. (2011). Does mindfulness training improve cognitive abilities? A systematic review of neuropsychological findings. *Clinical Psychology Review, 31*, 449–464. doi:10.1016/j.cpr.2010.11.003.

Chiesa, A., & Serretti, A. (2009). Mindfulness-based stress reduction for stress management in healthy people: A review and meta-analysis. *The Journal of Alternative and Complementary Medicine, 15*, 593–600. doi:10.1089/acm.2008.0495.

Cole, P. M., Martin, S. E., & Dennis, T. A. (2004). Emotion regulation as a scientific construct: Methodological challenges and directions for child development research. *Child Development, 75*, 317–333. doi:10.1111/j.1467-8624.2004.00673.x.

Cowan, N. (1988). Evolving conceptions of memory storage, selective attention, and their mutual constraints within the human information-processing system. *Psychological Bulletin, 104*, 163. doi:10.1037/0033-2909.104.2.163.

Craik, F. I., & Tulving, E. (1975). Depth of processing and the retention of words in episodic memory. *Journal of Experimental Psychology: General, 104*, 268. doi:10.1037/0096-3445.104.3.268.

Davidson, R. J. (2010). Empirical explorations of mindfulness: Conceptual and methodological conundrums. *Emotion, 10*, 8–11. doi:10.1037/a0018480.
Davidson, R. J., Kabat-Zinn, J., Schumacher, J., Rosenkranz, M., Muller, D., Santorelli, S. F., ... Sheridan, J. F. (2003). Alterations in brain and immune function produced by mindfulness meditation. *Psychosomatic Medicine, 65*, 564–570. doi:10.1097/01.PSY.0000077505.67574.E3.
de Vibe, M., Solhaug, I., Tyssen, R., Friborg, O., Rosenvinge, J. H., Sørlie, T., & Bjørndal, A. (2013). Mindfulness training for stress management: A randomised controlled study of medical and psychology students. *BMC Medical Education, 13*, 107. doi:10.1186/1472-6920-13-107.
Etkin, A., Egner, T., & Kalisch, R. (2011). Emotional processing in anterior cingulate and medial prefrontal cortex. *Trends in Cognitive Sciences, 15*, 85–93. doi:10.1016/j.tics.2010.11.004.
Farb, N. A., Anderson, A. K., Mayberg, H., Bean, J., McKeon, D., & Segal, Z. V. (2010). Minding one's emotions: Mindfulness training alters the neural expression of sadness. *Emotion, 10*, 25–33. doi:10.1037/a0017151.
Fitzpatrick, C., McKinnon, R. D., Blair, C. B., & Willoughby, M. T. (2014). Do preschool executive function skills explain the school readiness gap between advantaged and disadvantaged children? *Learning and Instruction, 30*, 25–31. doi:10.1016/j.learninstruc.2013.11.003.
Flavell, J. H., Miller, P. H., & Miller, S. A. (1985). *Cognitive development*. Englewood Cliffs, NJ: Prentice-Hall.
Flook, L., Smalley, S., Kitil, J., Galla, B., Kaiser-Greenland, S., Locke, J., & Kasari, C. (2010). Effects of mindful awareness practices on executive functions in elementary school children. *Journal of Applied School Psychology, 26*(1), 70–95. doi.10.1080/15377900903379125.
Giedd, J. N., Blumenthal, J., Jeffries, N. O., Castellanos, F. X., Liu, H., Zijdenbos, A., ... Rapoport, J. L. (1999). Brain development during childhood and adolescence: A longitudinal MRI study. *Nature Neuroscience, 2*, 861–863. doi:10.1038/13158.
Golan, M., & Crow, S. (2004). Targeting parents exclusively in the treatment of childhood obesity: Long-term results. *Obesity Research, 12*, 357–361. doi:10.1038/oby.2004.45.
Goldin, P. R., & Gross, J. J. (2010). Effects of mindfulness-based stress reduction (MBSR) on emotion regulation in social anxiety disorder. *Emotion, 10*, 83–91. doi:10.1037/a0018441.
Graziano, P. A., Reavis, R. D., Keane, S. P., & Calkins, S. D. (2007). The role of emotion regulation in children's early academic success. *Journal of School Psychology, 45*, 3–19. doi:10.1016/j.jsp.2006.09.002.
Greenberg, M. T., & Harris, A. R. (2012). Nurturing mindfulness in children and youth: Current state of research. *Child Development Perspectives, 6*, 161–166. doi:10.1111/j.1750-8606.2011.00215.x.
Gross, J. J. (1998). Antecedent-and response-focused emotion regulation: Divergent consequences for experience, expression, and physiology. *Journal of Personality and Social Psychology, 74*, 224. doi:10.1037/0022-3514.74.1.224.
Gross, J. J. (2002). Emotion regulation: Affective, cognitive, and social consequences. *Psychophysiology, 39*, 281–291. doi:10.1017/S0048577201393198.
Grossman, P., Niemann, L., Schmidt, S., & Walach, H. (2004). Mindfulness-based stress reduction and health benefits: A meta-analysis. *Journal of Psychosomatic Research, 57*, 35–43. doi:10.1016/S0022-3999(03)00573-7.
Hamre, B. K. & Pianta, R. C. (2006). Student-teacher relationships. In: Bear, George G. and Minke, Kathleen M. (Ed). Children's needs III: Development, prevention, and intervention, (pp. 59–71). Washington, DC, US: National Association of School Psychologists.
Hawn Foundation. (2011). *The MindUP curriculum: Brain-focused strategies for learning and living*. New York, NY: Scholastic.
Hofmann, S. G., Sawyer, A. T., Witt, A. A., & Oh, D. (2010). The effect of mindfulness-based therapy on anxiety and depression: A meta-analytic review. *Journal of Consulting and Clinical Psychology, 78*, 169. doi:10.1037/a0018555.
Hölzel, B. K., Carmody, J., Vangel, M., Congleton, C., Yerramsetti, S. M., Gard, T., & Lazar, S. W. (2011). Mindfulness practice leads to increases in regional brain gray matter density. *Psychiatry Research: Neuroimaging, 191*, 36–43. doi:10.1016/j.pscychresns.2010.08.006.
Hölzel, B. K., Ott, U., Hempel, H., Hackl, A., Wolf, K., Stark, R., & Vaitl, D. (2007). Differential engagement of anterior cingulate and adjacent medial frontal cortex in adept meditators and non-meditators. *Neuroscience Letters, 421*, 16–21. doi:10.1016/j.neulet.2007.04.074.
Hölzel, B. K., Carmody, J., Evans, K. C., Hoge, E. A., Dusek, J. A., Morgan, L., & Lazar, S. W. (2010). Stress reduction correlates with structural changes in the amygdala. *Social Cognitive and Affective Neuroscience, 5*(1), 11–17. http://doi.org/10.1093/scan/nsp034.
Huppert, F. A., & Johnson, D. M. (2010). A controlled trial of mindfulness training in schools: The importance of practice for an impact on well-being. *The Journal of Positive Psychology, 5*, 264–274. doi:10.1080/17439761003794148.
Huttenlocher, P. R. (2009). *Neural plasticity*. Cambridge, MA: Harvard University Press.
Jha, A. P., Krompinger, J., & Baime, M. J. (2007). Mindfulness training modifies subsystems of attention. *Cognitive, Affective, & Behavioral Neuroscience, 7*, 109–119.
Jha, A. P., Stanley, E. A., Kiyonaga, A., Wong, L., & Gelfand, L. (2010). Examining the protective effects of mindfulness training on working memory capacity and affective experience. *Emotion, 10*, 54. doi:10.1037/a0018438.

Johnson, A. E., Forston, J. L., Gunnar, M. R., & Zelazo, P. D. (2011). *A randomized controlled trial of mindfulness meditation training in preschool children.* Poster presented at the Biennial Meeting of the Society for Research in Child Development, Montreal, QC.

Kabat-Zinn, J. (2003). Mindfulness-based interventions in context: Past, present, and future. *Clinical Psychology: Science and Practice, 10*, 144–156. doi:10.1093/clipsy.bpg016.

Kaiser-Greenland, S. (2010). *The mindful child: How to help your kid manage stress and become happier, kinder, and more compassionate*. New York, NY: Simon and Schuster.

Kilpatrick, L. A., Suyenobu, B. Y., Smith, S. R., Bueller, J. A., Goodman, T., Creswell, J. D., … Naliboff, B. D. (2011). Impact of mindfulness-based stress reduction training on intrinsic brain connectivity. *NeuroImage, 56*, 290–298. doi:10.1016/j.neuroimage.2011.02.034.

Klingberg, T. (2010). Training and plasticity of working memory. *Trends in Cognitive Sciences, 14*, 317–324. doi:10.1016/j.tics.2010.05.002.

Koutakis, N., Stattin, H., & Kerr, M. (2008). Reducing youth alcohol drinking through a parent–targeted intervention: The Örebro Prevention Program. *Addiction, 103*, 1629–1637. doi:10.1111/j.1360-0443.2008.02326.x.

Kozasa, E. H., Sato, J. R., Lacerda, S. S., Barreiros, M. A., Radvany, J., Russell, T., … Amaro, E. (2012). Meditation training increases brain efficiency in an attention task. *NeuroImage, 59*, 745–749. doi:10.1016/j.neuroimage.2011.06.088.

Kuyken, W., Weare, K., Ukoumunne, O. C., Vicary, R., Motton, N., Burnett, R., … Huppert, F. (2013). Effectiveness of the mindfulness in schools programme: Non-randomised controlled feasibility study. *The British Journal of Psychiatry, 203*, 126–131. doi:10.1192/bjp.bp.113.126649.

Ledesma, D., & Kumano, H. (2009). Mindfulness-based stress reduction and cancer: A meta-analysis. *Psycho-Oncology, 18*, 571–579. doi:10.1002/pon.1400.

Modinos, G., Ormel, J., & Aleman, A. (2010). Individual differences in dispositional mindfulness and brain activity involved in reappraisal of emotion. *Social Cognitive and Affective Neuroscience, 5*, 369–377. doi:10.1093/scan/nsq006.

Moffitt, T. E., Arseneault, L., Belsky, D., Dickson, N., Hancox, R. J., Harrington, H., … Caspi, A. (2011). A gradient of childhood self-control predicts health, wealth, and public safety. *Proceedings of the National Academy of Sciences, 108*, 2693–2698. doi:10.1073/pnas.1010076108.

Mrazek, M. D., Franklin, M. S., Phillips, D. T., Baird, B., & Schooler, J. W. (2013). Mindfulness training improves working memory capacity and GRE performance while reducing mind wandering. *Psychological Science, 24*, 776–781. doi:10.1177/0956797612459659.

Munakata, Y., Herd, S. A., Chatham, C. H., Depue, B. E., Banich, M. T., & O'Reilly, R. C. (2011). A unified framework for inhibitory control. *Trends in Cognitive Sciences, 15*, 453–459. doi:10.1016/j.tics.2011.07.011.

Napoli, M., Krech, P. R., & Holley, L. C. (2005). Mindfulness training for elementary school students: The attention academy. *Journal of Applied School Psychology, 21*, 99–125. doi:10.1300/J370v21n01_05.

Neville, H. J., & Bavelier, D. (1998). Neural organization and plasticity of language. *Current Opinion in Neurobiology, 8*, 254–258. doi:10.1016/S0959-4388(98)80148-7.

Oberle, E., Schonert-Reichl, K. A., Lawlor, M. S., & Thomson, K. C. (2012). Mindfulness and inhibitory control in early adolescence. *The Journal of Early Adolescence, 32*, 565–588. doi:10.1177/0272431611403741.

Ochsner, K. N., Bunge, S. A., Gross, J. J., & Gabrieli, J. D. (2002). Rethinking feelings: An FMRI study of the cognitive regulation of emotion. *Journal of Cognitive Neuroscience, 14*, 1215–1229. doi:10.1162/089892902760807212.

Passolunghi, M. C., & Siegel, L. S. (2004). Working memory and access to numerical information in children with disability in mathematics. *Journal of Experimental Child Psychology, 88*, 348–367. doi:10.1016/j.jecp.2004.04.002.

Perkins, D. N., & Salomon, G. (1989). Are cognitive skills context-bound? *Educational Researcher, 18*, 16–25. doi:10.3102/0013189X018001016.

Rees, B. (2011). Overview of outcome data of potential meditation training for soldier resilience. *Military Medicine, 176*, 1232–1242.

Roeser, R. W., & Peck, S. C. (2009). An education in awareness: Self, motivation and self-regulation in contemplative perspective. *Educational Psychologist, 44*, 119–136. doi:10.1080/00461520902832376.

Roeser, R. W., & Zelazo, P. D. R. (2012). Contemplative science, education and child development: Introduction to the Special Section. *Child Development Perspectives, 6*, 143–145. doi:10.1111/j.1750-8606.2012.00242.x.

Rosenzweig, M. R., & Bennett, E. L. (1996). Psychobiology of plasticity: Effects of training and experience on brain and behavior. *Behavioural Brain Research, 78*, 57–65. doi:10.1016/0166-4328(95)00216-2.

Rubia, K., Taylor, E., Smith, A. B., Oksannen, H., Overmeyer, S., & Newman, S. (2001). Neuropsychological analyses of impulsiveness in childhood hyperactivity. *The British Journal of Psychiatry, 179*, 138–143. doi:10.1192/bjp.179.2.138.

Rubin, K. H., Coplan, R. J., Fox, N. A., & Calkins, S. D. (1995). Emotionality, emotion regulation, and preschoolers' social adaptation. *Development and Psychopathology, 7*, 49–62. http://dx.doi.org/10.1017/S0954579400006337.

Segal, Z. V., Teasdale, J. D., & Williams, J. M. G. (2004). Mindfulness-based cognitive therapy: Theoretical rationale and empirical status. In S. C. Hayes, V. M. Follette, & M. M. Linehan (Eds.), *Mindfulness and acceptance: Expanding the cognitive-behavioral tradition* (pp. 45–65). New York, NY: Guilford Press.

Semple, R. J., Lee, J., Rosa, D., & Miller, L. F. (2010). A randomized trial of mindfulness-based cognitive therapy for children: Promoting mindful attention to enhance social-emotional resiliency in children. *Journal of Child and Family Studies, 19*, 218–229. doi:10.1007/s10826-009-9301-y.

Shapiro, S. L., Astin, J. A., Bishop, S. R., & Cordova, M. (2005). Mindfulness-based stress reduction for health care professionals: Results from a randomized trial. *International Journal of Stress Management, 12*, 164. doi:10.1037/1072-5245.12.2.164.

Shapiro, S. L., Lyons, K. E., Miller, R. C., Butler, B., Vieten, C., & Zelazo, P. D. (2015). Contemplation in the classroom: A new direction for improving childhood education. *Educational Psychology Review, 27*, 1–30. doi:10.1007/s10648-014-9265-3.

Shiffrin, R. M., & Schneider, W. (1977). Controlled and automatic human information processing: II. Perceptual learning, automatic attending and a general theory. *Psychological Review, 84*, 127. doi:10.1037/0033-295X.84.2.127.

Shonin, E., Van Gordon, W., Slade, K., & Griffiths, M. D. (2013). Mindfulness and other Buddhist-derived interventions in correctional settings: A systematic review. *Aggression and Violent Behavior, 18*, 365–372. doi:10.1016/j.avb.2013.01.002.

Sibinga, E., Perry-Parrish, C., Chung, S. E., Johnson, S. B., Smith, M., & Ellen, J. M. (2013). School-based mindfulness instruction for urban male youth: A small randomized controlled trial. *Preventive Medicine, 57*, 799–801. doi:10.1016/j.ypmed.2013.08.027.

Singh, N. N., Lancioni, G. E., Winton, A. S., Karazsia, B. T., & Singh, J. (2013). Mindfulness Training for Teachers Changes the Behavior of Their Preschool Students. *Research in Human Development, 10*(3), 211–233 DOI: 10.1080/15427609.2013.818484.

Swanson, H. L., & Sachse-Lee, C. (2001). Mathematical problem solving and working memory in children with learning disabilities: Both executive and phonological processes are important. *Journal of Experimental Child Psychology, 79*, 294–321. doi:10.1006/jecp.2000.2587.

Tan, L. B., & Martin, G. (2012). Mind full or mindful: A report on mindfulness and psychological health in healthy adolescents. *International Journal of Adolescence and Youth*, 1–11. doi:10.1080/02673843.2012.709174.

Tang, Y. Y., Lu, Q., Fan, M., Yang, Y., & Posner, M. I. (2012). Mechanisms of white matter changes induced by meditation. *Proceedings of the National Academy of Sciences, 109*, 10570–10574. doi:10.1073/pnas.1207817109.

Tang, Y. Y., Lu, Q., Geng, X., Stein, E. A., Yang, Y., & Posner, M. I. (2010). Short-term meditation induces white matter changes in the anterior cingulate. *Proceedings of the National Academy of Sciences, 107*, 15649–15652. doi:10.1073/pnas.1011043107.

Tang, Y. Y., Ma, Y., Wang, J., Fan, Y., Feng, S., Lu, Q., … Posner, M. I. (2007). Short-term meditation training improves attention and self-regulation. *Proceedings of the National Academy of Sciences, 104*, 17152–17156. doi:10.1073/pnas.0707678104.

Tang, Y. Y., & Posner, M. I. (2009). Attention training and attention state training. *Trends in Cognitive Sciences, 13*, 222–227. doi:10.1016/j.tics.2009.01.009.

Teasdale, J. D., Segal, Z. V., Williams, J. M. G., Ridgeway, V. A., Soulsby, J. M., & Lau, M. A. (2000). Prevention of relapse/recurrence in major depression by mindfulness-based cognitive therapy. *Journal of Consulting and Clinical Psychology, 68*, 615. doi:10.1037/0022-006X.68.4.615.

Ursache, A., Blair, C., & Raver, C. C. (2012). The promotion of self-regulation as a means of enhancing school readiness and early achievement in children at risk for school failure. *Child Development Perspectives, 6*, 122–128. doi:10.1111/j.1750-8606.2011.00209.x.

Van de Weijer-Bergsma, E., Formsma, A. R., de Bruin, E. I., & Bögels, S. M. (2012). The effectiveness of mindfulness training on behavioral problems and attentional functioning in adolescents with ADHD. *Journal of Child and Family Studies, 21*, 775–787. doi:10.1007/s10826-011-9531-7.

Van der Oord, S., Bögels, S. M., & Peijnenburg, D. (2012). The effectiveness of mindfulness training for children with ADHD and mindful parenting for their parents. *Journal of Child and Family Studies, 21*, 139–147. doi:10.1007/s10826-011-9457-0.

Zelazo, P. D., & Carlson, S. M. (2012). Hot and cool executive function in childhood and adolescence: Development and plasticity. *Child Development Perspectives, 6*, 354–360. doi:10.1111/j.1750-8606.2012.00246.x.

Zelazo, P. D., Carlson, S. M., & Kesek, A. (2008). The development of executive function in childhood. In C. A. Nelson & M. Luciana (Eds.), *Handbook of developmental cognitive neuroscience* (pp. 553–574). Cambridge, MA: MIT Press.

Zelazo, P. D., & Lyons, K. E. (2012). The potential benefits of mindfulness training in early childhood: A developmental social cognitive neuroscience perspective. *Child Development Perspectives, 6*, 154–160. doi:10.1111/j.1750-8606.2012.00241.x.

Zoogman, S., Goldberg, S. B., Hoyt, W. T., & Miller, L. (2015). Mindfulness interventions with youth: A meta-analysis. *Mindfulness, 6*(2), 290–302. doi:10.1007/s12671-013-0260-4.

Zylowska, L., Ackerman, D. L., Yang, M. H., Futrell, J. L., Horton, N. L., Hale, S. G., … Smalley, S. L. (2008). Mindfulness meditation training in adults and adolescents with ADHD: A feasibility study. *Journal of Attention Disorders, 11*, 737–746. doi:10.1177/1087054707308502.

18 Promoting Caring: Mindfulness- and Compassion-Based Contemplative Training for Educators and Students

Brooke D. Lavelle Heineberg

Introduction

There is a need in education to nurture the development of students' capacities for self-care and compassion in order to enhance their well-being and promote their ethical sensitivities and civic engagement. Teachers also need to be provided with support and methods to enhance their own prosocial capacities for care so that they may enhance their own well-being and in turn provide safe, supportive environments in which students can most effectively learn and grow.

Research shows that social connectedness and prosocial qualities like compassion have demonstrable effects on psychological and physiological health and well-being (Cacioppo & Hawkley, 2009; Pace et al., 2009). Caring relationships are also foundational to well-being and provide the nurturing support, safety, and motivation necessary to foster learning and student achievement (Wentzel, Battle, Russell, & Looney, 2010). Such relationships also provide opportunities for students and teachers to realize their natural capacities for care and compassion by helping them learn to care for and empathize with others in the way that others have cared for them (Noddings, 1984).

Research suggests that the capacities for care and compassion are present early in development (Warneken, 2013) and that they can be trained through adolescence and adulthood (Lutz, Brefczynski-Lewis, Johnstone, & Davidson, 2008; Pace et al., 2009). Teams of educators and researchers have been working to develop and deliver contemplative-based programs for teachers and students, as recent research suggests that certain forms of meditation training may enhance health, well-being, and prosocial behavior, such as helping and cooperation (Grossman, Niemann, Schmidt, & Walach, 2004; Pace et al., 2009), and altruistic action (Condon, Desbordes, Miller, & DeSteno, 2013; Leiberg, Klimecki, & Singer, 2011; Weng et al., 2013). Many of these programs, which are drawn from distinct yet related mindfulness- and compassion-based contemplative models, build upon the foundational work of the social-emotional learning (SEL) programs and include specific contemplative methods that support the systematic cultivation of self-regulatory skills and prosocial capacities like compassion.

Mindfulness- and contemplative-based interventions generally assume that humans are endowed with a natural capacity for prosociality that can be cultivated and developed. Mindfulness interventions tend to emphasize that these qualities

B.D. Lavelle Heineberg (✉)
Mind and Life Institute, 4 Bay Road, Suite 101, Hadley, MA 01035, USA
e-mail: brooke.dodson.lavelle@gmail.com

K.A. Schonert-Reichl, R.W. Roeser (eds.), *Handbook of Mindfulness in Education*, Mindfulness in Behavioral Health, DOI 10.1007/978-1-4939-3506-2_18

can be awakened and drawn out through practices that foster mindfulness, presence, openness, and self-regulatory skills. By learning to get in touch with our own natural capacity for compassion, we learn to remain open to and sensitive to others. Compassion interventions tend to build on these foundational mindfulness practices and emphasize the need for skills and practices that support the development of discernment and analytical faculties that help people overcome obstacles or blocks to enacting compassion and care. This chapter provides an overview of the theoretical underpinnings of three secular mindfulness- and compassion-based interventions—namely Mindfulness-Based Stress Reduction (MBSR), Cognitively-Based Compassion Training (CBCT), and Sustainable Compassion Training (SCT)—that have been adapted for use in educational settings. The current status and direction of these projects will be discussed, followed by suggestions for further research and development.

Mindfulness- and Compassion-Based Contemplative Interventions

Interest in contemplative practices has grown in recent years, yet a majority of the research to date primarily has assessed the efficacy of MBSR programs in alleviating stress in adult clinical populations. In the last several years, however, numerous mindfulness-based programs also have been adapted for use in educational and other contexts. More recently, compassion-based contemplative approaches, including CBCT and SCT, have been selected for scientific study. Preliminary research on these programs suggests that such approaches may be of benefit in clinical, nonclinical, and educational settings (Condon et al., 2013; Pace et al., 2009; Reddy et al., 2013). All three approaches aim to foster self-regulatory and prosocial skills, yet little attention has been paid to the theoretical frameworks that underpin these programs and the differences between their respective approaches. Here I provide an overview of these contemplative models as well as a brief summary of their application and research.

Mindfulness-Based Stress Reduction

MBSR, developed by Jon Kabat-Zinn, is one of the best-known and most commonly researched secular contemplative-based interventions designed to help individuals reduce stress (Kabat-Zinn, 2000). The program, which was influenced and inspired by Japanese Zen, Tibetan Dzogchen, and modern *vipassanā* traditions, primarily offers participants training in mindfulness. Such training involves the training of attention as well as the cultivation of a particular stance toward the world as a way of helping participants come to terms with reality as it is. It is understood that through this "coming to terms" with things as they are, without trying to change them, that self-healing takes place (Kabat-Zinn, 2011). Mindfulness practice therefore involves learning to become more present to stress, pain, illness, and the challenges in one's life while discovering stability and peace within these very challenges.

Mindfulness as a way of being is often described as a means of "waking up" (Kabat-Zinn, 2005). In terms of contemplative practice, mindfulness is operationally defined as the act of "paying attention in a particular way: on purpose, in the present moment, and non-judgmentally" (Kabat-Zinn, 1994, p. 4). As the definition suggests, the practice of mindfulness involves not only attentional training, but also a particular way of seeing the world that is facilitated by the cultivation of a certain set of attitudes. These are: (1) non-judging; (2) patience; (3) beginner's mind; (4) trust; (5) non-striving; (6) acceptance; and (7) letting go (Kabat-Zinn, 2000).

Non-judging refers to an attitude of impartiality; a way of bearing witness to one's experience without the veil of implicit biases or preferences. Patience refers to the ability to abide in this moment and to allow all things—including one's own healing—to unfold in their own time. Beginner's mind involves approaching each moment with an innocent, child-like curiosity. It encourages one to try to see things as if for the first time, which affords flexibility in perceiving and responding to situations. Trust concerns developing one's intuition and learning to rely on one's own experience and capacity for self-care. Non-striving refers to the paradox of non-doing: The act of trying to achieve a particular goal undermines the cultivation of mindfulness, the willingness to abide in the present moment. The attitude of acceptance pushes this notion further: One is encouraged to open to the present moment and embrace all it contains. Learning to see things as they are is the first step in allowing the process of change to begin. The final attitude of letting go, or non-attachment, is the practice of putting aside the tendency to want things to be a certain way. It involves letting go of thoughts of the past or future, or the tendency to cling to certain aspects of experience while rejecting others (Kabat-Zinn, 2000).

Taken together, these attitudes create the frame for practice and ethical engagement. Through practice, one can learn to re-perceive stressful situations and thought patterns in a more open, non-reactive way. This affords the practitioner the capacity to learn to interrupt automatic, habitual reactive patterns, and to develop cognitive and emotional flexibility in responding to situations (Shapiro, Carlson, Astin, & Freedman, 2006). A key feature of mindfulness practice also involves learning to relate differently to one's thoughts rather than changing the specific content of thoughts. In fact, increasing evidence supports the idea that mindfulness practice has potential to reduce stress and enhance resilience, likely by breaking the interrupting automatic, habitual ways that individuals react to stressful or emotionally charged situations (Williams, 2010). This particular approach might also reduce the negative impact of recurrent distressing and self-focused thoughts (Ortner, Kilner, & Zelazo, 2007). Put another way, mindfulness practice may work by interrupting simulations of past or future events that serve to exacerbate stress and instead encourage one to be more present (Farb et al., 2007). Research has also shown that this way of learning to attend to and relate to one's own experience can enhance self-compassion and empathy (Shapiro, Schwartz, & Bonner, 1998; Singer & Lamm, 2009). MBSR has been applied and evaluated in a range of settings. See, for example, Grossman et al. (2004) for a review. Below I highlight several adaptations of MBSR in educational settings.

Cognitively-Based Compassion Training

CBCT was first developed in 2005 by Geshe Lobsang Tenzin Negi to help Emory University undergraduates deal with depression. The CBCT model draws from the *lojong* or "mind training" tradition of Tibetan Buddhism (Negi, 2009; Ozawa-de-Silva and Negi, 2013) but has been adapted for use in a variety of secular settings. In this model, compassion is understood as the heartfelt wish that others be free from suffering combined with the readiness to act on their behalf. It arises from a deep sense of affection for others, together with insight into the causes of their suffering and the recognition that their suffering can be alleviated (Negi, 2009; Ozawa-de Silva, Dodson-Lavelle, Raison, & Negi, 2011).

CBCT theory assumes that people are able to empathize readily with members of their own family or in-group, but generally find it more difficult to empathize with strangers, members of other social groups, and especially those who have harmed or threatened them in some way. Despite this tendency, CBCT views compassion as a trainable skill that is developed through the cultivation of impartiality and affection. To cultivate impartiality, one reflects deeply on the dangers inherent in bias and stereotype, and considers the construction of categories such as "friend" or "enemy" to be superficial and changeable. To enhance feelings of closeness and affection to others, one learns to cultivate gratitude for others by reflecting on their kindness and the countless ways in which we depend on others to survive.

Cultivating impartiality and affection can help foster empathy for others (Emmons & McCullough, 2003; Otake, Shimai, Tanaka-Matsumi, & Otsui, 2006; Singer & Lamm, 2009). Feeling moved or concerned by others' suffering is not necessarily the same as compassion, however. Sometimes witnessing the suffering of others can overwhelm one or cause empathic distress or burnout. Thus CBCT also provides strategies and practices for helping participants cultivate inner strength and emotional stability. One gains this strength in part by deepening insight into the causes of stress and suffering, and recognizing that it can be overcome. When one realizes that suffering can be transformed, one gains confidence and sets the determination to do so. This step, in which one gains insight into the causes of suffering, recognizes that they can be overcome, and sets a determination to overcome these causes is called self-compassion.

These three keys—affection, impartiality, and self-compassion—are central components of the CBCT program. They are taught systematically in ordered steps, typically over the course of 8 weeks. The steps are: (1) developing attention and stability of mind; (2) cultivating insight into the nature of mental experience; (3) cultivating self-compassion; (4) developing impartiality; (5) developing appreciation and gratitude; (6) developing affection and empathy; (7) generating aspirational compassion; and (8) realizing active compassion. Classes typically include presentations of pedagogical material, discussion, and guided analytical meditation.

Although mindfulness programs encourage the reduction of cognitive simulations, CBCT programs actively encourage participants to simulate more positive and constructive ways of relating to oneself and others. The program is "cognitively based," therefore, in that it relies on analytical meditations that encourage participants to gain insight into the ways they of and relate to others in sometimes biased, hostile, and limiting ways. These insights are then deepened through repeated reflection and practice until they transform the ways in which one relates to and treats others.

Research on CBCT has shown that college students who were taught and practiced CBCT displayed reduced emotional upset in response to psychosocial stress as well as less activation of autonomic and immune pathways that have been implicated in the development of a host of chronic, stress-related illnesses (Pace et al., 2009, 2010). Results from a study of a CBCT program for adolescent girls in foster care (ages 13–16) showed that participation in a 6-week CBCT program was associated with increased hopefulness and a trend in decreased general anxiety (Reddy et al., 2012 as described in Ozawa-de Silva & Dodson-Lavelle, 2011) as well as reduced markers for stress and immune system hyperactivity (Pace et al., 2010). Practicing CBCT also has been shown to enhance empathic accuracy (Mascaro, Rilling, Negi, & Raison, 2012). The program is currently being adapted and developed for teachers and students, survivors of trauma and domestic violence, and women in prison.

Sustainable Compassion Training

In 2008, John Makransky of Boston College began teaching a secularized version of his SCT Program, which draws from Dzogchen and Mahāmudrā practices from the Tibetan Nyingma and Kagyü traditions (Makransky, 2007). SCT was designed primarily to help those in social service professions become more compassionate, present, and resilient, and to avoid burnout often associated with prolonged exposure to stress and trauma, or empathy-fatigue.

In the SCT model, compassion is understood as a form of love and empathic concern that wishes for someone who is suffering to be free from stress and pain. According to this model, compassion has five aspects: (1) affection; (2) empathic concern; (3) the wish for others to be free from stress and suffering; (4) compassionate action; and (5) wisdom or insight. Affection here refers to sensing others as worthy of unconditional love and respect, including not only to those whom one finds it easy to care for, but also to those who fall outside of one's ingroup, or who challenge one in some way. Empathic concern involves becoming aware of the suffering of another and sensing this suffering as similar to one's own. Getting in touch with one's own difficult experiences helps one to sense more deeply what it is like for another to undergo such experiences. The wish for others to be free from suffering reflects one's natural capacity for care and compassion that is evoked when they witness someone they love in pain and discomfort. Through training, one learns to extend this natural capacity—which is often held back—to others. Wisdom or insight involves recognizing that others are more than just one's limited, shifting, biased thoughts or perceptions of them. Learning to sense the worth and potential of others more deeply helps draw out one's natural capacity of care for them. Compassionate action naturally follows from the cultivation of the components of care above, and it can also emerge naturally from a firm sense of security as well as a responsibility for the well-being of others (Makransky, 2007).

This program also aims to address common impediments to cultivating compassion, including: (1) reducing others to one's limited, stereotypical thoughts of them, and relating to them in biased ways; (2) strong feelings of self-dislike prevalent in American culture that make one feel unworthy of receiving compassion; (3) aversion to or inability to bear witness to one's own feelings; (4) a rigid sense of self that is independent from others; and (5) a tendency to experience distressing feelings and sufferings as all consuming (Makransky, 2007).

Although SCT draws on similar analytical reflections utilized in CBCT, this approach assumes a more relational view as foundational to the cultivation of compassion. SCT rests on the assumption that one needs to experience themself as an object worthy of care and compassion in order to see others as objects worthy care and compassion (Makransky, 2011). By recalling and connecting with caring figures in one's life, one is empowered to access and develop trust in their innate capacity for care and compassion. Such practices for receiving love and compassion are mutually supported and reinforced by practices for deepening and relaxing into this caring capacity, and for extending this care and compassion to others (Makransky, 2007, 2011).

Research on a compassion program adapted in connection to SCT showed compassion training increases compassionate responses to others' suffering (Condon et al., 2013). SCT is currently being adapted for use with nursing students and college students suffering with body image issues. SCT also serves as the contemplative foundation for Mind and Life Institute's new program for teachers and students, *A Call to Care* (see D. Lavelle Heineberg, Makransky and Seigle, 2015, www.mindandlife.org), and also courageofcare.org), described below.

Mindfulness and Compassion Training in Education

MBSR, CBCT, and SCT have all been adapted for use with teachers and students in educational settings, yet research and development of these and other contemplative-based trainings in education is still in its early stages. To date, much of the research has focused primarily on assessing mindfulness-based interventions for students, with far less attention to compassion-based interventions and programs for teachers. Here I briefly highlight results from a few studies that have examined the effects of mindfulness training with children and teachers. I then describe efforts underway to implement compassion-based programs in educational settings. Several recent reviews offer more comprehensive overviews of the current status of mindfulness-based programs in education than is possible here (Meiklejohn et al., 2012; Zenner, Herrnleben-Kurz, & Walach, 2014; Zoogman, Goldberg, Hoyt, & Miller, 2015).

Mindfulness-Based Programs for Teachers

Flook, Goldberg, Pinger, Bonus, and Davidson (2013) evaluated the effects of a modified 8-week MBSR (mMBSR) program for teachers. The program was adapted from the standard MBSR format to include school-related activities and specific strategies for incorporating mindfulness skills in the classroom. The intervention group showed significant reductions in psychological symptoms and burnout and increases in self-compassion and attention as compared to a wait-list control group. Results also showed that mMBSR training positively impacted observer-rated classroom behavior, suggesting that such programs for teachers may have tangible benefits to students and the classroom climate.

Several other mindfulness-based programs have been developed and implemented with teachers including Stress Management and Relaxation Techniques (SMART) in Education (http://www.smart-in-education.org/),

Cultivating Awareness and Resilience in Educators (CARE) (http://www.care4teachers.org/), and Mindfulness, Courage, and Reflection for Educators (also known as The Aware Teacher; see http://www.couragene.org/tat). Research on these and other related programs for educators suggests that mindfulness-based training may improve teachers' well-being and efficacy, and reduce stress and burnout (Jennings, Frank, Snowberg, Coccia, & Greenberg, 2013; Kemeny et al., 2012; Roeser et al., 2013).

Mindfulness-Based Programs for Students

Flook et al. (2010) conducted an RCT of an 8-week Inner Kids mindfulness program for second- and third-grade students. Results showed that children with weaker executive function skills at the outset of the study showed significant improvement on overall executive function following the training compared to controls. Napoli, Krech, and Holley (2005) conducted and RCT with first- to third-grade students which demonstrated that participation in the mindfulness and attention intervention yielded decreases in self-reported test anxiety as well as improvements in teacher-rated and behavioral measures of attention. Research by Schonert-Reichl and Lawlor (2010) on the effects of Mindful Education (ME) training for fourth- to seventh-grade students showed that students who received this training reported increased optimism. These students were rated by their teachers as less aggressive and oppositional, and more likely to act prosocially toward others compared to wait-list controls. Broderick and Metz (2009) conducted a nonrandomized study to assess the efficacy of mindfulness training program, Learning to BREATHE, for adolescents. Students who received the training showed significant reduction in self-reported negative affect and increases in emotion regulation, calmness, and self-acceptance as compared to controls.

Though more work remains to be done in this area, preliminary evidence suggests that mindfulness programs can be adapted in developmentally appropriate ways and can offer students methods for self-care and regulation. Researchers at Center for Investigating Healthy Minds (http://www.investigatinghealthyminds.org/) are currently assessing the efficacy of a mindfulness-based prosocial skills training program, the Kindness Curriculum, with preschoolers, while also offering classroom teachers the opportunity to receive training in MBSR. This focus on combined teacher and student interventions addresses a gap in this area, and also addresses the need to attend to and evaluate the prosocial effects of mindfulness training.

Compassion-Based Programs for Teachers

The Mind and Life Institute together with a network of advisors and collaborators developed *A Call to Care*, an interdisciplinary program for fostering care and compassion in teachers and students (D. Lavelle Heineberg et al., 2015). The program draws heavily from SCT and integrates SEL and other skills-based training to support learning, health, and well-being, and to foster ethical sensitivity. The program is organized around three modes of care: receiving care, self-care, and extending care. Each mode is divided further into four investigations: why care is important, learning how to care, overcoming obstacles to care, and deepening our capacity for care. This model is intended to enhance experiences of nurturing and interconnection by emphasizing the interdependence of receiving and extending care, and the importance of supportive relationships to well-being and development more generally.

Many teachers find it difficult to imagine themselves as the object of care. Yet, in the absence of supportive, loving relationships, a fundamental sense of self-respect, or appreciation of one's own worth, attempts to care for students and others is built on a fragile base. The core skills and practices of the receiving care mode are therefore designed to help teachers and students learn to re-experience moments of interconnection, warmth, affection, and inner safety in relationship with caring figures in their lives from which they can learn to see, welcome, and care for others more deeply.

The self-care mode offers teachers and students mindfulness, deep relaxation, and body-centered strategies to cultivate their capacity to become attuned to the wisdom of their bodies, learn to manage stress and difficult emotions, and promote cognitive flexibility and openness to experience. The ability to receive care empowers and is empowered by the extension of care to others. The extending care mode aims to expand the circle of care beyond in-group and out-group boundaries by targeting the biased, stereotypical, and reductive thoughts that hold these boundaries in place.

This program is currently being developed and piloted with teams of educators in the USA as well as international partners abroad. Subgroups of these educators are also developing a corresponding curriculum for students, with the hopes of eventually designing programs for parents and other community members. This work is still in its very early stages, yet it addresses a need to develop and assess integrated compassion-based programs for educational contexts.

Compassion-Based Programs for Students

Researchers and contemplatives at Emory University have adapted their CBCT program for use with elementary school children (Ozawa-de Silva & Dodson-Lavelle, 2011). The program, designed for children ages 5–9, offers methods for helping children cultivate compassion through practices of self-compassion, impartiality, empathy, affection, and engaged compassion for others. Evaluation of the effects of this program on prosocial behavior, bullying, social exclusion, stereotyping, and bias are ongoing at local schools in Atlanta, GA. The team is also currently developing a training program for teachers.

Conclusions and Future Directions

Although research on mindfulness- and compassion-based programs is still in its early phases, the programs and research described above are promising. The rate of interest in and growth of programs in this field in the past few years is also impressive. Still, much work needs to be done to evaluate the most effective and developmentally appropriate ways to help teachers and students learn both why and how to be more caring and compassionate.

The three distinct, yet related, approaches for cultivating mindfulness and compassion described above all show promise as potentially effective educational interventions. Much more rigorous research in this area is needed, however, to evaluate the effects of different theories and styles of programs on teachers' and students' health, well-being, and prosocial capacities. Attention to the details of these interventions, as well as the benefits of different styles of practice, need to be more clearly articulated, and eventually research comparing these programs needs to be initiated. There is also a clear need to develop new measures to assess the effects of these programs and mindfulness and compassion more broadly. These interventions are relatively new, yet little attention is paid to these issues in the literature. The field could therefore benefit from more theoretical work on these interventions, as well as a compendium of practices relevant to educators to help others orient to the field. The development of a more broad theoretical framework that address the need for mindfulness- and compassion-based interventions in education could also provide an organizing framework for the field that connects contemplative interventions with established SEL programs and other skills-based trainings, including behavioral and other psychological interventions.

In addition to evaluating overall efficacy of different contemplative approaches to cultivating mindfulness and compassion, interventionists and researchers need to attend more closely to the potential limits within contemporary meditation programs. Generally speaking, most of these programs focus primarily on the individual and his or her intra-personal processes, thereby missing the focus on inter-personal process and practices so central to healthy relationships and prosocial development and behavior. SCT attempts to address this limitation; still more work needs to be done to develop and integrate group work and practice in these interventions. Similarly, more work could be done to develop integrated programs for teachers, students, and school communities.

Another set of challenges related to the successful implementation of these practices in educational settings is that of teacher training and sustainability. We know that teacher development and well-being is critical to the effectiveness of any school-based program (e.g., Durlak & DuPre, 2008; Ransford, Greenberg, Domitrovich, Small, & Jacobson, 2009). Many educators, however, have not been adequately prepared to create the types of caring and supportive classroom environments that recent research has shown as critical for student learning and well-being. Finding high-quality, in-depth means of supporting and training teachers in ways that are caring and nourishing, and not burdensome, remains a challenge. Developing plans for sustainability, including school-wide and community engagement, inclusion, and training is also essential. Discovering ways of sharing these materials in more accessible, cost-effective, and culturally sensitive ways is also of primary importance. Programs that provide principles or frameworks for practice and that encourage participation from educators in their design, development, and implementation seem like a promising way to empower communities and nurture sustainability.

Research also has shown that it is essential to ensure teacher buy-in and openness to programming before implementing new programs in classrooms, as teachers who are resistant and/or lack delivery skills may actually *hinder* students' social-emotional competencies (see, for example Reyes, Brackett, Rivers, Elbertson, & Salovey, 2012). Administrative support is also key. Issues related to buy-in and support raise broader concerns about systematic support for this kind of work in general. Such issues also call for deeper investigations into other obstacles or blocks to this work. Most educators and parents recognize the need for programs that nurture and support their students' emotional, social, and ethical development, and yet what are the forces at play that keep us from doing this work more deeply and on a wider scale? This is not merely a systemic issue, though obviously related. How else might educators, administrators, parents and others be avoiding this invitation to deeper personal investigation and growth? And, how can we safely and lovingly invite more educators into a community of care to engage and share this work with integrity and confidence?

References

Broderick, P. C., & Metz, S. (2009). Learning to BREATHE: A pilot trial of a mindfulness curriculum for adolescents. Advances in School Mental Health Promotion, 2(1), 35–46.

Cacioppo, J. T., & Hawkley, L. C. (2009). Perceived social isolation and cognition. *Trends in Cognitive Sciences, 13*, 447–454.

Condon, P., Desbordes, G., Miller, W. B., & DeSteno, D. (2013). Meditation increases compassionate responses to suffering. *Psychological Science, 24*, 2125–2127.

D. Lavelle Heineberg, B., Makransky, J., & Seigle, P. (2015). *A call to care: Professional development guide* (Unpublished manual).

Durlak, J. A., & DuPre, E. P. (2008). Implementation matters: A review of research on the influence of implementation on program outcomes and the factors affecting implementation. *American Journal of Community Psychology, 41*, 327–350.

Emmons, R. A., & McCullough, M. E. (2003). Counting blessings versus burdens: An experimental investigation of gratitude and subjective well-being in daily life. *Journal of Personality and Social Psychology, 84*, 377–389.

Farb, N. A. S., Segal, Z. V., Mayberg, H., Bean, J., McKeon, D., Fatima, Z., & Anderson, A. K. (2007). Attending to the present: Mindfulness meditation reveals distinct neural modes of self-reference. *Social Cognitive and Affective Neuroscience, 2*, 313–322.

Flook, L., Goldberg, S. B., Pinger, L., Bonus, K., & Davidson, R. J. (2013). Mindfulness for teachers: A pilot study to assess effects on stress, burnout and teaching efficacy. *Mind, Brain, and Education, 7*, 182–195. doi:10.1111/mbe.12026.

Flook, L., Smalley, S. L., Kitil, M. J., Galla, B. M., Kaiser-Greenland, S., Locke, J, … Kasari, C. (2010). Effects of mindful awareness practices on executive functions in elementary school children. *Journal of Applied School Psychology, 26*, 70–95. doi:10.1080/15377900903379125.

Grossman, P., Niemann, L., Schmidt, S., & Walach, H. (2004). Mindfulness-based stress reduction and health benefits: A meta-analysis. *Journal of Psychosomatic Research, 57*, 35–43.

Jennings, P. A., Frank, J. L., Snowberg, K. E., Coccia, M. A., & Greenberg, M. (2013). Improving classroom learning environments by Cultivating Awareness and Resilience in Education (CARE): Results of a

randomized controlled trial. *School Psychology Quarterly, 28*, 374–390.
Kabat-Zinn, J. (1994). *Mindfulness meditation for everyday life*. New York, NY: Hyperion.
Kabat-Zinn, J. (2000). *Full catastrophe living: Using the wisdom of your body and mind to face stress, pain, and illness*. New York, NY: Bantam Dell.
Kabat-Zinn, J. (2005). *Coming to our senses*. New York, NY: Bantam Dell.
Kabat-Zinn, J. (2011). Some reflections on the origins of MBSR, skillful means, and the trouble with maps. *Contemporary Buddhism, 12*, 281–306. http://dx.doi.org/10.1080/14639947.2011.564844.
Kemeny, M. E., Foltz, C., Cavanagh, J. F., Cullen, M., Giese-Davis, J., Jennings, P., & Ekman, P. (2012). Contemplative/emotion training reduces negative emotional behavior and promotes prosocial responses. *Emotion, 12*, 338–350.
Leiberg, S., Klimecki, O., & Singer, T. (2011). Short-term compassion training increases prosocial behavior in a newly developed prosocial game. *PLoS One, 6*, e17798. doi:10.1371/journal.pone.0017798.
Lutz, A., Brefczynski-Lewis, J., Johnstone, T., & Davidson, R. J. (2008). Regulation of the neural circuitry of emotion by compassion meditation: Effects of meditative expertise. *PLoS One, 3*, e1897. doi:10.1371/journal.pone.0001897.
Makransky, J. (2007). *Awakening through love: Unveiling your deepest goodness*. Boston, MA: Wisdom.
Makransky, J. (2011). Compassion beyond fatigue: Contemplative training for people who serve others. In J. Simmer-Brown & F. Grace (Eds.), *Meditation and the classroom* (pp. 85–94). New York, NY: SUNY Press.
Mascaro, J. S., Rilling, J. K., Negi, L. T., & Raison, C. L. (2012). Compassion meditation enhances empathic accuracy and related neural activity. *Social Cognitive and Affective Neuroscience, 8*, 48–55. doi:10.1093/scan/nss095.
Meiklejohn, J., Phillips, C., Freedman, M. L., Griffin, M. L., Beigel, G., Roach, A., … Saltzman, A. (2012). Integrating mindfulness training into K-12 education: Fostering the resilience of teachers and students. *Mindfulness, 3*, 291–307. doi:10.1007/s12671-012-0094-5.
Noddings, N. (1984). Caring: A feminist approach to ethics and education: University of California Press: Berkeley CA.
Napoli, M., Krech, P. R., & Holley, L. C. (2005). Mindfulness training for elementary school students: The attention academy. *Journal of Applied School Psychology, 21*, 99–125.
Negi, L.T. (n.d.) Cognitively-Based Compassion Training: A Manual. Unpublished manuscript.
Ortner, C. N. M., Kilner, S. J., & Zelazo, P. D. (2007). Mindfulness meditation and reduced emotional interference on a cognitive task. *Motivation and Emotion, 31*, 271–283.
Otake, K., Shimai, S., Tanaka-Matsumi, J., & Otsui, K. (2006). Happy people become happier through kindness: A counting kindnesses intervention. *Journal of Happiness Studies, 7*, 361–375.
Ozawa-de Silva, B., & Dodson-Lavelle, B. (2011). An education of heart and mind: Practical and theoretical issues in teaching cognitively-based compassion training to children. *Practical Matters, 4*, 1–28.
Ozawa-de Silva, B., Dodson-Lavelle, B., Raison, C. L., & Negi, L. T. (2011). Compassion and ethics: Scientific and practical approaches to the cultivation of compassion as a foundation for ethical subjectivity and well-being. *Journal of Healthcare, Science and the Humanities, 2*, 145–161.
Ozawa-de Silva, B., & Negi, L. T. (2013). Cognitively-based compassion training: Protocol and key concepts. In T. Singer & M. Bolz (Eds.), *Compassion: Bridging theory and practice* (pp. 416–437). Leipzig, Germany: Max Planck Institute for Human Cognitive and Brain Sciences.
Pace, T. W. W., Negi, L. T., Adame, D. D., Cole, S. P., Sivili, T. I., Brown, T. D., … Raison, C. L. (2009). Effect of compassion meditation on neuroendocrine, innate immune and behavioral responses to psychosocial stress. *Psychoneuroendocrinology, 34*, 87–98.
Pace, T. W. W., Negi, L. T., Sivili, T. I., Issa, M. J., Cole, S. P., Adame, D. D., & Raison, C. L. (2010). Innate immune neuroendocrine and behavioral responses to psychosocial stress do not predict subsequent compassion meditation practice time. *Psychoneuroendocrinology, 35*, 310–315.
Ransford, C. R., Greenberg, M. T., Domitrovich, C. E., Small, M., & Jacobson, L. (2009). The role of teachers' psychological experiences and perceptions of curriculum supports on the implementation of a social and emotional learning curriculum. *School Psychology Review, 38*, 510–532.
Reddy, S. D., Negi, L. T., Dodson-Lavelle, B., Ozawa-de Silva, B., Pace, T. W. W., Cole, S. P., … Craighead, L. W. (2013). Cognitive-based compassion training: A promising prevention strategy for at-risk adolescents. *Journal of Child and Family Studies, 22*, 219–230.
Reyes, M. R., Brackett, M. A., Rivers, S. E., Elbertson, N. A., & Salovey, P. (2012). The interaction effects of program training, dosage, and implementation quality on targeted student outcomes for the RULER approach to social and emotional learning. *School Psychology Review, 41*, 82–99.
Roeser, R. W., Schonert-Reichl, K. A., Jha, A., Cullen, M., Wallace, L., Wilensky, R., … Harrison, J. (2013). Mindfulness training and reductions in teacher stress and burnout: Results from two randomized, waitlist-control field trials. *Journal of Educational Psychology, 105*, 787–804. doi:10.1037/a0032093.
Roeser, R. W., Skinner, E., Beers, J., & Jennings, P. A. (2012). Mindfulness training and teachers' professional development: An emerging area of research and practice. *Child Development Perspectives, 6*, 167–173.
Schonert-Reichl, K. A., & Lawlor, M. S. (2010). The effects of a mindfulness-based education program on pre-and early adolescents' well-being and social and emotional competence. *Mindfulness, 1*(3), 137–151.

Shapiro, S. L., Carlson, L. E., Astin, J. A., & Freedman, B. (2006). Mechanisms of mindfulness. *Journal of Clinical Psychology, 62*, 373–386.

Shapiro, S. L., Schwartz, G. E., & Bonner, G. (1998). Effects of mindfulness-based stress reduction on medical and premedical students. *Journal of Behavioral Medicine, 21*, 581–599.

Singer, T., & Lamm, C. (2009). The social neuroscience of empathy (The year in cognitive neuroscience 2009). *Annals of the New York Academy of Sciences, 1156*, 81–96.

Warneken, F. (2013). The development of altruistic behavior: Helping in children and chimpanzees. *Social Research, 80*, 431–442.

Weng, H. Y., Fox, A. S., Shackman, A. J., Stodola, D. E., Caldwell, J. Z. K., Olson, M. C., … Davidson, R. J. (2013). Compassion training alters altruism and neural responses to suffering. *Psychological Science, 24*, 1171–1180.

Wentzel, K. R., Battle, A., Russell, S., & Looney, L. (2010). Social supports from teachers and peers as predictors of academic and social motivation. *Contemporary Educational Psychology, 35*, 193–202.

Williams, M. (2010). Mindfulness and psychological stress. *Emotion, 10*, 1–7.

Zenner, C., Herrnleben-Kurz, S., & Walach, H. (2014). Mindfulness-based interventions in schools—A systematic review and meta-analysis. *Frontiers in Psychology, 5*, 1–20. doi:10.3389/fpsyg.2014.00603.

Zoogman, S., Goldberg, S. B., Hoyt, W. T., & Miller, L. (2015). Mindfulness interventions with youth: A meta-analysis. *Mindfulness, 6*(2), 290–302. doi:10.1007/s12671-013-0260-4.

Mindfulness Training to Promote Self-Regulation in Youth: Effects of the Inner Kids Program

19

Brian M. Galla, Susan Kaiser-Greenland, and David S. Black

The mind, hard to control,
Flighty—alighting where it wishes—
One does well to tame.
The disciplined mind brings happiness.

~Buddha
Dhammapada

...Set your mind to concentrate.
For those whose minds are slack and wandering
Are caught between the fangs of the afflictions.

~Shantideva
The Way of the Bodhisattva

Introduction

Self-regulation research has seen enormous growth in the past decade due, no doubt, to a growing recognition of self-regulation as an important feature of human health and development. Prospective longitudinal studies confirm that children with higher self-regulation are more prepared to learn when they enter kindergarten (Blair, 2002; Blair & Razza, 2007), earn higher grades throughout the schooling years (Duckworth & Carlson, 2013), are more likely to graduate from high school (Galla et al., 2014), and are more likely to earn a college degree by age 25 (McClelland, Acock, Piccinin, Rhea, & Stallings, 2012). The benefits of self-regulation extend beyond the classroom. Children who are better able to regulate their attention, emotion, and behavior display better social functioning (Kochanska, Murray, & Harlan, 2000; Spinrad et al., 2006), are more physically healthy (Tsukayama, Toomey, Faith, & Duckworth, 2010), and have fewer mental health problems (Eisenberg, Hofer, & Vaughan, 2007). Children with higher self-regulation also go on to earn higher incomes, save more for retirement, and are less likely to have a history of incarceration as young adults (Moffitt et al., 2011).

Yet, despite its importance, people appear to struggle mightily with self-regulation. In a large international survey, adults from 50 different countries endorsed "self-discipline" as among their lowest strengths of character (Park, Peterson, & Seligman, 2006). It is therefore not surprising that repeated failures of self-regulation constitute a major public health challenge, as these failures are linked with addiction as well as physical and mental health problems (Baumeister, Heatherton, & Tice, 1994). Given its association to so many consequential life outcomes, researchers and policymakers alike are eager to find ways to promote self-regulation during childhood and adolescence.

B.M. Galla (✉)
School of Education, University of Pittsburgh, Pittsburgh, PA, USA
e-mail: gallabri@pitt.edu

S. Kaiser-Greenland
The Inner Kids Program, Los Angeles, CA, USA
e-mail: skaiserg@me.com

D.S. Black
Keck School of Medicine, University of Southern California, Los Angeles, CA, USA
e-mail: davidbla@usc.edu

K.A. Schonert-Reichl, R.W. Roeser (eds.), *Handbook of Mindfulness in Education*, Mindfulness in Behavioral Health, DOI 10.1007/978-1-4939-3506-2_19

Mindfulness training offers one approach to promote self-regulation, and potentially, to improve long-term developmental outcomes. Although mindfulness training programs are geared primarily for adults, there have been advancements in the development of programs designed for children and adolescents. In this chapter, we focus on one mindfulness training program called Inner Kids (Kaiser-Greenland, 2010) and the impact it might have on self-regulation and other important health constructs. The aims of this chapter are to: (a) define self-regulation and consider its relation to other conceptually similar constructs and its developmental trajectory across childhood and adolescence; (b) provide a brief overview of mindfulness; and (c) offer a discussion of how mindfulness training might promote self-regulation. We then turn to a discussion of Inner Kids, as well as to results of a randomized controlled trial testing the program's beneficial effect on self-regulation in second- and third-grade children. We conclude with specific recommendations for future research.

Defining and Conceptualizing Self-Regulation

We define self-regulation as the process of voluntarily regulating attention, emotion, and behavior in the service of personally valued, higher-order goals (Baumeister et al., 1994). For the sake of clarity, we elaborate upon several features of this definition. First,because higher-order goals incline behavior toward rewards that are temporally, spatially, or more psychologically distant (Fujita, 2011), they often come into conflict with other goals that incline behavior toward immediately rewarding objects or experiences but which do not advance higher-order goals. Successful self-regulation will therefore often require self-control, which entails overriding these conflicting response tendencies (Mischel, Shoda, & Rodriguez, 1989). This may involve the inhibition of a strong but maladaptive response, the activation of a weak but adaptive response, or the substituting of one process for another (Baumeister et al., 1994). For example, a dieter would rely on self-control in order to refrain from eating a slice of cheesecake despite a strong urge to do so. Similarly, a child may draw upon self-control in order to stay focused on a boring, but important, homework assignment instead of watching online videos. Second, and as the name implies, self-regulation is self-initiated and is therefore distinct from merely complying with external rules and authority. For example, it would not be an instance of self-regulation for a teenager to start cleaning her room only because her parents demanded it. Third, we distinguish self-regulation from more involuntary, impulsive forms of action control, which typically entail inflexible reactions to the environment based on biologically endowed differences (Derryberry & Rothbart, 1997) or previous learning histories (Dickinson, 1985).

Self-regulation is conceptually related to an aspect of temperament called effortful control, which has been defined as "the ability to inhibit a dominant response to perform a subdominant response, to detect errors, and to engage in planning" (Rothbart & Rueda, 2005, p. 169). In terms of the Big Five taxonomy of personality, self-regulation is a facet of conscientiousness, which also encompasses the traits dependability, punctuality, and orderliness, among others (MacCann, Duckworth, & Roberts, 2009). Self-regulation can be considered the conceptual opposite of impulsivity, or the tendency to act spontaneously, without planning or considering the consequences of acting (Sharma, Markon, & Clark, 2013). Exercising self-regulation depends in part upon the executive functions, a suite of higher-level cognitive processes, including working memory, response inhibition, and attention shifting, which collectively enable top-down, goal-directed control over lower-level impulses (Diamond, 2012).

Extensive behavioral and neurobiological research suggests that self-regulation ability emerges in the first year of life followed by rapid development during the early childhood years (Diamond, 2002; Garon, Bryson, & Smith, 2008; Waber et al., 2007; Welsh, Pennington, & Groisser, 1991). Adolescence marks another period of maturation in the prefrontal cortex signaling further increases in the efficiency of higher-order cognitive abilities and behavioral control, such as responsible decision-making (Casey, Tottenham, Liston, & Durston, 2005; Giedd, 2004; Giedd et al., 1999). Such periods of developmental plasticity suggest that early childhood and adolescence may represent windows of opportunity to intervene and promote self-regulation, and hence, healthy development (Blair & Diamond, 2008; Moffitt et al., 2011).

Mindfulness and Mindfulness Training

Mindfulness is defined as a nonreactive awareness of present moment experience (Analayo, 2003; Kabat-Zinn, 2003). Mindfulness denotes a presence of mind (Brown, Ryan, & Creswell, 2007), one that is alert, receptive, and absent of distraction (Analayo, 2003; Bodhi, 2011). In the psychological literature, mindfulness has been operationalized to include two major components: awareness of present moment experience through the regulation of attention, and an attitude of curiosity, openness, and acceptance (Bishop et al., 2004). Regarding the attention component, mindfulness involves the sustained moment-to-moment awareness of ongoing sensory, affective, and cognitive experience. In this way, mindfulness enables a continuous discernment of ongoing experience that functions to provide greater sensory clarity and to reduce biases of information processing (Vago & Silbersweig, 2012). The acceptance component of mindfulness implies that when experience is met with mindful awareness, there are no attempts made to control, suppress, or get involved with it; mindfulness simply reveals what is occurring in any given moment of experience in a receptive, nonreactive manner (Bishop et al., 2004). A mindful mode of information processing can be contrasted to a conceptually driven mode of processing, in which thoughts, emotions, and behavior are filtered through habitual evaluations, emotional reactions, and expectations (Brown et al., 2007).

Mindfulness is most commonly trained in the context of contemplative practices, such as meditation and yoga. For our purposes here, we focus on two broad styles of meditation that are widely acknowledged for cultivating the capacity for mindfulness (Brown & Ryan, 2004; Lutz, Dunne, & Davidson, 2007; Lutz, Slagter, Dunne, & Davidson, 2008). The first style of meditation practice is called focused attention (FA) and involves engaging and sustaining moment-to-moment attention on a mental or physical object, such as the rhythmic movement of the belly or chest during breathing. Here, no attention is given to the sensory experiences that fall outside of this limited focus; all other objects of experience are treated as distractions from the primary object. When the attention strays, it is refocused back to the chosen object. The goal of FA training is to stabilize and unify the mind so that it becomes free of distraction and tiredness (Vago & Silbersweig, 2012). Mindfulness is cultivated during FA to the degree that this training involves a sustained moment-to-moment metacognitive monitoring of the location and quality of attention (Lutz et al., 2008).

The second style of meditation practice used to establish and cultivate mindfulness is called open monitoring (OM) (Lutz et al., 2008). OM practice is typically integrated into mindfulness training programs following initial experience in cultivating focused attention. During OM, the attentional field is widened to include any experiences that enter conscious awareness. In this way, awareness is brought to bear on the moment-by-moment unfolding of experience—including sense impressions, mental and emotional states, and so on—without the need to focus on any one object in particular (Brown & Ryan, 2004). Maintaining undistracted awareness of sensory experience enables greater recognition into how moment-to-moment experience is typically overlaid with habitual emotional reactions, evaluations, and attempts to escape or perpetuate the experience based on its emotional tone. Once recognized, these implicit features of subjective experience can be investigated, rather than reacted upon or suppressed, allowing for the development of metacognitive insight into their constantly fluctuating nature (Analayo, 2003). Such insights gradually reinforce a degree of "de-automatization" from heretofore unseen conditioned reactions to sensory input (Kang, Gruber, & Gray, 2013), which also provides the basis for altering or even reducing compulsive mental habits that reinforce psychological suffering (Bishop et al., 2004).

Mindfulness and Executive Function

The skills learned during FA and OM training map conceptually onto the executive function capacities underlying self-regulation (Black, Semple, Pokhrel, & Grenard, 2011). During concentration practice, for example, individuals must work to keep in mind the goal to sustain attention on a present moment experience (working memory), monitor for deviations from that goal (conflict monitoring), inhibit elaborative processing of distracting stimuli (inhibitory control), and redirect attention as needed (attention shifting). Indeed, multiple studies show that brief mindfulness training is associated with improvements in executive function. For example, a study by Zeidan, Johnson, Diamond, David, and Goolkasian (2010) showed that 4 days of 20-min FA training improved working memory compared to a control group who listened to an audio book recording. Studies involving more intensive mindfulness training have also shown training-related improvements in components of executive function, including inhibitory control (Sahdra et al., 2011), working memory (Chambers, Lo, & Allen, 2008; Jha, Stanley, Kiyonaga, Wong, & Gelfand, 2010; Mrazek, Franklin, Phillips, Baird, & Schooler, 2013), perceptual sensitivity (MacLean et al., 2010), and sustained attention (Lutz et al., 2009).

In addition to research involving mindfulness training, studies also show that dispositional mindfulness—or individual differences in the general tendency to be mindful in daily life—is associated with executive function ability. Dispositional mindfulness is typically measured using self-report scales that tap various aspects of mindfulness, including present-moment attention and awareness, nonreactivity to inner experience, and nonjudgmental acceptance of experience (Baer, Smith, & Allen, 2004; Baer, Smith, Hopkins, Krietemeyer, & Toney, 2006; Baer et al., 2008; Black, Sussman, Johnson, & Milam, 2012a; Brown & Ryan, 2003). Individuals who score higher on various aspects of dispositional mindfulness have been shown to have better inhibitory control (Galla, Hale, Shrestha, Loo, & Smalley, 2012; Moore & Malinowski, 2009) and sustained attention (Galla et al., 2012; Mrazek, Smallwood, & Schooler, 2012; Schmertz, Anderson, & Robins, 2009).

While published research on children and adolescents is noticeably sparse (for a review, see Black, Milam, & Sussman, 2009), there are several studies that suggest it is possible to improve executive function via mindfulness training. In a study of third-grade children, Linden (1973) found that children who participated in an 18-week, twice weekly program of mindfulness practices were better able to find target objects amidst a distracting background (Children's Embedded Figures Test) relative to two control groups who showed no improvement. In another study, Napoli, Krech, and Holley (2005) found that elementary school-age children who completed a 24-week, bi-monthly mindfulness training program improved in selective, but not sustained, attention compared to a wait-list control condition.

Mindfulness and Emotion Regulation

The majority of research on mindfulness and self-regulation falls into the category of emotion regulation, defined broadly as "the processes by which individuals influence which emotions they have, when they have them, and how they experience and express these emotions" (Gross, 1998, p. 275). The links between mindfulness and emotion regulation are fairly straight forward given that mindfulness involves a nonreactive awareness and acceptance of present moment experience. By learning to observe and accept unpleasant experiences, for example, mindfulness training may help individuals learn to disengage from habitual ruminative thoughts (Greeson, Garland, & Black, 2014). Mindfulness training may also reduce the need to change, escape, or suppress unpleasant experiences that often have the paradoxical effect of making the unpleasant experience more salient (Wegner, 1994).

There is now a wealth of scientific evidence attesting to the benefits of mindfulness training in adults for emotion regulation, and hence psychological well-being (Baer, 2003; Brown et al., 2007; Grossman, Niemann, Schmidt, & Walach, 2004; Hofmann, Sawyer, Witt, & Oh, 2010). Research with children and adolescents also suggests that mindfulness training can benefit the self-regulation of emotion. For example, a recent study tested whether mindfulness training could improve emotion regulation in a sample of urban, economically disadvantaged fourth- and fifth-grade students (Mendelson et al., 2010). Over the course of 12 weeks, students received mindfulness training for 45 min, 4 days per week. Relative to a wait-list control condition, mindfulness training was associated with significant reductions in involuntary responses to stress, including rumination and intrusive thoughts.

Dispositional mindfulness is also related to emotion regulation in children and adolescents. In a study by Greco, Baer, and Smith (2011), adolescents who scored higher on a self-report measure tapping both awareness (e.g., "It's hard for me to pay attention to only one thing at a time") and acceptance (e.g., "I get upset with myself for having certain thoughts" [reverse-scored]) also reported less thought suppression, or the tendency to push away or escape unpleasant thoughts (e.g., "There are things that I try not to think about"). A recent naturalistic study also showed the benefits of dispositional mindfulness for day-to-day emotion regulation (Ciesla, Reilly, Dickson, Emanuel, & Updegraff, 2012). In this study, 78 high-school students first completed the Five Factor Mindfulness Questionnaire (FFMQ; Baer et al., 2008), a widely used self-report measure of mindfulness. The FFMQ assesses five aspects of mindfulness: awareness of actions, observation of present moment experience, nonreactivity to inner experience, nonjudgmental acceptance of experience, and the ability to describe experience. Next, students completed self-report measures of daily hassles, sadness, and rumination each night for a week. Students with higher levels of nonreactivity, nonjudgment, and awareness of actions reported less sadness and rumination in their daily lives. Moreover, nonreactivity and nonjudgment moderated the effect of daily stress on sadness and rumination. That is, daily stress predicted increases in sadness and rumination for students with lower levels of nonreactivity and nonjudgment, but not for students with higher levels of nonreactivity and nonjudgment. Together, these correlational data suggest that mindfulness may buffer the negative effects of stress on psychological well-being by protecting against maladaptive emotion regulation strategies, including rumination.

Mindfulness and Self-Regulation of Desires, Impulses, and Behavior

Although most research exploring the links between mindfulness and self-regulation has involved either executive function or emotion regulation, research is beginning to examine the effect of mindfulness training on the self-regulation of maladaptive desires and urges, and hence, the prevention of maladaptive behaviors. In fact, one of the central aims of mindfulness training in traditional Buddhist doctrine is to reduce problematic desires that serve to perpetuate psychological suffering (Analayo, 2003). Research examining the links between mindfulness training and reductions in craving and maladaptive impulses typically builds upon dual process models of information processing. Dual process models—ubiquitous to psychology and cognitive science—suggest that behavior is the result of an interplay between impulsive and controlled processes (Strack & Deutsch, 2004). Impulsive processes describe a set of mental operations that can be carried out quickly with little to no conscious awareness. Controlled processes, on the other hand, describe a set of higher-order mental operations that enable deliberate judgments and appraisals and can be used to guide behavior toward intended goals (Hofmann et al., 2009). Reflective processes are flexible, but computationally intensive, whereas impulsive processes are computationally efficient, but relatively inflexible. As such, the fast response stemming from impulsive processing may not always be appropriate or consistent with goal standards. For example, the mere perception of a cigarette might automatically trigger the impulse to smoke even though this impulse conflicts with the higher-order goal to abstain. The ability to successfully adjudicate conflicts that arise between impulsive and reflective processes is at the root of successful self-control (Hofmann et al., 2009). Mindfulness training has the potential to influence both the impulsive, bottom-up processing system and the controlled, top-down system.

Because mindfulness involves increased monitoring and awareness of interoceptive cues, increasing this capacity might promote earlier recognition of automatically activated desires before intense craving can occur (Teper, Segal, & Inzlicht, 2013). For example, a series of studies by Papies, Barsalou, and Custers (2011) showed that a brief mindfulness induction reduced automatic impulses toward attractive stimuli. Impulsive approach tendencies, measured using an implicit approach-avoidance task, were eliminated among participants who were trained to view reactions to external stimuli as passing mental events. Mindfulness training has also been shown to "decouple" the link between impulsive processes and self-regulation failure. For example, a study by Ostafin, Bauer, and Myxter (2012) showed that mindfulness training moderated the relationship between implicit alcohol motivations and drinking behavior. Among participants who received three mindfulness training sessions, automatic alcohol motivations (measured using an implicit association test) did not predict self-reported drinking behavior. For participants who did not receive training, implicit alcohol motivations strongly predicted drinking behavior.

In addition to disrupting the early stages of impulsive processes, mindfulness training also shows promise as one way to reduce the experience of craving in a number of health-related domains (Black, 2014; O'Reilly, Cook, Spruijt-Metz, & Black, 2014). For example, research with adults suggests that mindfulness training is effective for dealing with cravings toward unhealthy food (Alberts, Mulkens, Smeets, & Thewissen, 2010), as well as smoking cigarettes (Elwafi, Witkiewitz, Mallik, Thornhill, & Brewer, 2012; Witkiewitz & Bowen, 2010).

Regarding controlled mental processes, mindfulness may improve the ability to maintain valued goals in working memory (Jha et al., 2010) and to better act on these goals. For example, dispositional mindfulness—measured using the Mindful Awareness Attention Scale (MAAS; Brown & Ryan, 2003)—moderated the relationship between intentions to exercise and self-reported exercise behavior (Chatzisarantis & Hagger, 2007). Specifically, intentions to exercise predicted actual exercise behavior among individuals with higher dispositional mindfulness. For less mindful individuals, intentions to exercise did not predict behavior.

Research with adolescent samples also suggests that mindfulness can counteract the effects of the impulsive system on self-regulation failures, as well as buffer against maladaptive behavioral intentions. In a series of studies, Black and colleagues analyzed data from a nationally representative longitudinal study of Chinese adolescents relating dispositional mindfulness to cigarette smoking. Study participants completed the MAAS in addition to self-reporting the number of days during the last month in which they smoked cigarettes. In one study, dispositional mindfulness indirectly reduced smoking frequency through its effect on negative affect and perceived stress (Black, Milam, Sussman, & Johnson, 2012). Specifically, adolescents with higher dispositional mindfulness experienced lower levels of negative affect and perceived stress, which in turn mediated the association between dispositional mindfulness and frequency of smoking cigarettes. In a second study, dispositional mindfulness moderated the effect of intentions to smoke on smoking frequency (Black, Sussman, Johnson, & Milam, 2012b). That is, intentions to smoke cigarettes predicted higher frequency of cigarette smoking for adolescents with lower dispositional mindfulness; intentions did not predict smoking frequency for adolescents with higher mindfulness. Together, these two studies suggest that mindfulness can shield against self-regulation failure (i.e., cigarette smoking) by protecting against negative affective states and by countering maladaptive intentions.

Adapting Mindfulness Training for Children: Inner Kids

The studies highlighted above suggest that improving the capacity for mindfulness may be an effective means for promoting self-regulation. However, less is known about the specifics and effectiveness of child-friendly adaptations of mindfulness training, and further, what effect these adaptations may have for improving self-regulation ability. In this section, we first discuss the Inner Kids program as one model for how to adapt mindfulness training for children and adolescents. Then, we describe results of a randomized controlled trial examining the effect of Inner Kids to promote self-regulation in elementary school-age youth.

Modeled after classical mindfulness training for adults, Inner Kids is a semi-structured curriculum that teaches secular and age-appropriate mindfulness exercises to youth (Kaiser-Greenland, 2010). In broad terms, the Inner Kids program focuses on the development of three areas that are also emphasized in classical mindfulness training: attention, emotional balance, and compassion. Inner Kids has been developed in two formats to suit children as young as 4 (preschool) and as old as 18 (twelfth grade) with a flexible length and frequency that varies according to the students' ages and the facilitators' objectives. The first format (stand alone drop-in activities) is designed so that parents and professionals can integrate relatively brief (under 10 min) mindfulness-based activities into their routines at home, work, or school. Transitions—for instance, when children are standing in line, sitting at the kitchen table, getting ready to leave the house, waiting their turn or waiting to go to lunch, recess or the next class—are opportunities to integrate mindfulness activities into daily life. In the second format (life-skills classes), the same activities are sequenced together to create longer, stand-alone classes that challenge children and teens with longer periods of mindfulness practice and group process. This second, life-skills class format is the course structure that was used in the study described below where young children (ages 4–9) typically receive Inner Kids training in 30-min sessions twice a week for 8 weeks. For older children, the course usually meets once a week for 45–60 min, for 10–12 weeks.

Each Inner Kids life-skills class is divided into three main sections. The first section involves a sitting introspective practice, and the closing third section involves another introspective period (often lying down). Unlike the first and third sections of each class, the middle section includes goal-directed, relational activities and games directed toward a specific learning objective. At the beginning of the program, the first and third sections are relatively brief, but over the course of the 8- to 12-week program these sections are gradually extended as students develop a capacity to engage in introspective practices for longer periods of time.

Inner Kids activities are designed to help youth "develop and strengthen their ability to pay attention to their inner and outer experiences" (Goodman & Greenland, 2009, p. 418) in an objective and friendly manner. In addition to games, songs, and activities that develop awareness of oneself and others (collectively referred to as "Awareness Practices"), Inner Kids activities also emphasize other fundamental elements of classical meditation training (collectively referred to as "Kindness Practices") in an age-appropriate manner, including: (1) the cultivation of kindness, compassion, and an ethic of service toward oneself, others, and the broader community; (2) an understanding that all actions, large or small, have consequences that one cannot always anticipate; (3) an understanding that thoughts, emotions, and physical sensations come, go, and that they change; (4) an understanding that people, places, and things are connected in ways one might not expect; (5) an understanding that there is a way to view inner and outer experience with a clear-headed perspective even when one is overly excited or upset; and (6) an understanding that many life events do not fit neatly into a category of right or wrong, and/or black or white.

The multi-lesson curriculum is divided into four equal-length units (one to four lessons each), with each unit containing lessons that include both Awareness and Kindness Practices. In addition, each unit will target one or more age-appropriate, real life applications of mindfulness. For example, students learn that breath awareness can help them calm, focus, and concentrate, or that mindful awareness can help them clearly see and better understand what is happening in, to, and around them.

Because attention serves as the foundation for all the later practices in the program, the first of the four units is designed to help kids become more familiar with the process of their attention (e.g., how it always wanders, that we can consciously control it) and to help them learn how to focus and stabilize it with greater ease. The first unit is also devoted to allowing children to become aware of their present moment experience and developing a visceral understanding of breath and sensory awareness, specifically awareness of sound. To promote FA, this unit introduces students to various mindful breathing and mindful listening activities as children sit, move, stand, and lie down. The breath awareness activities focus on the sensation of breath as it moves in, out, and through the body, thus grounding the child in a visceral, body-based experience as opposed to the more cerebral stance often taken when a child "tries" to pay attention. In addition to mindful breathing and mindful listening, in the first unit students are also introduced to Kindness Practices that encourage both FA and kindness to self. Students are given opportunities to develop a present-moment and visceral experience of kindness by extending friendly wishes toward oneself (e.g., through visualizing themselves in a safe place, and actively wishing happiness, safety, and health for themselves or giving themselves a hug). An example of a mindful breathing, a mindful listening, and a kindness activity are set forth in the Appendix below.

Once children have received FA instructions and have had some formal practice focusing and sustaining their attention on the sensations of breathing and listening, the second unit leads students through a group of exercises aimed at deepening their clarity and awareness regarding inner experience. The second unit expands the objects of awareness from breath and sound to include their inner experience of the five common main sensory systems, as well as the vestibular sensory system (awareness of physical balance) and the proprioceptive sensory system (awareness of one's body in space). A common exercise to train FA using the senses is to ring a very resonant chime and ask the children to raise their hands when they can no longer hear the sound. In Inner Kids classes for young children, this exercise is immediately preceded by a playful, movement sequence. Engaging in purposeful and lively activities prior to more formal attention training has a number of functions, not the least of which being that they are fun. Movement prior to introspection often makes it easier for children to concentrate while encouraging them to temporarily "drop" an analytic mindset and approach the mindfulness-based exercise from a different, more experiential perspective.

In this unit, children are also given instructions on developing the capacity for more mindful presence by: (1) observing their sensory experiences impartially by noticing and identifying sensory experience as it occurs; and (2) by using mindful awareness to calm their minds and bodies prior to reflecting on their experiences so that they are able to view what is happening as objectively as possible. If students notice that there is an "emotional charge" connected with their experience, the object is not to "get rid of" the emotion but rather to become aware of it and reflect on how it might affect their capacity to see the experience impartially.

New Awareness Practices, such as eating meditations and mindfulness of movement, are also introduced in this unit. The Kindness Practices are extended in unit 2 and provide children with opportunities to develop a sense for extending kindness toward others as well as themselves through aspirations that both self and other are safe, happy, healthy, and living in peace (e.g., "may I be happy," "may you be happy," "may everyone be happy").

The third unit builds on the sense of self-awareness and self-management that is weaved throughout the first two units. Children are taught strategies and skills for becoming more familiar with how their minds and bodies react to inner and outer experiences. This unit emphasizes awareness of thoughts, emotions, and physical sensations and teaches children about how the three are inter-connected. In addition, activities in this unit promote an experiential understanding that actions tend to follow from these thoughts, emotions, and sensations and that they have consequences. For example, children are introduced to the "Awareness Meter" (see Fig. 19.1), "Pinky Pointing," (see Appendix), and similar techniques that help them notice, identify, and then gauge how certain experiences result in feelings that are pleasant, unpleasant, and neutral (e.g., an argument with a parent feels unpleasant, having fun with a friend on the playground feels pleasant). The Awareness Meter and Pinky Pointing are concrete tools used in this unit to help children notice, identify, and connect how these various feelings are often accompanied by other inner experiences (e.g., thoughts and/or physical sensations, for instance a stomach ache) and/or urges to act in a particular way. Children are also encouraged to become more aware of how they habitually tend to react to and respond to various situations, which might then provide opportunities for a larger discussion about different and more flexible ways of responding. The Kindness Practices in unit 3 are designed, among other things, to help children become acquainted with the experience of offering compassion to people who are experiencing some kind of suffering, in addition to feeling joy and happiness for people who are experiencing good fortune.

The fourth and final unit is designed to help children become more aware of themselves as interdependent members of a community. The

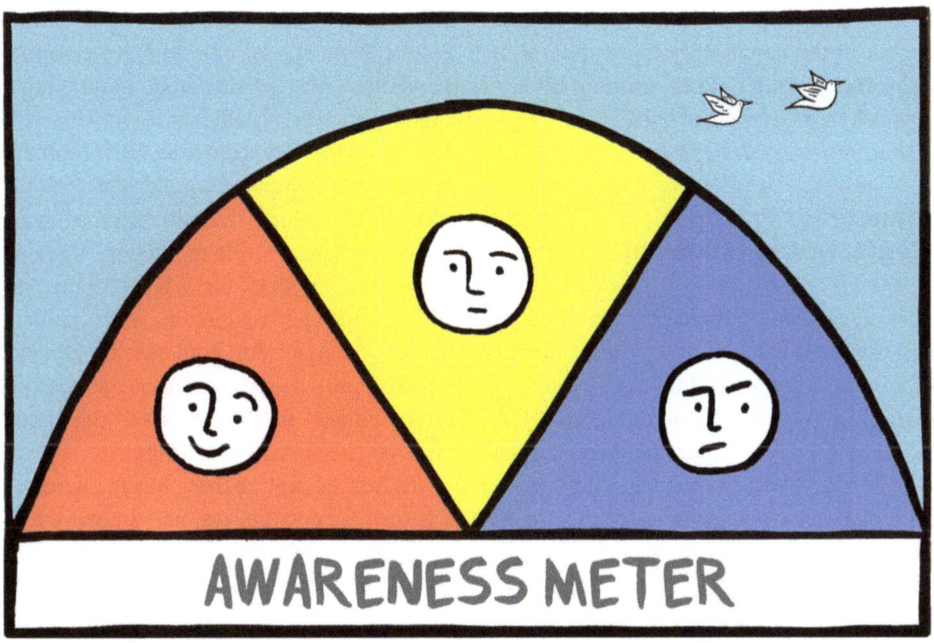

Fig. 19.1 The Awareness Meter is a visual aid that offers children a playful way to reflect on a life experience and communicate to you whether it is pleasant, unpleasant, or neutral. © Susan Kaiser Greenland, 2013 | www.innerkids.com | *The materials provided are authored and copyrighted by Susan Kaiser Greenland. They are intended for the sole use of Inner Kids training participants and may not be duplicated without the express permission of the author. Artist: Lindsay DuPont*

"clear seeing" of inner experience developed in the earlier units is now used to help children become more aware of and connected to their outer experiences, notably through an awareness of other people and the environment. Awareness Practices that help children become more attuned to others, such as mirroring the physical movements of their peers, are developed to help foster a sense of community and teamwork among children. Kindness Practices in this unit also promote awareness and a visceral understanding of interconnectedness. For instance, children can be led through an exercise where they visualize the entire life cycle of a piece of fruit—from seed to stomach. The child can imagine the progressive trajectory of a raisin, from the grape seed being planted and tended to, to the fruit being harvested, dried, and shipped to the grocery, and finally to the raisin being purchased by the child's family and packaged into their lunch. In this way, the children can gain a greater sense of the many people involved in bringing the fruit to them, as well as how this awareness shifts their perspectives. Cultivation of this type of awareness can open doors for discussions about gratitude and ways to act in the community that supports the environment (e.g., older children might think to start a recycling program at school).

Does Inner Kids Promote Self-Regulation in Children?

With this description of Inner Kids in mind, we now turn to a short discussion of recent efforts to study the effect of Inner Kids to promote self-regulation. In this study (Flook et al., 2010), 64 second- and third-grade children attending a university laboratory school were randomized to either a mindfulness training condition or an active control condition. Children in the mindfulness training condition met with an Inner Kids facilitator (S.K.G.) twice per week for 8 consecutive weeks. Children in the control condition engaged in a period of quiet reading. Each session was 30 min long and all activities took place at school. Self-regulation ability was measured using the Behavior Rating Inventory of Executive Function (BRIEF; Gioia, Isquith, Guy, & Kenworthy, 2000). The BRIEF is an adult-report questionnaire that assesses multiple aspects of self-regulation and executive function utilized in everyday life. For example, parents and teachers can report on children's ability to resist impulses and problematic urges (inhibitory control), their ability to plan and manage current and future task demands (plan/organize), and their ability to monitor performance on a task as well as to monitor how their actions might affect others (monitor). The eight subscales can be combined to form a Global Executive Composite (GEC) score. The BRIEF was designed to be a more comprehensive, ecologically valid measure of self-regulation compared to behavioral measures that typically only measure discrete aspects of self-regulation and executive function (Isquith, Gioia, & Espy, 2004). In the current study, teachers and parents assessed children's self-regulation immediately before and after the 8-week intervention period.

Results indicated that Inner Kids training was particularly effective in promoting self-regulation for children who began the program with lower self-regulation (for full results, see Flook et al., 2010). That is, children with lower initial self-regulation who participated in the Inner Kids training showed significant improvement in self-regulation (as indexed by the GEC score) following training compared to children in the control group. For children initially rated as average or above-average on self-regulation, there was no discernible effect of Inner Kids training on their post-training self-regulation. A similar pattern of change emerged for both teacher-reported and parent-reported self-regulation, suggesting that improvements in children's self-regulation generalized to non-school settings.

To further explore these results, we also tested whether Inner Kids training improved specific components of self-regulation on the BRIEF. Based on both teacher and parent reports, children with initial lower self-regulation who received training in Inner Kids showed significant improvement in their ability to initiate tasks, to shift between tasks, and to monitor performance on tasks. Interestingly, improvements in these three domains may reflect the set of skills practiced during mindfulness training, which included focusing attention on a physical sensation (initiate), sustaining focus over time (monitor), and redirecting attention back to the sensation following any lapses (shifting). While the results of this study are preliminary, they do provide interesting evidence that mindfulness training may be particularly beneficial for otherwise healthy youth who have relatively low self-regulatory abilities.

Future Directions and Conclusion

The scientific evidence on the efficacy of mindfulness training for children and adolescents is considerably small compared to the research literature on adults (Black, 2015; Black et al., 2009). However, the research surveyed in this chapter suggests that mindfulness training with youth is both feasible and may foster skills and mindsets related to successful self-regulation. Looking forward, attending to the methodological rigor of studies is a primary concern. Ensuring true random assignment to groups is an important methodological component, especially given the normative development and growth in self-regulation. Designing active control groups that involve comparable activities (e.g., relaxation-training, group support) to the treatment will also be an important future step in teasing out potential active ingredients and controlling for important confounds. Monitoring implementation fidelity and training dosage will be helpful for determining how often and how much mindfulness practice is necessary for measurable effects to emerge. Including long-term follow-up assessments, beyond the immediate post-intervention assessment, is crucial to determine the sustained influence of mindfulness training on trajectories of self-regulation. Specifically, regarding self-regulation as the target of mindfulness training, incorporating reliable and objective measures into the assessment battery is critical. It will also be crucial to examine whether gains in self-regulation due to mindfulness training mediate changes observed in other areas of social–emotional or academic functioning (for an example, see Jha et al., 2010).

Appendix: Inner Kids Sample Practices

Pinky Pointing

A playful way for children to notice and identify what they are thinking and how they are feeling and communicate what they learn to you without using words.

Sequence for Pinky Pointing

- Suggest that sometimes it is hard to put feelings into words, but that it is important to find ways to notice feelings and communicate them. Pinking Pointing can help when it is hard to describe feelings with words.
- Explain that you are going to ask a question, and children will respond with a pinkies-up, pinkies-down, or a pinkies-sideways. Ask children to wait to respond until they hear the word "Go" as in "1-2-3-Go!"
- Ask a simple, concrete question (for instance, is it easy or hard to sit still right now), and invite children to answer using their pinkies (pinkies up if it is easy, pinkies down if it is hard, pinkies sideways if it is in-between). "1-2-3-Go!"
- Ask children to keep their pinkies in the air and look around.
- Point out that not everyone feels the same way. Now that is interesting!
- Repeat with one or more clear, concrete questions.

Notes

- It is common for children to check how their friends respond before responding themselves. To avoid this, make sure children wait to give their pinkies up, down, or sideways until they hear the words "1-2-3-Go!"
- After children answer a question, ask them to keep their pinkies in the air and check to see how others responded. This reminds them that they are not alone in how they are feeling, and the flip side, that not everyone feels the same way that they feel.
- There are no right or wrong answers, and one answer is not "better" than another, the object is simply to notice and identify what is happening, in the present moment.

The Awareness Meter

The Awareness Meter is a visual aid that offers children a playful way to reflect on a life experience and communicate to you whether it is pleasant, unpleasant, or neutral. The sequence for using the Awareness Meter is similar to the sequence for playing Pinky Pointing.

Sequence for Awareness Meter

- Check to make sure that children understand the meaning of the words "pleasant," "unpleasant," and "neutral" by asking for examples of pleasant, unpleasant, and neutral experiences.
- Suggest that it is helpful to pay attention to the quality of our life experiences by noticing which ones feel pleasant, unpleasant, or neutral.
- Ask a simple, concrete question (for instance, what is it like to stop and feel your breathing) and invite children to answer using the Awareness Meter (pointing to the red triangle for pleasant, the blue triangle for unpleasant, and the yellow triangle for neutral).
- Ask children to keep pointing to the appropriate triangle on the Awareness Meter while they look around to see where their friends are pointing.
- If working with a group of children, there will usually be different opinions.
- If there are different opinions, ask for volunteers to describe the pleasant, unpleasant, or neutral qualities of their experiences.
- Brainstorm about ways that noticing these different qualities can help children navigate life's ups and downs.

Notes

- The object of the activity, in the first instance, is for children to notice and identify the quality of a life experience. A pleasant experience is not necessarily better than an unpleasant or a neutral one.

Counting Breaths

Counting breaths develops concentration (focused attention) and helps students quiet busy thoughts by narrowing their field of concentration. Sometimes referred to as training wheels for meditation, it is one of the first formal introspective practices we teach children.

Sequence for Counting Breaths

- Ask children to define concentration. For instance, concentration is paying attention to one thing and nothing else.
- Ask students to define a distraction. For instance, a distraction is something that makes it difficult to pay attention to one thing and nothing else.
- Ask children to offer examples of things that are easy to focus on (a favorite video game, for instance) and things that are hard to focus on (homework that feels boring, for instance).
- Explain that counting breaths is one way to practice concentrating and that the more we practice, the easier it becomes to concentrate on one thing and ignore distractions.
- Encourage children to sit (or stand) like a mountain with their spines straight and their muscles relaxed.
- Raise one finger and suggest that children keep the number one in their minds (silently think the number 1) when they breathe-in and relax when they breathe-out.
- Raise a second finger and suggest that children silently think the number 2 when they breathe-in and relax when they breathe-out.
- Raise a third finger and suggest that children silently think the number 3 when they breathe-in and relax when they breathe-out.
- Continue counting from 1 to 3 using hand motions (no words) for the remainder of the introspective period.

Notes

- Children can lead the class in counting breaths either out loud or by raising a finger with each inhale (one finger, then two fingers, then three fingers).
- Group students in pairs or small groups and ask them to take turns leading three breaths together by raising a finger with each inhale.

Listening on Purpose

Even when a room seems quiet, there's sound around us. If you take a minute to listen carefully, you might be surprised at all that you hear.

Sequence for Listening on Purpose

- Encourage children to sit (or stand) like a mountain with their spines straight and muscles relaxed.
- Invite children to close their eyes and remind them you will keep yours open.
- Lead a brief progressive muscle relaxation starting at the top of the head and moving down by first relaxing the muscles in their faces, then their chins, necks and shoulders, upper arms, lower arms, hands, fingers, chests, bellies, rears, upper legs, lower legs, ankles, feet, toes.
- With spines straight and muscles relaxed, encourage children to listen normally, making no special effort. Remind them not to be surprised if soon their minds wander. The moment children notice that their minds have wandered is a moment of mindful awareness!
- After *listening on purpose* for a few minutes, ask children how they feel. Many children say they feel more relaxed or focused or calm. Reflect on times that listening on purpose could be helpful outside of mindfulness class—at home, at school, or in the community.

Notes

- When working with a group, start with a few minutes of listening on purpose and extend the length of time as children become more comfortable with the activity.
- Pace the activity based on how long the least comfortable child can practice.
- Transitions, or times that children are waiting, are opportunities to *listen on purpose*.
- You can use a bell, tone bar, water feature, or CD to better control the ambient sound.

Imaginary Hugs

Children practice concentrating as they picture themselves in a safe place where they are happy, healthy, and having a lot of fun. Children bring to mind pictures of other people too and visualize images of themselves, their families, their friends, and eventually everyone and everything having a lot of fun as they live happily, safely, and peacefully together.

Sequence for Imaginary Hugs

- Ask children what it feels like to get a hug and give someone a hug.
- Check to make sure that young children understand the words "pretend" and "imagine" by asking them what it means to imagine that they are doing something else or to pretend that they are in someplace else.
- Invite children to imagine a peaceful place. If working with a group, ask children to put one hand on their heads when they have a peaceful place in mind so that you will know when everyone is ready.
- Once children have a peaceful place in mind, ask them to pretend they can feel, see, touch, hear, taste, or smell something in that peaceful place.
- Encourage children to give themselves a hug and send themselves a friendly wish picturing themselves in a peaceful place where they are having fun and feeling happy.
- Next invite children to give an imaginary hug to a friend or family member and send that person a friendly wish. Ask children to put one hand on their head when they have chosen the friend or family member.
- Once all the children have a hand on their head, encourage them to hold their arms away from their chests in a circle and pretend they are hugging that friend or family member picturing him or her in a peaceful place where they are happy, safe, and having fun.
- Children can give even more people imaginary hugs by bringing them to mind too as they make their arms wide enough to hug all of them in their imaginations while silently sending them friendly wishes.
- Close by encouraging children to stretch their arms out wide and imagine that they can hug the entire planet as they imagine a world where everyone and everything is happy, healthy, safe, and peaceful.

Notes

- We only invite children to close their eyes, we do not insist on it, and we remind them that our eyes will be open and watching the room when their eyes are closed.

- We do not ask children to ignore or change their feelings about what is happening in their lives when they picture the world as a kind and happy place. Nor do we ask them to change their feelings about people they know by asking them to like someone whom they don't already like.

References

Alberts, H. J. E. M., Mulkens, S., Smeets, M., & Thewissen, R. (2010). Coping with food cravings. Investigating the potential of a mindfulness-based intervention. *Appetite, 55*, 160–163.

Analayo, B. (2003). *Satipatthana: The direct path to realization*. Birmingham, England: Windhorse.

Baer, R. A. (2003). Mindfulness training as a clinical intervention: A conceptual and empirical review. *Clinical Psychology: Science and Practice, 10*, 125–143.

Baer, R. A., Smith, G. T., & Allen, K. B. (2004). Assessment of mindfulness by self-report: The Kentucky inventory of mindfulness skills. *Assessment, 11*, 191–206.

Baer, R. A., Smith, G. T., Hopkins, J., Krietemeyer, J., & Toney, L. (2006). Using self-report assessment methods to explore facets of mindfulness. *Assessment, 13*, 27–45.

Baer, R. A., Smith, G. T., Lykins, E. L. B., Button, D., Krietemeyer, J., Sauer, S., … Williams, J. M. (2008). Construct validity of the five facet mindfulness questionnaire in meditating and nonmeditating samples. *Assessment, 15*, 329–342.

Baumeister, R. F., Heatherton, T. F., & Tice, D. M. (1994). *Losing control: How and why people fail at self-regulation*. San Diego, CA: Academic Press.

Bishop, S. R., Lau, M., Shapiro, S., Carlson, L., Anderson, N. D., Carmody, J., … Devins, G. (2004). Mindfulness: A proposed operational definition. *Clinical Psychology: Science and Practice, 11*, 230–241.

Black, D. S. (2014). Mindfulness-based interventions: An antidote to suffering in the context of substance use, misuse, and addiction. *Substance Use & Misuse, 49*, 487–491.

Black, D. S. (2015). Mindfulness training for children and adolescents: A state-of-the-science review. In K. W. Brown, R. M. Ryan, & J. D. Creswell (Eds.), *Handbook of mindfulness: Theory and research (pp. 283-310)*. New York, NY: Guilford Press.

Black, D. S., Milam, J., & Sussman, S. (2009). Sitting-meditation interventions among youth: A review of treatment efficacy. *Pediatrics, 124*, e532–e541.

Black, D. S., Milam, J., Sussman, S., & Johnson, C. A. (2012). Testing the indirect effect of trait mindfulness on adolescent cigarette smoking through negative affect and perceived stress mediators. *Journal of Substance Abuse, 17*, 417–429.

Black, D. S., Semple, R. J., Pokhrel, P., & Grenard, J. L. (2011). Component processes of executive function-mindfulness, self-control, and working memory-and their relationships with mental and behavioral health. *Mindfulness, 2*, 179–185.

Black, D. S., Sussman, S., Johnson, C. A., & Milam, J. (2012a). Psychometric properties of the mindful awareness attention scale (MAAS) among Chinese adolescents. *Assessment, 19*, 40–50.

Black, D. S., Sussman, S., Johnson, C. A., & Milam, J. (2012b). Trait mindfulness helps shield decision-making from translating into health-risk behavior. *Journal of Adolescent Health, 51*, 588–592.

Blair, C. (2002). School readiness: Integrating cognition and emotion in a neurobiological conceptualization of children's functioning at school entry. *American Psychologist, 57*, 111–127.

Blair, C., & Diamond, A. (2008). Biological processes in prevention and intervention: The promotion of self-regulation as a means of preventing school failure. *Development and Psychopathology, 20*, 899–911.

Blair, C., & Razza, R. P. (2007). Relating effortful control, executive function, and false belief understanding to emerging math and literacy ability in kindergarten. *Child Development, 78*, 647–663.

Bodhi, B. (2011). What does mindfulness really mean? A canonical perspective. *Contemporary Buddhism, 12*, 19–39.

Brown, K. W., & Ryan, R. M. (2003). The benefits of being present: Mindfulness and its role in psychological well-being. *Journal of Personality and Social Psychology, 84*, 822–848.

Brown, K. W., & Ryan, R. M. (2004). Perils and promise in defining and measuring mindfulness: Observations from experience. *Clinical Psychology: Science and Practice, 11*, 242–248.

Brown, K. W., Ryan, R. M., & Creswell, J. D. (2007). Mindfulness: Theoretical foundations and evidence for its salutary effects. *Psychological Inquiry, 18*, 211–237.

Casey, B. J., Tottenham, N., Liston, C., & Durston, S. (2005). Imaging the developing brain: What have we learned about cognitive development. *Trends in Cognitive Sciences, 9*, 104–110.

Chambers, R., Lo, B. C. Y., & Allen, N. B. (2008). The impact of intensive mindfulness training on attentional control, cognitive style, and affect. *Cognitive Therapy and Research, 32*, 303–322.

Chatzisarantis, N. L. D., & Hagger, M. S. (2007). Mindfulness and the intention-behavior relationship within the theory of planned behavior. *Personality and Social Psychology Bulletin, 33*, 663–676.

Ciesla, J. A., Reilly, L. C., Dickson, K. S., Emanuel, A. S., & Updegraff, J. A. (2012). Dispositional mindfulness moderates the effects of stress among adolescents: Rumination as a mediator. *Journal of Clinical Child and Adolescent Psychology, 41*, 760–770.

Derryberry, D., & Rothbart, M. K. (1997). Reactive and effortful processes in the organization of temperament. *Development and Psychopathology, 9*, 633–652.

Diamond, A. (2002). Normal development of prefrontal cortex from birth to young adulthood: Cognitive functions, anatomy, and biochemistry. In D. T. Stuss & R. T. Knight (Eds.), *Principles of frontal lobe function* (pp. 466–503). London, UK: Oxford University Press.

Diamond, A. (2012). Executive functions. *Annual Review of Psychology, 64*, 135–168.

Dickinson, A. (1985). Actions and habits: The development of behavioural autonomy. *Philosophical Transactions of the Royal Society of London. Series B, Biological Sciences, 308*, 67–78.

Duckworth, A. L., & Carlson, S. M. (2013). Self-regulation and school success. In B. W. Sokol, F. M. E. Grouzet, & U. Müller (Eds.), *Self-regulation and autonomy: Social and developmental dimensions of human conduct* (pp. 208–230). New York, NY: Cambridge University Press.

Eisenberg, N., Hofer, C., & Vaughan, J. (2007). Effortful control and its socioemotional consequences. In J. J. Gross (Ed.), *Handbook of emotion regulation*. New York, NY: Guilford.

Elwafi, H. M., Witkiewitz, K., Mallik, S., Thornhill, T. A., & Brewer, J. A. (2012). Mindfulness training for smoking cessation: Moderation of the relationship between craving and cigarette use. *Drug and Alcohol Dependence, 130*, 222–229.

Flook, L., Smalley, S. L., Kitil, J., Galla, B. M., Kaiser-Greenland, S., Locke, J., …, Kasari, C. (2010). Effects of mindful awareness practices on executive functions in elementary school children. *Journal of Applied School Psychology, 26*, 70–95.

Fujita, K. (2011). On conceptualizing self-control as more than the effortful inhibition of impulses. *Personality and Social Psychology Review*, 15, 352–366.

Galla, B. M., Hale, T. S., Shrestha, A., Loo, S. K., & Smalley, S. L. (2012). The disciplined mind: Associations between the Kentuck inventory of mindfulness skills and attention control. *Mindfulness, 3*, 95–103.

Galla, B. M., Plummer, B. D., White, R. E., Meketon, D., D'Mello, S. K., & Duckworth, A. L. (2014). The Academic Diligence Task (ADT): Assessing individual differences in effort on tedious but important schoolwork. *Contemporary Educational Psychology, 39*(4), 314–325.

Garon, N., Bryson, S. E., & Smith, I. M. (2008). Executive function in preschoolers: A review using an integrative framework. *Psychological Bulletin, 134*, 31–60.

Giedd, J. N. (2004). Structural magnetic resonance imaging of the adolescent brain. *Annals of the New York Academy of Sciences, 1021*, 77–85.

Giedd, J. N., Blumenthal, J., Jeffries, N. O., Castellanos, F. X., Liu, H., Zijdenbos, A., … Rapoport, J. L. (1999). Brain development during childhood and adolescence: A longitudinal MRI study. *Nature Neuroscience, 10*, 861–863.

Gioia, G. A., Isquith, P. K., Guy, S. C., & Kenworthy, L. (2000). *Behavior rating inventory of executive function*. Lutz, FL: Psychological Assessment Resources.

Goodman, T. A., & Greenland, S. K. (2009). Mindfulness with children: Working with difficult emotions. In F. Didonna (Ed.), *Clinical handbook of mindfulness* (pp. 417–429). New York, NY: Springer.

Greco, L. A., Baer, R. A., & Smith, G. T. (2011). Assessing mindfulness in children and adolescents: Development and validation of the Child and Adolescent Mindfulness Measure (CAMM). *Psychological Assessment, 23*, 606–614.

Greeson, J., Garland, E., & Black, D. S. (2014). Mindfulness: A transtherapeutic approach for transdiagnostic mental processes. In A. Ie, C. Ngnoumen, & E. Langer (Eds.), *The Wiley Blackwell handbook of mindfulness* (Vol. 2). Oxford, England: Wiley.

Gross, J. J. (1998). The emerging field of emotion regulation: An integrative review. *Review of General Psychology, 2*, 271–299.

Grossman, P., Niemann, L., Schmidt, S., & Walach, H. (2004). Mindfulness-based stress reduction and health benefits: A meta-analysis. *Journal of Psychosomatic Research, 57*, 35–43.

Hofmann, W., Friese, M., & Strack, F. (2009). Impulse and self-control from a dual-systems perspective. *Perspectives on Psychological Science, 4*, 462879.

Hofmann, S. G., Sawyer, A. T., Witt, A. A., & Oh, D. (2010). The effect of mindfulness-based therapy on anxiety and depression: A meta-analytic review. *Journal of Consulting and Clinical Psychology, 78*, 169–183.

Isquith, P. K., Gioia, G. A., & Espy, K. A. (2004). Executive function in preschool children: Examination through everyday behavior. *Developmental Neuropsychology, 26*, 403–422.

Jha, A. P., Stanley, E. A., Kiyonaga, A., Wong, L., & Gelfand, L. (2010). Examining the protective effects of mindfulness training on working memory and affective experience. *Emotion, 10*, 54–64.

Kabat-Zinn, J. (2003). Mindfulness-based interventions in context: Past, present, and future. *Clinical Psychology: Science and Practice, 10*, 144–156.

Kaiser-Greenland, S. (2010). *The mindful child: How to help your kid manage stress and become happier, kinder, and more compassionate*. New York, NY: Free Press.

Kang, Y., Gruber, J., & Gray, J. R. (2013). Mindfulness and de-automatization. *Emotion Review, 5*, 192–201.

Kochanska, G., Murray, K. T., & Harlan, E. T. (2000). Effortful control in early childhood: Continuity and change, antecedents, and implications for social development. *Developmental Psychology, 36*, 220–232.

Linden, W. (1973). Practicing of meditation by school children and their levels of field dependence-independence, test anxiety, and reading achievement. *Journal of Consulting and Clinical Psychology, 41*, 139–143.

Lutz, A., Dunne, J. D., & Davidson, R. J. (2007). Meditation and the neuroscience of consciousness. In

P. D. Zelazo, M. Moscovitch, & E. Thompson (Eds.), *The Cambridge handbook of consciousness*. Cambridge, NY: Cambridge University Press.
Lutz, A., Slagter, H. A., Dunne, J., & Davidson, R. J. (2008). Attention regulation and monitoring in meditation. *Trends in Cognitive Sciences, 12*, 163–169.
Lutz, A., Slagter, H., Rawling, N., Francis, A., Greischar, L. L., & Davidson, R. J. (2009). Mental training enhances attentional stability: Neural and behavioral evidence. *Journal of Neuroscience, 29*, 13418–13427.
MacCann, C., Duckworth, A. L., & Roberts, R. D. (2009). Empirical identification of the major facets of conscientiousness. *Learning and Individual Differences, 19*, 451–458.
MacLean, K. A., Ferrer, E., Aichele, S. R., Bridwell, D. A., Zanesco, A. P., Jacobs, T. L., … Saron, C. D. (2010). Intensive meditation training improves perceptual discrimination and sustained attention. *Psychological Science, 21*, 829–839.
McClelland, M. M., Acock, A., Piccinin, A., Rhea, S. A., & Stallings, M. C. (2012). Relations between preschool attention span-persistence and age 25 educational outcomes. *Early Childhood Research Quarterly, 28*, 314–324.
Mendelson, T., Greenberg, M. T., Dariotis, J. K., Gould, L. F., Rhoades, B. L., & Leaf, P. J. (2010). Feasibility and preliminary outcomes of a school-based mindfulness intervention for urban youth. *Journal of Abnormal Child Psychology, 38*, 985–994.
Mischel, W., Shoda, Y., & Rodriguez, M. L. (1989). Delay of gratification in children. *Science, 244*, 933–938.
Moffitt, T. E., Arseneault, L., Belsky, D., Dickson, N., Hancox, R. J., Harrington, H. L., … Caspi, A. (2011). A gradient of childhood self-control predicts health, wealth, and public safety. *Proceedings of the National Academy of Sciences, 108*(7), 2693–2698.
Moore, A., & Malinowski, P. (2009). Meditation, mindfulness and cognitive flexibility. *Consciousness and Cognition, 18*, 176–186.
Mrazek, M. D., Franklin, M. S., Phillips, D. T., Baird, B., & Schooler, J. W. (2013). Mindfulness training improves working memory capacity and GRE performance while reducing mind wandering. *Psychological Science, 24*, 776–781.
Mrazek, M. D., Smallwood, J., & Schooler, J. W. (2012). Mindfulness and mind-wandering: Finding convergence through opposing constructs. *Emotion, 12*, 442–448.
Napoli, M., Krech, P. R., & Holley, L. C. (2005). Mindfulness training for elementary school students: The Attention Academy. *Journal of Applied School Psychology, 21*, 99–125.
O'Reilly, G. A., Cook, L., Spruijt-Metz, D., & Black, D. S. (2014). Mindfulness-based interventions for obesity-related eating behaviours: A literature review. *Obesity Reviews, 15*, 453–461.
Ostafin, B. D., Bauer, D. J., & Myxter, P. (2012). Mindfulness decouples the relation between automatic alcohol motivation and heavy drinking. *Journal of Social and Clinical Psychology, 31*, 729–745.
Papies, E. K., Barsalou, L. W., & Custers, R. (2011). Mindful attention prevents mindless impulses. *Social Psychological and Personality Science, 3*, 291–299.
Park, N., Peterson, C., & Seligman, M. E. P. (2006). Character strengths in fifty-four nations and the fifty US states. *Journal of Positive Psychology, 1*, 118–129.
Rothbart, M. K., & Rueda, M. R. (2005). The development of effortful control. In U. Mayr, E. Awh, & S. W. Keele (Eds.), *Developing individuality in the human brain: A tribute to Michael I. Posner* (pp. 167–188). Washington, DC: American Psychological Association.
Sahdra, B. K., MacLean, K. A., Ferrer, E., Shaver, P. R., Rosenberg, E. L., Jacobs, T. L., … Saron, C. D. (2011). Enhanced response inhibition during intensive meditation training predicts improvements in self-reported adaptive socio-emotional functioning. *Emotion, 11*, 299–312.
Schmertz, S. K., Anderson, P. L., & Robins, D. L. (2009). The relation between self-report mindfulness and performance on tasks of sustained attention. *Journal of Psychopathology and Behavioral Assessment, 31*, 60–66.
Sharma, L., Markon, K. E., & Clark, L. A. (2013). Toward a theory of distinct types of "impulsive" behaviors: A meta-analysis of self-report and behavioral measures. *Psychological Bulletin, 140*, 374–408.
Spinrad, T. L., Eisenberg, N., Cumberland, A., Fabes, R. A., Valiente, C., Shepard, S. A., … Guthrie, K. (2006). Relation of emotion-related regulation to children's social competence: A longitudinal study. *Emotion, 6*, 498–510.
Strack, F., & Deutsch, R. (2004). Reflective and impulsive determinants of social behavior. *Personality and Social Psychology Review, 8*, 220–247.
Teper, R., Segal, Z. V., & Inzlicht, M. (2013). Inside the mindful mind: How mindfulness enhances emotion regulation through improvements in executive control. *Current Directions in Psychological Science, 22*, 449–454.
Tsukayama, E., Toomey, S. L., Faith, M. S., & Duckworth, A. L. (2010). Self-control protects against overweight status in the transition to adolescence. *Archives of Pediatrics and Adolescent Medicine, 164*, 631–635.
Vago, D. R., & Silbersweig, D. A. (2012). Self-awareness, self-regulation, and self-transcendence (S-ART): A framework for understanding the neurobiological mechanisms of mindfulness. *Frontiers in Neuroscience, 6*, 1–30.
Waber, D. P., De Moor, C., Forbes, P. W., Almi, C. R., Botteron, K. N., Leonard, G., … Brain Development Cooperative Group. (2007). The NIH MRI study of normal brain development: Performance of a population based sample of healthy children aged 6 to 18 years on a neuropsychological battery. *Journal of*

the International Neuropsychological Society, 13, 729–746.

Wegner, D. M. (1994). Ironic processes of mental control. *Psychological Review, 101*, 34–52.

Welsh, M. C., Pennington, B. F., & Groisser, D. B. (1991). A normative-developmental study of executive function: A window on prefrontal function in children. *Developmental Neuropsychology, 7*(2), 131–149.

Witkiewitz, K., & Bowen, S. (2010). Depression, craving, and substance use following a randomized trial of mindfulness-based relapse prevention. *Journal of Consulting and Clinical Psychology, 78*, 362–374.

Zeidan, F., Johnson, S. K., Diamond, B. J., David, Z., & Goolkasian, P. (2010). Mindfulness meditation improves cognition: Evidence of brief mental training. *Consciousness and Cognition, 19*, 597–605.

A Mindfulness-Based Social and Emotional Learning Curriculum for School-Aged Children: The MindUP Program

20

Jacqueline E. Maloney, Molly Stewart Lawlor, Kimberly A. Schonert-Reichl, and Jenna Whitehead

Mindfulness-Based Interventions and Social and Emotional Learning

Mindfulness-based interventions (MBIs) are secular programs that employ practices adapted from primarily Buddhist contemplative traditions with the goal of promoting holistic development and well-being (Cullen, 2011; Roeser, 2014). MBIs offer a specific type of mental training with the aim of cultivating *mindful awareness*. Simply defined, mindful awareness is an unbiased present-centered awareness that is accompanied by states of clarity, compassion, and equanimity (Kabat-Zinn, 2003; Roeser, 2013; Young, this volume). Mindful awareness is cultivated through specific training techniques practiced with an attitude of open-heartedness, curiosity, kindness, patience, perseverance, and acceptance of what unfolds during practice (Grossman, 2015). Mindful awareness can be cultivated by practicing moment-to-moment awareness of objects, sensations, and emotions, accepting them as they arise without attempting to evaluate, change, or control the experience.

Over the last 30 years, there has been a convergence of evidence demonstrating that participation in MBIs increases psychological well-being and leads to greater satisfaction with life in both clinical and non-clinical adult populations (for a review see Keng, Smoski, & Robins, 2011). Albeit less conclusive, preliminary evidence suggests that mindfulness training with adults may also improve cognitive abilities, such as attention, working memory, and inhibitory control (Chiesa, Calati, & Serretti, 2011; Jha et al., 2010) and may encourage prosocial action (Condon et al., 2013).

Recently, there has been increasing interest in whether mindfulness-based practices can offer similar benefits to children and adolescents. Although promising, the research is preliminary, and methodological limitations temper conclusions and generalizations to greater populations (Greenberg & Harris, 2012). Moreover, much of the research has focused on *reducing* symptoms related to ill-being, such as rumination, depression, anxiety, and "problem" behaviors (e.g., Biegel, Brown, Shapiro, & Schubert, 2009; Van de Weijer-Bergsma, Langenberg, Brandsma, Oort, & Bögels, 2014). Studies that look at MBIs as potential for *increasing* mental well-being in young people are few in number. Furthermore, few have explored the role of mindful awareness

J.E. Maloney (✉) • M.S. Lawlor
K.A. Schonert-Reichl • J. Whitehead
University of British Columbia,
Vancouver, BC, Canada
e-mail: jacqueline.maloney@alumni.ubc.ca;
northshoremolly@gmail.com;
kimberly.schonert-reichl@ubc.ca;
jenna.whitehead@alumni.ubc.ca

K.A. Schonert-Reichl, R.W. Roeser (eds.), *Handbook of Mindfulness in Education*,
Mindfulness in Behavioral Health, DOI 10.1007/978-1-4939-3506-2_20

in social and emotional competencies, an area of development which has been linked not only to greater well-being, but also to increased prosocial behavior and better school performance (Durlak, Weissberg, Dymnicki, Taylor, & Schellinger, 2011).

Social and emotional learning (SEL) is a growing field in education that aims to foster core social and emotional competencies, such as self-awareness, self-regulation, initiating and maintaining healthy relationships, and treating others with respect and care (see Lawlor, this volume). Durlak et al. (2011) have suggested that:

> Over time mastering SEL competencies results in a developmental progression that leads to a shift from being predominantly controlled by external factors to acting increasingly in accord with internalized beliefs and values, caring and concern for others, making good decisions, and taking responsibility for one's choices and behaviors (Bear & Watkins, 2006, p. 406).

Because mindfulness practices are theorized to enhance one's ability to observe external factors and internal reactions and foster the self-control to be able to pause and reflect before taking conscious action (MLERN, 2012), they may potentially enhance school-based SEL programs by offering a practical way to cultivate social–emotional skills rather than simply learn about them conceptually or through talk.

Researchers in the field of mindfulness have expressed concern that some MBIs have decontextualized the practices from their traditional ethical framework (for discussions, see Greenberg & Mitra, 2015; Grossman, 2015; Monteiro, Musten, & Compson, 2015). Situating MBIs in an SEL framework in which ethics of social responsibility and care are emphasized may be one way to teach secular mindfulness in a clear ethical framework, which, some argue, is critical for mindfulness training to lead to transformation for those beyond the self (e.g., Grossman, 2015). Research in this area, however, is scant. Investigating mindfulness-based SEL programs that incorporate ethics and mindfulness can, therefore, shed light on this important potential synergy.

Mindfulness Education during Pre- and Early Adolescence

It is still unknown when it is developmentally appropriate, prudent, and effective to introduce young people to mindfulness practices in schools. Transitional periods in development may be a particularly important time to implement mindfulness education programs. Transitional periods have been defined as phases in the life span in which developmental challenges and demands are intensified and can be considered phases of heightened vulnerability or risk where events that have the potential to alter behavior, affect, cognition, or context can result in lifelong changes (Graber & Brooks-Gunn, 1996; Pickles, Rutter, & Torestad, 1991). Thus, transitional periods like early adolescence may be thought as "windows of opportunity"—times in the life cycle in which positive development can be cultivated and fostered through opportunities provided to individuals in their environment that promote success and serve as protective factors that move the individual toward competence (Roeser & Zelazo, 2012). Pre- and early adolescence (i.e., the "tween" years—ages 9–12 approximately) is one such transitional period in development due to the nature and rapid pace of changes that occur in such a short-time span. Indeed, few developmental periods are characterized by many changes at many levels, including changes due to puberty, cognitive, and emotional development, and social changes which include an increasing focus on the peer group and changes in the nature of parent–child and adult–child relationships (Eccles & Roeser, 2011). These years are also characterized by increases in various mental health problems (Roeser & Eccles, 2014). Thus, pre- and early adolescence is an especially important time to implement interventions to promote social and emotional competencies and optimal cognitive function and prevent related psychopathology (Schonert-Reichl et al., 2013). Based on preliminary research with children and adolescents, MBIs show potential as universal preventative interventions to promote healthy development during this transitional developmental period and beyond (for reviews, see Felver, Celis-de Hoyos, Tezanos, & Singh, 2015; Zoogman, Goldberg, Hoyt, & Miller, 2015). One such program that we describe in more detail that was developed for students of this age period is the MindUp Program by the Hawn Foundation.

Program Development and Process Evaluations

Development of MindUP Curriculum

The development of the lessons that comprise the MindUP program and exploration of ways to provide program training and implementation were both iterative processes that took place over a decade. Specifically, the development of the program was informed by leading experts in the fields of cognitive developmental neuroscience, SEL, and positive psychology as well as from feedback provided by educators and students who participated in earlier versions of the MindUP curriculum. Some of the key components of the current program include: (1) universal participation of all students; (2) tools for creating an atmosphere of an *optimistic classroom* that emphasizes mindful awareness of one's self and others, embracing differences among classmates, and personal growth; (3) a manualized curriculum that is evidence-based, classroom-tested, and meets several prescribed learning outcomes; (4) in-service teacher training; and (5) extension of the concepts and skills learned in the program to other areas of the classroom curriculum and to daily life outside of the classroom (see http://thehawnfoundation.org). In each lesson, students are introduced to key concepts and offered the opportunity to practice skills related to the concepts. Each of the lessons are linked to research on neuroscience with the goal of helping students develop a sophisticated understanding of how the nervous system operates and the role that the brain plays in emotions, behavior, decision making, and learning.

Description of MindUP Curriculum

Theory of Change The MindUP program is a fully developed and manualized program. The lessons that comprise the program are informed from theory and research in cognitive developmental neuroscience (Diamond, 2009, 2012; Zelazo & Lyons, 2012), contemplative science and mindfulness (Roeser & Zelazo, 2012), SEL (Greenberg et al., 2003), and positive psychology (Layous & Lyubomirsky, 2013; Lyubomirsky, Sheldon, & Schkade, 2005).

The MindUP program's approach is similar to other effective SEL programs and also includes activities aimed at developing SEL competencies such as self-awareness, self-management, social awareness, relationship skills, and responsible decision-making (Collaborative for Academic, Social and Emotional Learning, Weissberg & Cascarino, 2013). The core components of program lessons include mindfulness attention awareness practices that have been identified as those that promote children's executive functions (EFs—cognitive control abilities depending on the prefrontal cortex (PFC) that organize, sequence, and regulate behavior), regulation of stress, well-being, and prosociality (see Fig. 20.1). Additionally, the MindUP lessons draw from research and theory in positive psychology which suggests that practicing gratitude and performing acts of kindness bolster one's sense of well-being and happiness (e.g., Emmons & McCullough, 2003; Layous & Lyubomirsky, 2014; Lyubomirksy & Layous, 2013). Also incorporated in the MindUP model is an ecobehavioral systems orientation (Weissberg, Caplan, & Sivo, 1989) in which teachers generalize the curriculum-based skills throughout the school day and support the students' use and internalization of skills to support a positive classroom environment.

Each lesson incorporates mindfulness practices with activities that provide students with opportunities to learn about their brain, understand how their thoughts and feelings affect their actions, and learn strategies to become a caring and altruistic person. Based on teacher feedback from pilot studies, three age-appropriate versions of the MindUP curriculum were created to be calibrated to children at different grade levels:

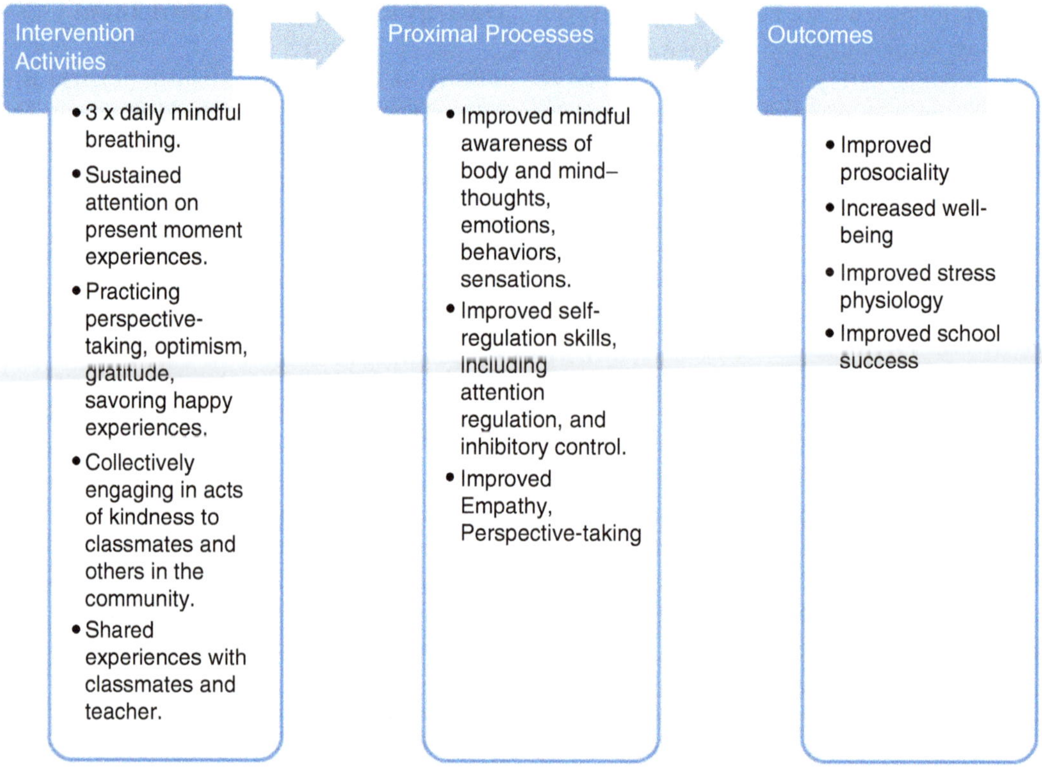

Fig. 20.1 MindUP Theory of Change

grades K-2, 3–5, and 6–8. Each manual was written to be developmentally appropriate for the target age groups and includes detailed lesson plans that can be broken into 10- and 15-min portions, as well as teaching scripts and worksheets to aid in implementation. The manuals contain myriad extension activities and literature suggestions that can be integrated into regular classroom curricula, including math, language arts, science, and social and emotional learning. They also link lesson themes to life outside of the classroom. Manuals for these grades were published by Scholastic books in 2011, and the program is currently being offered in hundreds of classrooms across the United States, Canada, China, Hong Kong, Serbia, Australia, Uganda, Portugal, Finland, the U.K., and in various countries throughout Latin America.[1]

[1] See http://thehawnfoundation.org/mindup/mindup-international/

MindUP Program Practices and Units

The MindUP curriculum includes 15 lessons and each component of the program builds on previous skills learned, moving children from focusing on internal experiences (e.g., mindful smelling, mindful tasting) to cognitive experiences (e.g., taking others' perspectives), to students practicing gratitude, and ending with students enacting acts of kindness to others in their home, classroom, and community. The 15 lessons in the current MindUP curriculum are divided into four main units. The first unit, entitled "Getting Focused," introduces students to brain structure and function and the concept of mindful awareness, "attending to the here and now—other people, the environment, a concern or challenge—in a considerate, nonjudgmental way" (The Hawn Foundation, 2011, p. 34). At the end of Unit 1, students are introduced to the *Core Practice*, a mindfulness practice in which students focus on the resonant sound of a chime that marks the opening and closing of the practice. After the sound of the opening chime dissipates, students practice focusing on their breathing. They are encouraged to notice when their mind wanders away from the object of observation and to bring it back to it without judging their performance. The curriculum suggests that students engage in the Core Practice for 1–3 min at a time, three times a day.

Grounded in the latest research and theory in neuroscience, students first learn how training their focused awareness might affect their brain and nervous system, giving them a self-regulatory strategy to calm down when they are stressed out or overwhelmed by emotions. For example, students learn that their amygdala act similarly to a security guard, sometimes overreacting to situations that are not in fact dangerous. Students are then taught about the concept of mindfulness in Lesson 2 and given an opportunity to practice. The Core Practice, introduced in Lesson 3, allows them to experience first-hand how focusing their attention on their breathing may help "engage" the prefrontal cortex, described as their *wise leader*. Doing so can help students calm down so that they are able to pause before making decisions instead of reacting mindlessly.

Unit two, "Sharpening Your Senses," introduces students to the practice of *mindful sensing* in which students concentrate on one of their senses in order to practice focused, present-centered awareness. Lessons include mindful listening, mindful seeing, mindful smelling, mindful tasting, and mindful movement. For example, students practice mindful tasting by engaging all of their senses while slowly eating something. They look at the food very carefully and take time to smell it; they notice the sensation of the morsel in their mouths and the taste of it on their tongues; they notice the sound made by biting into the food when they take their first small bite and pause to savor the flavor. Continuing the process very slowly, students notice that the sensations they experience with each bite are different and unique.

Unit three, "It's All about Attitude," aims to foster a positive mindset in students with the goal of preparing the mind for learning and building positive relationships through the application of mindful awareness to improve social and emotional skills. Lessons are based on research in SEL and positive psychology. Students learn about and practice perspective-taking, optimism, and savoring happy experiences. For example, students learn to "make a happy movie" by focusing their minds on an experience that brings up pleasurable emotions. They explore how focusing on a happy memory makes them feel both physically and emotionally.

The last unit, "Taking Action Mindfully," offers students the opportunity to put mindful awareness into action by practicing gratitude, performing random acts of kindness, and collaboratively planning a social action project to benefit their larger community or the world. Students also practice introspection to notice how they feel when they pay attention to the positive things they have in their lives, no matter how small or seemingly insignificant.

Learning to Deliver MindUP Program in Classrooms

The Hawn Foundation currently offers in-service teacher training and continual learning support via an online portal, webinars, and mentorship programs for the MindUP Program. Training includes a full-day, interactive training session. Teachers learn about the theory and research guiding each unit and its lessons and participate in interactive discussions on SEL and the developmental characteristics of children's social and emotional competence. The training also includes experiential learning in mindfulness practice. Teachers are given strategies that guide the introduction of mindfulness to the classroom with considerations for engaging students (e.g., by invitation), and how to work with common challenges to practice (e.g., restlessness). Teachers learn through lecture, video, readings, and role-plays of curriculum instructional techniques. Additional support is provided via a web-learning portal where teachers can participate in Webinars, see additional teaching tips, view videos, access an e-library of related materials, ask questions, and share best practices. To ensure the program is being implemented with fidelity, The Hawn Foundation offers a booster session approximately 4 months after the initial training. Teachers can request this in the form of another workshop or a mentoring session. To become an accredited MindUP teacher or school, after the first year of implementation, schools must conduct an evaluation (using a predesigned evaluation kit) to assess teacher and student satisfaction and better understand how teachers are actually implementing the program in order for MindUP to provide additional recommendations and/or coaching if need be. MindUP recommends hosting a refresher workshop the following year.

Program Evaluation

Over the past several years, the MindUP program has been evaluated via both formative/process and outcome evaluations utilizing both qualitative and quantitative methodologies. See Fig. 20.1 for a summary of these evaluations. Equally important to outcome evaluations in understanding the effectiveness of MBIs are program *process evaluations* that examine the implementation fidelity of the program (i.e., the degree to which the program was implemented as designed). Domitrovich and Greenberg (2000) noted that one major shortcoming of many, if not most, preventive intervention studies are that investigators do not report on aspects of implementation. It is not enough to understand *if* a program works; researchers must also investigate the "hows," "whys," and contexts for optimal program effectiveness (Harachi, Abbott, Catalano, Haggerty, & Fleming, 1999). Moreover, practitioners intending to implement the program need to be informed of the most effective ways to introduce the program in natural contexts in order to ensure evidenced-based programs are equally as effective as found to be in research studies (Domitrovich & Greenberg, 2000). Thus, it is essential to move beyond a "black box approach" to evaluating programs that focus only on outcomes in order to better understand the mechanisms that may influence outcomes (Harachi et al., 1999). For each study conducted on MindUP (e.g., Schonert-Reichl et al., 2015; Schonert-Reichl & Lawlor, 2010), researchers have included a process evaluation, which has been essential in the iterative development of the curriculum, as well as study design. The first quasi-experimental study took place in 2005. Since then, Schonert-Reichl and colleagues have conducted four subsequent studies with a fifth longitudinal follow-up study currently underway (see Fig. 20.2).

Formative Evaluation

Following the quasi-experimental study described below (Schonert-Reichl & Lawlor, 2010), Lawlor (2007) conducted a formative evaluation of the MindUP curriculum (then called Focus Mind) to inform the development of the next iteration of the program. Through teacher questionnaires, focus groups, student satisfaction surveys, and implementation lesson tracking, Lawlor obtained qualitative and quantitative data to investigate feasibility, program integrity, and participant responsiveness of the program. Participants included nine teachers, one administrator, and 110 students from kindergarten to grade 6 across three sites.

Overall, both teachers and students reported some satisfaction with the program. All teachers rated the program positively with ratings of four (positive) or five (very positive) on a five-point Likert scale ($M=4.5$). Students reported mid to high levels of enjoyment of the program, and teachers reported mid to high levels of student engagement for each lesson. Three key findings emerged from qualitative data that were considered in future revisions and implementation of the program: (1) Primary grade teachers identified a need for age-appropriate lesson plans for younger students. These comments supported the work to create a primary curriculum in the current iteration of the program. (2) Although teachers reported the manual as largely, "easy to use, well-organized and written," 87.5 % of those teachers felt the training they received was not

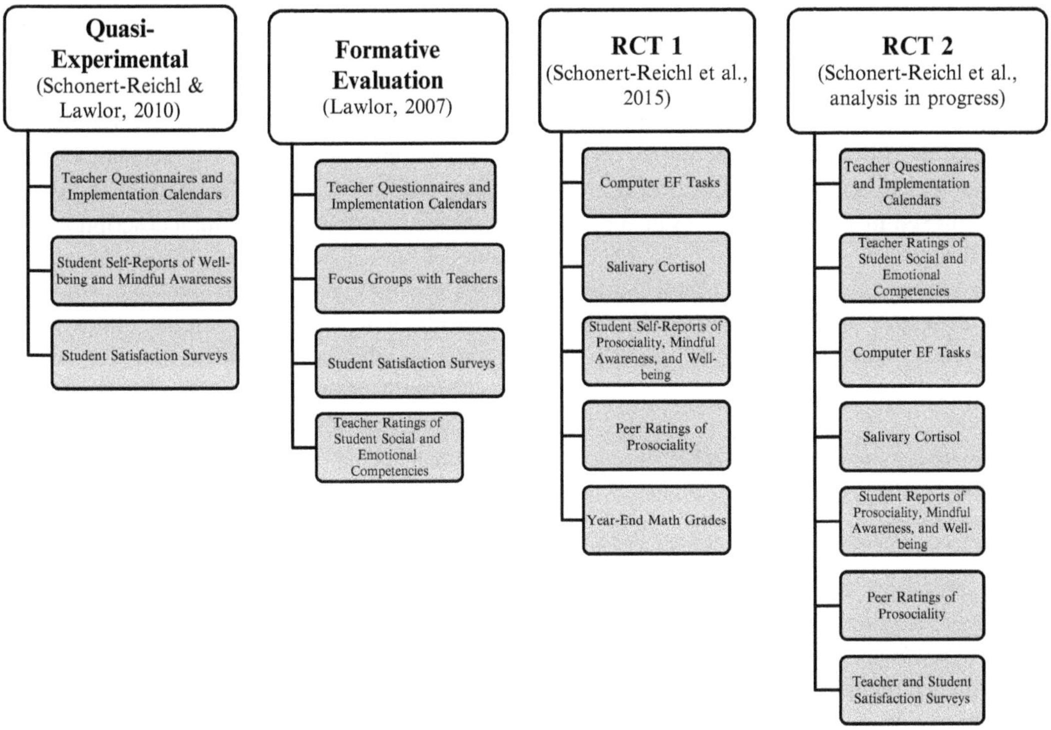

Fig. 20.2 Summary of studies on MindUP conducted by Schonert-Reichl and colleagues. *Notes:* The Quasi-Experimental Study was conducted in 2005. The formative process evaluation (Lawlor, 2007) followed. RCT 1 was conducted in 2008. It compared MindUP to an active control group, which received a social responsibility program. RCT 2 was conducted in 2011–2012 and had several conditions: (1) teachers who participated in a mindfulness-based SEL program for themselves Stress Management and Relaxation Techniques in Education (SMART-in-Education) before being trained and implementing MindUP; (2) teachers who did not participate in SMART, but were trained and implemented MindUP; (3) teachers who participated in SMART but did not implement MindUP, teaching a district-mandated social responsibility program instead, and (4) teachers who neither participated in SMART, nor implemented MindUP, but taught the social responsibility program. The data on students' perceptions of MindUP (Maloney et al., 2014) were from RCT 2. Quantitative analyses are underway

sufficient to feel comfortable to implement the program. Based on these findings, the protocol for teacher training was reformatted to include more time to learn about mindfulness, more information on particular techniques, and more time to practice and role-play to facilitate comfort level with the program. (3) Results indicated a need to improve the program's ability to be embedded into existing required subject areas. To improve the program's implementation, sustainability, and growth, the Focus Mind curriculum was modified so that the core practices, approaches, and lessons could be easily transferable to what teachers are already doing within their classrooms, resulting in the current MindUP curriculum (see description above).

Triangulating Data: Investigating Multiple Outcomes Using Multiple Methods

Over the last decade, Schonert-Reichl et al. (2015; Schonert-Reichl & Lawlor, 2010) have evaluated iterations of the MindUP program, examining multiple outcomes from multiple perspectives in order to provide an in-depth understanding of student changes related to participation in the program. Doing so helps account for potential errors or biases that may be present when conducting a single-method study, for example, relying solely on studies employing self-report measures. These studies have included quantitative measures of outcomes, including social and emotional competencies through teacher-, self-, and peer-reports; third-person objective assessments of executive functions; and biological measures of stress via diurnal cortisol. Schonert-Reichl and colleagues have also conducted mixed-method process evaluations in order to better understand the implementation fidelity and acceptability of the MindUp program (e.g., Lawlor, 2007; Maloney, Whitehead, Lawlor, & Schonert-Reichl, 2014).

Measuring Social and Emotional Competencies from Multiple Perspectives

Along with investigating changes in mindful awareness, a primary focus of the research on MindUP has been the examination of changes in social and emotional competencies as a result of participating in MindUP, such as perspective-taking, empathy, and prosocial behavior. To gain an in-depth understanding of changes in social and emotional competencies from multiple perspectives, Schonert-Reichl et al. (2015; Schonert-Reichl & Lawlor, 2010) have employed reports from three different perspectives: teachers, individual students, and peers. Especially important to understanding changes in students' behaviors as a result of the MindUP curriculum is peer-report data from the perspective of the students' classmates in order to triangulate data and provide a balanced perspective. For example, self-reports may be biased due to social desirability (Crandall, Crandall, & Katkovsky, 1965). Teacher reports may also be biased because the teachers in the MindUP studies are not blind to condition, having implemented the program themselves. Collecting data from peers is one way to address these issues because the peer nomination approach has the unique advantage that observations of the same behaviors are provided by many different observers. Given that 20–30 students in the classroom may be providing information about the target participant (see Quiggle, Garber, Panak, & Dodge, 1992), no single rater can unduly influence the target participant's final score (Huesmann, Eron, Guerra, & Crawshaw, 1994).

Peer assessment instruments involve the use of peer nominations in which students are presented with a list of their classmates participating in the study. For each behavioral description, students are asked to "circle the names of the students in your classroom who are kind; who help other children when they have a problem; who cooperate; who break the rules; who take the perspectives of others," etc. Peers are participant observers that can provide an important glimpse into the behaviors of their classmates that do not occur when adults are present, and hence peer reports can be more comprehensive than adult reports as they are more likely to garner reports of both positive and antisocial behaviors (Pepler & Craig, 1995). In this vein, peer reports provide an effective way to determine how students are perceived by their peers (Hoza et al., 2005). We speculate here that peers' ratings of classmates' behaviors would be less likely than teachers to be influenced by knowledge of the intervention status given that it is unlikely that children would be able to generate the hypothesis of the study. However, we have no data to support such a claim, and future investigations of the MindUP program would benefit from collecting data from observers blind to intervention status in order to allow for a less biased assessment of children's classroom behaviors.

Objective Measures of Outcomes Related to Social and Emotional Competencies

In addition to report measures, Schonert-Reichl et al. (2015) have also employed third-person objective measures of outcomes related to social and emotional competencies, namely executive functions and the diurnal function of the stress hormone cortisol. Executive functions (EF) refer to higher cognitive processes utilized in problem solving, reasoning, and planning (Diamond & Lee, 2011), and thus are intertwined with social and emotional competencies, especially with the core competency of self-management (Lawlor, this volume). Another important part of social and emotional learning is developing the capacity to cope with stress in a healthy way (Weissberg & Cascarino, 2013). One way to observe this is to examine activity in the hypothalamic-pituitary-adrenocortical (HPA) axis via diurnal cortisol rhythms (Miller, Chen, & Zhou, 2007). Interpretation of these results must be done with caution, however. There are no clear existing guidelines for healthy cortisol patterns and patterns seem to vary with different populations (O' Leary, O'Neill, & Dockray, 2015). Nevertheless, there is theoretical and limited empirical support that mindfulness practices may affect HPA functioning (O' Leary et al., 2015; Vago & Silbersweig, 2012), which, therefore, warrants its investigation in studies of MBIs. These measures, by examining prefrontal self-regulatory function and the HPA axis around stress reactivity, afford an objective complement to self- and other-reported measures of students' social–emotional competencies.

Importance of Including Students' Voices in Program Evaluations

A shortcoming in evaluations of preventative interventions for children and adolescents is that researchers frequently do not ask students for feedback regarding the program. Despite the recent proliferation of research on universal school-based MBIs, relatively little is known about children and adolescents' subjective experiences with mindfulness training, particularly in school settings. In general, studies examining both young people's well-being, as well as outcomes of school-based interventions, typically utilize observations or other raters as evaluators (e.g., teachers, parents; Ben-Arieh, 2005). There is a tendency in outcome research to treat young people as if they are "passive objects who are acted on by the adult world" (Ben-Arieh, 2007, p. 7).

There has been a growing appreciation, however, on the role of children and adolescent perspectives in evaluating programs targeting their own well-being (Ben-Arieh, 2008; Mason & Danby, 2011). Young participants should be seen as valued contributors to the research process (Ben-Arieh, 2005). Research supports the validity and reliability of children's self-reports of their experiences, such as subjective well-being, finding children's reports of well-being to be highly correlated with more "objective" measures of well-being, such as family's and friend's observations and reports (Sandvik, Diener, & Seidlitz, 1993). Moreover, asking young people about well-being has also drawn attention to issues in the field of which researchers were previously unaware, giving new meaning to findings (Fattore, Mason, & Watson, 2007, 2009). Further, research studies have shown that adult and children perspectives on services can vary dramatically (Stüntzner-Gibson, Koren, & DeChillo, 1995). Therefore, it is important to include children's and adolescents' perspectives in order to gather a holistic understanding of any program. Asking young people about their perceptions of a program can help researchers and educators understand students' perceived benefits and challenges, assisting in the refinement of program content and implementation to better fit students' needs. It is imperative to understand whether students themselves find mindfulness education programs acceptable and useful, considering it is their well-being and growth that is the target of the interventions.

An additional motivation to accessing young people's voices is honoring their need for belonging and feeling heard (Lind, 2007). There is both a social and a legal obligation for program evaluation to represent the views of participants. According to Article 12 of the United Nations Convention on the Rights of the Child, "Parties shall assure to the child who is capable of forming his or her own views the right to express those views freely in all matters affecting the child, the views of the child." Thus, there is both an empirical and social obligation for researchers to move beyond outcome evaluations to include more descriptive accounts of students' experiences with mindfulness education programs (e.g., Maloney et al., 2014).

Overview of Efficacy Evaluations on MindUP

In addition to process evaluations, Schonert-Reichl and her colleagues have conducted several iterative investigations on the efficacy of the MindUP program. We summarize these studies in the following section.

Quasi-Experimental Study

A quasi-experimental control group pretest/posttest design was used to evaluate program outcomes and implementation fidelity in a pilot study of the first iteration of the MindUP curriculum (Schonert-Reichl & Lawlor, 2010). This evaluation included 246 fourth- to seventh-grade children drawn from 12 classrooms (six program classrooms and six comparison classrooms) attending public elementary schools in Vancouver, BC. The student sample represented a range of socioeconomic statuses and cultural backgrounds (82 % participation rate). Students were administered questionnaires at both pretest and posttest on a series of instruments designed to assess dimensions of their social and emotional understanding (emotional awareness, reflection, and rumination), mindful attention and awareness, optimism, and self-concept. Teachers rated students at pretest and posttest on dimensions of social and emotional competence and aggressive behaviors.

Results revealed that students who participated in the program, compared to those who did not, showed significant improvements on all four dimensions of teacher-rated school behaviors, including attentional control, aggression, behavioral dysregulation, and social competence. Significant improvements were also found for students' self-reported optimism and mindful attention. Although positive statistical trends in positive affect were observed for MindUP students in comparison to control students, no differences were observed in negative effect. Preadolescents (grades 4 and 5) who participated in MindUP also demonstrated significant improvements from pre- to posttest in general self-concept compared to those in the control group, who experienced significant decreases. Interestingly, the reverse was found for early adolescents (grades 6 and 7): Whereas the control condition increased in self-concept from pre- to posttest, the MindUP group *decreased* in self-concept, a finding to be further explored in the analysis of Schonert-Reichl and colleagues' latest study on MindUP (see RCT 2 Fig. 20.2).

Randomized Controlled Trial

Next, a collaborative study was conducted in order to assess outcomes of an earlier version of the MindUP program in a randomized controlled trial (RCT; Schonert-Reichl et al., 2015). Drawn from four classrooms (two program classrooms, two comparison classrooms) in British Columbia, Canada, 99 fourth- and fifth-grade classrooms were randomly assigned to receive a 12-week version of the MindUP program or serve as an active control, which implemented a "business as usual" social responsibility program. This research included assessments of students' EF, stress physiology (obtained via diurnal salivary cortisol), and year-end math grades as rated by teachers. Additionally, students filled out questionnaires that included peer-reports of prosociality and self-reports of well-being, social and emotional competencies, school self-concept, and mindful attention and awareness. Both MindUP and comparison teachers completed program implementation calendars to keep a daily record of study-related activities completed in class.

Analyses of student- and peer-report data indicated that after exposure to MindUP, participants had significant increases in optimism, emotional control, empathy, perspective taking, prosocial goals, and mindful attention, along with decreased depressive symptoms compared to those in the active control group. Conversely, the control group demonstrated significant decreases in scores on each of these measures. MindUP participants were also more likely to improve than control group on peer-rated sociality with significant improvements in sharing, trustworthiness, helpfulness, and taking others' perspectives, and significant decreases in aggressive behavior, as rated by classmates. As predicted, both MindUP and control groups improved on self-reported social responsibility, demonstrating no significant difference between groups at posttest. Regarding academic-related outcomes, in comparison to control groups, MindUP participants had a significant increase in self-reported school self-concept (i.e., perceived academic abilities and interest and enjoyment thereof) and demonstrated a 15 % gain in teacher-reported math achievement.

On EF tasks, students in MindUP had significantly shorter response times (RTs) on average, while maintaining equal accuracy compared to control children on tasks that required inhibition, working memory, and selective attention, suggesting MindUP participants were better able to pay attention and inhibit distractions during these computer tasks. Furthermore, researchers found that the MindUP participants' diurnal cortisol patterns maintained a steep slope throughout the school year. Conversely, control children demonstrated changes from a steeper diurnal pattern to a flatter, blunter pattern. This change may have indicated greater allostatic load in control students over time (i.e., an inefficient response to stressors that creates negative health effects over time; Gunnar & Vazquez, 2001). Interestingly, the MindUP participants had significantly *higher* morning cortisol than the control group at posttest, despite their overall steeper pattern, indicating a need for future studies to investigate the nuances of MBIs on cortisol functioning, and the association with other indicators of stress (i.e., students' perceived stress, health functioning).

Study of Students' Perceptions of MindUP

To address the gap in the literature regarding pre- and early adolescents' perceptions of MBIs, Maloney et al. (2014) sought to understand participants' perceptions of the MindUP program and the application of the program to other areas of their lives by analyzing responses from a post-program participant satisfaction survey. The survey was administered to 189 grade 4–7 students (52 % female) drawn from eight classrooms across seven schools in British Columbia as part of a larger RCT conducted by Schonert-Reichl and her colleagues (data currently under analysis). The goal was to learn about students' perceptions of specific program components, any skills they perceived to have gained from participating in the program, and their experiences with mindfulness practices in their own words. Thus, in addition to close-ended yes/no or Likert-Scale questions, the participant satisfaction survey included several open-ended questions to which children were encouraged to write their opinions.

Descriptive statistics (frequencies) were performed to summarize students' responses to the close-ended questions. The data from each individual open-ended question were coded by independent raters via a six-step thematic analysis (Braun & Clarke, 2006). Themes were refined over the cycles of coding until the two coders achieved a 90 % inter-rater reliability on a subsample of data (Hruschka et al., 2004). Next, the entire data set was independently coded by the two coders and subsequently compared. Any discrepancies in the final round of coding were discussed until the coders reached consensus.

Students' Perceptions of the General Program

> The best part about the MindUP Program was learning about things that can help other people to calm down and think positive.[2]—Grade 7 Girl

Overall, 88 % of the participants found the program acceptable with 43 % reporting they

[2] A note on quotations: This study included many children new to Canada; therefore, English language skills varied among participants. No participants' comments were excluded from the study based on language ability unless we could not understand them. The quotations here appear exactly as written on student surveys unless we felt that spelling might hinder understanding. In those cases, words are placed in brackets.

"liked it a lot," 35 % "liked it," and 10 % reporting the program was "OK." Of the 148 students who answered the open-ended question, "Was there anything you liked about MindUP?," many cited mindfulness activities as the part of the program that they enjoyed the most ($n=79$, 53 %[3]). Specifically, students enjoyed the mindful sensing activities ($n=55$, 37 %), especially mindful eating ($n=37$; 25 %). Many participants cited the Core Practice as being their favorite aspect of the program ($n=29$; 20 %). For example, one participant commented, "I liked the breathing exercises, it helped me calm down in situations and also calm down my amygdala." Another remarked enjoying the "moments of silence." The neuroscience component was also popular among participants ($n=15$, 10 %). Several other students mentioned other favorite program components, including optimism ($n=8$, 5 %), and prosocial components, such as acts of kindness and perspective taking ($n=6$, 4 %) and gratitude ($n=3$, 2 %).

In addition to program components, several themes arose related to outcomes students perceived as a result of participating in MindUP. Many students mentioned that they appreciated the increased sense of well-being that they gained from participating in the program ($n=27$, 18 %). For example, several participants reported that the program helped them feel calm and relaxed. Some specific comments included, "We can have about 10 min everyday that we can use to calm down," "after PE, it feels really good and relaxed," and MindUP was "a calming period in some hectic days." One student mentioned that participating in the program "ma[d]e me feel more positive about myself." Others reported gains in mindful awareness of one's self and others ($n=12$, 8 %). A few students made comments related to self-awareness, including "the ability it gave me to calm down and to understand myself and others," and "you can learn a lot about yourself."

Some participants also reported that they appreciated the improvement in their self-regulation skills, such as the ability to calm down when experiencing overwhelming emotions and feeling overly excited ($n=8$, 5 %). For example, one student wrote, "I liked that I can now be calm in a minute or 2 as opposed to an hour or so." Another noted appreciating to be able to go "from [hyper] and energetic to mindful and calm." Yet another remarked enjoying "the calming down part because I am really impatient when I am waiting." One participant noticed the effect the practice had on the class: "I thought that it really had a positive energy and a good affect on everyone, making some of the more energetic students calmer."

Less frequently mentioned outcomes that students appreciated were improved focus, concentration, and memory ($n=5$, 3 %). One student remarked, "It got everyone focused at the beginning of the day." Another stated, "I liked that it teaches you how to pay attention to what you're doing." Two students mentioned that they found the program helpful for schoolwork. For example, one stated, "I could finish and do works efficiently and more happily than before I learned about mindfulness."

In answer to the closed-ended yes/no question, "Was there anything you did not like about MindUP," 29 % of students reported that there was an aspect of the MindUP program that they did not like. Remarkably, in response to the open-ended question regarding what students did not like, there were more mentions of positive experiences with the program ($n=48$, 55 %) than negative ($n=39$, 45 %).

Some participants found aspects of the program boring ($n=15$, 17 %) or too time-consuming ($n=6$, 7 %). Of these students, four of the students who mentioned it was boring and two who mentioned it wasted time had taken part in the MindUP program previously. The most frequently mentioned activity that students did not like was the Core Practice, some finding it boring while others too challenging ($n=8$, 9 %). For example, one student mentioned, "sometimes I would get bored or I couldn't calm down enough." Yet another child reported not liking "closing my eyes and breathing because after I want[ed] to fall asleep." Another did not like "[d]eep breathing. It

[3] Note that percentages are calculated based on the number of students who answered the question, not the entire sample of 189 students.

seemed ridiculous how you could find a complete mental stillness in your mind, even after weeks of practice." This observation may indicate that if the Core Practice is introduced or perceived as a method for finding mental stillness, rather than a non-judgmental observational practice, it could undermine young people's desire to explore and investigate their inner lives.

There were quite a few comments made regarding the implementation of the program ($n=11$, 13 %). Some reported finding the behavior of other students during the program disruptive. For example, one participant stated, "Lots of others disturbed and judged the way I did my mindfulness. Others act disrespectfully (read, laugh, play on phone or iPod, etc.)." There were a few mentions of not liking how teachers implemented the program, for example reports that the lessons went on too long, that the breathing practice was offered too frequently or was taking away from other activities in class, and that some of the lessons were given for homework. One student offered insight into how the Core Practice was taught: "I didn't like how in the middle of meditating, [my teacher] started giving us instructions even though [the teacher] said we should ignore everything we hear."

Some positive comments reiterating what children did like in response to this question were: "The things we learned are all helpful in life," "I loved everything because it fits the situation I was stuck in and helped me a lot," "It helps you express your feelings about you and your friends," and "I liked doing everything because it helped me be happy."

Children's Reports of Learning

> I learnt how to be alot more self-aware and to be able to understand myself. I also liked how we learnt to enjoy things.—Grade 6 Boy

Overall, 96 % of students reported they learned something new in the program. Children were asked to evaluate what they had learned in specific program components by reporting whether the MindUP program helped them learn about: the brain, mindfulness, being mindful of the senses, perspective taking and being mindful of others, gratitude, acts of kindness, how to be more optimistic, how to help themselves be happy, and how to focus their attention and calm down. They responded using a four-point Likert scale (1=*not at all true*, 2=*a little bit true*, 3=*true most of the time*, and 4=*true all of the time*). The most frequent response across all 10 questions was "true most of the time." See Table 20.1 for a summary of the results.

In response to the open-ended question regarding what students had learned in the program, 117 children provided specific responses that expanded upon the close-ended questions. Similar to the open-ended question about what children liked, children reported learning skills that promoted their well-being ($n=53$, 45 %), self-regulation ($n=35$, 30 %), and mindful awareness ($n=22$, 19 %). Learning specific mindfulness practices ($n=19$, 16 %), such as breathing and mindful sensing, was also mentioned frequently, as well as learning about the brain and nervous system ($n=39$, 31 %).

Developing a Practice in Life

> I learned how to do mindfulness by myself and now every morning I do it when I wake up.—Grade 6 Girl

In response to a close-ended question, the majority of students (40 %) reported using "a few things" outside of the program (e.g., in their school or home life), while 24 % of students reported using "quite a few things" and 14 % of students reported using "a lot." Only 6 % of students reported that they did not use the skills learned in MindUP outside of the program. Participants were also asked whether they tried to help others more often since participating in the MindUP program. The response was an overwhelming "yes" (n =83 %), with 30 % students reporting that "it was a little bit true" that they tried to help others more often after participating in the program, 37 % participants reporting it was true for them "most of the time," and 17 % children reporting that it was "true all of the time."

Table 20.1 Student reports of learning program components in MindUP (closed-ended)

Program Components	Responses in percentages			
	Not at all true	A little bit true	True most of the time	True all of the time
Brain	6	29	46	19
Mindfulness	3	19	43	35
Mindful of my senses	7	21	45	28
Perspective-taking	7	23	50	20
Optimism and Thinking Positively	9	27	38	26
How I Can Help Myself to be Happy	14	26	41	19
Savoring (Making a Happy Movie in my Mind)	16	29	38	17
Gratitude	8	31	35	26
Acts of Kindness	5	24	46	25
Focus my Attention and Calm down	9	24	37	30

Throughout the survey, there were some individual comments that offered unique insight into the program. One child wrote, "It teaches you something that you can't really explain." Another stated, "It made my life sort of easier." One student remarked, "I find that MindUP has helped me see life differently." Teacher observations echoed those of students (see Table 20.2).

Discussion

The studies presented here have attempted to build on current strengths in the field of mindfulness education and address some of the limitations (see Felver et al., 2015; Greenberg & Harris, 2012). One shortcoming in the field has been the paucity of replication studies on existing interventions; the majority of published studies have evaluated different mindfulness education programs with a variety of components, making it difficult to compare results across studies (Felver et al., 2015). The studies presented here have focused on one program that has changed and evolved over time informed by the results of previous studies.

The reviewed studies have included both process and outcome evaluations employing experimental designs. They included multiple informants (teachers, students, and peers), as well as multiple methods (questionnaires, computer tasks, cortisol, participant satisfaction surveys, math grades, and implementation calendars). Triangulating data in this way contributes to reliability and validity of the findings presented.

Overall, these findings suggest that participating in MindUP may offer several benefits to grade 4–7 Canadian students, including: increased mindful awareness; improved social and emotional competencies; increased proficiency in EF; better relationships with teachers and peers; improved academic achievement and engagement; and improved psychological and physiological well-being. MindUP has proven to be an acceptable and effective universal mindfulness-based SEL program that was successfully implemented in public elementary schools across neighborhoods made up of culturally diverse populations, ranging from low to high social economic statuses. Similarly, classroom teachers included in these studies came from a range of cultural backgrounds, had various years of experience teaching, and differed in prior exposure to and experience with contemplative practices. These encouraging findings from two cities with diverse populations warrant further investigation of the effectiveness and acceptability of the MindUP program with other populations.

Several similar themes were identified from student and teacher responses to participant satisfaction surveys that corroborate quantitative findings. Both teachers and students made frequent mentions of students learning *self-regulation skills* in the program; that is "self-control of thought, action, and emotion" (Zelazo & Lyons, 2012, p. 154). Students made comments concerning all three of these aspects of self-regulation. In particular, many mentioned that they learned how to quickly find calm after experiencing overwhelming emotions so that they could think before acting. Similar findings have been reported by older adolescents in previous qualitative investigations of mindfulness practices (e.g.,

Table 20.2 Teachers' Perceptions of MindUP

Theme	Comments
Program Components	"The core breathing is very well received by the students and I truly believe it has helped all the students… It especially helped them after recess/lunch when there was a wild soccer match"
	"The sensory activities and optimism lessons were well received. They really enjoyed learning about the brain"
	"Sometimes they felt bored by the lessons as they had done something similar before (i.e., smelling, tasting, etc.). They enjoyed the brain lessons and most of them, the Core Practice"
	Students "appreciated the sophisticated yet accessible background information. They felt guided and respected"
	"They LOVED our mindfulness practices. We now have a 'do not disturb, we are practicing mindfulness' [sign] at our door"
Observations of Student Behavior	"Mindful behavior in general was a positive method to avoid classroom conflicts for some students"
	"One boy who had a major melt-down in September listened intently every lesson, for him it was an epiphany! No more meltdowns!"
	"MindUP leads to better work ethic, kindness, better learners, happy kids"
	"Great program for all classrooms. Mindful kids → Peaceful schools"
Challenges	"It was difficult to explain the 2 aspects of mindfulness: paying close attention was easy, but being non-judgmental was hard. I used empathy instead"
	"I feel that MindUP has the potential to be very powerful in a child's learning. However, to be implemented effectively, I feel that teachers need more time, training, and resources"
Extensions into Regular Curriculum and Classroom Life	"We used the mindfulness terminology and philosophy across the board. In English, French, and Math. [We used mindfulness practices] as a calming tool/strategy before tests"
	"I noticed how I quickly went further and deeper and followed my own inspiration when guiding breathing exercises. I was able to do a lot of classroom management and address problems and difficulties"

Milligan, Badali, & Spiroiu, 2013; Monshat et al., 2012; Wisner, 2014). These findings are in line with the theoretical and empirical literature that suggests mindfulness training may improve emotion regulation and EF (Diamond, 2012; Lyons & Delange, this volume; MLERN, 2012). The findings that MindUP participants were significantly more proficient at objective EF tasks than controls (Schonert-Reichl et al., 2015) lend further support to this theory.

A related theme that emerged was *well-being*. This included mentions of mental well-being, such as increased positive affect, optimism, and gratitude, as well as fewer experiences of anger and impatience. Quantitative self-report measures supported these findings. Additionally, students commented on improved physical well-being, such as feeling calmer and more relaxed after practicing mindfulness. Also relevant are students' mentions of finding a sense of calm more quickly after experiencing emotional or physical distress, following their participation in the MindUP program. Not only do these results coincide with previous findings in the literature (e.g., Kuyken et al., 2013), but they also provide qualitative support for the theory that mindfulness practices may have a balancing effect on the autonomic nervous system (i.e., homeostasis; Tang, Yang, Leve, & Harold, 2012; Vago & Silbersweig, 2012).

Perhaps the most frequent theme that appeared across the participant satisfaction surveys was that students experienced increases in *mindful attention and awareness*. Many reported gaining an understanding of the importance of mindful awareness. Some students talked about an increased ability to pay attention and concentrate on what was going on in the present moment. Others discussed a newfound awareness of themselves, of their surroundings, and of the consequences of their actions, especially in relation to interactions with family and friends. A few students mentioned the importance of not judging their experiences, but being open and grateful for every moment. These findings indicate that students gained a comprehensive understanding and appreciation of the somewhat intangible experience of mindfulness, something that, as one student and one teacher noted, can be challenging to describe.

These students' descriptions of their experience of mindfulness fall in line with current working definitions of the construct mindfulness (see Cullen, 2011). This finding provides support that mindfulness practices, such as mindful breathing and mindful sensing, are accessible and developmentally suitable throughout pre- and early adolescence when introduced within a SEL framework. This finding is further corroborated by significant improvement in MindUP students' self-reported mindful attention and awareness compared to controls as measured by an adaptation of the Mindful Attention Awareness Scale appropriate for this age group (Lawlor, Schonert-Reichl, Gadermann, & Zumbo, 2013).

Students and teachers consistently mentioned increases in *prosocial behavior* throughout the consumer satisfaction surveys, noting that participating in the program made them kinder, more respectful of others, better able to understand other people's perspectives, and more likely to help others. Peer-, teacher- and self-reports corroborated these findings. Increased prosocial behavior is linked to mindfulness practices in both theoretical and empirical research (see MLERN, 2012). The findings from the presented studies suggest that integrating mindfulness practices into an SEL program may be an effective way to cultivate secular ethics as a basis for mindfulness.

Equally important as investigating the perceived benefits of the program are reported dissatisfaction and challenges with the program. Similar to the recent studies on mindfulness practices for adolescents (Britton et al., 2014; Milligan et al., 2013), the most frequent comment among the students who disliked components of the program was that they found aspects of the program boring, particularly the Core Practice of watching the breath.

Encountering boredom seems to be part and parcel of mindfulness practice: Even experienced adults who have practiced mindfulness meditation for years report finding the practice boring at times (Lomas, Cartwright, Edginton, & Ridge, 2014). In fact, a fundamental aspect of mindfulness practice is being able to develop a clarity of awareness that enables the practitioner to recognize and embrace obstacles, such as restlessness, and notice their impermanence (Monteiro et al., 2015). For example, with guidance and practice, students may recognize that while practicing mindfulness, they experience moments of boredom and moments of engagement, rather than perceiving the activity as uniformly boring. The question is: How can we engage these students in practice in order to help them sit with boredom rather than disengage from practice? Future studies should address this phenomenon through qualitative inquiry with participants. Additionally, observational data of program implementation (e.g., videotaping lessons) could investigate whether specific instructional strategies are related to student engagement and their willingness to explore the experience of boredom.

It is noteworthy that participants mentioned no iatrogenic effects in relation to mindfulness practices; that is, there were no mentions of mindfulness training causing harm or distress. In studies of MBIs for adults and older adolescents, participants have mentioned feeling distressed or overwhelmed when first introduced to mindfulness training (e.g., Lomas et al., 2014; Mason & Hargreaves, 2001; Monshat et al., 2012). It should be noted, however, that students in the present study were not asked whether their perceptions of mindfulness practices changed throughout the program. Future studies should investigate pre- and early adolescents' experiences with mindfulness practice over time.

Future Directions

The research conducted on MindUP inspires several potential areas of investigation for future studies on MindUP and other mindfulness-based SEL programs.

Physiological Effects and Mechanisms: Given teachers' and students' mention of mindfulness practices contributing to recovery from emotional and physical stress and post-practice feelings of calm and relaxation, future studies should explore potential neurobiological mechanisms underlying this phenomenon by employing other physical measures to monitor autonomic nervous system (ANS) activity, such as heart rate, respiratory rate, oxygen intake, oxytocin, and skin conductance, especially in relation to stress. Having additional measures of ANS activity would contribute to a better understanding of how mindfulness practices may affect stress responses during this transitional developmental period. Additionally, students frequently mentioned that practicing the core breathing practice helped them experience a sense of calm and relaxation. Such mentions may point to a causal relationship between mindful breathing and activation of the parasympathetic nervous system (i.e., the "rest and digest" system). Future experimental studies should explore the effects of deep belly breathing and observing the breath on the nervous system to illuminate a potential mechanism for reported sensations of calm.

Variation Among Individuals and Specific Populations: Research is needed that specifically explores the effects of mindfulness-based SEL programs on different populations of students, for example those with different personalities (e.g., big five personality traits), from special populations (e.g., students living with mood disorders, students diagnosed with attention deficit and hyperactivity, students on the autism spectrum, students with developmental delays), and with special learning needs (e.g., students with learning differences). It is unclear whether specific mindfulness practices may be more or less suitable for students with different needs and personalities. For example, some articles have suggested that practicing mindfulness may not be appropriate for people experiencing extreme anxiety and that some mindfulness practices, such as observing one's thoughts and feelings, can exacerbate symptoms of anxiety (Lomas et al., 2014). Because school-based MBIs are intended for universal populations, it is important to explore whether the programs are appropriate for <u>all</u> students to ensure that they do no harm, a fundamental ethical guideline for mindfulness practice.

Motivation and Autonomy: Students' motivations for practice and their relations to program acceptability and efficacy also need to be explored. Whereas outside of institutions people generally have the autonomy to choose whether they would like to take part in mindfulness practices or not, one of the cautions of integrating mindfulness practices into regular school curricula is that it could result in students not being given a choice whether to take part in mindfulness practices or not. Similarly, it is conceivable that, similar to other SEL programs, MindUP could become mandated at a school or district level, requiring that teachers implement the program. Autonomy is both theoretically and empirically linked to motivation (Ryan & Deci, 2000). Research should investigate whether offering students autonomy in relation to mindfulness practices (e.g., whether they wish to participate or not, choosing the type of mindfulness practice, choosing the length of practice, choosing when to practice) has an effect on their engagement with mindfulness practices and/or the outcomes of practice. Similarly, program efficacy in relation to teacher autonomy should also be explored. Further investigation into the dissemination and implementation of MindUP as it is currently being employed in schools is also necessary to understand how the program is being applied in schools outside of monitored intervention research, and how implementation under "real world" conditions affects acceptability and efficacy of the program.

Training and Experience: The results presented here provide some insight into the discussion of how much training and experience with mindfulness practices teachers require to successfully introduce mindfulness practices to students. As Felver et al. (2015) noted, "the amount of training and experience needed to implement MBI[s] with full fidelity has yet to be determined. It could be that more simplistic MBI[s] require less extensive training than a more comprehensive MBI such as MBSR" (p. 8). It is helpful to know that even teachers who have had no previous experience with mindfulness practices (as was the case with several teachers across these studies) were able to safely and effectively implement mindfulness practices in their classroom with minimal training and a detailed, evidence-based curriculum. However, several teachers commented over the studies that they would have preferred more training. Future studies on MindUP should examine the length of training and the types of on-going support needed for individual teachers to be able to feel secure in effectively implementing the program. Further, studies that observe teacher implementation could provide valuable information on best practices for introducing mindfulness practices in schools. To date, we know of no published studies that have examined this important topic.

Because the published MindUP curriculum is now publically available without training, new contexts and questions for investigation have arisen: Are teachers likely to seek out training and on-going support in addition to the manual? Is additional training necessary to successfully implement the program? Do teachers need their own mindfulness practice to be able to effectively implement the program? Do teachers need to embody specific qualities associated with mindfulness (e.g., kindness, compassion, caring, openness, acceptance, present-centered focus, patience, calm) to be able to effectively implement the program? These important questions remain to be empirically explored. To investigate some of these questions, Schonert-Reichl and colleagues are currently analyzing data from RCT 2 (see Fig. 20.1) that examined the implementation and efficacy of MindUP among teachers who participated in a mindfulness-based SEL program designed specifically for educators—Stress Management And Relaxation Training-in-Education (SMART; see Roeser, this volume; Roeser et al., 2013)—compared to those who did not. Longitudinal observational studies of MindUP that include teachers with various amounts of training and personal experience with contemplative practices are also essential.

Effects Over Time: Longitudinal studies are necessary to better understand potential long-term developmental effects of practice and to determine whether there are any sleeper effects from mindfulness training as have been observed in some recent studies on MBIs in schools (Kuyken et al., 2013; Van de Weijer-Bergsma et al., 2014). Additionally, it is important to know whether students continue to use the practices even after they are no longer practicing mindfulness training at school given that the immediate benefits associated with mindfulness training appear to come with consistent and frequent practice (Tang et al., 2012).

Qualitative Inquiry: The studies on MindUP described here investigated student perceptions solely through written responses to participant satisfaction surveys. Future studies should include other methods of obtaining participant insights, including focus groups and one-on-one interviews. Doing so could illuminate many currently unanswered questions concerning whether particular practices are more effective for different populations of youth, what young people experience during mindfulness practice, and how their experiences with and perceptions of mindfulness practice may change with repeated practice. Neurophenomenological studies that employ think-aloud descriptions of participants' experiences during and immediately following mindfulness practices in conjunction with measurements of neurobiology could further illuminate underlying neurological mechanisms related to mindfulness practice.

Conclusion

The question of whether mindfulness practices are suitable as universal preventative interventions in schools has been raised by researchers, mindfulness practitioners, and educators. In this chapter, we overviewed studies that have found myriad beneficial outcomes to individuals participating in a mindfulness-based SEL program. The vast majority of students and teachers in the studies presented here reported favorable impressions of the MindUP program, providing support that schools may indeed be a suitable venue for introducing mindfulness practices. Our findings also provide support that, when combined, mindfulness practices and SEL can lead to positive improvements in social relations. Thus, MBIs that also teach secular ethics, such as kindness, perspective-taking, and gratitude, may offer benefits that transcend the individual and extend to others as well. Research on mindfulness education, however, is still in its infancy, and much work has yet to be done before any conclusions regarding generalizability of programs can be made.

References

Bear, G. G., & Watkins, J. M. (2006). Developing self-discipline. In G. G. Bear & K. M. Minke (Eds.), *Children's needs III: Development, prevention, and intervention* (pp. 29–44). Bethesda, MD: National Association of School Psychologists.

Ben-Arieh, A. (2005). Where are the children? Children's role in measuring and monitoring their well-being. *Social Indicators Research, 74*, 573–596. http://doi.org/10.1007/s11205-004-4645-6.

Ben-Arieh, A. (2007). The child indicators movement: Past, present, and future. *Child Indicators Research, 3–16*. http://doi.org/10.1007/s12187-007-9003-1.

Biegel, G. M., Brown, K. W., Shapiro, S. L., & Schubert, C. M. (2009). Mindfulness-based stress reduction for the treatment of adolescent psychiatric outpatients: A randomized clinical trial. *Journal of Consulting and Clinical Psychology, 77*(5), 855–866. http://doi.org/10.1037/a0016241.

Braun, V., & Clarke, V. (2006). Using thematic analysis in psychology. *Qualitative Research in Psychology, 3*(2), 77–101. http://doi.org/10.1191/1478088706qp063oa.

Britton, W. B., Lepp, N. E., Niles, H. F., Rocha, T., Fisher, N. E., & Gold, J. S. (2014). A randomized controlled pilot trial of classroom-based mindfulness meditation compared to an active control condition in sixth-grade children. *Journal of School Psychology, 52*, 263–278. http://doi.org/10.1016/j.jsp.2014.03.002.

Chiesa, A., Calati, R., & Serretti, A. (2011). Does mindfulness training improve cognitive abilities? A systematic review of neuropsychological findings. *Clinical Psychology Review, 31*, 449–464. http://doi.org/10.1016/j.cpr.2010.11.003.

Condon, P., Desbordes, G., Miller, W., DeSteno, D., Hospital, M. G., & DeSteno, D. (2013). Meditation increases compassionate responses to suffering. *Psychological Science, 24*, 2125–2127. http://doi.org/10.1177/0956797613485603.

Crandall, V. C., Crandall, V. J., & Katkovsky, W. (1965). A children's social desirability questionnaire. *Journal of Consulting Psychology, 29*, 27–36. http://doi.org/10.1037/h0020966.

Cullen, M. (2011). Mindfulness-based interventions: An emerging phenomenon. *Mindfulness, 2*, 186–193. http://doi.org/10.1007/s12671-011-0058-1.

Diamond, A. (2009). The interplay of biology and the environment broadly defined. *Developmental Psychology, 45*, 1–8. http://doi.org/10.1037/a0014601.

Diamond, A. (2012). Activities and programs that improve children's executive functions. *Current Directions in Psychological Science, 21*, 335–341. http://doi.org/10.1177/0963721412453722.

Diamond, A., & Lee, K. (2011). Interventions shown to aid executive function development in children 4 to 12 years old. *Science, 333*, 959–964. http://doi.org/10.1126/science.1204529.

Domitrovich, C. E., & Greenberg, M. T. (2000). The study of implementation: Current findings from effective programs that prevent mental disorders in school-aged children. *Journal of Educational and Psychological Consultation, 11*, 193–221. http://doi.org/10.1207/s1532768xjepc1102_04.

Durlak, J. A., Weissberg, R. P., Dymnicki, A. B., Taylor, R. D., & Schellinger, K. B. (2011). The impact of enhancing students' social and emotional learning: A meta-analysis of school-based universal interventions. *Child Development, 82*(1), 405–432. http://doi.org/10.1111/j.1467-8624.2010.01564.x.

Eccles, J. S., & Roeser, R. W. (2011). Schools as developmental contexts during adolescence. *Journal of Research on Adolescence, 21*, 225–241. doi:10.1111/j.1532-7795.2010.00725.x.

Emmons, R. A., & McCullough, M. E. (2003). Counting blessings versus burdens: An experimental investigation of gratitude and subjective well-being in daily life. *Journal of Personality and Social Psychology, 84*, 377–389.

Fattore, T., Mason, J., & Watson, E. (2007). Children's conceptualisation(s) of their well-being. *Social*

Indicators Research, 80, 5–29. http://doi.org/10.1007/s11205-006-9019.

Fattore, T., Mason, J., & Watson, E. (2009). When children are asked about their well-being: Towards a framework for guiding policy. *Child Indicators Research, 2*, 57–77. http://doi.org/10.1007/s12187-008-9025-3.

Felver, J. C., Celis-de Hoyos, C. E., Tezanos, K., & Singh, N. N. (2015). A systematic review of mindfulness-based interventions for youth in school settings. *Mindfulness*. Retrieved from http://doi.org/10.1007/s12671-015-0389-4.

Graber, J. A., & Brooks-Gunn, J. (1996). Transitions and turning points: Navigating the passage from childhood through adolescence. *Developmental Psychology, 32*, 768–776. http://doi.org/10.1037//0012-1649.32.4.768.

Greenberg, M. T., & Harris, A. R. (2012). Nurturing mindfulness in children and youth: Current state of research. *Child Development Perspectives, 6*, 161–166. http://doi.org/10.1111/j.1750-8606.2011.00215.x.

Greenberg, M. T., & Mitra, J. L. (2015). From mindfulness to Right Mindfulness: The intersection of awareness and ethics. *Mindfulness, 6*, 74–78. http://doi.org/10.1007/s12671-014-0384-1.

Greenberg, M. T., Weissberg, R. P., O'Brien, M. U., Zins, J. E., Fredericks, L., Resnik, H., & Elias, M. J. (2003). Enhancing school-based prevention and youth development through coordinated social, emotional, and academic learning. *American Psychologist, 58*, 466–474. doi:10.1037/0003-066X.58.6- 7.466

Grossman, P. (2015). Mindfulness: Awareness informed by an embodied ethic. *Mindfulness, 6*, 17–22. http://doi.org/10.1007/s12671-014-0372-5.

Gunnar, M. R., & Vazquez, D. M. (2001). Low cortisol and a flattening of expected daytime rhythm: Potential indices of risk in human development. *Development and Psychopathology, 13*, 515–538. doi:10.1017/s0954579401003066.

Harachi, T. W., Abbott, R. D., Catalano, R. F., Haggerty, K. P., & Fleming, C. B. (1999). Opening the black box: Using process evaluation measures to assess implementation and theory building. *American Journal of Community Psychology, 27*, 711–731.

Hoza, B., Mrug, S., Gerdes, A. C., Hinshaw, S. P., Bukowski, W. M., Gold, J. A., … Arnold, L. E. (2005). What aspects of peer relationships are impaired in children with Attention-Deficit/Hyperactivity Disorder? *Journal of Consulting and Clinical Psychology, 73*, 411–423. http://doi.org/10.1037/0022-006X.73.3.411.

Hruschka, D. J., Schwartz, D., John, D. C. S., Picone-Decaro, E., Jenkins, R. A., & Carey, J. W. (2004). Reliability in coding open-ended data: Lessons learned from HIV behavioral research. *Field Methods, 16*, 307–331. http://doi.org/10.1177/1525822x04266540.

Huesmann, L. R., Eron, L. D., Guerra, N. G., & Crawshaw, V. B. (1994). Measuring children's aggression with teachers' predictions of peer nominations. *Psychological Assessment, 6*, 329–336. http://doi.org/10.1037/1040-3590.6.4.329.

Jha, A.P., Stanley, E.S., Kiyonaga, A., Wong, L., Gelfand, L. (2010). Examining the protective effects of mindfulness training on working memory capacity and affective experience. *Emotion, 10*, 54–64. doi: 10.1037/a0018438

Kabat-Zinn, J. (2003). Mindfulness-based interventions in context: Past, present, and future. *Clinical Psychology: Science and Practice, 10*, 144–156. http://doi.org/10.1093/clipsy.bpg016.

Keng, S.-L., Smoski, M. J., & Robins, C. J. (2011). Effects of mindfulness on psychological health: A review of empirical studies. *Clinical Psychology Review, 31*, 1041–1056. http://doi.org/10.1016/j.cpr.2011.04.006.

Kuyken, W., Weare, K., Ukoumunne, O. C., Vicary, R., Motton, N., Burnett, R., … Huppert, F. (2013). Effectiveness of the Mindfulness in Schools programme: Non-randomised controlled feasibility study. *The British Journal of Psychiatry, 203*, 126–131. http://doi.org/10.1192/bjp.bp.113.126649.

Lawlor, M. S. (2007). *The Hawn Foundation Mindfulness Education curriculum: Process evaluation of the Focus Mind/Mindful Matters program* (Report prepared for The Hawn Foundation).

Lawlor, M. S., Schonert-Reichl, K. A., Gadermann, A. M., & Zumbo, B. D. (2013). A validation study of the Mindful Attention Awareness Scale Adapted for children. *Mindfulness, 5*, 730–741. http://doi.org/10.1007/s12671-013-0228-4.

Layous, K., & Lyubormirsky, S. (2013). How do simple positive activities increase well-being? *Current Directions in Psychological Science, 22*, 57–62. doi: 10.1177/0963721412469809.

Layous, K., & Lyubomirsky, S. (2014). Benefits, mechanisms, and new directions for teaching gratitude to children. *School Psychology Review, 43*, 153–159.

Lind, C. (2007). The power of adolescent voices: Co-researchers in mental health promotion. *Educational Action Research, 15*(3), 371–383.

Lomas, T., Cartwright, T., Edginton, T., & Ridge, D. (2014). A qualitative summary of experiential challenges associated with meditation practice. *Mindfulness*. Retrieved from http://doi.org/0.1007/s12671-014-0329-8.

Lyubomirksy, S., & Layous, K. (2013). How do simple positive activities increase well-being? *Current Directions in Psychological Science, 22*, 57–62.

Lyubomirsky, S., Sheldon, K. M., & Schkade, D. (2005). Pursuing happiness: The architecture of sustainable change. *Review of General Psychology, 9*, 111–131. http://doi.org/10.1037/1089-2680.9.2.111.

Maloney, J. E., Whitehead, J. K., Lawlor, M. S., & Schonert-Reichl, K. A. (2014, October). *Children's perceptions of the MindUP program.* Poster presented at the International Symposium for Contemplative Studies, Boston, MA.

Mason, J., & Danby, S. (2011). Children as experts in their lives: Child inclusive research. *Child Indicators Research, 4*, 185–189. http://doi.org/10.1007/s12187-011-9108-4.

Mason, O., & Hargreaves, I. (2001). A qualitative study of mindfulness-based cognitive therapy for depression. *British Journal of Medical Psychology, 74*, 197–212. http://doi.org/10.1348/000711201160911.

Miller, G. E., Chen, E., & Zhou, E. S. (2007). If it goes up, must it come down? Chronic stress and hypothalamic-pituitary-adrenocortical axis in humans. *Psychological Bulletin, 133*(1), 25–45. http://doi.org/10.1037/0033-2909.133.1.25.

Milligan, K., Badali, P., & Spiroiu, F. (2013). Using Integra Mindfulness Martial Arts to address self-regulation challenges in youth with learning disabilities: A qualitative exploration. *Journal of Child and Family Studies, 24*(3), 562–575. doi: 10.1007/s10826-013-9868-1.

Mind and Life Education Research Network (MLERN); Davidson, R., Dunne, J., Eccles, J. S., Engle, A., Greenberg, M., Jennings, P., … Vago, D. (2012). Contemplative practices and mental training: Prospects for American education. *Child Development Perspectives, 6*, 146–153. doi: 10.1111/j.1750-8606.2012.00240.x.

Monshat, K., Khong, B., Hassed, C., Vella-Brodrick, D., Norrish, J., Burns, J., & Herrman, H. (2012). "A conscious control over life and my emotions:" Mindfulness practice and healthy young people. A qualitative study. *Journal of Adolescent Health, 52*, 572–577. http://doi.org/10.1016/j.jadohealth.2012.09.008.

Monteiro, L. M., Musten, R. F., & Compson, J. (2015). Traditional and contemporary mindfulness: Finding the Middle Path in the tangle of concerns. *Mindfulness, 6*, 1–13. http://doi.org/10.1007/s12671-014-0301-7.

O' Leary, K., O'Neill, S., & Dockray, S. (2015). A systematic review of the effects of mindfulness interventions on cortisol. *Journal of Health Psychology*. doi: 10.1177/1359105315569095.

Pepler, D. J., & Craig, W. M. (1995). A peek behind the fence: Naturalistic observations of aggressive children with remote audiovisual recording. *Developmental Psychology, 31*, 548–553.

Pickles, A., Rutter, M., & Torestad, B. (1991). Statistical and conceptual models of "turning points" in developmental processes. In D. Magnusson, L. R. Bergman, & G. Rudinger (Eds.), *Problems and methods in longitudinal research: Stability and change* (pp. 133–165). Cambridge: Cambridge University Press.

Quiggle, N. L., Garber, J., Panak, W. F., & Dodge, K. A. (1992). Social information processing in aggressive and depressed children. *Child Development, 63*, 1305–1320. http://doi.org/10.2307/1131557.

Roeser, R. W. (2013). Mindfulness and human development: A commentary on the special issue. *Research in Human Development, 10*, 273–283. http://doi.org/10.1080/15427609.2013.818490.

Roeser, R.W. (2014). The emergence of mindfulness-based interventions in educational settings, in S.A. Karabenick & T.C. Urdan (Eds.) *Motivational interventions: Advances in motivation and achievement* (pp. 379–419). Bingley, UK: Emerald Group Publishing Limited doi: 10.1108/S0749-742320140000018010.

Roeser, R.W., & Eccles, J.S. (2014). Schooling and the mental health of children and adolescents in the United States. In M. Lewis & K.D. Rudolph (Eds.) *Handbook of developmental psychopathy* (pp. 163–184). New York, NY: Springer. doi: 10.1007/978-1-4614-9608-3_9.

Roeser, R. W., Schonert-Reichl, K. A., Jha, A., Cullen, M., Wallace, L., Wilensky, R., Harrison, J. (2013). Mindfulness training and reductions in teacher stress and burnout: Results from two randomized wait-list control field trials. *Journal of Educational Psychology, 105*, 787–804. http://doi.org/10.1037/a0032093.

Roeser, R.W., & Zelazo, P. D. (2012). Contemplative science, education and child development: Introduction to the special section. *Child Development Perspectives, 6*, 143–145. doi: 10.1111/j.1750- 8606.2012.00242.x.

Ryan, R. M., & Deci, E. L. (2000). Self-determination theory and the facilitation of intrinsic motivation, social development, and well-being. *American Psychologist, 55*, 68–78. http://doi.org/10.1037110003-066X.55.1.68.

Safran, S. P. (1995). Peers' perceptions of emotional and behavioral disorders: What are students thinking? *Journal of Emotional and Behavioral Disorders, 3*(2), 66–75. http://doi.org/10.1177/106342669500300201.

Sandvik, E., Diener, E., & Seidlitz, L. (1993). Subjective well-being: The convergence and stability of self-report and non-self-report measures. *The Journal of Personality, 61*, 317–342. http://doi.org/10.1007/978-90-481-2354-4_6.

Schonert-Reichl, K. A., Guhn, M., Gadermann, A. M., Hymel, S., Sweiss, L., & Hertzman, C. (2013). Development and validation of the Middle Years Development Instrument (MDI): Assessing children's well-being and assets across multiple contexts. *Social Indicators Research, 114*, 345–369. http://doi.org/10.1007/s11205-012-0149-y.

Schonert-Reichl, K. A., & Lawlor, M. S. (2010). The effects of a mindfulness-based education program on pre- and early adolescents' well-being and social and emotional competence. *Mindfulness, 1*, 137–151. doi:10.1007/s12671-010-0011-8.

Schonert-Reichl, K. A., Oberle, E., Lawlor, M. S., Abbott, D., Thomson, K., Oberlander, T. F., & Diamond, A. (2015). Enhancing cognitive and social-emotional development through a simple-to administer mindfulness-based school program for elementary school children: A randomized controlled trial. *Developmental Psychology, 51*, 52–66. http://doi.org/10.1037/a0038454.

Stüntzner-Gibson, D., Koren, P. E., & DeChillo, N. (1995). The Youth Satisfaction Questionnaire: What kids think of services. *Families in Society, 76*, 616–624.

Tang, Y.-Y., Yang, L., Leve, L. D., & Harold, G. T. (2012). Improving executive function and its neurobiological mechanisms through a mindfulness-based intervention: Advances within the field of developmental neuroscience. *Child Development Perspectives, 6*(4), 361–366. http://doi.org/10.1111/j.1750-8606.2012.00250.x.

The Hawn Foundation. (2011). *The MindUP curriculum: Brain-focused strategies for learning and living*. New York: Scholastic.

Vago, D. R., & Silbersweig, D. A. (2012). Self-awareness, self-regulation, and self-transcendence (S-ART): A framework for understanding the neurobiological mechanisms of mindfulness. *Frontiers in Human Neuroscience, 6*, 1–30. http://doi.org/10.3389/fnhum.2012.00296.

Van de Weijer-Bergsma, E., Langenberg, G., Brandsma, R., Oort, F. J., & Bögels, S. M. (2014). The effectiveness of a school-based mindfulness training as a program to prevent stress in elementary school children. *Mindfulness, 5*, 238–248. http://doi.org/10.1007/s12671-012-0171-9

Weissberg, R. P., Caplan, M. Z., & Sivo, P. J. (1989). A new conceptual framework for establishing school-based social competence promotion programs. In L. A. Bond & B. E. Compas (Eds.), *Primary prevention and promotion in the schools* (pp. 255–296). Newbury Park, CA: Sage.

Weissberg, R.P., & Cascarino, J. (2013). Academic learning + social-emotional learning = national priority. *Phi Delta Kappan, 95*, 8–13. doi:10.1177/003172171309500203.

Wisner, B. L. (2014). An exploratory study of mindfulness meditation for alternative school students: Perceived benefits for improvig school climate and student functioning. *Mindfulness, 5*, 626–638. http://doi.org/10.1007/s12671-013-0215-9.

Zelazo, P. D., & Lyons, K. E. (2012). The potential benefits of mindfulness training in early childhood: A developmental social cognitive neuroscience perspective. *Child Development Perspectives, 6*, 154–160. http://doi.org/10.1111/j.1750-8606.2012.00241.x.

Zoogman, S., Goldberg, S. B., Hoyt, W. T., & Miller, L. (2015). Mindfulness interventions with youth: A meta-analysis. *Mindfulness, 6*, 290–302. http://doi.org/10.1007/s12671-013-0260-4.

Two Universal Mindfulness Education Programs for Elementary and Middle-School Students: Master Mind and Moment

21

Alison E. Parker and Janis B. Kupersmidt

"Something in modern life is still making many young people feel overwhelmed and anxious" (Twenge, 2011, p. 471). This issue is of great concern for parents and educators because children and adolescents continue to experience anxiety levels that are higher than same-aged youth decades ago (Twenge, 2000, 2011). Despite the fact that elementary school is a time when children's social–emotional (e.g., emotion regulation) and cognitive skills (e.g., executive functioning) are growing (e.g., Anderson, 2002; Denham, 1998; Pons, Lawson, Harris, & de Rosnay, 2003), high levels of stress and anxiety may negatively impact skills development, resulting in a wide range of possible negative consequences for youth. For example, children's academic performance may suffer, which has implications not only for elementary school but also for making a successful transition to middle school (e.g., McClelland, Acock, & Morrison, 2006; Sabol & Pianta, 2012). In addition, experiencing stress and negative affect on a daily basis can also put children at risk for developing and utilizing unhealthy coping methods and ineffective decision-making skills in risky situations (e.g., Mason, Hitch, & Spoth, 2009; Skeer, McCormick, Normand, Buka, & Gilman, 2009; Wills, Sandy, Yaeger, Cleary, & Shinar, 2001). If children do not possess the skills and resources to cope with environmental demands, it can take a large toll on their physical, mental, and academic well-being (Compas, Conner-Smith, Saltzman, Thomsen, & Wadsworth, 2001; Jacobson, Williford, & Pianta, 2011; Konishi & Hymel, 2009). Thus, there is a need for evidence-based, universal education programs that will provide all children with the skills and resources they need to help them manage everyday demands and foster the growth of self-regulatory abilities to enhance their academic success and healthy decision-making. One approach to building these skills in youth is through the teaching and utilization of daily mindfulness practices introduced systematically to students in a school-based setting.

Mindfulness has been conceptualized as being attentive to and aware of the present moment and accepting each moment without judgment (Kabat-Zinn, 1994, 2003). When experiencing a thought or emotion, one learns to observe and reflect on the experience rather than react automatically or impulsively (e.g., Shapiro, Carlson, Astin, & Freedman, 2006). As posited by Zelazo and Lyons (2012), participation in mindfulness training may facilitate children's development of self-regulation because it may reduce emotionally arousing influences (e.g., anxiety) and, at the same time, cultivate more deliberate, top-down processes (e.g., cognitive flexibility). Self-regulation, or the ability to modulate one's emotions, thoughts, and behaviors, is an important

A.E. Parker (✉) • J.B. Kupersmidt
Innovation Research and Training, Durham, NC, USA
e-mail: aparker@irtinc.us; jkupersmidt@irtinc.us

K.A. Schonert-Reichl, R.W. Roeser (eds.), *Handbook of Mindfulness in Education*,
Mindfulness in Behavioral Health, DOI 10.1007/978-1-4939-3506-2_21

predictor of academic success (e.g., Blair & Diamond, 2008) and healthy decision-making (e.g., Mason et al., 2011).

There are already a growing number of studies investigating the benefits of mindfulness practice for children and adolescents. Some of these benefits include improvements in attention, behavior and emotion regulation, effective stress responses, executive functioning (EF), and social–emotional competence as well as decreases in sleep problems, depression, anxiety, feelings of discomfort, and externalizing behaviors (e.g., Biegel, Brown, Shapiro, & Schubert, 2009; Bootzin & Stevens, 2005; Broderick & Metz, 2009; Mendelson et al., 2010; Metz et al., 2013; Napoli, Krech, & Holley, 2005; Oberle, Schonert-Reichl, Lawlor, & Thomson, 2012; Parker, Kupersmidt, Mathis, Scull, & Sims, 2014; Saltzman & Goldin, 2008; Schonert-Reichl & Lawlor, 2010; Sibinga et al., 2011).

Given the growing evidence of there being multiple benefits associated with youth engaging in regular mindfulness practice, we developed and evaluated two universal, school-based, mindfulness education programs: The Master Mind program was developed for use with late elementary-school students with the goal of preventing risky decision-making around smoking and drinking. The Moment program was created for use with middle-school students with the goal of enhancing academic outcomes. The main goal of this chapter is to describe the conceptual approaches and procedures used in the development and evaluation of both programs. Specifically, five main topics will be discussed in the chapter about the two programs: (1) the theory of change used to guide program development; (2) developmental issues to consider regarding mindfulness practice and education by youth; (3) translation of prevention science findings into recommendations for effective, school-based mindfulness curricula; (4) description of scope and sequence, activities, and instructional materials; and (5) program evaluation results.

Theory of Change

The theory of change model described below provides the theoretical underpinnings for our mindfulness education programs (Fig. 21.1).

Mindfulness practice is hypothesized to increase three proximal outcomes, namely, attention, behavior regulation, and emotional regulation. In turn, increases in these proximal outcomes are hypothesized to improve the more distal outcomes of academic achievement and healthy decision making (e.g., making choice to not use cigarettes or alcohol). The empirical research findings supporting the hypothesized relationships between mindfulness practice and positive outcomes are described next.

Attention

The ability to pay attention and concentrate in the classroom is a strong and stable predictor of children's academic achievement (Preston, Heaton, McCann, Watson, & Selke, 2009; Rueda, Checa, & Rothbart, 2010). Being easily or frequently distracted may interfere with direct instruction resulting in gaps in learning and understanding. Likewise, lack of attention and concentration skills may result in incomplete or missing assignments and poor grades. In fact, children who are

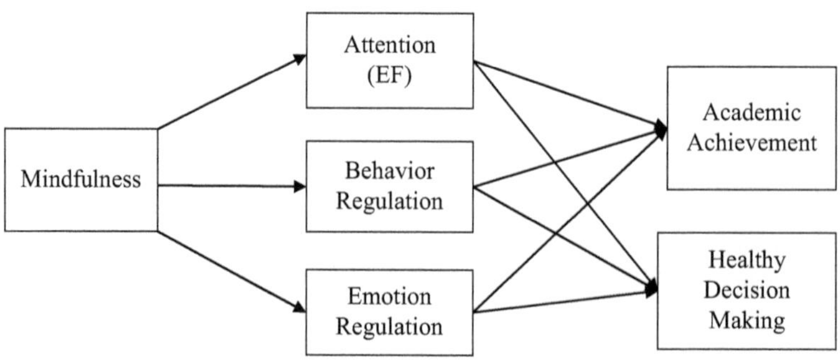

Fig. 21.1 Theory of change model guiding mindfulness education program development

better able to sustain their concentration during class time are more likely to maintain higher academic performance in comparison to students who are not able to maintain their concentration (Rabiner, Murray, Schmid, & Malone, 2004). EF is also positively associated with children's academic achievement throughout the school years (Blair & Diamond, 2008; Blair & Razza, 2007; Bull, Espy, & Wiebe, 2008; Jacobson et al., 2011).

Attentional problems can also influence social interactions with peers. For example, children who do not pay attention to social cues in their environment may have more difficulty successfully establishing and maintaining friendships than children who can attend to and respond to social cues (e.g., Eisenberg et al., 2003; Murphy, Laurie-Rose, Brinkman, & McNamara, 2007). Peer problems resulting from attention problems may put children at risk for making unhealthy and risky decisions, possibly because they do not have all the information needed to make informed choices. Children as young as 9 years of age with poor EF are at greater risk for smoking or drinking than children with higher EF skills (Riggs, Spruijt-Metz, Chou, & Pentz, 2012).

Learning to be aware and attentive of what is going on inside and outside of the self, which can build attention skills, is an important part of mindfulness. This is becoming evident in mindfulness training with youth. For example, school-aged children who participated in mindfulness programs displayed increases in their attention abilities (e.g., Napoli et al., 2005; Saltzman & Goldin, 2008; Schonert-Reichl, & Lawlor, 2010) and reductions in parent-reported ADHD symptoms (van der Oord, Bögels, & Peijnenburg, 2012). Mindfulness training also has the potential to improve EF, more broadly. For example, elementary-school-aged children's self-reported mindful awareness was positively associated with higher scores on a performance task of EF skills (Oberle et al., 2012). In another study, participation in a mindfulness training program resulted in improvements in parent- and teacher-rated EF scores for children with EF difficulties (Flook et al., 2010). Thus, mindfulness education in schools has the potential to enhance children's attention as well as a broader set of EF skills.

Behavior Regulation

Children's ability to monitor and regulate their behavior has implications for their everyday lives. An important type of behavior regulation is self-control. There has been a call to target self-control in intervention efforts based on a three-decade longitudinal study by Moffitt et al. (2011), who claimed that individuals with high self-control in childhood had better physical health, higher socioeconomic status and income, and lower levels of criminal offending in adulthood than those with poor self-control in childhood (Moffitt et al., 2011).

Children's ability to regulate their behavior is associated with success in school (Ponitz, McClelland, Matthews, & Morrison, 2009; Valiente, Lemery-Chalfant, Swanson, & Reiser, 2008). In contrast, an inability to monitor and regulate one's behaviors (e.g., aggression, delinquency) may disturb academic learning and achievement from childhood into adolescence (Masten et al., 2005). Additionally, good behavioral self-control may act as a buffer, protecting youth from engaging in risky activities, such as using alcohol, tobacco, or other drugs (e.g., Wills, Pokhrel, Morehouse, & Fenster, 2011; Wills, Sandy, & Yaeger, 2002). Overall, these findings support a call to action to develop programs that facilitate the development of healthy behavior regulation in youth.

Mindfulness training is one way to respond to this call. Mindfulness training provides the opportunity to become more aware and reflective of one's thoughts, which may enhance the ability to resist reflexive, impulsive reactions to those thoughts. For example, children who participated in a mindfulness education program, compared to those who did not, exhibited fewer problem behaviors (i.e., aggressive and oppositional) as reported by their teachers (Schonert-Reichl & Lawlor, 2010). Similarly, in another study, late elementary-school students experienced less teacher-reported social and aggressive problems as a function of participating in a mindfulness education program (Parker, Kupersmidt, & Mathis et al., 2014). Thus, engaging in mindfulness practice may positively influence students' behaviors in and outside of the classroom.

Emotion Regulation

Children experience and express a variety of positive and negative emotions on a daily basis and the ability to be aware of and regulate these emotions in socially appropriate ways is important (Halberstadt, Denham, & Dunsmore, 2000). It is well-known that the development of emotion regulation is beneficial to youth. Studies of elementary- and middle-school-aged children have found positive associations between emotion regulation and academic success and classroom productivity (Graziano, Reavis, Keane, & Calkins, 2007; Trentacosta & Izard, 2007). Conversely, an inability to be aware of or regulate emotions may have a negative impact on children's success in school (Whitted, 2010). For example, experiencing negative effect (i.e., anxiety, frustration) toward school work can result in poor academic performance (e.g., Gumora & Arsenio, 2002). Additionally, young children's poor regulation of emotions also predicted high levels of externalizing behaviors in school (Rydell, Berlin, & Bohlin, 2003). An inability to regulate negative affect may also put youth at risk for engaging in risky behaviors such as using alcohol or tobacco. For example, youth who experience or express negative effect (e.g., anger) are more likely to make decisions to use substances than youth who are better able to control their emotions (Eftekhari, Turner, & Larimer, 2004; Mason et al., 2009). However, being equipped with the ability to deal with stressful feelings or events may protect youth from participating in risky activities (e.g., Wills et al., 2001).

Mindfulness practice provides opportunities to learn how to be aware and accepting of one's feelings as well as to learn that these feelings can pass without the need to react to them. These practices may help children to become more aware of and help them better cope with negative feelings. In fact, in two separate studies, participation by high-school students in a mindfulness education program resulted in improvements in emotion regulation skills (Broderick & Metz, 2009; Metz et al., 2013). In another study, fourth- to seventh-grade students demonstrated increases in dimensions of social–emotional competence as a function of participating in a school-based mindfulness program (Schonert-Reichl & Lawlor, 2010). In addition, participation by urban-, elementary-, and middle-school students in a mindfulness-based yoga intervention resulted in reductions in problematic responses to stress (e.g., rumination; Mendelson et al., 2010). Thus, mindfulness training in the classroom may facilitate the growth of emotion awareness and regulation.

In summary, current research suggests that mindfulness training has the capacity to enhance children's attention and emotion and behavior regulation abilities that are most often tied to academic success and healthy decision-making. Cultivating these abilities in youth will then pave a path for improved daily functioning during the elementary and middle-school years.

Developmental Considerations Associated with Mindfulness Abilities in Youth

To be aware of one's body, feelings, and thoughts requires the availability of certain cognitive and emotional abilities. Some people question whether youth possesses the cognitive and emotional capabilities to learn and understand mindfulness. However, this question is becoming less of an issue given the growing number of studies illustrating the benefits of mindfulness education and practice for youth. What then are the abilities that a youth must have in order to be able to learn and practice mindfulness? Some of the abilities are: to be able to pay attention, follow directions, sit still or hold a pose, and think flexibly and abstractly. Young people must also have the meta-cognitive awareness of one's own thoughts and emotions. Children and adolescents do, in fact, possess the cognitive and emotional competencies to learn, understand, and utilize mindfulness in their daily lives. For example, during late childhood and adolescence, attention (e.g., Kim, Deater-Deckard, Mullineaux, & Allen, 2010) and EF, which includes working memory, inhibitory control, and cognitive flexibility, are becoming more fully developed (e.g., Anderson, Anderson, Northam, Jacobs, & Catroppa, 2001; Blakemore & Choudhury, 2006; Boelema et al., 2014; Jones, Rothbart, & Posner, 2003). Late childhood and early adolescence have been shown to be periods of maturation and consolidation of these core abilities. Notably, these observed improvements in skills such as decision-making, effortful self-control, and working memory coincide with the ongoing development of the pre-frontal cortex (e.g., Blakemore & Choudhury, 2006; Lewis & Stieben, 2004).

Youth's emotional abilities are also emerging during the school years. Elementary-school-aged children can recognize, experience, and express a variety of primary and self-conscious emotions as well as experience and distinguish among multiple or blended emotions (Bosacki & Moore, 2004; Camras et al., 1988; Denham, 1998; Larsen, To, & Fireman, 2007; Russell & Widen, 2002). Children also display a good understanding of their own and others' emotions (Dunn & Hughes, 1998; Pons et al., 2003) and are developing emotion regulatory strategies to successfully manage their emotional arousal (e.g., Fabes & Eisenberg, 1992; Waters & Thompson, 2014).

Overall, youth do have the cognitive and emotional abilities to engage in mindfulness practice. It is, however, important to keep in mind that these cognitive and emotional capabilities are still developing; hence, program content and methods need to be tailored to be developmentally appropriate and accessible to these young minds (Fodor & Hooker, 2008). The lessons and activities in the Master Mind and Moment programs were developed to be developmentally appropriate for their respective target populations. For example, we tailored the language used in all of the instructional materials to meet the developmental expectations of a fifth-grade reading level or less. We also included definitions for all new terms to provide the students and teachers with a common vocabulary. Slogans and short titles for skills (e.g., "Take a Pause") were also used to provide a common means of communication between teachers and students as well as to provide verbal cues to facilitate students' recall of specific mindfulness practices. Concrete examples (e.g., illustrations in the Master Mind program or photographs in the Moment program of being mindful versus not mindful) and metaphors (e.g., thoughts as clouds) for teaching abstract concepts about mindfulness to students are incorporated throughout both programs. In addition, because children's attention spans increase in length throughout the school years (Kim et al., 2010), elementary- and middle-school-aged youth can be expected to meditate for shorter periods of time than that of adults. Thus, the mindful journeys in each program were created to last between 2 and 5 min in length.

Translation of Prevention Science Findings into Recommendations for Effective, School-Based Mindfulness Curricula

The Master Mind and Moment programs were carefully designed to incorporate principles from research on the most effective prevention programs that have resulted in the greatest impact and fidelity of implementation (e.g., Botvin, Griffin, & Nichols, 2006; Ennett et al., 2003; Greenberg et al., 2003; Nation et al., 2003). Below we describe some examples.

Interactive Activities

The inclusion of highly interactive activities and teaching methods in prevention programs has been associated with better outcomes for children and adolescents, as well as greater implementation fidelity (Ennett et al., 2003; Tobler et al., 2000). For example, in a meta-analysis of 207 substance abuse prevention programs, Tobler et al. (2000) identified a small 6 % reduction in the rate of prevalence of substance use in programs that lacked interactivity, whereas prevention programs that included interactive activities showed a 34 % reduction rate in prevalence of substance use. Interactivity among students in the classroom may include exchanging of ideas, role-playing, or providing feedback on the newly acquired skills, or discussing possible ways to handle challenging situations inside or outside of the classroom (Tobler et al., 2000).

Based upon these findings on the importance of prevention programs being highly interactive, every lesson in the Master Mind and Moment programs includes at least one experiential or interactive activity. These activities are designed to increase student engagement as well as provide opportunities for guided and regular mindfulness practice. One method used to integrate interactivity into the programs is to have students participate in group discussions rather than listen to lectures by a teacher. Some examples of discussion topics include key mindfulness concepts and thinking about the application of new mindfulness practices to coping with everyday stressful experiences.

A second method that was used to create interactive lessons involves the demonstration and practice of kinesthetic or mindful movements as well as guided mindful meditation. Students repeatedly practice a variety of mindfulness skills both in class and at home in both programs. These efforts to have students engage in consistent daily mindfulness practice across the week may help them to build their skills. The daily practice was hypothesized to result in students spending enough time engaged in mindfulness so that they may quickly observe some of the anticipated benefits of regular mindfulness practice such as feeling more aware, focused, and calm. By experiencing these short-term beneficial outcomes, students may increase their desire and motivation to sustain their mindfulness practice when the program is completed. As part of both programs, teachers and students also develop plans for how to continue their daily mindfulness practice, both as a class and on their own, after the program has ended.

Peer-Led Activities

An important feature of effective prevention programs is the inclusion of peer-led as opposed to teacher-led activities (e.g., Cuijpers, 2002). In both the Master Mind and Moment programs, yoga poses are referred to as mindful movements. They are taught and demonstrated to students in brief videos led by same-aged instructors. The child or adolescent actors who provide instruction vary in their sex, race, and ethnicity. In addition to these videos, students lead their classmates through designing and acting out role plays of how they will use their new mindfulness skills in dealing with daily stressful experiences in school or at home.

Teacher Preparation

Findings from the mental health and substance abuse fields suggest that in order for a teacher to effectively learn and implement an intervention program, the teacher must be well-prepared (e.g., Ennett et al., 2003; Payne & Eckert, 2010). This means that the goals, objectives, theory of change, and instructions of a program must be manualized and instructors must be trained, preferably by the program developers. Consistent with these recommendations, both the Master Mind and Moment programs are fully manualized for use by teachers and teachers may enroll in in-person teacher training workshops. The 20-lesson manuals contain goals, objectives, and lesson plans for each lesson (see section on Program Description for examples). A professional graphic design artist designed the materials with input from psychologists, teachers, and instructional designers to create the layout and content of the instructional materials used in each program. As a result of these collaborative efforts, easy-to-interpret visual cues and icons are used to help guide teachers in easily locating what they need to successfully teach each lesson with fidelity.

Teacher training consists of a 1-day, instructor-led workshop that lasts approximately 8 h that is completed prior to the implementation of either program. In these training workshops, teachers learn about mindfulness, the theory of change model for each program, the scope and sequence of topics included in each program, and the contents of each lesson plan. Teachers are also offered tips for teaching each lesson. Throughout the training day, teachers are also provided with multiple opportunities to practice and experience the mindfulness skills included in each program.

Lesson Length

According to a recent report, less than half of the research-based programs reviewed were implemented with adequate implementation fidelity (U.S. Department of Education, Planning, Policy Development, & Policy and Program Studies Services, 2011). Teachers have many competing demands on them during the typical school day. Thus, despite the many benefits that mindfulness was expected to have on enhancing youth's self-regulatory and academic abilities, it was thought that teachers may believe that they do not have the time to add a non-required subject to their already demanding, full school day. With findings on problems with fidelity of implementation and the pressures on teachers in mind, we created the unique structure of both mindfulness programs. Creating a program with short, daily lessons that can be easily integrated into teaching curricula and schedules may have a positive impact on implementation fidelity. Thus, unlike many prevention programs that are designed to fit a typical class period of 45–50 min, the lessons in both programs were designed to be brief so that they could be completed in 15 min. In this way, teachers could implement the Master Mind or Moment programs and still have time during a class period to teach other content. Also, we recommended to teachers that they teach the program during a natural transition point in the school day such as when the students first arrive to school in the morning or when they return to class after lunch, recess, or physical education. Integrating mindfulness education and practice into natural transition points between unstructured and instructional time during the school day was expected to help students pay more attention and successfully adapt their behavior. These assumptions were verified. Multiple teachers reported that they appreciated the brief length of lessons and noticed that their students settled down more quickly after the mindfulness lessons. We believe that these factors contributed to teachers' enthusiastic adoption and faithful implementation of both programs (further described in the Evaluation section below).

Lesson Goals and Objectives

In addition to considering factors such as program length in the design of each program, most teachers also have to meet certain curriculum objectives for each grade level. If teachers create one or more instructional objectives that do not meet their grade-level standards, then they have less time available to teacher core and required objectives. One of our aims was to be sure that when teachers taught Master Mind or Moment, they did not worry that they were teaching skills that were inconsistent with grade-level standards or wasting core instructional time. Thus, when we developed the lessons, we considered the appropriate Common Core Standards for K-12 education (e.g., Language Arts) for each program and then created a document for teachers that aligned the goals and objectives of each lesson with the Common Core Standards. This integration provided teachers with additional instructional materials and tools to use to complement their existing curricula while being able to also teach and practice mindfulness with their students. This type of mapping, such that lessons were designed to meet multiple goals, may have also enhanced program adoption and implementation.

In short, the literature from child and adolescent development and prevention science informed the iterative development and instructional design of both mindfulness education programs and contributed to positive reviews of the programs by students and teachers in focus groups and efficacy studies.

Program Description: The Master Mind and Moment Programs

Our proposed theoretical model, developmental considerations, and best practices in prevention program implementation guided the development of the content and design of the Master Mind and Moment programs. The Master Mind program was designed to be taught to fourth- and fifth-grade students with the goal of promoting healthy decision-making in risky situations (e.g., smoking or drinking). The Moment program was designed for use with sixth- and seventh-grade students with the goal of promoting academic achievement. Both programs seek to build children and adolescents' self-regulatory abilities by training and practice in mindfulness. The core mindfulness activities, scope and sequence, and instructional materials for each program are described below.

Core Mindfulness Activities

Embedded within the programs are five sets of activities that are taught to and practiced by students including (1) mindful breathing, (2) mindful meditations, (3) mindful movements, (4) real-world applications, and (5) daily practices. Individually, these components have been associated with beneficial outcomes and it is expected that together, they will positively contribute to students' mindfulness practice and the growth of self-regulatory abilities.

Mindful Breathing Awareness of breathing is fundamental to mindfulness practice and is considered to be an anchor to the present moment (Kabat-Zinn, 1990). Furthermore, mindful breathing exercises have been associated with reduced depression or rumination (Burg & Michalak, 2011). Learning how to become aware of the breath is a fundamental step in developing mindfulness and is integral to both the Master Mind and Moment programs. Mindful breathing is highlighted in many of the activities in both programs.

Mindful Meditations Various forms of meditation (e.g., mindfulness meditation) practiced in schools have resulted in a number of benefits to students, such as improvements in coping and self-control abilities, as well as reductions in stress and anxiety (e.g. Wisner, Jones, & Gwin, 2010). The purpose of teaching and practicing mindful meditations with students is to guide them through various brief meditations and visualizations. Specifically, these meditations provide students with the experience of becoming more aware of their bodily sensations, feelings, and thoughts. Some meditations were adapted from the adult Mindfulness-Based Stress Reduction course (Kabat-Zinn, 2003) to be developmentally appropriate for elementary- or middle-school-aged children. The audiotaped, guided mindful meditations were renamed for the students as journeys, a word that is more developmentally accessible to students than the word meditation. Additionally, the meditations, or journeys, were shortened in length to 2–5 min in order to account for the shorter attention span during these developmental periods.

Mindful Movements Performing mindful movements (e.g., yoga poses) has the potential to improve children's ability to cope with stress (Mendelson et al., 2010; White, 2012). Thus, the goal of teaching students mindful movements is to provide them with opportunities to become aware of their bodies, movement, and breathing. The mindful movements taught to each age group were carefully selected by a certified yoga instructor such that they were developmentally appropriate to learn in class and could be practiced independently. Some examples include the sitting twist (i.e., twisting at the waist), lemon squeeze (i.e., tensing and releasing body parts), or tree pose (i.e., balancing on one leg). In addition, the movements were also selected so that they could be completed easily either at or next to students' desks.

Real-World Applications of Mindfulness Practice Providing opportunities for students to observe and practice their newly learned skills is a key characteristic that makes a preventive intervention program work successfully (e.g., Nation et al., 2003). Thus, at the end of each week of lessons, which also represents the end of a unit on each foundation of mindfulness, students consider how they can apply their new mindfulness skills to handling everyday hassles or stressors. Students are presented with hypothetical stories of fellow peers experiencing a problem or challenge, and as a class, the students are asked to use their new mindfulness skills to solve the problems. Focus groups with elementary- and middle-school-aged students were conducted to ensure that the hypothetical situations included in the programs represented common experiences of youth in each age group. These experiences spanned across a range of situations that commonly induce stress and anxiety in youth including academics (e.g., taking a test or speaking in front of others or balancing school, home, and extracurricular activities); peers (e.g., making new friends, arguing with friends); and making healthy choices (e.g., ignoring friends' requests to skip school).

Daily Practice of Mindfulness Skills Higher frequency of engagement in mindfulness practice is related to increases in positive outcomes for adults (e.g., Carmody & Baer, 2008; Carson, Carson, Gil, & Baucom, 2004). Thus, providing opportunities for regular mindfulness practice may also be beneficial for children and adolescents (e.g., MLERN, 2012). In both programs, students practice mindfulness daily in their classrooms and nightly with at-home practice assignments. These activities provide students with the opportunity to have consistent, daily practice in school and at home with the goals of establishing daily mindfulness routines and increasing positive youth outcomes.

Scope and Sequence

The Master Mind and Moment programs are organized into 4 units consisting of 5 lessons per unit for a total of 20 lessons. Each unit represents one of the four foundations of mindfulness (Nhat Hanh, 1990). One foundation is taught in each unit during each week across a 4-week period. The four foundations are (1) awareness of the body, (2) awareness of feelings, (3) awareness of thoughts, and (4) awareness of objects of the mind (we narrowed the scope of the fourth foundation to focus on relationships with the self and with others). We describe the main goals for each week with respect to each foundation. In addition, we provide at least one description of a lesson activity for each program. It is important to note that there is some overlap in the specific mindfulness practices that are taught and practiced in each program (e.g., stop and take three breaths, mindful movements, thoughts are not facts, etc.). In this chapter, we provide a variety of illustrative examples from each program. We also describe how the lessons were created so that they are developmentally appropriate for the target age group.

Week 1: Awareness of the Body This week focuses on teaching students how to be more aware of their bodies and their bodily sensations. For example, Master Mind program involves students learning and practicing the "Take a Pause" skill, which includes taking three deep breaths when exposed to a stressful situation. The skill is easy to teach involving clear, direct instructions and easy for a late elementary-school student to learn. It is practiced when students are asked to consider a variety of everyday, common elementary social and school stressors such as having an argument with a friend or taking a test. In the Moment program, middle-school students learn and practice several types of mindful movements including both sitting and standing yoga poses. Several movements require multiple instructions and students learn to make these mindful movements, hold the pose, and focus their thoughts on their breathing. By the end of the week for both programs, students should be more aware of the present moment, their breathing, and their entire bodies.

Week 2: Awareness of Feelings This week focuses on teaching students how to be aware of pleasant and unpleasant feelings. For example, in the Master Mind program students write entries in a journal about pleasant emotions that they may experience during the week. As a group, students share their experiences with the class and discuss ways to cultivate these emotions in their lives. The space for writing the entry is small with specific questions (e.g., "How did your body feel during the pleasant event?") to answer to reduce the burden, real or perceived, on elementary students to write lengthy journal entries. Before students complete the activity on their own, they generate examples in a guided discussion with their teacher as a group to help make the task more concrete and achievable. In the Moment program, students learn and practice healthy ways to express emotions. Students first learn how to identify a range of emotions both in themselves and others (e.g., facial and bodily expressions of emotions). Building on this, students discuss how feelings can influence one's thoughts and mind, which requires middle-school students to think abstractly about the difference between emotions and behaviors. Students then discuss ways to express feelings and view videotaped examples of same-aged peers expressing emotions in healthy and unhealthy ways. In a group discussion format, students compare and contrast these video experiences. By the end of the week, students should be more aware of different types of emotions and healthy strategies for expressing emotion and practice cultivating positive emotions and letting go of negative emotions.

Week 3: Awareness of Thoughts This week focuses on teaching students how thoughts work and drive one's actions. In the Master Mind program, students learn that thoughts are not facts. This is a very abstract idea for elementary-school students requiring the metacognitive ability to distinguish different forms of cognitions. We use both metaphors and visual illustrations to help students understand, internalize, and accept this idea. For example, students are presented with an illustrated example of a social event that might happen during the school day. In this example, students are asked to imagine greeting a peer in the hallway at school and being ignored by him or her. Teachers then solicit reasons from their students about why this negative social experience may have happened ranging from benign (e.g., distracted by something) to hostile intent (e.g., he doesn't like me) of the ignoring peer. Students are then asked to generate other examples of times when what they thought might not necessarily have been true. Although the "thoughts are not facts" activity is also taught to students in the Moment program, this activity is enhanced with a discussion about how this type of judgmental thinking can influence their own behaviors. As another example, students in the Moment program are taught a more complex practice which includes learning to be aware of having a mind that is not fully in the present or a "bored mind." In this activity, students consider the broader concept of their minds and that there may be different states of minds. Students learn ways to be aware of a bored mind, how to bring themselves back to the present moment, which includes being aware of what is going on inside themselves and around them, and why this is important. By the end of this week, students should become more aware of their own thoughts and busy minds, recognize how to view their thoughts in a non-judgmental manner, and practice letting thoughts go.

Week 4: Awareness of Relationships This focuses on teaching students to be aware of their relationships with themselves and with others. For example, students in the Master Mind program learn about self-compassion in a guided, concrete way. They participate in a mindful journey that builds upon the Take a Pause breathing skill (described above) that they learned earlier in the program. In this activity, teachers guide students to think about kind or positive words about themselves (i.e., happy, healthy). Students then participate in a mindful journey, repeating the positive words—one for each of the three breaths. Students discuss different times they might want to use this new mindful journey in their daily lives. In the Moment program, the concept of relationships is taught in a more abstract way, focusing on the idea that everything is interdependent and influences one another. Students are asked to think about the types of relationships in their lives (e.g., parents, friends, or acquaintances) and how these relationships might influence them in different ways. This helps students to become more aware of their interactions with others. By the end of this week, students should be more aware of different types of relationships, understand how to show compassion toward themselves and others, and communicate effectively with others, particularly in situations that might be stressful or upsetting.

Instructional Materials

The Master Mind and Moment programs include a complete set of instructional materials for teachers to help them implement the program. For both programs, teachers are provided with a teacher manual, student workbooks, and a multimedia software application. The multimedia software includes instructional materials for teaching each lesson such as audio files for guiding the mindful meditations, videotaped scenes providing instruction and demonstrations of mindful movements, and infographics and illustrations to provide more concrete visual examples of many mindfulness concepts. In both programs, during the final lesson in each week, we focus on applying mindfulness practices to real-world situations. Students are presented with social dilemmas that are commonly faced by same-aged peers. In the Master Mind program, students read letters written by same-aged peers to their mindfulness teacher that are printed in their workbooks. In contrast, in the Moment program, students are presented with videotaped dilemmas of peer-aged actors to watch and discuss. Students watch the first half of a videotaped scene during which a peer-aged actor is experiencing a challenge or stressor. The class then works as a group to discuss how mindfulness might help in that situation. Then, the students watch the second half of the video to see how the peer-aged actor coped with the situation by using a mindfulness practice.

Teachers and students can also access each program's website. Both websites host audio files of mindful meditations and videos demonstrating mindful movements designed to facilitate students' practices at home. Specific to the Moment program website, daily practice assignments are available for students to complete at home or at their leisure. Teachers have access to a dashboard that allows them to enroll students in the practice assignments and monitor their progress in completing them. The dashboard includes additional functionality of compiling all of the students' responses into a downloadable report for the teacher that can be printed or saved.

In the Master Mind program, students are enrolled into the Master Mind Academy on the first day of the program and introduced to the overall program. They are told that in the Academy, they will be taking a journey together across four connected mountains and that each mountain represents the four parts of the Master Mind program: body, feelings, thoughts, and relationships. As they travel over each mountain, students receive a sticker badge when they complete each part (i.e., week) of the program. At the conclusion of the program, students are told that they will get a sticker badge to symbolize that they have become a Master Mind and graduated from Master Mind Academy. As students participate in the program, they have two character guides who help to teach the mindfulness skills: Pax, a monkey, and Paws, a panda. Paws (named for taking a "pause" and breathing) has completed the Master Mind program and provides examples of the benefits of mindfulness to Pax. In contrast, Pax (named for *paix* or peace) is learning alongside the students about how to become more mindful. One of the developmental challenges in mindfulness education with children is to provide concrete examples of abstract concepts. As can be seen in the example in Fig. 21.2, students are introduced to the complex idea of what it means to be mindful through a guided discussion with their teacher and classmates utilizing this image with four illustrations.

In contrast to the Master Mind program, the Moment program does not include illustrated animal characters, given that it is developed for older students in middle school. Instead, the Moment program utilizes photographs and videos of peer-aged actors who provide direct instruction of and model program practices. In addition, there are also illustrations of students in real-world scenarios that supplement the videos of the program practices. As can be seen in Fig. 21.3, students can refer to a comic strip that illustrates the real-world example of a same-aged peer stopping and taking three breaths, when feeling nervous in front of the class.

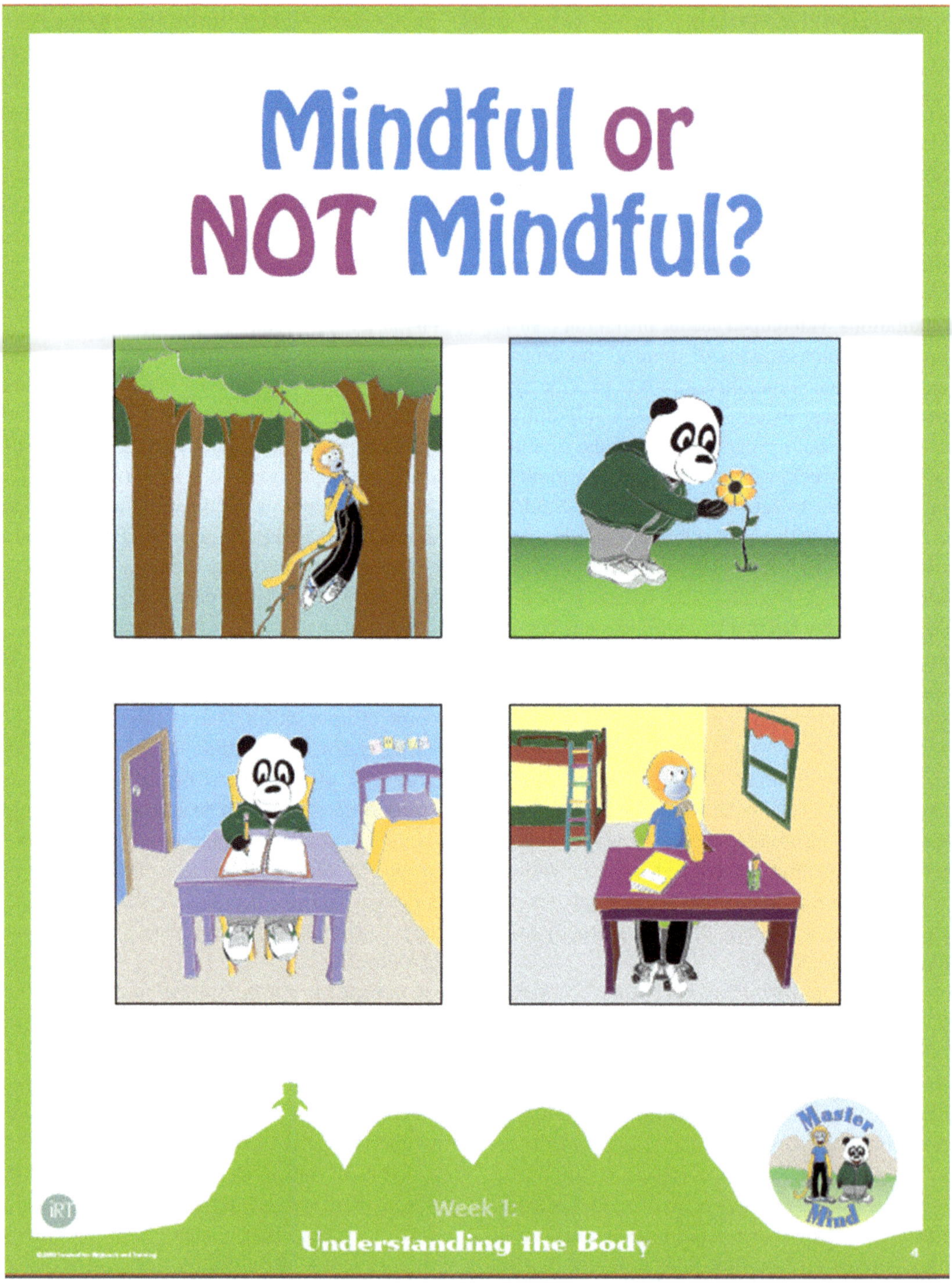

Fig. 21.2 Example of classroom activity in the Master Mind Program. Published herein with the permission of the author

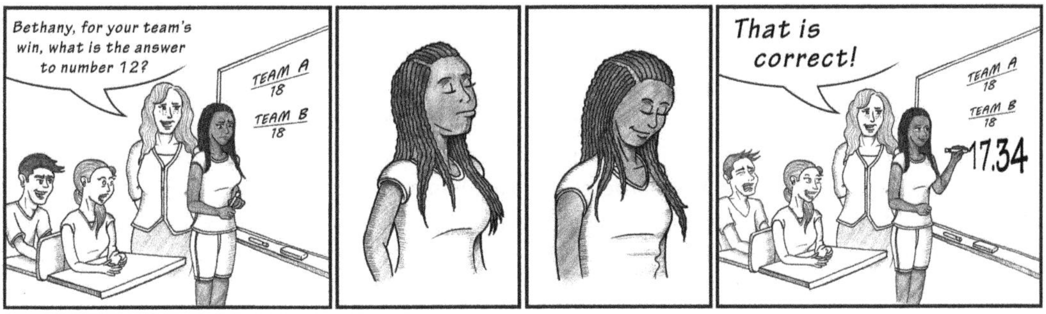

Fig. 21.3 Example of classroom activity in the Moment Program. Published herein with the permission of the author

Program Evaluation Results

The Master Mind and Moment programs were evaluated in small efficacy trials, each using a randomized wait-list controlled group design. The goal for each study was to evaluate the effectiveness of the program for changing youth outcomes as well as the fidelity and feasibility of the program.

In the Master Mind evaluation, we investigated the impact of the Master Mind program on students' behavior regulation, EF, and intentions to use substances (see Parker, Kupersmidt, Mathis et al., 2014). There were a total of 111 elementary-school students (M age = 10.09, SD = .51) who participated in the study with 71 students in the intervention and 40 students in the wait-list control group. In the Moment evaluation, we investigated the impact of the Moment program on students' behavior regulation, EF, and academic functioning (see Parker, Kupersmidt, & Willoughby, 2014). In this study, there were 118 middle-school students (M age = 11.70; SD = .65) who participated with 72 students in the intervention and 46 students in wait-list control group.

The procedures used in conducting each study were similar to one another. Prior to implementing each program, teachers participated in an 8-h training workshop that was conducted by the program developer. The intervention teachers implemented their respective mindfulness education program in their classrooms for approximately 4 weeks. The wait-list control group teachers went about "business as usual" and followed their regular education curriculum. Teachers in the intervention group received a Teacher Manual containing 20 scripted lessons as well as additional instructional resources. At pre- and post-test intervention time points, students completed self-report questionnaires and a brief computer task designed to measure EF. In addition, at both time points, teachers completed rating scale questionnaires about their students' behaviors. Intervention students and teachers also completed questionnaires to assess program feasibility.

Main Outcome Findings

Master Mind Program Efficacy Findings Parker, Kupersmidt, Mathis, et al. (2014) reported that students who participated in the Master Mind program had higher EF skills at the posttest compared to students in the wait-list control group. In addition, students in the intervention group had lower teacher-rated social problems and aggression problems in contrast to students in the wait-list control group.

Gender moderated some of the outcomes. Specifically, girls who participated in the Master Mind program had lower teacher-rated anxiety compared to girls in the wait-list control group. Although only marginally significant, boys in the intervention group had better teacher-rated self-control in comparison to boys in the control group. There were no significant changes in teacher-rated attention or student-reported intentions to use alcohol or tobacco as a function of participating in the Master Mind program. Notably, reports by students in the sample regarding intent to use substances were uniformly low suggesting a possible floor effect.

Moment Program Efficacy Findings Parker, Kupersmidt, and Willoughby (2014) found that students who participated in the Moment program experienced decreases in teacher-reported attention problems as well as teacher-reported aggression problems. Students who participated in the Moment program, compared to students in the wait-list control group, were rated by teachers as having less EF dysfunction related to behavior regulation and metacognition.

Among accurate performers on an EF performance task (i.e., those who were correct at least 85% of the time), students who participated in the Moment program had faster reaction times (RT) than students in the wait-list control group.

Conclusions from Program Evaluation Efficacy Studies Despite the fact that the two programs were implemented with different age groups with one consisting of children and the other consisting of early adolescents, the findings across the two efficacy studies were similar. The findings for each study, including effect sizes (Cohen's *d*), are summarized in Table 21.1. Both studies found that measures representing different aspects of EF showed effects of mindfulness education and practice. In addition, aspects of behavioral regulation, such as aggression problems, seemed to be positively affected by these programs. Although one might consider these findings as preliminary, given that they used relatively small samples, the robust, consistent nature of the results suggests that even with relatively low power, mindfulness education implemented in school-based setting using daily brief practices has a potentially powerful impact on some youth outcomes.

Table 21.1 Main outcome findings for Master Mind and Moment programs

Construct	Master Mind	Moment
Executive functioning		
Performance	.42**[a]	.74*[b]
Behavior Regulation: Teacher-report	n/a	.74**
Metacognition: Teacher-report	n/a	1.22**
Attention: Teacher-report	.16	.64**[c]
Aggression: Teacher-report	.54**	1.21**
Social problems: Teacher-report	.41*	n/a
Anxiety: Teacher-report	.62* (girls)	n/a
Self-control: Teacher-report	.56^{+} (boys)	n/a
Intentions to use substances: student-report	-.16	n/a

$^{+}p<.10$, $^{*}p<.05$, $^{**}p<.01$.
Note: n/a = not applicable, a = Accuracy; b = Reaction Time, c = Mean effect size of two teacher-report measures

Program Feasibility Findings

In addition to assessing program efficacy, students and teachers in the intervention groups were asked to provide consumer satisfaction and feasibility feedback about the Master Mind and Moment programs, respectively.

Master Mind Program Feasibility Findings In the Master Mind program, all teachers reported that they enjoyed teaching the lessons to their students and found the lessons easy to prepare and teach. Teachers also reported that the length of time it took to teach each lesson made it feasible to integrate them into the regular school day. Teachers also reported that they would continue to use some of the mindfulness skills with students in their classrooms during the school year. Importantly, teachers also reported that they would probably implement the Master Mind program in future school years.

Most students reported that they enjoyed participating and learning new information in the Master Mind program. Several students reported that the Master Mind program helped them to be more mindful in their everyday lives. They also reported particularly liking the "Taking a Pause" (i.e., stopping to pause and take three breaths) activity.

Moment Program Feasibility Findings Similar to the Master Mind program, teachers reported that they enjoyed implementing the Moment program in their classrooms and found the lessons easy to prepare and teach. Teachers also reported that they would continue to use some of the mindfulness skills in their classrooms during the school year. In addition, teachers reported that they would likely implement the Moment program in the future.

Students reported that they enjoyed and learned from the Moment program. Students reported that the most important thing that they learned in the Moment program was stopping and taking three breaths ("Take 3") and recognizing that thoughts are not facts.

Implementation Fidelity Findings

For both Master Mind and Moment programs, the intervention classrooms were observed by trained members of the research team. The goal was to observe 75 % or more of the lessons in the program taught in each of the intervention classrooms, meaning that the goal was to observe 15 lessons per intervention class. Each lesson can be further divided into sections, based upon the discrete activities included in the lesson. Observers utilized a Fidelity Checklist that reflected this dosage information such that each section was rated in terms of its completeness of implementation. The Likert ratings ranged from a low of 1 representing "not at all taught" to a high of 4 representing "thoroughly taught." A mean score for the observed sections was calculated for each class, and then, the mean score was calculated across the intervention classrooms.

For the Master Mind program, the mean score for implementation dosage was 3.99, suggesting that all the sections of the program were thoroughly taught to students. For the Moment program, the mean score across intervention classrooms was also 3.99, again suggesting that the program was thoroughly taught to students. In the Moment program evaluation, teachers in the wait-list control group also recorded their daily regular education activities. No comparable mindfulness activities were taught to students in the wait-list control classrooms during the 4-week program evaluation period.

Recommendations for Future Research

There are a number of directions for future research in the area of mindfulness education that are suggested by these two efficacy studies. First, there is a need for additional efficacy trials to more fully understand the long-term impact of mindfulness education on a range of youth outcomes across age groups. These studies would allow for the empirical examination of developmental differences in the impact of mindfulness education. Consistent with these goals, the next steps for both the Master Mind and Moment programs are to examine program efficacy of the programs in adequately powered, large-scale, randomized controlled trials including immediate posttest assessments as well as longer-term follow-up evaluations of youth outcomes.

Second, once outcome effectiveness is established, unpacking complex programs to determine their effective ingredients is needed to develop the most parsimonious programs while maintaining maximal impact on outcomes. Paring programs down to their essential elements will contribute to them being more ready for universal and widespread dissemination. Given the unique structure of the Master Mind and Moment programs that consist of brief daily lessons, one question of interest concerns whether massed (e.g., daily) or spaced (e.g., weekly) lessons would produce significantly better youth outcomes.

Consistent with recommendations made by Greenberg and Harris (2012), we also recommend that future studies should examine the potential mediating mechanisms that may explain the relationship between mindfulness and positive youth outcomes. Identifying significant mediators will advance understanding of the active ingredients operating in mindfulness education and mindfulness practice. For example, EF may mediate the relationship between mindfulness and children's academic achievement. If so, then programs which aim to promote academic success should aim to include mindfulness practices designed to improve EF and assess growth in these abilities over time.

In addition to exploring potential mediators, the examination of potential moderators may also be of interest. Replicating common prevention program moderators such as implementation dosage and quality for their differential impact on youth should be tested. In addition, the frequency of mindfulness practice at home may be an important moderator of the effectiveness of mindfulness education programs for achieving positive youth outcomes.

Furthermore, an investigation into the factors affecting fidelity of implementation of mindfulness education in school settings is also needed. As mentioned previously, instructors, who are not the program developers, often do not teach prevention programs with fidelity, thereby potentially diluting the effectiveness of evidence-based programs (Ennett et al., 2003). Thus, it is critical for the prevention field to determine how to design and package mindfulness educations programs in order to increase implementation fidelity and quality.

Teacher training is also an important area of interest for research. As recommended in the prevention science literature, teachers need to be trained; however, the parameters around training are not well-defined. For example, it is unclear how many hours of training are actually needed for teachers to effectively implement the programs with fidelity. In addition, it is also unknown if it would be beneficial for youth outcomes if teachers first participated in their own mindfulness training prior to implementing mindfulness education programs in their classrooms. Furthermore, mindfulness education for teachers may have an effect on their teaching performance, more generally. Research that examines the effects of the dosage, modality, and content of teacher training of mindfulness programs on quality of teacher implementation and student outcomes is needed.

Recommendations for Educational Practice

Observing classrooms participating in our two mindfulness-based programs has provided us with a wealth of knowledge regarding factors that may facilitate universal program adoption and full implementation of mindfulness education programs as well as directions for future mindfulness educational practices. As we had originally hypothesized, program and lesson length were important factors that appeared to facilitate delivery of full implementation dosage. Specifically, teachers in both evaluation studies thoroughly implemented almost 100 % of the activities in each lesson in each program. We concluded from teacher comments and feedback that this high level of fidelity is partly attributable to the brief length of each lesson as well as our suggestion to teachers that they implement the programs following a natural transition time.

In addition, students appeared to enjoy participating in the wide range of activities included in the programs, especially those that involved mindful movement. Given that some children do not have the opportunity for daily physical activity in school and the recent campaigns to reduce childhood obesity, teachers considered the inclusion of mindful movements to be a central part of each program. The integration of mindfulness and movement provided children with the opportunity to not only become aware of their bodies and breathing, but also to have the opportunity to develop and increase flexibility, strength, and balance.

We also recommend aligning all prevention programs, including mindfulness curricula, with each state's or country's standard course of study objectives for the appropriate grade levels. By aligning each program activity with academic standards (e.g., language arts, science, healthful living), greater buy-in is obtained from key decision makers in the school system including administrators, principals, and teachers. In this way, by implementing either the Master Mind or Moment programs, teachers were able to meet required objectives rather than implementing an ancillary program that took time away from instructional activities that did meet these objectives.

Finally, teachers participated in an 8-h, in-person training workshop for each program, and they were provided with several resources to assist them in teaching the lessons. Observations of teacher quality of implementation suggested that the length of training that we provided seemed to be sufficient for accomplishing the goals of introducing teachers to the importance of mindfulness education, the theory of change underlying each program, the content of each lesson, and opportunities to practice mindfulness skills. However, because the mindful meditations were led by recorded voices and mindful movements were led by videotaped child actors, it is not clear if teachers could have adequately led these practices on their own without completing additional training or having supplemental mindfulness experiences. The use of these supporting instructional materials made it possible for full and effective program implementation by teachers following attendance at a relatively short training workshop and time for personal program review. It is important to note that some lessons appeared to include content that was relatively more challenging for teachers to teach based upon our observations of greater variability in teacher performance. These more challenging lessons involved teachers' facilitation of open-ended classroom discussions, particularly those discussions that generated a wide range of emotional reactions or thoughts from their students. Thus, additional training and/or consulting may be needed to fully train some teachers to be effective in using these kinds of pedagogical methods.

Conclusion

This chapter explains how developmental and prevention science research findings have been translated to influence the development of universal, school-based, mindfulness education programs for use with elementary- and middle-school students. The integration and incorporation of research findings and practice recommendations into the content, pedagogy, and instructional design of the Master Mind and Moment programs can provide the foundation for achieving both positive youth outcomes and the tools needed for broad dissemination. Findings from two small evaluation studies provided support for mindfulness education programs taught by regular education teachers in the classroom, and at the same time, provided a call for more research on factors associated with the successful implementation and dissemination of effective mindfulness education programs.

Acknowledgments The content described in this chapter was supported by Award Number R43 DA024508 (Parker) from the National Institute on Drug Abuse and Award Number R305A090175 (Parker) from the Institute of Education Sciences (IES). The content is solely the responsibility of the authors and does not necessarily represent the official views of the National Institute on Drug Abuse, the National Institutes of Health, Institute of Education Sciences, or the Department of Education.

References

Anderson, P. (2002). Assessment and development of executive function (EF) during childhood. *Child Neuropsychology, 8*, 71–82. doi:10.1076/chin.8.2.71.8724.

Anderson, V., Anderson, P., Northam, E., Jacobs, R., & Catroppa, C. (2001). Development of executive functions through late childhood and adolescence in an Australian sample. *Developmental Neurology, 20*, 385–406.

Biegel, G., Brown, K., Shapiro, S., & Schubert, C. (2009). Mindfulness-based stress reduction for the treatment of adolescent psychiatric outpatients: A randomized clinical trial. *Journal of Consulting and Clinical Psychology, 77*, 855–866.

Blair, C., & Diamond, A. (2008). Biological processes in prevention and intervention: The promotion of self-regulation as a means of preventing school failure. *Development and Psychopathology, 20*, 899–911.

Blair, C., & Razza, R. (2007). Relating effortful control, executive function, and false belief understanding to emerging math and literacy ability in kindergarten. *Child Development, 78*(2), 647–663. doi:10.1111/j.1467-8624.2007.01019.x.

Blakemore, S. J., & Choudhury, S. (2006). Development of the adolescent brain: Implications for executive function and social cognition. *Journal of Child Psychology and Psychiatry, 47*(3–4), 296–312.

Boelema, S. R., Harakeh, Z., Ormel, J., Hartman, C. A., Vollebergh, W. M., & van Zandvoort, M. E. (2014). Executive functioning shows differential maturation from early to late adolescence: Longitudinal findings from a TRAILS study. *Neuropsychology, 28*(2), 177–187. doi:10.1037/neu0000049.

Bootzin, R. R., & Stevens, S. J. (2005). Adolescents, substance abuse, and the treatment of insomnia and daytime sleepiness. *Clinical Psychology Review, 25*, 629–644.

Bosacki, S. L., & Moore, C. (2004). Preschoolers' understanding of simple and complex emotions: Links with gender and language. *Sex Roles, 50*, 659–675.

Botvin, G. J., Griffin, K. W., & Nichols, T. (2006). Preventing youth violence and delinquency through a universal school-based prevention approach. *Prevention Science, 7*(4), 403–408. doi:10.1007/s11121-006-0057-y.

Broderick, P. C., & Metz, S. (2009). Learning to BREATHE: A pilot trial of a mindfulness curriculum for adolescents. *Advances in School Mental Health Promotion, 2*, 35–46.

Bull, R., Espy, K., & Wiebe, S. A. (2008). Short-term memory, working memory, and executive functioning in preschoolers: Longitudinal predictors of mathematical achievement at age 7 years. *Developmental Neuropsychology, 33*(3), 205–228. doi:10.1080/87565640801982312.

Burg, J. M., & Michalak, J. (2011). The healthy quality of mindful breathing: Associations with rumination and depression. *Cognitive Therapy and Research, 35*(2), 179–185. doi:10.1007/s10608-010-9343-x.

Camras, L. A., Ribordy, S., Hill, J., Martino, S., Spaccarelli, S., & Stefani, R. (1988). Recognition and posing of emotional expressions by abused children and their mothers. *Developmental Psychology, 24*, 776–781.

Carmody, J., & Baer, R. A. (2008). Relationships between mindfulness practice and levels of mindfulness, medical and psychological symptoms and well-being in a mindfulness-based stress reduction program. *Journal of Behavioral Medicine, 31*(1), 23–33. doi:10.1007/s10865-007-9130-7.

Carson, J. W., Carson, K. M., Gil, K. M., & Baucom, D. H. (2004). Mindfulness-based relationship enhancement. *Behavior Therapy, 35*(3), 471–494. doi:10.1016/S0005-7894(04)80028-5.

Compas, B. E., Conner-Smith, J. K., Saltzman, H., Thomsen, A. H., & Wadsworth, M. E. (2001). Coping with stress during childhood and adolescence: Problems, progress, and potential in theory and research. *Psychological Bulletin, 127*, 87–127.

Cuijpers, P. (2002). Peer-led and adult-led school drug prevention: A meta-analytic comparison. *Journal of Drug Education, 32*(2), 107–119. doi:10.2190/LPN9-KBDC-HPVB-JPTM.

Denham, S. A. (1998). *Emotional development of young children*. New York, NY: Guildford Press.

Dunn, J., & Hughes, C. (1998). Young children's understanding of emotions within close relationships. *Cognition and Emotion, 12*, 171–190.

Eftekhari, A., Turner, A. P., & Larimer, M. E. (2004). Anger expression, coping, and substance use in adolescent offenders. *Addictive Behaviors, 29*, 1001–1008.

Eisenberg, N., Valiente, C., Fabes, R. A., Smith, C. L., Reiser, M., Shepard, S. A., … Cumberland, A. J. (2003). The relations of effortful control and ego control to children's resiliency and social functioning. *Developmental Psychology, 39*, 761–776.

Ennett, S. T., Ringwalt, C. L., Thorne, J., Rohrbach, L. A., Vincus, A., Simons-Rudolph, A., & Jones, S. (2003). A comparison of current practice in school-based substance use prevention programs with meta-analysis findings. *Prevention Science, 4*, 1–14.

Fabes, R., & Eisenberg, N. (1992). Young children's coping with interpersonal anger. *Child Development, 63*, 116–128.

Flook, L., Smalley, S. L., Kitil, M., Galla, B. M., Kaiser-Greenland, S., Locke, J., … Kasari, C. (2010). Effects of mindful awareness practices on executive functions in elementary school children. *Journal of Applied School Psychology, 26*(1), 70–95. doi:10.1080/15377900903379125.

Fodor, I. E., & Hooker, K. E. (2008). Teaching mindfulness to children. *Gestalt Review, 12*, 75–91.

Graziano, P. A., Reavis, R. D., Keane, S. P., & Calkins, S. D. (2007). The role of emotion regulation in children's early academic success. *Journal of School Psychology, 45*, 3–19.

Greenberg, M. T., & Harris, A. R. (2012). Nurturing mindfulness in children and youth: Current state of research. *Child Development Perspectives, 6*(2), 161–166. doi:10.1111/j.1750-8606.2011.00215.x.

Greenberg, M. T., Weissberg, R. P., O'Brien, M. U., Zins, G. E., Fredericks, L., Resnik, H., & Elias, M. J. (2003). Enhancing school-based prevention and youth development through coordinated social, emotional, and academic learning. *American Psychologist, 58*, 466–474.

Gumora, G., & Arsenio, W. F. (2002). Emotionality, emotion regulation, and school performance in middle school children. *Journal of School Psychology, 40*, 395–413.

Halberstadt, A. G., Denham, S. A., & Dunsmore, J. C. (2000). Affective social competence. *Social Development, 10*, 79–119.

Jacobson, L. A., Williford, A. P., & Pianta, R. C. (2011). The role of executive function in children's competent adjustment to middle school. *Child Neuropsychology, 17*(3), 255–280. doi:10.1080/09297049.2010.535654.

Jones, L., Rothbart, M. K., & Posner, M. I. (2003). Development of executive attention in preschool children. *Developmental Science, 6*(5), 498–504. doi:10.1111/1467-7687.00307.

Kabat-Zinn, J. (1990). *Full catastrophe living: Using the wisdom of your body and mind to face stress, pain and illness*. New York, NY: Delacorte.

Kabat-Zinn, J. (1994). *Wherever you go, there you are: Mindfulness meditation in everyday life*. New York, NY: Hyperion.

Kabat-Zinn, J. (2003). Mindfulness-based interventions in context: Past, present, and future. *Clinical Psychology: Science and Practice, 10*, 144–156.

Kim, J., Deater-Deckard, K., Mullineaux, P. Y., & Allen, B. (2010). Longitudinal studies of anger and attention span: Context and informant effects. *Journal of Personality, 78*(2), 419–440. doi:10.1111/j.1467-6494.2010.00621.x.

Konishi, C., & Hymel, S. (2009). Bullying and stress in early adolescence: The role of coping and social support. *The Journal of Early Adolescence, 29*(3), 333–356. doi:10.1177/0272431608320126.

Larsen, J. T., To, Y. M., & Fireman, G. (2007). Children's understanding and experience of mixed emotions. *Psychological Science, 18*(2), 186–191. doi:10.1111/j.1467-9280.2007.01870.x.

Lewis, M. D., & Stieben, J. (2004). Emotion regulation in the brain: Conceptual issues and directions for developmental research. *Child Development, 75*, 371–376.

Mason, W. A., Hitch, J. E., & Spoth, R. L. (2009). Longitudinal relations among negative affect, substance use, and peer deviance during the transition from middle to late adolescence. *Substance Use and Misuse, 44*, 1142–1159. doi:10.1080/10826080802495211.

Mason, W., Toumbourou, J. W., Herrenkohl, T. I., Hemphill, S. A., Catalano, R. F., & Patton, G. C. (2011). Early age alcohol use and later alcohol problems in adolescents: Individual and peer mediators in a bi-national study. *Psychology of Addictive Behaviors, 25*(4), 625–633. doi:10.1037/a0023320.

Masten, A. S., Roisman, G. I., Long, J. D., Burt, K. B., Obradović, J., Riley, J. R., ... Tellegen, A. (2005). Developmental cascades: Linking academic achievement and externalizing and internalizing symptoms over 20 Years. *Developmental Psychology, 41*(5), 733–746. doi:10.1037/0012-1649.41.5.733.

McClelland, M. M., Acock, A. C., & Morrison, F. J. (2006). The impact of kindergarten learning-related skills on academic trajectories at the end of elementary school. *Early Childhood Research Quarterly, 21*(4), 471–490. doi:10.1016/j.ecresq.2006.09.003.

Mendelson, T., Greenberg, M. T., Dariotis, J. K., Gould, L., Rhoades, B. L., & Leaf, P. J. (2010). Feasibility and preliminary outcomes of a school-based mindfulness intervention for urban youth. *Journal of Abnormal Child Psychology, 38*(7), 985–994. doi:10.1007/s10802-010-9418-x.

Metz, S. M., Frank, J. L., Reibel, D., Cantrell, T., Sanders, R., & Broderick, P. C. (2013). The effectiveness of the Learning to BREATHE program on adolescent emotion regulation. *Research in Human Development, 10*(3), 252–272. doi:10.1080/15427609.2013.818488.

Mind and Life Education Research Network (MLERN). (2012). Contemplative practices and mental training: Prospects for American education. *Child Development Perspectives, 6*(2), 146–153.

Moffitt, T. E., Arseneault, L., Belsky, D., Dickson, N., Hancox, R. J., Harrington, H., ... Caspi, A. (2011). A gradient of childhood self-control predicts health, wealth, and public safety. *PNAS Proceedings of the National Academy of Sciences of the United States of America, 108*(7), 2693–2698. doi:10.1073/pnas.1010076108.

Murphy, L., Laurie-Rose, C., Brinkman, T. M., & McNamara, K. A. (2007). Sustained attention and social competence in typically developing preschool-aged children. *Early Child Development and Care, 177*(2), 133–149. doi:10.1080/03004430500349559.

Napoli, M., Krech, P. R., & Holley, L. C. (2005). Mindfulness training for elementary school students: The Attention Academy. *Journal of Applied School Psychology, 21*, 99–125.

Nation, M., Crusto, C., Wandersman, A., Kumpfer, K. L., Seybolt, D., Morrissey-Kane, E. & Davino, K. (2003). What works in prevention: Principles of effective prevention programs. *American Psychologist, 58*, 449–456.

Nhat Hanh, T. (1990). *Transformation and healing: Sutra on the four establishments of mindfulness*. New York, NY: Parallax Press.

Oberle, E., Schonert-Reichl, K. A., Lawlor, M. S., & Thomson, K. C. (2012). Mindfulness and inhibitory control in early adolescence. *Journal of Early Adolescence, 34*, 45–51. doi:10.1177/0272431611403741.

Parker, A. E., Kupersmidt, J. B., Mathis, E. T., Scull, T. M., & Sims, C. (2014). The impact of mindfulness education on elementary school students: Evaluation of the *Master Mind* Program. *Advances in School Mental Health Promotion, 7*(3), 184–204. doi:10.1080/1754730X.2014.916497.

Parker, A. E., Kupersmidt, J. B., & Willoughby, M. T. (2014). An investigation of mindfulness education and self-regulation in middle school classrooms. Unpublished manuscript.

Payne, A. A., & Eckert, R. (2010). The relative importance of provider, program, school, and community predictors of the implementation quality of school-based prevention programs. *Prevention Science, 11*, 126–141.

Ponitz, C., McClelland, M. M., Matthews, J. S., & Morrison, F. J. (2009). A structured observation of behavioral self-regulation and its contribution to kindergarten outcomes. *Developmental Psychology, 45*(3), 605–619. doi:10.1037/a0015365.

Pons, F., Lawson, J., Harris, P., & de Rosnay, M. (2003). Individual differences in children's emotion understanding: Effects of age and language. *Scandinavian Journal of Psychology, 44*, 347–353.

Preston, A. S., Heaton, S. C., McCann, S. J., Watson, W. D., & Selke, G. (2009). The role of multidimensional attentional abilities in academic skills of children with ADHD. *Journal of Learning Disabilities, 42*(3), 240–249. doi:10.1177/0022219408331042.

Rabiner, D. L., Murray, D. W., Schmid, L., & Malone, P. S. (2004). An exploration of the relationship between ethnicity, attention problems, and academic achievement. *School Psychology Review, 33*, 498–509.

Riggs, N. R., Spruijt-Metz, D., Chou, C., & Pentz, P. (2012). Relationships between executive cognitive function and lifetime substance use and obesity-related behaviors in fourth grade youth. *Child Neuropsychology, 18*, 1–11.

Rueda, M., Checa, P., & Rothbart, M. K. (2010). Contributions of attentional control to socioemotional and academic development. *Early Education and Development, 21*(5), 744–764. doi:10.1080/10409289.2010.510055.

Russell, J. A., & Widen, S. C. (2002). Words versus faces in evoking preschool children's knowledge of the causes of emotions. *International Journal of Behavioral Development, 26*, 97–103.

Rydell, A., Berlin, L., & Bohlin, G. (2003). Emotionality, emotion regulation and adaptation among 5- to 8-year-old children. *Emotion, 3*, 30–47.

Sabol, T. J., & Pianta, R. C. (2012). Patterns of school readiness forecast achievement and socio-emotional development at the end of elementary school. *Child Development, 83*(1), 282–299. doi:10.1111/j.1467-8624.2011.01678.x.

Saltzman, A., & Goldin, P. (2008). Mindfulness based stress reduction for school-age children. In S. C. Hayes & L. A. Greco (Eds.), *Acceptance and mindfulness interventions for children adolescents and families* (pp. 139–161). Oakland, CA: Context Press/New Harbinger.

Schonert-Reichl, K. A., & Lawlor, M. S. (2010). The effects of a mindfulness-based education program on pre- and early adolescents' well-being and social and emotional competence. *Mindfulness, 1*(3), 137–151. doi:10.1007/s12671-010-0011-8.

Shapiro, S. L., Carlson, L. E., Astin, J. A., & Freedman, B. (2006). Mechanisms of mindfulness. *Journal of Clinical Psychology, 62*, 373–386.

Sibinga, E. S., Kerrigan, D., Stewart, M., Johnson, K., Magyari, T., & Ellen, J. M. (2011). Mindfulness-based stress reduction for urban youth. *The Journal of Alternative and Complementary Medicine, 17*(3), 213–218. doi:10.1089/acm.2009.0605.

Skeer, M., McCormick, M. C., Normand, S. T., Buka, S. L., & Gilman, S. E. (2009). A prospective study of familial conflict, psychological stress, and the development of substance use disorders in adolescence. *Drug and Alcohol Dependence, 104*, 65–72.

Tobler, N. S., Roona, M. R., Ochshorn, P., Marshall, D. G., Streke, A. V., & Stackpole, K. M. (2000). School-based adolescent drug prevention programs: 1998 meta-analysis. *The Journal of Primary Prevention, 20*, 275–336.

Trentacosta, C. J., & Izard, C. E. (2007). Kindergarten children's emotion competence as a predictor of their academic competence in first grade. *Emotion, 7*(1), 77–88. doi:10.1037/1528-3542.7.1.77.

Twenge, J. M. (2000). The age of anxiety? The birth cohort change in anxiety and neuroticism, 1952-1993. *Journal of Personality and Social Psychology, 79*, 1007–1021.

Twenge, J. M. (2011). Generational differences in mental health: Are children and adolescents suffering more, or less? *American Journal of Orthopsychiatry, 81*(4), 469–472. doi:10.1111/j.1939-0025.2011.01115.x.

U.S. Department of Education, Office of Planning, Evaluation and Policy Development, Policy and Program Studies Services. (2011). *Prevalence and implementation fidelity of research-based prevention programs in public schools: Final report*. Washington, DC. Retrieved from http://www2.ed.gov/about/offices/list/opepd/index.html?src=oc

Valiente, C., Lemery-Chalfant, K., Swanson, J., & Reiser, M. (2008). Prediction of children's academic competence from their effortful control, relationships, and classroom participation. *Journal of Educational Psychology, 100*(1), 67–77. doi:10.1037/0022-0663.100.1.67.

van der Oord, S., Bögels, S. M., & Peijnenburg, D. (2012). The effectiveness of mindfulness training for children with ADHD and mindful parenting for their parents. *Journal of Child and Family Studies, 21*(1), 139–147. doi:10.1007/s10826-011-9457-0.

Waters, S. F., & Thompson, R. A. (2014). Children's perceptions of the effectiveness of strategies for regulating anger and sadness. *International Journal of Behavioral Development, 38*(2), 174–181.

White, L. (2012). Reducing stress in school-age girls through mindful yoga. *Journal of Pediatric Health Care, 26*(1), 45–56. doi:10.1016/j.pedhc.2011.01.002.

Whitted, K. S. (2010). Understanding how social and emotional skill deficits contribute to school failure. *Preventing School Failure, 55*, 10–16.

Wills, T. A., Pokhrel, P., Morehouse, E., & Fenster, B. (2011). Behavioral and emotional regulation and adolescent substance use problems: A test of moderation effects in a dual-process model. *Psychology of Addictive Behaviors, 25*(2), 279–292. doi:10.1037/a002287.

Wills, T. A., Sandy, J. M., Yaeger, A. M., Cleary, S. D., & Shinar, O. (2001). Coping dimensions, life stress, and adolescent substance use: A latent growth analysis. *Journal of Abnormal Psychology, 110*, 309–323.

Wills, T. A., Sandy, J. M., & Yaeger, A. M. (2002). Moderators of the relation between substance use level and problems: Test of a self-regulation model in middle adolescence. *Journal of Abnormal Psychology, 111*, 3–21.

Wisner, B. L., Jones, B., & Gwin, D. (2010). School-based meditation practices for adolescents: A resource for strengthening self-regulation, emotional coping, and self-esteem. *Children & Schools, 32*, 150–159.

Zelazo, P., & Lyons, K. E. (2012). The potential benefits of mindfulness training in early childhood: A developmental social cognitive neuroscience perspective. *Child Development Perspectives, 6*(2), 154–160. doi:10.1111/j.1750-8606.2012.00241.x.

Working on the Inside: Mindfulness for Adolescents

22

Patricia C. Broderick and Stacie M. Metz

In our twenty-first century world, the pace of change has gathered steam, and the requirements for student success have become increasingly demanding and complex (Collaborative for Academic, Social, and Emotional Learning [CASEL], 2008; Garner & Shonkoff, 2012). The knowledge explosion of the previous century, rapid technological innovations, and social forces such as globalization have created unprecedented challenges for educators not only in equipping students with the knowledge and skills they need to succeed but also in selecting the content and skills to be learned (Harsh & Mallory, 2013; McCarthy, Giardina, Harewood, & Jin-Kyung, 2003). Educators face the daunting task of leaving no child behind in a race to the top. Amidst this information overload and the stress it engenders, we can lose sight of the fact that certain social and emotional skills and dispositions are essential for the kinds of flexible decision-making, stress-hardiness, life-long learning, and innovation that will certainly be required if we wish to maintain prosperity and civility in a rapidly changing world (CASEL, 2008).

Social and emotional skills provide the foundation for learning how to manage life effectively, from learning to channel attention and sustain motivation when work becomes demanding, to working well with others, to coping with inevitable frustrations, to avoiding behaviors that put health at risk (Roeser, Vanderwolf, & Strobel, 2001). Decades of research have consistently shown that well-designed and implemented classroom-based prevention programs can reduce conduct problems while building skills for mental health, interpersonal relationships, and academic achievement (Durlak et al., 2007; Greenberg et al., 2003; Payton et al., 2008). This is especially important during adolescence given it is a stress-sensitive period of development. As we discuss below, emotional distress appears to be heightened by virtue of the developmental stage of adolescence regardless of preexisting vulnerabilities. Thus, we need to prioritize the teaching of effective emotion regulation (distress tolerance) skills to all adolescents, not just to those at increased risk of problems, as part of comprehensive social-emotional learning (SEL) programming. Mindfulness may be uniquely suited to this task (e.g., Broderick & Metz, 2009; Roeser & Peck, 2009). In the following sections, we review certain strengths and vulnerabilities of

P.C. Broderick (✉)
Bennett Pierce Prevention Research Center, The Pennsylvania State University, University Park, PA, USA
e-mail: pcb13@psu.edu

S.M. Metz
West Chester University of PA, West Chester, PA, USA
e-mail: SMetz@wcupa.edu

K.A. Schonert-Reichl, R.W. Roeser (eds.), *Handbook of Mindfulness in Education*, Mindfulness in Behavioral Health, DOI 10.1007/978-1-4939-3506-2_22

the adolescent period and address how teaching mindfulness to youth can support resilience during this time of life.

Adolescent Strengths and Vulnerabilities

Adolescence is associated with major cognitive advances and gains in physical strength and vitality (Steinberg, 2008, 2014). However, this period is also notable for the onset of many physical and mental health problems that are *preventable* and that persist into adulthood, interfering with educational achievement and work productivity in long-lasting ways (Costello, Foley, & Angold, 2006; Spear, 2000). A recent Centers for Disease Control and Prevention (CDC) report (2010) confirms that behaviors which pose a physical and mental health risk across the life span often have their beginnings in childhood and adolescence and should be addressed by means of school health and other programmatic interventions to potentially reverse this trend. Demands for interpersonal, stress management, and problem-solving skills increase as students progress through the school years (Resnick et al., 1997). Yet, while there are many evidenced-based programs for younger children (e.g. PATHS; Greenberg, Kusche, Cook, & Quamma, 1995), far fewer well-established evidence-based programs exist for adolescents. Moreover, the tightly compacted schedule of academic courses found in most traditional comprehensive high schools often makes school-based SEL programs challenging to accommodate. This state of affairs represents a significant educational gap when we consider the importance of social-emotional skills to health and productivity. Mindfulness appears to strengthen foundational skills in self-awareness and self-regulation and supports the cognitive skills needed for learning. These are skills for *all* adolescents, given the opportunities and challenges of their stage of development. Because schools are the places where adolescents spend much of their time, school-based interventions may offer the best hope of a positive universal initiative.

Clearly, the dimensions of need are great, and evidence from large-scale epidemiological studies suggests the global scope of this problem (Patel, Flisher, Hetrick, & McGorry, 2007). Conduct problems have increased significantly over successive cohorts in the UK since 1958 (Collishaw, Maughan, Goodman, & Pickles, 2004). In Australia, affect-related disorders, including substance abuse disorders, contribute 60–70 % of the disease burden in young people (Public Health Group, 2005). The US Surgeon General's report (2000) concludes that one out of five children and adolescents in the USA suffers from significant social, emotional, and behavioral problems that place them at risk for school failure. A 1993 report by the American Academy of Pediatrics (AAP) that contained a list of threats to adolescent well-being was updated in 2001 to include the following items: school problems (including learning disabilities and attention difficulties); mood and anxiety disorders; adolescent suicide and homicide; firearms in the home; school violence; drug and alcohol abuse; HIV/AIDS; and the effects of media on violence, obesity, and sexual activity (AAP, 2001). These were called the "new morbidities." As Dahl (2004) observes, most of these threats derive from emotional and behavioral dysregulation.

A Perfect Storm

Adolescence is known to be a stressful period. Adolescents report high levels of school-related stress associated with homework, tests, expectations for achievement, and interactions with teachers (Jacobshagen, Rigotti, Semmer, & Mohr, 2009; Ystgaard, 1997). The time pressures that challenge so many adults also affect the younger generation. Melman, Little, and Akin-Little (2007) reported a linear relationship between number of regularly scheduled activities in which adolescents were involved and their self-reported levels of anxiety. Frustration with impersonal schooling in the context of minimal support can lead to dropping out in large numbers, especially for minority youth (Bridgeland, DiIulio, & Morison, 2006). Although increasing needs for autonomy are normative and energizing, concerns about the future can translate into additional pressure (Luthar & Sexton, 2004).

Overall, these challenges require emotion regulation skills to be met successfully.

What is it about the adolescent period that makes it both a time of developmental opportunity and risk? Contemporary adolescents face a host of developmental challenges that can threaten their physical and emotional well-being, including increasing psychological, emotional, and behavioral autonomy from parents (Darling, Cumsille, & Martinez, 2008), a stage-environment mismatch between adolescents and their schools (Eccles et al., 1993) that is linked to a decline in academic orientation and disengagement from schools starting in the early adolescent years (Archambault, Janosz, Morizot, & Pagani, 2009; Gutman, Sameroff, & Cole, 2003), and self-consciousness about bodily changes (Rodriguez-Tome et al., 1993), increasing susceptibility to peer influence (Sim & Koh, 2003), and pressures of romantic relationships (Collins, 2003) associated with the onset of puberty. In addition, adolescent development may also be affected by youth participation in antisocial or risky behaviors (Reyna & Farley, 2006) or heavy exposure to media which may supersede behavioral expectations of the family and community (Comstock & Scharrer, 2006; Kaiser Family Foundation, 2010). The provision of supportive learning environments wherein competence and autonomy are enhanced can reverse threats to physical and mental well-being (see Eccles & Roeser, 2011). Mindfulness, concentration, and stress-reduction tools can be important components to positive youth development.

Neurobiological Changes of Adolescence

In addition to these developmental challenges, evidence is mounting that adolescence is a *sensitive period for stress* because of puberty-related changes in hormones and dramatic plasticity in the structure and function of the brain (Blakemore & Frith, 2005; Huttenlocher, 1979; Romeo, 2010). Appropriate environmental stimulation during a sensitive period is critical to normal brain development, and its absence during a particularly vulnerable period can produce enduring modifications (Hubel & Wiesel, 1962). Although conditions for optimal brain development at adolescence are still unclear, evidence is beginning to demonstrate that adolescence is a period of particular vulnerability to social and emotional input from the environment based on studies of emotional information processing, emotion and behavior regulation, and stress reactivity.

Adolescents process emotional information in ways that are different from prepubertal children and adults. Mid to late pubertal adolescents show greater pupil dilation to emotion-related words, rate themselves as higher in negative affect, and tend to remember more emotion-related words in delayed recall tasks than younger children, suggesting increased limbic reactivity at puberty (Silk et al., 2009). While adults show increased amygdala responses only to images of fearful faces, adolescents show greater amygdala activation to both fearful and neutral faces (Thomas et al., 2001). Findings for adolescents of exaggerated startle reflex (a measure of fear processing) (Quevedo, Benning, Gunnar, & Dahl, 2009) and stronger interference effects from emotional stimuli on task completion (Hare et al., 2008) lend further support to the proposition that the adolescent brain is particularly reactive to emotional information (Blakemore, 2008; Casey, Jones, & Hare, 2008).

Changes in the brain over the course of adolescence occur primarily in the frontal and parietal cortices, which are the site of executive functions, a general term used to describe higher-order cognitive and socioemotional processes. At puberty, a period of synaptogenesis in these regions accounts for a peak in gray matter volume that is followed by a gradual decline as the cortex is fine-tuned (Giedd et al., 1999). Synaptic pruning largely occurs in areas which play a role in judgment, impulse control, planning, and emotion regulation (Casey, Giedd, & Thomas, 2000). Some social and cognitive functions show a temporary decline in early puberty as this synaptic reorganization process begins (Chodhury, 2010; Huttenlocher, 1979). Myelination of the frontal cortex, which allows for smooth and efficient operations, proceeds continuously over the course of adolescence but is not complete until early adulthood. This neural rewiring project follows a dyssynchronous developmental trajectory. For example, brain circuits that are involved in reward-seeking (e.g., nucleus accumbens) mature earlier than circuits that monitor and assess consequences of risk-taking (e.g., prefrontal cortex) (Casey, Getz, & Galvan, 2008; Fuster, 2002). Thus, it is hypothesized that adolescents' appetitive pull toward risky behavior is not sufficiently kept in check by a well-functioning internal monitor, a situation described by Dahl as "turbo-charging the engines of a fully mature car belonging to an unskilled driver" (2004, p. 18). Strengthening the executive capacities of the developing brain could go a long way towards risk reduction in adolescence.

Effects of Stress in Adolescence

In the context of such rapid neurobiological changes, the adolescent period may be uniquely sensitive to the effects of stress, although the precise mechanisms for this phenomenon are still unclear (Eiland & Romeo, 2013; Romeo, 2010). In general, the perception of threat or stress (i.e., feeling stressed-out) is accompanied by a cascade of endocrinological events, primarily the release of catecholamine and glucocorticoid hormones. Although the human stress response is adaptive in short bursts and helps mobilize energy reserves for goal-directed purposes, stress can negatively affect health, learning, and productivity when it is prolonged or when the stress response is dysregulated (McEwen, 2003). Attention and learning capacities as well as cardiovascular, gastrointestinal, immune, reproductive, and other bodily systems are negatively impacted by chronic stress (Romero & Butler, 2007). Cortisol, one of the glucocorticoid hormones, is released from the adrenal cortex as an end result of hypothalamic–pituitary–adrenocortical (HPA) axis activation and has been implicated in much of the aforementioned impacts. Glucocorticoids increase levels of glucose in the blood, alter immunity, and contribute to many chronic physical and mental illnesses (Miller & Blackwell, 2006). Executive functions, such as the ability to direct attention and solve problems efficiently, show clear stress-induced disruptions, particularly when control over stressors is perceived to be lacking (Arnsten & Shansky, 2004). In the case of learning, mild stress can enhance memory, but chronic or excessive stress can result in damage to parts of the brain critical for new learning and memory consolidation to the point of killing hippocampal neurons (Sapolsky, 1999) and suppressing neurogenesis (Andersen & Teicher, 2008). Glucocorticoids also bind to stretches of DNA and act as gene transcription factors serving important functions of gene activation and suppression (Romero & Butler, 2007).

Given the potentially dire consequences of a chronically activated stress system, it is critically important to consider the effects of stress on adolescents' developing brains when such consequences can extend over a lifetime. Accumulating evidence from animal and some human studies that measure changes in stress-related hormones and autonomic functions at puberty supports the argument that adolescence is a stress-sensitive period. Basal cortisol levels in humans and animals have been found to rise over the transition to adolescence (Stroud et al., 2009). Animal studies confirm periods (infancy, childhood) of hyporesponsivity to stress hormones, presumably as protection for the developing brain, which are dramatically reversed at puberty when the brain becomes more sensitized to the effects of gonadal and stress-related hormones (Lee, Brandy, & Koenig, 2003; McEwen, 2005). Hormones are instrumental in laying down new neural pathways at adolescence, so overexpression of and increased sensitivity to cortisol during this period of rapid brain reorganization may signal a window of vulnerability for development of psychopathology (Spear, 2009).

Several recent human experimental studies have demonstrated that normally developing adolescents, compared to younger and older groups, display heightened stress reactivity on cortisol and other autonomic nervous system (ANS) measures during challenging situations. Stroud et al. (2009) assessed HPA axis and cardiac functions in a group of children (7–12) and adolescents (13–17) randomly exposed to two psychological stressors. Performance stress was assessed by requiring participants to make a 5-min speech, answer mental arithmetic questions, and copy a picture from its mirror image in front of a small audience. Social stress was induced by means of a social rejection interaction involving confederates who gradually excluded the participant during conversation. Although no significant differences were noted between age groups in self-reported distress, adolescents showed consistently more pronounced physiological responsiveness on all stress-related measures. Cortisol levels were highest in response to the performance stressors.

Several recent studies have considered the physiological effects that mental anticipation of a stressor and memories about past stressors have on stress reactivity in normal adolescents. Sumter, Bokhorsta, Miersa, Van Pelt, and Westenberg (2010) investigated this question in a large sample of 9–17 year old boys and girls during the period prior to making a public presentation as well as during the actual task. Strongest cortisol rises were shown for adolescents during the anticipatory period, highlighting the potentially important role that perceptions of stress play in activating the stress response at adolescence (Folkman & Lazarus, 1988). A large prospective study of Dutch adolescents (Oldehinkel et al., 2010) also reported that level of perceived stress was positively associated with cardiac and cortisol measurements.

Adam (2006) investigated the normal fluctuations in emotional experience of adolescents' day-to-day lives using diary methods and cortisol sampling. Cortisol fluctuations covaried with momentary emotional states. When adolescents reported feeling angry or worried, their cortisol levels were significantly higher than what would normally be predicted for the individuals based on their typical daily patterns. The physiological impact is also substantial when stressors involve peer-rejection. Sebastian, Viding, Williams, and Blakemore (2009) asked young (11–13) and mid (14–15) adolescent female participants to play a 3-min computer game called "cyberball" which manipulated inclusion and ostracism conditions as a function of being "thrown' the ball or ignored by two other players. Compared to adult studies using this manipulation, adolescents reported greater negative mood in both age groups, and younger adolescents also showed significant increases in distress. Even a short experience of social stress showed marked effects on affect. Considering the convergences of these factors, the "intersection of stress and the developing adolescent brain may represent a 'perfect storm' in the context of dysfunctional emotional development" (Romeo, 2010, p. 249). Alternatively, consistent with practices in indigenous cultures around the world, adolescence also has been seen as a key time for mental training and the cultivation of virtue. We believe that mindfulness training might capitalize on biological opportunities in ways that Western culture more often than not fails to do today (Larson, 2000).

The Importance of Emotion Regulation

The strategies used to motivate behavior and manage distress in order to respond to different situations or to achieve certain goals, such as those involved in learning, may be broadly defined as emotion regulation (Campos, Frankel, & Camras, 2004). Emotion regulation processes can include identification and acceptance of emotional experiences, capacity to sustain wholesome emotional and motivational states, prioritization among competing goals, management of distress and modulation of excitement, and adaptive adjustment of behavioral responses. Emotion regulation, as a overarching construct for these various processes, is viewed by contemporary researchers as a foundation for well-being, academic achievement, and positive adjustment throughout the life span (Eisenberg, Spinrad, & Eggum, 2010). Adolescents who possess more flexible regulatory skills are more resilient and less susceptible to emotional and behavioral disorders (Gross, 1998). Difficulties in emotion regulation represent a core feature of many adolescent-onset emotional and behavioral problems including depression, anxiety, conduct problems, deliberate self-injury, disordered eating, substance use, and abuse (Beato-Fernández,

Rodríguez-Cano, Pelayo-Delgado, & Calaf, 2007; Cisler, Olatunji, Felder, & Forsyth, 2010; Gross & Munoz, 1995; Laye-Gindhu & Schonert-Reichl, 2005).

Of great significance to educators is the fact that heightened emotional distress is predictive of behavior problems and academic failure (Needham, Crosnoe, & Muller, 2004). MacPherson et al. (2010) reported a link between distress tolerance and risky behavior in a large prospective study of adolescents. Adolescents with low distress tolerance were significantly more likely to have engaged in harmful risk-taking behavior than those with greater capacity for distress tolerance despite similar risk-taking propensity. Young adolescents' levels of school-related distress predicted their academic performance (Gumora & Arsenio, 2002), and levels of school-related strain mediated psychosomatic symptoms in a large group of Swiss secondary students (Jacobshagen et al., 2009). Roeser et al. (2009) suggested that emotional distress disrupts the learning process via several mechanisms including the reduction of self-regulatory efficacy and academic motivation and the amplification of experiential avoidance.

One of the tenets of SEL is that many problem behaviors have the same root causes (Weissberg & O'Brien, 2004). Negative emotionality, or emotional distress, has been identified as a causal risk factor for emotional, behavioral, and academic problems and not just the consequence (Daughters et al., 2009). The inability to manage distress (distress intolerance) leads to diminished goal-directed efforts and dysfunctional coping strategies that can ultimately reinforce avoidance by maladaptive means (Hayes, Wilson, Gifford, Follette, & Strosahl, 1996).

The Contribution of Mindfulness for Training Attention and Emotion Regulation

"Mindfulness" is a term used to describe a certain kind of attention that is characterized by several attributes: intentionality, present moment focus, and non-evaluative, compassionate observation of experience (Kabat-Zinn, 1994). Mindfulness can also refer to the act of paying attention in this way (e.g., being mindful). All of these attributes can be practiced by intentionally directing and maintaining attention on narrow (such as breath) or broad (such as a range of sensory phenomena) targets as is done in meditation or mindful awareness practice. Attention is purposefully and voluntarily directed to phenomena as they occur in the present moment and is marked by curiosity and openness to the nature of the experience as well as the quality of the attention itself. Nonjudgment refers to the dual capacity to notice that one's attention is captured by cognitive and emotional triggers related to experience and to counter this automatic tendency by intentionally exploring the experience without preconceptions or reflexive self-judgment. Practicing mindfulness does not imply entering a "zone" or some dreamlike, relaxed mental state, nor is it related to any specific mental content. Rather, mindfulness is full and engaged attention to whatever is occurring and is related to executive processes crucial to learning and self-regulation (Flook et al., 2010).

Over time, behaviors can become automatic and operate outside of conscious awareness in response to particular triggers (Berkowitz, 2008). Maladaptive behaviors (e.g., aggression, procrastination) may thus become impulsive automatic responses to emotional distress (e.g., anger, anxiety) or perceptions of unpleasantness (e.g., boredom). Practice of an attentive and non-reactive attitude toward impulses may "increase the gap between impulse and action" (Ekman, as cited in Boyce, 2005, p. 40). It is precisely to these automatic processes, often referred to as "automatic pilot," that mindful attention is directed. Mindfulness practice may allow elements of conscious and less conscious experience to be perceived from a de-centered, de-contextualized, and more accepting stance. This approach disrupts reactivity, strengthens attention and openness, and brings problem-solving behavior under more conscious and reflective regulation (Zelazo & Cunningham, 2007).

Research on the effects of mindfulness training with adults has shown an array of benefits. These include enhanced interoceptive awareness (Lazar et al., 2005), and improved attention (Jha, Kropinger, & Baime, 2007; Jha, Stanley, Kiyonaga, Wong, & Gelfand, 2010) especially in advanced meditators (van den Hurk, Giommi, Gielen, Speckens, & Barendregt, 2010) but also after a brief period of meditation training (Tang et al., 2009; Zeidan, Johnson, Diamond, David, & Goolkasian, 2010). Benefits also include increases in positive mood and immune system functioning (Davidson et al., 2003), reductions in depressive relapse (Ma & Teasdale, 2004), enhanced empathy (Shapiro & Brown, 2007), reductions in substance abuse (Ostafin & Marlatt, 2008), and reduced stress (Chiesa & Serreti, 2009). Mindfulness meditation practice has been effective in reducing chronic pain (Grossman, Tiefenthaler-Gilmer, Raysz, & Kesper, 2007), aiding weight loss (Tapper et al., 2008), increasing telomerase activity (Jacobs et al., 2010), and protecting against age-related loss of gray matter (Pagnoni & Cekic, 2007).

Although research with children and youth is more limited, studies have documented improvements in attention skills (Napoli, Krech, & Holley, 2005; Zylowska et al., 2008), sleep quality (Bootzin & Stevens, 2005; Britton, Haynes, Fridel, & Bootzin, 2010), well-being in adolescent boys (Huppert & Johnson, 2010), reduced depressive symptoms (Kuyken et al., 2013; Raes, Griffith, van der Geuth, & Williams, 2014), improved executive functions, well-being and prosociality (Schonert-Reichl, Oberle, Lawlor, Abbott, & Thomson, 2015), and reductions in symptoms in clinic-referred adolescents (Biegel, Brown, Shapiro, & Schubert, 2009; Bogels, Hoogstad, vanDun, deSchutter, & Restifo, 2008; Semple, Lee, Rosa, & Miller, 2010). A recent meta-analysis (Zoogman, Goldberg, Hoyt, & Miller, 2015) reported small to moderate effects of mindfulness compared to active controls in nonclinical samples but larger effects for clinical groups. Presently, there is a need for more research on mindfulness interventions using rigorous experimental designs to assess effects of these approaches among diverse groups across multiple settings. More research is also needed to explore the integration of mindfulness into ongoing school curricula as universal prevention. Learning to BREATHE is a mindfulness-based classroom program that was developed for this purpose.

Learning to BREATHE: A Universal Prevention Program

Learning to BREATHE (L2B; Broderick, 2013) is a developmentally appropriate universal prevention program that can be integrated into secondary education settings. The program is designed to increase emotion regulation, stress management, compassion and executive functions in order to promote well-being and support learning. L2B uses themes from Mindfulness-Based Stress Reduction (MBSR) developed by Kabat-Zinn (1990) and incorporates them into a program that is shorter, more accessible to students, and compatible with school curricula. The program includes instruction in the practice of mindful awareness and self/other compassion and provides opportunities to practice these skills in a group setting. L2B objectives are explicitly linked to standards for health, counseling, and other professional areas so that the L2B program may be incorporated into existing curricula and assessment plans.

The themes that form the core of the curriculum may be adapted for various student groups, including those in clinical settings, and may be presented in 6, 12, or 18 sessions within a health, school counseling, or other curriculum. Each lesson includes a short introduction to the theme, several activities for group participation and discussion to engage students in the lesson, and an opportunity for in-class mindfulness practice. Mindfulness practice, as used here, refers to the practice of training the mind to pay attention in a particular way: on purpose, in the present moment, and with openness (Kabat-Zinn, 1994). Several short mindfulness practices are taught as part of the program, including body scan, awareness of thoughts, awareness of feelings, and loving-kindness and gratitude practices. Loving-kindness practice is a technique that supports self-compassion and compassion for others (see Fredrickson, Cohn, Coffey, Pek, & Finkel, 2008). Workbooks and audio files for home mindfulness practice are provided to students as part of this program.

Six major themes are built around the BREATHE acronym: B (Body) body awareness; R (Reflections) understanding and working with thoughts; E (Emotions) understanding and working with feelings; A (Attention) integrating awareness of thoughts, feelings, and bodily sensations; T ("Tenderness/Take it as it is") reducing harmful self-judgments and increasing acceptance of self and others; and H (Healthy habits of mind) cultivating positive emotions and integrating mindfulness into daily life. The overall goal of the program is to cultivate emotional balance and inner empowerment (E) through the practice of mindfulness, an advantage referred to as gaining the "inner edge." This curriculum has versions for younger and older adolescents. Classroom adaptations may be made to meet the needs of groups, and other informal mindfulness practice is encouraged between sessions.

Clearly, attempts to bring mindful awareness practices into educational settings must take into consideration the needs of the entire system: administration, teachers, staff, etc. Therefore, it is very important for teachers and administrators to understand the nature and benefits of mindfulness practice themselves in order to support students and model mindfulness for them. The practice of mindful awareness offers a way to perceive every experience and task of the day with full attention, interest, and compassion. Mindfulness is not something that can be learned like a list of facts from a teacher, book, or curriculum manual. To be authentic and useful, mindfulness practice must be tried, experienced, applied, and incorporated into one's day-to-day life. Thus, every moment of every day in the classroom is an opportunity to practice being mindful. Learning to BREATHE is best conceptualized as one contribution to a coordinated mindful SEL program.

Theory of Change and Developmental Assumptions

The L2B program assumes that the practice of mindful awareness will impact student academic and behavioral outcomes by reducing stress and increasing distress tolerance, strengthening executive functions, increasing emotional balance and behavioral regulation, cultivating acceptance of self and others, and ultimately supporting academic goals (Blair & Diamond, 2008). For the purposes of this model, stress is defined as the experience of conscious or nonconscious emotions and patterns of reactivity (e.g., anxiety, boredom, irritation, impulsivity) that cause regulatory processes to break down and impede goal-directed behavior. Figure 22.1 illustrates a model in which typical reactions to stress (distress) trigger pathways to emotional regulation or chronic dysregulation.

First, the perception of distress can be triggered by internal or external conditions or some combination of the two. Poor stress management (emotion and behavioral dysregulation) can interfere with accomplishments in important areas of adolescent functioning. Second, maladaptive response patterns generally take the form of avoidance of or over-engagement with the distressing object or condition in an effort to reduce distress. For example, adolescents may seek to "numb" feelings of social rejection by disengaging from school or, more seriously, by drinking, taking drugs, or cutting. Distress is temporarily blunted, relief is provided in the short-term, and the maladaptive behavior acquires reinforcing properties that strengthen dysfunctional patterns.

Not only do the maladaptive behaviors provide transient relief (positive reinforcement), but they also serve to permit escape from emotional pain (negative reinforcement). Alternatively, adolescents might become preoccupied with their distress in ways that strengthen the associations between automatic thoughts and negative affect. An example of this pattern is obsessive worry or rumination, which is constant reexamination or reexperiencing of distressing conditions or events in a misguided effort to resolve problems and regulate emotions.

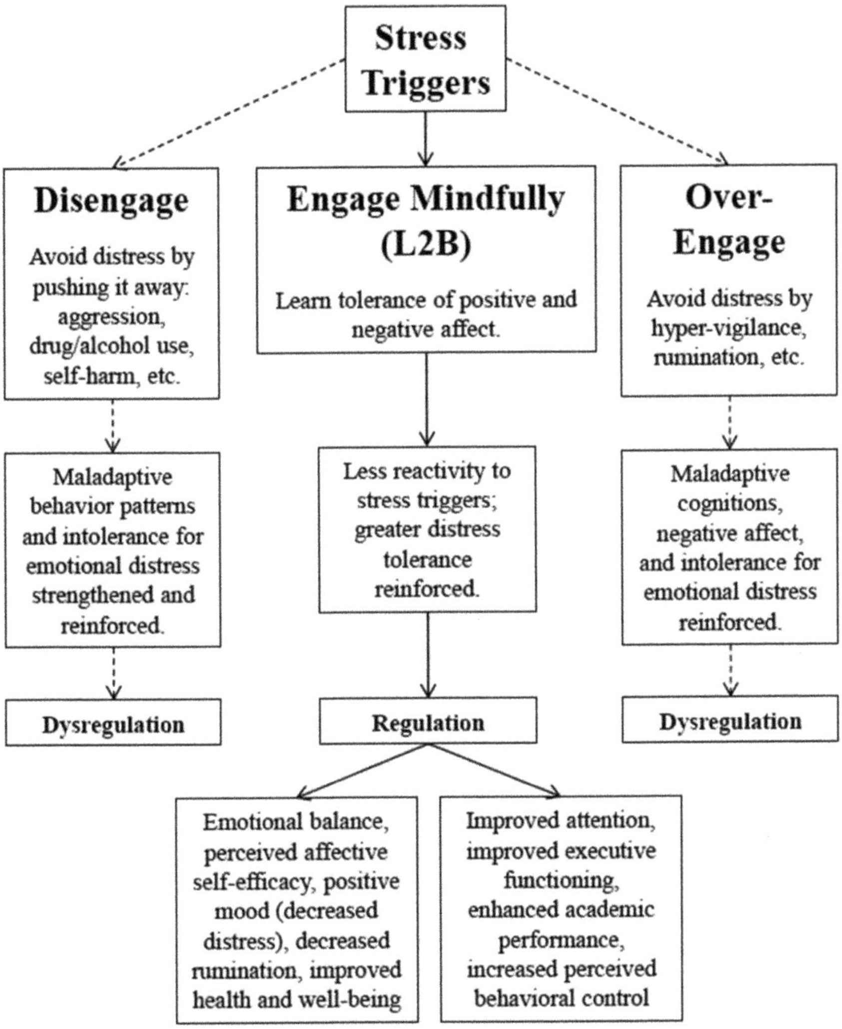

Fig. 22.1 Conceptual model of L2B

Rumination heightens attention to distress cues, amplifies rather than attenuates distress, and reduces the capacity of working memory to effectively engage in learning (Lyubomirsky & Tkach, 2004).

The practice of mindfulness may increase meta-cognitive awareness of mental processes that contribute to emotion dysregulation and offers a means of restoring balance when strong emotions arise. Emotions are not static. Therefore, to train in the skills of emotion awareness, identification, and management, it is useful to practice noticing emotions "on the spot." This practice offers the opportunity to develop resilience in the face of uncomfortable feelings that otherwise might provoke a harmful behavioral response. Mindfulness practice also strengthens attention by voluntarily and repeatedly orienting attention to a specific object of focus while letting go of distractions. Mindfulness practice includes establishing an intention to "pay attention" in a certain way, thus strengthening the executive skill of keeping a plan in mind while inhibiting distractions and shifting attention from irrelevant to relevant stimuli. Through mindfulness practice, automatic, non-reflective processes may come under more conscious control, fostering reflective decision-making and reducing impulsive reactions. The practice of orienting to experience with curiosity, patience, and nonjudgment strengthens tolerance for distress and may reduce the threat appraisal that the adolescent brain is prone to make, providing a potential protective factor against stressors that abound in the environment. The practice of tolerating experience as it arises without engaging in automatic, possibly impulsive, reactions may strengthen resilience and support a sense of affective regulatory self-efficacy, control and self-compassion. Perception of control is an important criterion of effective stress management (Sapolsky, 2004), and learning skills to deal with feelings constructively could strengthen perceptions of personal efficacy.

Certain assumptions about adolescent development provide a framework for this approach to introducing mindfulness to adolescents (Broderick & Blewitt, 2014). Adolescents are involved at a deep psychological level with constructing an identity and developing autonomy from adults, a task that can become overwhelming and confusing. Although adolescents' ability to understand and manage emotions can advance, training in this area has often been neglected in school settings. The school-based format of Learning to BREATHE provides support for the exploration of mindfulness-based emotion regulation strategies and invites students to consider the usefulness of these strategies for their lives. The discussion and practice included in L2B complement adolescents' increased capacity for introspection while maintaining sensitivity to adolescents' internal pressure for social conformity and tendency to social comparison. Non-intrusive discussion of general stressors facilitates self-discovery in the peer context and reduces isolation. Information about how the mind works, i.e., the common tendency to be distracted or to hold onto thoughts that may not be helpful, can bolster the individual adolescent's realization that she or he is not alone. Finally, the active participation of students in practice, in-class, and at home supports integration of program content.

Research on Learning to BREATHE

A pilot study of the L2B program was conducted in a private high school for girls in suburban Pennsylvania (Broderick & Metz, 2009). All seniors ($n = 120$) participated in the six-session program as part of their health curriculum. Program sessions were delivered one to two times per week during seniors' health classes over a period of approximately 5 weeks. Class sessions ranged from 32 to 43 min each. A small group of juniors served as the control ($n = 33$).

No demographic characteristics or pretest subscale scores, except age, were significantly different between the program participants completing both assessments ($n = 105$) and controls ($n = 17$). Mean gain scores (posttest–pretest scores) were compared between groups to assess program effectiveness. In comparison to the control group, the program participants demonstrated a significant reduction in negative affect, mean gain score −2.51 vs. 1.63, $t(120) = 2.34$, $p < .05$, and a significant increase in feeling calm/relaxed/self-accepting, mean gain score of .90 vs. −.65, $t(120) = -2.06$, $p < .05$. No other mean gain scores demonstrated significant differences between the program and control groups.

Due to the very small sample size of the control group, there was low power to detect significant differences between program and control groups, if they existed. As a result, paired t-tests were computed within the mindfulness program group to examine differences from pretest to posttest across the multiple measures. Program participants, on the Positive and Negative Affect Scale (PANAS; Watson, Clark, & Tellegen, 1988) displayed a statistical reduction from pretest to posttest in negative affect, $t(103) = 3.89$, $p < .01$, and a significant increase in feeling calm/relaxed/self-accepting $t(103) = -3.21$, $p < .01$. They also demonstrated a significant decline from pretest to posttest in the total score on the Difficulties in Emotion Regulation Scale (DERS; Gratz & Roemer, 2004), $t(103) = 2.77$, $p < .01$, lack of emotional awareness (DERS subscale), $t(103) = 3.12$, $p < .01$, and lack of emotional clarity (DERS subscale), $t(103) = 2.16$, $p < .05$. No significant changes from pretest to posttest ($p > .05$) were found within the Ruminative Response Scale (RRS; Nolen-Hoeksema & Morrow, 1991); whereas in the Somatization Index of the Child Behavior Checklist (SICBC; Achenbach, 1991), program participants demonstrated a significant reduction from pretest to posttest in feeling overtired, $t(104) = 2.95$, $p < .01$, and complaints of aches/pains (not headaches or stomach aches), $t(104) = 1.99$, $p < .05$.

The process evaluation revealed that 87 % of program participants were satisfied or very satisfied with the L2B program, with 65 % of participants practicing mindfulness techniques outside of class during the length of the program. Specifically, the in-class program activities rated most useful included in-class meditation practice, body scan meditation, and a music and emotions activity; the activity rated the least useful was in-class discussion. Approximately half of all participants reported that the most important skill they learned from the program was how to better deal with stressful thoughts and feelings.

Examples of free responses to the question, "What did you learn from the program?" include the following representative statements from students:

> I learned to relax myself at a very stressful moment so that I don't feel sick.

> I can now pay attention to something or someone for a longer period of time.

> I have learned that, although a problem may seem huge at first, it is actually the size of a grain of sand in relation to the universe. Also I should treat myself kindly and respect my body.

> I've learned that I can have space in my mind.

An unpublished pilot study by L. Pinger and L. Flook was implemented in two fifth grade classes in public schools in Madison, WI. Improvements in social competence for students receiving L2B were noted on teacher reports once the program was completed. Performance for L2B students on a computerized task of spatial working memory showed statistically significant improvements in strategy use and reductions in error rate. The L2B students also demonstrated less depressed and anxious symptoms and a greater internal locus of control after program completion. Fifth grade teachers reported that the students learned to pause, if only briefly, and "acknowledge their thoughts and feelings, something that set L2B apart from most social skills programs" (http://www.investigatinghealthyminds.org/cihmProjEducation.html).

In addition to the pilot trials reported above, L2B has been implemented in other sites (including public high schools, alternative high schools, residential treatment programs, residential private schools, and after school-programs) although research data are not available or incomplete for many settings at the time of this writing. A L2B implementation at a public high school was recently evaluated (Metz et al., 2013). The evaluation used a pretest-posttest comparison group design which included 216 traditional education students currently enrolled in a concert choir course elective in either the L2B treatment or the instruction-as-usual comparison high school. The 18 program sessions were delivered on average once per week during the first 15 to 25 min of the concert choir class sessions. The students participating in the L2B program reported significantly lower levels of *perceived stress*, $F(1, 211) = 8.075$, $p < .01$, *psychosomatic complaints*, $F(1, 211) = 4.131$, $p < .05$, and higher levels of *efficacy in affective regulation*, $F(1, 211) = 19.682$, $p < .01$. Students in the treatment condition also evidenced significant larger gains in several emotion regulation skills including *emotional awareness*, $F(1, 211) = 5.900$, $p < .05$; *access to regulation strategies*, $F(1, 211) = 4.1418$, $p < .05$; *emotional clarity*, $F(1, 211) = 3.924$, $p < .05$; and *overall emotion regulation*, $F(1, 211) = 5.441$, $p < .05$. Overall, participants found program content and activities to be highly acceptable and socially valid via the process evaluation.

All of these implementations of the L2B program were preceded by initial training from the program developer (PB) coupled with weekly or bi-weekly phone supervision. Accommodations were made for each setting and students' needs. In addition, regular classroom teachers had the opportunity to participate in mindfulness classes prior to and during the implementations in several settings. Feedback from these early implementations led to program refinements that reflect effective practice for youth of all genders in a range of settings. Overall, qualitative interview data suggest students understood the concepts taught in the lessons and valued the practical skills that they received through participation. In particular, students repeatedly mentioned feeling more aware of their emotions—more empowered and in-control because they had practiced self-regulation skills in the sessions. These benefits directly impacted their response to classroom learning and relationships with teachers.

Bluth et al. (2015) studied the effects of L2B in an alternative school that served students who had struggled in traditional public high school settings. A group of 27 ethnically diverse (54 % Hispanic, 24 % African-American, 18 % Caucasian, 3 % other) students who were primarily from low income families were randomly assigned to either L2B or the school's standard substance abuse prevention class. Teachers made various accommodations in L2B over the course of the 11 weeks of classes (50 min each), including changing the location from the classroom to a more private space in the gym and beginning each class session with either body scan or restorative yoga. Since the L2B teachers were not part of the school faculty, they made special efforts to attend student functions in order to build trust. Analyses indicated that L2B was associated with greater improvements in depression and anxiety relative to the control class and small to medium effects on social connectedness, perceived stress, and mindfulness. Interestingly, adolescents' perceptions of the meaningfulness of the mindfulness class changed over the course of the program. While L2B participants initially perceived their class to be less relevant compared to participants in the substance abuse prevention class, this trend shifted as the class progressed. By the end of the 11 weeks, L2B participants rated the class more credible and relevant while these same variables decreased for substance abuse prevention students.

Mindfulness in Schools: Where to Start?

Introducing the inner work of mindfulness in any setting, but particularly in education, is a unique challenge. Unlike most current educational activities, whether they are being evaluated by researchers or not, mindfulness is a personal and highly experiential way of knowing that does not fit neatly into a conceptualization of learning with a set of "correct" answers. Simply adding one more program to an already full academic roster, especially if that program offers "more of the same" (i.e., more information about stress or wellness), may not necessarily add more value. Nor will it shift the dynamic from knowledge overload to deep, meaningful inquiry (see Zajonc, 2015). Mindfulness offers opportunities for silence and reflection in classrooms strained to their limits by the weight of curricular objectives, student needs, and limited time. In the process, it allows for the felt experience of deep connections with self and others, which can serve as the mental/emotional infrastructure for learning. Teacher and students alike must settle into present moment awareness and practice a specific skill set for paying attention. Openness, flexibility, and presence on the part of the teacher are important elements for facilitation.

How can this work be assessed in the service of building empirical support for contemplative educational practices? We offer some thoughts on how to marry mindfulness research in education with existing evaluation criteria, although this relationship is clearly in its infancy and will benefit greatly from future well-designed projects. We use the acronym S.C.H.O.O.L.S. to illustrate elements to consider in mindfulness-based educational research, using L2B and other programs as examples when appropriate. Given the limits of this chapter, we also restrict these comments to mindfulness-based programs despite the importance of studying creative and informal applications of mindfulness in the day-to-day life of the classroom. Our fundamental assumption is that teachers themselves are the best “lessons” in mindfulness for their students. Therefore, opportunities to introduce and to practice mindfulness with teachers are of the utmost importance. This topic is addressed elsewhere in this volume.

S: Settings

A mindfulness program for adolescents may be delivered within a school-based curriculum, an after-school program, a mental health outpatient/inpatient setting, or a residential setting. The setting of program delivery (universal, selective, indicated) often determines the level of impact (Gordon, 1987). Universal interventions, targeted at the general population, have widespread coverage and are most effective if administered in a school-based setting. Selective interventions target youth at risk of academic, social, or emotional problems while indicated interventions target youth who present early symptoms such as truancy, aggressive behavior, and depressed affect. Like universal interventions, these programs can be offered in the school as in special education or life skills classes although many are delivered in mental health outpatient settings (Biegel et al., 2009; Bogels et al., 2008; Tan & Martin, 2013). *Although L2B is intended to be universally administered, it could be used as a selective or indicated intervention.*

The maximum number of adolescents, including those who have not yet developed problems, may be reached via universal prevention, thereby reducing the stigma sometimes observed in selective/indicated interventions (Tomb & Hunter, 2004). Universal programming also increases the likelihood of sustainability and consistent positive outcomes over time (Hawkins, Kosterman, Catalano, Hill, & Abbott, 2005). Implementation setting and targeted level of intervention are important considerations for researchers and program users alike with regard to program selection and adaptations needed to ensure success.

C: Curriculum

Mindful teaching certainly *does not* require a curriculum and should be supported in all its authentic manifestations. However, if research is to be done to investigate the effectiveness of mindfulness with youth, researchers need to replicate findings in order to build an evidence base. This is possible when curricula are available. In selecting a mindfulness-based program that matches the needs and capacity of the setting and the students, several elements might be considered: the existing evidence base for the program, developmental appropriateness of the program, availability of a well-designed instructor’s manual, and instructor training. The instructor’s manual should at minimum provide the conceptual model for the program, session objectives, and thematic activities. Supplementary materials (e.g., workbooks) should be age-appropriate. The curriculum choice is also tied to the selection of instructors. It is our view that teaching mindfulness requires instructors to have a personal, experiential understanding of mindfulness. Mindfulness training for classroom teachers and professional staff that precedes or runs concurrently with the intervention is strongly recommended as a way of preparing teachers, of supporting the goals of the program, and of infusing mindfulness into the life of the school (see chapters by Jennings, Roeser 2015). If the program includes experiential activities such as yoga, a room with additional floor space or minimal outside distractions may be important. The length of the program and the time needed for each session as well as cost of materials and training should be considered for ease of incorporation into existing school structure. If researchers choose to develop a curriculum, care should be taken to ground it theoretically in strong knowledge of adolescent development, mindfulness practice, and effective pedagogy. A program logic model for stakeholders such as parents and school administrators illustrating the program inputs, activities, output, and outcomes could ease the transition of such programs into schools (see Table 22.2 for a basic outline).

Table 22.1 Recently published adolescent mindfulness program evaluations

Study	Level of prevention	Program content	*N*	Participants	Program location	Length and frequency	Research design	Quantitative outcome variables	Main results/effect size
Beets and Mitchell (2010)	Universal	Yoga intervention	55	Rural U.S. pacific NW public high school students	Mandatory ninth grade physical education class in public high school	Four or five 45-min group sessions over 2 wks	2×2 crossover design with baseline assessment (random assignment to sequences)	Perceived stress (PSS); depressive symptoms (CES-D); health-related quality of life (KINDL)	*Acute effects*: Decreased PSS; increased KINDL subscales of physical health, general feelings, and self-esteem (pooled ES across all outcomes was 0.39 for sequence 1 and 0.46 for sequence 2) *Carryover effects (baseline to after removal of treatment)*: Increased KINDL subscales of physical health and self-esteem
Broderick and Metz (2009)	Universal	Learning to BREATHE mindfulness curriculum, (Broderick, 2010)	150	Female students aged 16–19y from a suburban PA private Catholic high school –93 % White	Senior health class in school	Six 40-min group sessions staggered over 5 wks	Pretest-Posttest Comparison Group Design [Intervention: 120 from entire senior class; Control: 30 juniors from same high school]	Positive and Negative Affect Schedule (PANAS); Difficulties in Emotion Regulation Scale (DERS); Ruminative Response Scale (RRS); Somatization Index of the Child Behavior Checklist (SICBC)	As compared to controls, mindfulness group decreased PANAS negative affect (ES = 0.57) and increased calm/relaxed/self-accepting score (ES = 0.53)
Beauchemin et al. (2008)	Selective	Mindfulness Meditation (Kabat-Zinn, 1994)	34	Youth aged 13–18y with learning disabilities from a private residential VT school –71 % male	Classes in school	5–10 min at beginning of each class period 5 days/wk for 5 consecutive wks	One-group pretest-posttest design	Social Skills Rating System (SSRS); State-Trait Anxiety Inventory (STAI)	Decreased trait anxiety and state anxiety STAI scores; improved student-reported SSRS social skills and teacher-reported SSRS social skills, student problem behavior and student academic achievement

Study	Level of prevention	Program content	*N*	Participants	Program location	Length and frequency	Research design	Quantitative outcome variables	Main results/effect size
Biegel et al. (2009)	Indicated	Mindfulness-based stress reduction (MBSR) training (Kabat-Zinn, 1990)	102	Adolescents aged 14–18y from current/past outpatient child and adolescent psychiatry department in a U.S. NE Kaiser Permanente hospital	Outpatient mental health facility	Eight 2-h group sessions, one per week	Pretest-posttest wait-list control group design [Intervention: 50 analyzed for intent-to-treat sample and 34 for completer; Control: 52 analyzed for intent-to-treat sample and 40 for completer]	DSM-IV-TR diagnostic changes; Perceived Stress Scale (PSS-10); State/Trait Anxiety Inventory (STAI); Hopkins Symptom Checklist 90 (Revised) (SCL-90-R); Rosenberg Self-Esteem Scale (SES)	As compared to controls, MBSR participation reduced self-reported anxiety, depressive, and somatization symptoms, and improved self-esteem, sleep quality, and DSM-IV-TR diagnostics (for completer and intent-to-treat samples)
				–73.5 % female					
				–45 % White, 28 % Hispanic, 27 % other					
Bogels et al. (2008)	Indicated	Mindfulness-based cognitive therapy (MBCT) (Segal et al., 2002)	14	Adolescents from The Netherlands aged 11–18 who were referred to a community mental health center with a diagnosis of ADHD, ODD/CD, or ASD	Community mental health center	Eight 1.5-h group sessions, one per wk	One-group pretest-posttest design including a	Several self-report scales measuring personal goals, symptoms, quality of life, and mindful awareness	Improved at posttest and 8-wk follow-up assessment on self-reported personal goals; Youth Self-Report/Child Behavior Checklist total symptoms score and subscales of externalizing symptoms and social problems; self-control; attention, happiness; mindful awareness (ES ranged from 0.5 to 1.5)
				–57 % male			8-wk follow-up assessment		

(continued)

Table 22.1 (Continued)

Study	Level of prevention	Program content	*N*	Participants	Program location	Length and frequency	Research design	Quantitative outcome variables	Main results/effect size
Huppert and Johnson (2010)	Universal	Mindfulness training (Kabat-Zinn, 1990)	155	UK male students aged 14–15y in independent (fee) boys' school – 95 % White British	Religious education classes in school	Four 40-min group classes, one per wk	Pretest-posttest comparison group design [Intervention: 6 classes with 78 with complete data; Control: 5 classes with 56 with complete data]	Cognitive and Affective Mindfulness Scale-Revised (CAMS-R); Ego-Resiliency Scale (ERS); Warwick-Edinburgh Mental Well-being Scale (WEMWBS); Ten-Item Personality Inventory (TIPI)	As compared to controls, mindfulness group increased in CAMS-R ($sr^2=.06$) and WEMWBS score ($sr^2=.05$)
Khalsa et al. (2013)	Universal	Modified Yoga Ed program for secondary schools	121	Adolescents aged 15–19y receiving regular education – 57.8 % male	Mass. rural secondary school	Two to three 30–40-min yoga sessions per wk for 11 wk	Pretest-posttest control group design [Intervention: 74 (4 classes); Control/ physical education as usual group: 47 (3 classes) from same school]	Self-Report of Personality Version of the Behavioral Assessment Survey for Children V2 (BASC-2); Profile of Mood States Short Form (POMS-SF); Resilience Scale (RS); Perceived Stress Scale (PSS); Inventory of Positive Psychological Attitudes-32R (IPPA)	As compared with physical-education-as-usual group, the treatment group demonstrated the statistical improvements in BASC-2 anger control (Std ES=0.48), POMS-SF fatigue/inertia (Std ES=0.48), and in resilience (RS) (Std ES=0.53) from pretest to posttest
Khalsa et al. (2013)	Indicated	Modified yoga Kripalu-style curriculum	135	Residential music students of a 6-wk summer program at university for advanced adolescent musicians – 43.7 % male – 73 % Caucasian – Mean age 16y	Mass. university residential summer program	Three 60-min Kripalu-style yoga classes each wk for 6 wk	Pretest-posttest control group design [Intervention: $n=84$; Control: $n=51$]	Performance Anxiety Questionnaire (PAQ); Music Performance Anxiety Inventory for Adolescents (MPAI-A); Performance-related Musculoskeletal Disorders Questionnaire (PRMD-Q)	As compared to the control group, the intervention group displayed statistical reductions from baseline to posttest in music performance anxiety in the group/solo subscales of the PAQ and also in the MPAI-A total scale score and subscales of somative/ cognitive and performance evaluation

Study	Level of prevention	Program content	*N*	Participants	Program location	Length and frequency	Research design	Quantitative outcome variables	Main results/effect size
Kuyken et al. (2013)	Universal	Mindfulness in Schools Programme (MiSP)	522	Adolescents aged 12–16 in 12 secondary schools in the UK	UK	Nine weekly lessons; student participation rate of varied across the schools from a single class within a single year group to all classes in a year group	Non-randomized controlled parallel group (MiSP programme vs. matched control group) study, with assessment of outcomes at baseline (pre-intervention), post-intervention and follow-up (3 months after baseline)	Warwick–Edinburgh Mental Well-being Scale (WEMWBS); Perceived Stress Scale (PSS); Center for Epidemiologic Studies Depression Scale (CES-D); Assessment of mindfulness practice	As compared to the comparison schools, students in the intervention schools reported fewer depressive symptoms (CES-D) at posttest and follow-up, lower perceived stress (PSS) at follow-up, and higher well-being (WEMWBS) at follow-up
Metz et al. (2013)	Selective	Learning to BREATHE mindfulness curriculum, (Broderick, 2010)	216	Adolescents in tenth to twelfth grade from two suburban PA public high schools in same school district – 34 % male	Concert choir course elective	Eighteen sessions 15–25 min at beginning of class sessions; typically once a wk over 16 wks	Pretest-posttest comparison group design [Experimental school: 6 classes with 129 with complete data; Comparison school: 3 classes with 87 with complete data]	Difficulties in Emotion Regulation Scale (DERS); Psychosomatic Complaints Scale; Affective Self-Regulatory Efficacy Scale; single-item of perceived stress level	As compared to comparison group, experimental group reported statistically lower levels of perceived stress (d=.40) and psychosomatic complaints (d=.28), and higher levels of efficacy in affective regulation (d=.62) and emotion regulation skills (d=.33) [including DERS subscales of emotional awareness (d=.34), access to regulation strategies (d=.30), emotional clarity (d=.28)]
Raes et al. (2014)	Universal	Mindfulness group program	408	Students aged 13–20y from five secondary schools (i.e., equivalent to American high schools)	Belgium	Eight weekly 100-min sessions	Pretest-posttest control group design (randomized controlled trial) with 6-month follow-up	Depression Anxiety Stress Scales (DASS-21)	As compared to the control group, the intervention group reported statistically greater reductions in depression (DASS-21-D) from pretest to posttest (*Cohen's* d=0.32) and from pretest to 6-month follow-up (*Cohen's* d=0.32)

(continued)

Table 22.1 (Continued)

Study	Level of prevention	Program content	*N*	Participants	Program location	Length and frequency	Research design	Quantitative outcome variables	Main results/effect size
Sibinga et al. (2011)	Selective	Mindfulness-based stress reduction (MBSR)	26	Youth aged 13–21y from a pediatric primary care clinic of an urban tertiary care hospital – 23 % male – 100 % African-American – Mean age of 16.8 y – 42 % HIV+	Pediatric primary care clinic of an urban tertiary care hospital	Nine sessions per wk over 8 wk	One group pretest posttest design	Child Health and Illness Profile—Adolescent Edition (CHIP-AE); Symptom Checklist-90 Revised (SCL-90R)	There were statistical reductions from pretest to posttest in the hostility SCL-90R subscale and in the CHIP-AE general discomfort subscale and in the general discomfort domain of emotional discomfort
Tan and Martin (2013)	Indicated	Taming the Adolescent Mind [Mindfulness-based cognitive therapy (MBCT)]	10	Adolescents aged 13–17y with a diagnosed mental health disorder (and parents) recruited from outpatient child and youth mental health service in Australia – 30 % male – 100 % Caucasian – Mean age of 15.7y	Outpatient Child and Youth Mental Health Service in Australia	5-wk, 1-h group intervention	One group pretest posttest design with a 3-month follow-up assessment	Youth: Depression Anxiety Stress Scale (DASS-21); Rosenberg Self-Esteem Scale; Children's Acceptance and Mindfulness Measure (CAMM); Avoidance and Fusion Questionnaire for Youth (AFQ-Y8) Parents: Child Behavior Checklist (CBCL)	Some subscales of the DASS-21 statistically showed improvement from pretest to the 3-month follow-up assessment including: total ($d=0.28$), stress ($d=0.36$), anxiety ($d=0.48$), and depression ($d=0.42$). There were also statistical improvements from pretest to the 3-month follow-up in self-esteem ($d=-0.42$), mindfulness (CAMM) ($d=-0.04$), psychological inflexibility (AFQ-Y8) ($d=.66$), and the parental CBCL score ($d=0.70$)

Study	Level of prevention	Program content	*N*	Participants	Program location	Length and frequency	Research design	Quantitative outcome variables	Main results/effect size
Zylowska et al. (2008)	Indicated	Mindfulness training: Mindful Awareness Practices (MAPs) (Kabat-Zinn, 1990; Segal et al., 2002)	8	Adolescents aged 15+ diagnosed with ADHD – 62.5 % female	Not specified	Eight weekly 2.5-h group sessions, daily at-home practice	One-group pretest-posttest design	Self-report scales of ADHD, depression, and anxiety symptoms; battery of cognitive tests	Negligible changes in depression and anxiety (no statistical testing performed due to small sample size)

Table 22.2 Basic program logic model

Inputs	Activities	Outputs	Outcomes
Resources for implementation and evaluation	Program strategies and procedures	Direct products of the program that help to monitor program reach or process	Benefits resulting from program
• Staff (and staff time)—for program facilitation and evaluation	• Training of program facilitators	• Number of teachers trained for program delivery	• Student self-report (knowledge, attitudes, values, behavior)
• Volunteers (and volunteer time)	• Number and length of sessions/modules	• Number of students reached	• Student behavior/performance (routinely collected school documentation)
• Money	• Example of activities	• Number of classes taught	• Physiological response (heart rate, cortisol, blood pressure)
• Fee for program use		• Number of objectives taught within each class	• System measures (teacher-reported classroom and school climate)
• Supplies/equipment		• Number of distributed educational materials	
• Space allocation		• Satisfaction surveys with students and teachers	
		• Number of volunteers recruited	

H: History of Program Approach

Some existing mindfulness-based programs for children and youth are derived from secular approaches such as MBSR, Mindfulness-Based Cognitive Therapy (MBCT), and positive psychology and are supported by recent advances in the neurosciences. A solid understanding of the theoretical foundations of existing programs can inform teachers' understanding of techniques, rationales, objectives, and assessments. The underlying assumptions about the mechanisms of change that serve as the program's foundation should be clear in order to make an informed decision. Despite the challenge of translating contemplative disciplines into contemporary educational language, it is very important not to lose their ethical character, wisdom, and experiential nature lest they become another rote activity. Current efforts to clarify components of mindfulness interventions from a psychological science perspective provide a useful approach for researchers and users of secular programs (see Baer, 2015).

O: Objectives

In educational settings, it is important to clearly define program objectives and link them to stated goals of schools, school districts, or national standards. For instance, the National Health Education Standards (NHES) provide expectations for what students should know and be able to do by grades 2, 5, 8, and 12 to promote personal, family, and community health (The Joint Committee on National Health Education Standards, 2007). Standard 7 indicates that students in grades 9–12 will demonstrate the ability to practice health-enhancing behaviors. Each of the six L2B program objectives linked to Standard 7, which made this program a good fit for a health class curriculum. For example, a L2B program objective was to increase body awareness. One way this standard was addressed was by means of the Body Scan activity. Instructors completed an activity completion checklist (process evaluation) and students completed a somatization questionnaire (outcome evaluation) in order to assess if the objective was met. Programs may stand a better chance of sustainability in educational settings if they can be clearly linked in some way to the objectives of the institution.

O: Outcomes

Outcomes are the benefits to program participants. Outcomes may be elicited via qualitative assessment (e.g., focus groups, unstructured interviews, journaling, or open-ended survey questions) and quantitative assessment (e.g., closed-ended item questionnaires from students or others, student school record extraction, or medical apparatus measurement of physiological responses). Often well-designed program evaluations use a mixed-methods approach, using the quantitative approach to compare results with other interventions and standardize them over time along with the qualitative approach to elicit unexpected outcomes. In the L2B program, several valid and reliable instruments as well as process evaluation measures were administered to assess program effects. In their work, Bogels et al. (2008) used both adolescent and parental reports of adolescent behavior. Physiological response measures can also be employed to assess the interaction between psychological and physiological health (Cicchetti & Gunnar, 2008). These measures include blood pressure, heart rate, respiratory sinus arrhythmia, cortisol levels, ANS reactivity, and hypothalamic–pituitary–adrenal (HPA) axis reactivity (Barnes, Davis, Murzynowski, & Treiber, 2004; Oldehinkel et al., 2010). For instance, Barnes et al. (2004) found a positive effect of meditation on the resting and ambulatory heart rate and blood pressure in middle school students. System outcomes such as teacher-reported classroom management or school climate surveys may also provide a school-wide measure of success. At minimum, outcomes should be assessed before and immediately after the program. Addition of a long-term follow-up assessment is a particularly helpful tool in building an evidence base for mindfulness in schools (see Kuyken et al., 2013).

Process evaluation data may help to explain why specific program components were effective at producing positive outcomes while others were not. Specifically, five implementation factors are used to structure a process evaluation (Grembowski, 2001; Israel et al., 1995): completeness (amount of implemented program activities), fidelity (extent to which program activities are implemented as intended), coverage (extent to which the target population received program activities), student reaction (target population's satisfaction with and reaction to program activities), and teacher reaction (teachers' satisfaction with and reaction to program activities). See Table 22.3 for an outline of possible process evaluation measures for teachers, students, and classroom observers.

Table 22.3 Process evaluation measures and purpose of data

Source	Measure	Purpose of collected data
Teachers		
	Post-training survey	Teachers reaction
	Teachers curriculum checklist (assesses content, method of delivery, and self-efficacy)	Completeness, fidelity, coverage, teacher reaction
	Post-implementation survey	Teacher reaction
	Focus groups	Teacher reaction
Classroom observer		
	Video-taping and reviewer checklist	Completeness, fidelity, coverage
	Classroom observer checklist	Completeness, fidelity, coverage
Students		
	Student curriculum checklist	Completeness, student reaction
	Student homework verification	Completeness, fidelity, coverage
	Forms	
	Post-program student satisfaction	Students reaction
	Survey	
	Focus groups	Student reaction

L: Layout or Design

The layout or design helps determines the effectiveness of a study. The randomized pretest-posttest control group design is the gold standard design in which a group is randomized into receiving or not receiving the program. Randomization minimizes the possibility that an extraneous factor is associated with the changes, but it is not always feasible in schools. Therefore, the nonrandomized pretest-posttest comparison group design is often used in which one school receives the program and pretest-posttest changes are compared to the pretest-posttest changes of a comparable group of students at another school who do not receive the program. The comparison group should be very similar to the program group in terms of basic demographics. At minimum, the one-group pretest-posttest design should be employed in which one group of students receives the program and outcomes are measured before and immediately after the program.

S: Sustainability

The active support of the school's mindfulness program is critical to its success and sustainability. Initially, a workgroup composed of teachers, counselors, psychologists, administrators, and parents who are interested in mindfulness might be formed to take responsibility for program implementation and evaluation and for proposing the initiative to school stakeholders such as parents and top-level administrators. Because mindfulness is a practice, opportunities to practice mindfulness (e.g., lunchtime meditation groups, workshops for parents, teen groups) might be built into the schedule and open to the whole school community. Ongoing training of instructors and regular in-service offerings help sustain interest and prepare teachers to expand programs. For research purposes, efforts should be made to integrate the outcome evaluation into the data monitoring or assessment system already in place which will feed directly into annual and long-term plans for the program. Partnerships with regional academic institutions that may supply free or low-cost evaluation services or with developers of research-based programs can aid in implementation and research. Program highlights should also be regularly communicated to parents and the outside community through annual reports, newsletters, and press releases that support contemplative educational innovations.

Conclusion

The purpose of this chapter was to present a rational for a universal approach to teaching mindfulness to adolescents and to describe an example of a program that was developed for this purpose. We reviewed some of the developmental opportunities and challenges of the adolescent period, with special attention to neurobiological changes. We also discussed the particular benefits of mindfulness, both as an antidote for stress and a trainable regulatory skill. The elements of Learning to BREATHE, a universal prevention program, were presented as an example of a mindfulness education program for school settings. Overall, existing data suggest the feasibility and efficacy of L2B as a form of universal prevention delivered in schools for adolescents with regard to the normative stresses of life during this time. Finally, we identify some important elements for researchers and educators to consider when selecting or implementing a mindfulness-based program.

In conclusion, current research is affirming what many people over the course of history have already discovered. Mindfulness practice has the power to help reduce distress, open the heart, and promote a deep sense of wellness. For contemporary adolescents, this is an urgent need. Thus, it is important for researchers, practitioners, and school professionals to work together within educational settings to support the well-being of all adolescents by means of effective empirically supported universal programming. Supporting the inner work of adolescents through mindfulness can have far-reaching consequences for the good of students at this stage of their development and beyond.

References

Achenbach, T. M. (1991). *Integrative guide for the 1991 CBCL/4-18, YSR, and TRF profiles*. Burlington, VT: University of Vermont, Department of Psychiatry.

Adam, E. K. (2006). Transactions among adolescent trait and state emotion and diurnal and momentary cortisol activity in naturalistic settings. *Psychoneuroendocrinology, 31*, 664–679.

American Academy of Pediatrics. (1993). The pediatrician and the "new morbidity". Committee on Psychosocial Aspects of Child and Family Health. *Pediatrics, 92*, 731–733.

American Academy of Pediatrics. (2001). The new morbidity revisited: A renewed commitment to the psychosocial aspects of pediatric care. Committee on Psychosocial Aspects of Child and Family Health. *Pediatrics, 108*, 1227–1230.

Andersen, S. L., & Teicher, M. H. (2008). Stress, sensitive periods and maturational events in adolescent depression. *Trends in Neuroscience, 31*, 183–191. doi:10.1016/j.tins.2008.01.004.

Archambault, A., Janosz, M., Morizot, J., & Pagani, L. (2009). Adolescent behavioural, affective, and cognitive engagement in school: Relationship to dropout. *Journal of School Health, 79*, 408–415. doi:10.1111/j.1746-1561.2009.00428.x.

Arnsten, A. F. T., & Shansky, R. M. (2004). Adolescent vulnerable period for stress-induced prefrontal cortical function? Introduction to part IV. *Annals of the New York Academy of Sciences, 1021*, 143–147.

Baer, R. (2015). Ethics, values, virtues, and character strengths in mindfulness-based interventions: A psychological science perspective. *Mindfulness, 6*, 956–969.

Barnes, V. A., Davis, H. C., Murzynowski, J. B., & Treiber, F. A. (2004). Impact of meditation on resting and ambulatory blood pressure and heart rate in youth. *Psychosomatic Medicine, 66*, 909–914.

Beato-Fernández, L., Rodríguez-Cano, T., Pelayo-Delgado, E., & Calaf, M. (2007). Are there gender-specific pathways from early adolescence psychological distress symptoms toward the development of substance use and abnormal eating behavior? *Child Psychiatry and Human Development, 37*, 193–203.

Beauchemin, J., Hutchins, T.L., & Patterson, F. (2008). Mindfulness meditation may lessen anxiety, promote social skills, and improve academic performance among adolescents with learning disabilities. *Complementary Health Practice Review,13*, 34–45. DOI: 10.1177/1533210107311624

Beets, M. W. & Mitchell, E. (2010). Effects of yoga on stress, depression, and health-related quality of life in a Nonclinical, Bi-Ethnic Sample of Adolescents: A Pilot Study. *Hispanic Health Care International, 8*, 47–53.

Berkowitz, L. (2008). On the consideration of automatic as well as controlled psychological processes in aggression. *Aggressive Behavior, 34*, 117–129. doi:10.1002/ab.20244.

Biegel, G. M., Brown, K. W., Shapiro, S. L., & Schubert, C. M. (2009). Mindfulness-based stress reduction for the treatment of adolescent psychiatric outpatients: A randomized clinical trial. *Journal of Consulting and Clinical Psychology, 77*, 855–866. doi:10.1037/a0016241.

Blair, C., & Diamond, A. (2008). Biological processes in prevention and intervention: The promotion of self-regulation as a means of preventing school failure. *Development and Psychopathology, 20*, 899–911. doi:10.1017/S095479408000436.

Blakemore, S. J. (2008). Development of the social brain during adolescence. *The Quarterly Journal of Experimental Psychology, 61*, 40–49.

Blakemore, S. J., & Frith, U. (2005). *The learning brain: Lessons for education*. Oxford, UK: Blackwell.

Bluth, K., Campo, R. A., Pruteanu-Malinici, S., Reams, A., Mullarkey, M., & Broderick, P. C. (2015). A school-based mindfulness pilot study for ethnically diverse at-risk adolescents. *Mindfulness*, 1–15. doi:10.1007/s12671-014-0376-1.

Bogels, S., Hoogstad, B., vanDun, L., deSchutter, S., & Restifo, K. (2008). Mindfulness training for adolescents with externalizing disorders and their parents. *Behavioural and Cognitive Psychotherapy, 36*, 193–209. doi:10.1017/S1352465808004190.

Bootzin, R. R., & Stevens, S. J. (2005). Adolescents, substance abuse, and the treatment of insomnia and daytime sleepiness. *Clinical Psychology Review, 25*, 629–644.

Boyce, B. (2005). Two sciences of the mind. *Shambhala Sun, 13*(34–43), 93–96.

Bridgeland, J. M., DiIulio, J. J., & Morison, K. B. (2006). *The silent epidemic*. A report by Civic Enterprises in association with Peter D. Hart Research Associates for the Bill & Melinda Gates Foundation.

Britton, W. B., Haynes, P. L., Fridel, K. W., & Bootzin, R. R. (2010). Polysomnographic and subjective profiles of sleep continuity before and after mindfulness-based cognitive therapy in partially remitted depression. *Psychosomatic Medicine, 72*, 539–548. doi:10.1097/PSY.0b013e3181dc1bad.

Broderick, P. C. (2013). *Learning to BREATHE: A mindfulness curriculum for adolescents*. Oakland, CA: New Harbinger.

Broderick, P. C., & Blewitt, P. (2014). *The life span: Human development for helping professionals* (4th ed.). New York, NY: Pearson.

Broderick, P. C., & Metz, S. (2009). Learning to BREATHE: A pilot trial of a mindfulness curriculum for adolescents. *Advances in School Mental Health Promotion, 2*, 35–46. doi:10.1080/1754730X.2009.9715696.

Campos, J. J., Frankel, C. B., & Camras, L. (2004). On the nature of emotion regulation. *Child Development, 75*, 377–394.

Casey, B. J., Getz, S., & Galvan, A. (2008). The adolescent brain. *Developmental Review, 28*, 62–77.

Casey, B. J., Giedd, J. N., & Thomas, K. M. (2000). Structural and functional brain development and its relation to cognitive development. *Biological Psychology, 54*, 241–257.

Casey, B. J., Jones, R. M., & Hare, T. A. (2008). The adolescent brain. *Annals of the New York Academy of Sciences, 1124*, 111–126. doi:10.1196/annals.1440.010.

Centers for Disease Control and Prevention. (2010). *School Health Programs: Improving the health of our nation's youth.* Retrieved from http://www.cdc.gov/chronicdisease/resources/publications/aag/pdf/2010/dash-2010.pdf

Chiesa, A., & Serreti, A. (2009). Mindfulness-based stress reduction for stress management in healthy people: A review and meta-analysis. *The Journal of Alternative and Complementary Medicine, 15*, 593–600. doi:10.1089/acm.2008.0495.

Chodhury, S. (2010). Culturing the adolescent brain: What can neuroscience learn from anthropology? *Social Cognitive and Affective Neuroscience, 5*, 159–167. doi:10.1093/scan/nsp030.

Cicchetti, D., & Gunnar, M. R. (2008). Integrating biological measures into the design and evaluation of preventive interventions. *Development and Psychopathology, 20*, 737–743. doi:10.1017/S0954579408000357.

Cisler, J. M., Olatunji, B. O., Felder, M. T., & Forsyth, J. P. (2010). Emotion regulation and the anxiety disorders. *Journal of Psychopathology and Behavioral Assessment, 32*, 68–82. doi:10.1007/s10862-009-9161-1.

Collaborative for Academic, Social, and Emotional Learning. (2008). *Social and emotional learning and student benefits: Implications for the Safe School/Healthy Students core elements.* Washington, DC: National Center for Mental Health Promotion and Youth Violence Prevention, Education Development Center.

Collins, W. A. (2003). More than myth: The developmental significance of romantic relationships during adolescence. *Journal of Research on Adolescence, 13*, 1–24. doi:10.1111/1532-7795.1301001.

Collishaw, S., Maughan, B., Goodman, R., & Pickles, A. (2004). Time trends in adolescent mental health. *Journal of Child Psychology and Psychiatry, 45*, 1350–1362. doi:10.1111/j.1469-7610.2004.00335.x.

Comstock, G., & Scharrer, E. (2006). Media and popular culture. In K. A. Renninger, I. E. Sigel, W. Damon, & R. M. Lerner (Eds.), *Handbook of child psychology* (Child psychology in practice 6th ed., Vol. 4, pp. 817–863). Hoboken, NJ: Wiley.

Costello, E. J., Foley, D., & Angold, A. (2006). A 10-year research update review: The epidemiology of child and adolescent psychiatric disorders. II. Developmental epidemiology. *Journal of the American Academy of Child and Adolescent Psychiatry, 45*, 8–25. doi:10.1097/01.chi.0000184929.41423.c0.

Dahl, R. E. (2004). *Adolescent brain development: Vulnerabilities and opportunities*. New York Academy of Sciences: New York, NY. Retrieved from http://search.proquest.com/docview/620449469?accountid=14971

Darling, N., Cumsille, P., & Martinez, M. L. (2008). Individual differences in adolescents' beliefs about the legitimacy of parental authority and their own obligation to obey: A longitudinal investigation. *Child Development, 79*, 1103–1118. doi:10.1111/j.1467-8624.2008.01178.x.

Daughters, S. B., Reynolds, E. K., MacPherson, L., Kahler, C. W., Danielson, C. K., Zvolensky, M., & Lejuez, C. W. (2009). Distress tolerance and early adolescent eternalizing and internalizing symptoms: The moderating role of gender and ethnicity. *Behaviour Research and Therapy, 47,* 198–205.

Davidson, R., Kabat-Zinn, J., Schumacher, J., Rosenkranz, M., Muller, D., Santorelli, S., … Sheridan, J. (2003). Alterations in brain and immune function produced by mindfulness meditation. *Psychosomatic Medicine, 65*(4), 564–570.

Durlak, J. A., Taylor, R. D., Kawashima, K., Pachan, M. K., DuPre, E. P., Celio, C. I., … Weissberg, R. P. (2007). Effects of positive youth development programs on school, family, and community systems. *American Journal of Community Psychology, 39*(3–4), 269–286. 10.1007/s10464-007-9112-5.

Eccles, J., Midgley, C., Buchanan, C., Wigfield, A., Reuman, D., & MacIver, D. (1993). Development during adolescence: The impact of stage/environment fit on young adolescents' experiences in schools and families. *American Psychologist, 48*, 90–101. doi:10.1037/0003-066X.48.2.90.

Eccles, J. S., & Roeser, R. W. (2011). Schools as developmental contexts during adolescence. *Journal of Research on Adolescence, 21*, 225–241. doi:10.1111/j.1532-7795.2010.00725.x.

Eiland, L., & Romeo, R. D. (2013). Stress and the developing adolescent brain. *Neuroscience, 249*, 162–171.

Eisenberg, N., Spinrad, T. L., & Eggum, N. D. (2010). Emotion-related self-regulation and its relationship to children's maladjustment. *Annual Review of Clinical Psychology, 6*, 495–525. doi:10.1146/annurev.clinpsy.121208.131208.

Flook, L., Smalley, S. L., Kitil, M. J., Galla, B. M., Kaiser-Greenland, S., Locke, J., … Kasari, C. (2010). Effects of mindful awareness practices on executive functions in elementary school children. *Journal of Applied School Psychology, 26*, 70–95. doi:10.1080/15377900903379125.

Folkman, S., & Lazarus, R. S. (1988). The relationship between coping and emotion: Implications for theory and research. *Social Science & Medicine, 26*, 309–317.

Fredrickson, B. L., Cohn, M. A., Coffey, K. A., Pek, J., & Finkel, S. M. (2008). Open hearts build lives: Positive emotions, induced through loving-kindness meditation, build consequential personal resources. *Journal of Personality and Social Psychology, 95*, 1045–1062. doi:10.1037/a0013262.

Fuster, J. M. (2002). Frontal lobe and cognitive development. *Journal of Neurocytology, 31*, 373–385.

Garner, A., & Shonkoff, J. (2012). Early childhood adversity, toxic stress, and the role of the pediatrician: Translating developmental science into lifelong health. *Pediatrics, 129*, e224–e231. doi:10.1542/peds.2011-2662.

Giedd, J. N., Blumenthal, J., Jeffries, N. O., Castellanos, F. X., Liu, H., Zijdenbos, A., … Rapoport, J. L. (1999). Brain development during childhood and adolescence: A longitudinal MRI study. *Nature Neuroscience, 2*(10), 861–863. doi:10.1038/13158.

Gordon, R. (1987). An operational classification of disease prevention. In J. A. Steinberg & M. M. Silverman (Eds.), *Preventing mental disorders*. Rockville, MD: Department of Health and Human Services. Retrieved from http://search.proquest.com/docview/617352424?accountid=14971.

Gratz, K. L., & Roemer, L. (2004). Multidimensional assessment of emotion regulation and dysregulation: Development, factor structure, and initial validation of the difficulties in emotion regulation scale. *Journal of Psychopathology & Behavioral Assessment, 26*(1), 41–54. Retrieved from http://search.proquest.com/docview/621640322?accountid=14971.

Greenberg, M. T., Kusche, C. A., Cook, E. T., & Quamma, J. P. (1995). Promoting emotional competence in school-aged children: The effects of the PATHS curriculum. *Development and Psychopathology, 7*, 117–136. Retrieved from http://search.proquest.com/docview/618690798?accountid=14971.

Greenberg, M. T., Weissberg, R. P., O'Brien, M. U., Zins, J. E., Fredericks, L., Resnik, H., & Elias, M. J. (2003). Enhancing school-based prevention and youth development through coordinated social, emotional, and academic learning. *American Psychologist, 58*, 466–474. doi:10.1037/0003-066X.58.6-7.466.

Grembowski, D. (2001). *The practice of health program evaluation*. Thousand Oaks, CA: Sage.

Gross, J. J. (1998). The emerging field of emotion regulation: An integrative review. *Review of General Psychology, 2*, 271–299. doi:10.1037/1089-2680.2.3.271.

Gross, J. J., & Munoz, R. F. (1995). Emotion regulation and mental health. *Clinical Psychology: Science and Practice, 2*, 151–164. Retrieved from http://search.proquest.com/docview/618800127?accountid=14971.

Grossman, P., Tiefenthaler-Gilmer, P., Raysz, A., & Kesper, U. (2007). Mindfulness training as an intervention for fibromyalgia: Evidence of post-intervention and 3-year follow-up benefits in well-being. *Psychotherapy and Psychosomatics, 76*, 226–233. doi:10.1159/000101501.

Gumora, G., & Arsenio, W. F. (2002). Emotionality, emotion regulation, and school performance in middle school children. *Journal of School Psychology, 40*, 395–413. doi:10.1016/S0022-4405(02)00108-5.

Gutman, L. M., Sameroff, A. J., & Cole, R. (2003). Academic trajectories from first to twelfth grades: Growth curves according to multiple risk and early child factors. *Developmental Psychology, 39*, 777–790.

Hare, T. A., Tottenham, N., Galvan, A., Voss, H. U., Glover, G. H., & Casey, B. J. (2008). Biological substrates of emotional reactivity and regulation in adolescence during an emotional go-nogo task. *Biological Psychiatry, 63*, 927–934. doi:10.1016/j.biopsych.2008.03.015.

Harsh, S., & Mallory, M. (2013). The future of education: Building capacity for success. *Delta Kappa Gamma Bulletin, 80*, 16–25.

Hawkins, J. D., Kosterman, R., Catalano, R. F., Hill, K. G., & Abbott, R. D. (2005). Positive adult functioning through social development intervention in childhood: Long-term effects from the Seattle Social Development Project. *Archives of Pediatrics & Adolescent Medicine, 159*(1), 25–31.

Hayes, S. C., Wilson, K. W., Gifford, E. V., Follette, V. M., & Strosahl, K. (1996). Emotional avoidance and behavioral disorders: A functional dimensional approach to diagnosis and treatment. *Journal of Consulting and Clinical Psychology, 64*, 1152–1168.

Hubel, D. N., & Wiesel, T. N. (1962). Receptive fields, binocular interactions and functional architecture in the cat's visual cortex. *Journal of Physiology, 160*, 106–154. Retrieved from http://search.proquest.com/docview/615421071?accountid=14971.

Huppert, F. A., & Johnson, D. M. (2010). A controlled trial of mindfulness training in schools: The importance of practice for an impact on well-being. *Journal of Positive Psychology, 5*, 264–274. doi:10.1080/17439761003794148.

Huttenlocher, P. R. (1979). Synaptic density in human frontal cortex—Developmental changes and effects of aging. *Brian Research, 163*, 195–205.

Israel, B. A., Cummings, K. M., Dignan, M. B., Heaney, C. A., Perales, D. P., Simons-Morton, B. G., & Zimmerman, M. A. (1995). Evaluation of health education programs: Current assessment and future directions. *Health Education Quarterly, 22*(3), 364–389. Retrieved from http://search.proquest.com/docview/618978536?accountid=14971

Jacobs, T. L., Epel, E. S., Lin, J., Blackburn, E. H., Wolkowitz, O. M., Bridwell, D. A., … Saron, C. D. (2010). Intensive meditation training, immune cell telomerase activity, and psychological mediatrso. *Psychoneuroendocrinology, 36*(5), 664–681. doi:10.1016/j.psyneuen.2010.09.010.

Jacobshagen, N., Rigotti, T., Semmer, N. K., & Mohr, G. (2009). Irritation at school: Reasons to initiate strain management earlier. *International Journal of Stress Management, 16*, 195–214. doi:10.1037/a0016595.

Jha, A. P., Kropinger, J., & Baime, M. (2007). Mindfulness training modifies subsystems of attention. *Cognitive, Affective, and Behavioral Neuroscience, 7*, 109–119. doi:10.3758/CABN.7.2.109.

Jha, A. P., Stanley, E. A., Kiyonaga, A., Wong, L., & Gelfand, L. (2010). Examining the protective effects of mindfulness training on working memory and affective experience. *Emotion, 10*, 54–64. doi:10.1037/a0018438.

Joint Committee on National Health Education Standards, (2007). *National health education standards: Achieving excellence* (2nd ed.). Atlanta, GA: American Cancer Society.

Kabat-Zinn, J. (1990). *Full catastrophe living: Using the wisdom of your body and mind to face stress, pain, and illness*. New York, NY: Delacorte.

Kabat-Zinn, J. (1994). *Wherever you go, there you are: Mindfulness meditation in everyday life*. New York, NY: Hyperion.

Kaiser Family Foundation. (2010). Generation M2: Media in the lives of 8- to 18-year-olds. Retrieved November 16, 2012, from http://www.kff.org/entmedia/upload/8010.pdf

Khalsa SB, Butzer B, Shorter SM, Reinhardt KM, & Cope S. (2013). Yoga reduces performance anxiety in adolescent musicians. *Altern Ther Health Medicine, 19*(2): 34–45.

Khalsa, S., Hickey-Schultz, L., Cohen, D., Steiner, N., & Cope, S. (2012). Evaluation of the mental health benefits of yoga in a secondary school: A preliminary randomized controlled trial. *The Journal of Behavioral Health Services & Research, 39*(1), 80–90. doi:10.1007/s11414-011--9249-8.

Kuyken, W., Weare, K., Ukoumunne, O. C., Vicary, R., Motton, N., Burnett, R., Huppert, F. (2013). Effectiveness of the mindfulness in schools programme: Non-randomised controlled feasibility study. *The British Journal of Psychiatry, 203*, 126–131. doi:10.1192/bjp.bp.113.126649.

Larson, R. W. (2000). Towards a psychology of positive youth development. *American Psychologist, 55*(1), 170–183.

Laye-Gindhu, A., & Schonert-Reichl, K. A. (2005). Nonsuicidal self-harm among community adolescents: Understanding the "whats" and "whys" of self-harm. *Journal of Youth and Adolescence, 34*, 447–457. doi:10.1007/s10964-005-7262-z.

Lazar, S. W., Kerr, C. E., Wasserman, R. H., Gray, J. R., Greve, D. N., Treadway, M. T., … Fischl, B. (2005). Meditation experience is associated with increased cortical thickness. *NeuroReport: For Rapid Communication of Neuroscience Research, 16*(17), 1893–1897. doi:10.1097/01.wnr.0000186598.66243.19.

Lee, P. R., Brandy, D., & Koenig, J. I. (2003). Corticosterone alters N-methyl-D-aspartate receptor subunit mRNA expression before puberty. *Molecular Brain Research, 115*, 55–62. doi:10.1016/S0169-328X(03)00180-3.

Luthar, S. S., & Sexton, C. C. (2004). The high price of affluence. In R. V. Kail (Ed.), *Advances in child development and behavior* (pp. 125–162). San Diego, CA: Elsevier.

Lyubomirsky, S., & Tkach, C. (2004). The consequences of dysphoric rumination. In C. Papageorgiou & A. Wells (Eds.), *Depressive rumination: Nature, theory and treatment* (pp. 21–42). West Sussex, England: Wiley.

Ma, S. H., & Teasdale, J. D. (2004). Mindfulness-based cognitive therapy for depression: Replication and exploration of differential relapse prevention effects. *Journal of Clinical and Consulting Psychology, 72*, 31–40.

MacPherson, L., Reynolds, E., Daughters, S., Wang, F., Cassidy, J., Mayes, L., & Lejuez, C. (2010). Positive and negative reinforcement underlying risk behavior in early adolescents. *Prevention Science: The Official Journal of the Society for Prevention Research, 11*(3), 331–342. doi:10.1007/s11121-010-0172-7.

McCarthy, C., Giardina, M. D., Harewood, S. J., & Jin-Kyung, P. (2003). Contesting culture: Identity and curriculum dilemmas in the age of globalization, postcolonialism, and multiplicity. *Harvard Educational Review, 73*, 449–465.

McEwen, B. S. (2003). Mood disorders and allostatic load. *Biological Psychiatry, 54*, 200–207.

McEwen, B. S. (2005). Glucocorticoids, depression, and mood disorders: Structural remodeling in the brain. *Metabolism, Clinical and Experimental, 54*, 20–23.

Melman, S., Little, S. G., & Akin-Little, A. (2007). Adolescent overscheduling: The relationship between levels of participation in scheduled activities and self-reported clinical symptomology. *The High School Journal, 90*, 18–30.

Metz, S. M., Frank, J. F., Reibel, D., Cantrell, T., Sanders, R., & Broderick, P. C. (2013). The effectiveness of the Learning to BREATHE program on adolescent emotion regulation. *Research in Human Development, 10*(3), 252–272. doi:10.1080/15427609.2013.818488.

Miller, G. E., & Blackwell, E. (2006). Turning up the heat: Inflammation as a mechanism linking chronic stress, depression, and heart disease. *Current Directions in Psychological Science, 15*, 269–272. doi:10.1111/j.1467-8721.2006.00450.x.

Napoli, M., Krech, P. R., & Holley, L. C. (2005). Mindfulness training for elementary school students: The attention academy. *Journal of Applied School Psychology, 21*, 99–125. doi:10.1300/J370v21n01_05.

Needham, B. L., Crosnoe, R., & Muller, C. (2004). Academic failure in secondary school: The inter-related role of health problems and educational context. *Social Problems, 51*, 569–586.

Nolen-Hoeksema, S., & Morrow, J. (1991). A prospective study of depression and posttraumatic stress symptoms after a natural disaster: The 1989 Loma Prieta earthquake. *Journal of Personality and Social Psychology, 61*, 115–121. doi:10.1037/0022-3514.61.1.115.

Oldehinkel, A. J., Ormel, J., Bosch, N. M., Bouma, E. M. C., VanRoon, A. M., Rosmalen, J. G. M., & Riese, H. (2010). Stressed out? Associations between perceived and psychological stress responses in adolescents: The TRAILS study. *Psychophysiology, 48*(4), 441–452. doi:10.1111/j.1469-8986.2010.01118.x.

Ostafin, B. D., & Marlatt, G. A. (2008). Surfing the urge: Experiential acceptance moderates the relation between automatic alcohol motivation and hazardous drinking. *Journal of Social and Clinical Psychology, 27*(4), 404–418. doi:10.1521/jscp.2008.27.4.404.

Pagnoni, G., & Cekic, M. (2007). Age effects on gray matter volume and attentional performance in Zen meditation. *Neurobiology of Aging, 28*(10), 1623–1627. doi:10.1016/j.neurobiolaging.2007.06.008.

Patel, V., Flisher, A. J., Hetrick, S., & McGorry, P. (2007). Mental health of young people: A global public health challenge. *The Lancet, 369*(9569), 1302–1313.

Payton, J., Weissberg, R. P., Durlak, J. A., Dymnicki, A. B., Taylor, R. D., Schellinger, K. B., & Pachan, M. (2008). *The positive impact of social and emotional learning for kindergarten to eighth-grade students: Findings from three scientific reviews*. Chicago, IL: Collaborative for Academic, Social, and Emotional Learning.

Public Health Group. (2005). *Victorian burden of disease study: Mortality and morbidity in 2001*. Melbourne, Victoria, Australia: Victorian Government Department of Human Services.

Quevedo, K., Benning, S. D., Gunnar, M. R., & Dahl, R. E. (2009). The onset of puberty: Effects on the psychophysiology of defensive and appetitive motivation. *Development and Psychopathology, 21*(1), 27–45. doi:10.1017/S0954579409000030.

Raes, P., Griffith, J. W., van der Geuth, K., & Williams, J. M. G. (2014). School-based prevention and reduction of depression in adolescence. A cluster-randomized controlled trial of a mindfulness group program. *Mindfulness, 5*(5), 477–486. doi:10.1007/s12671-013-0202-1.

Resnick, M. D., Bearman, P. S., Blum, R. W., Bauman, K. E., Harris, K. M., Jones, J., … Udry, J. R. (1997). Protecting adolescents from harm: Findings from the National Longitudinal Study on Adolescent Health. *Journal of the American Medical Association, 278*(10), 823–832.

Reyna, V. F., & Farley, F. (2006). Risk and rationality in adolescent decision making: Implications for theory, practice, and public policy. *Psychological Science in the Public Interest, 7*, 1–44.

Rodriguez-Tome, H., Bariaud, F., Zardi, M. F., Delmas, C., Jeanvoine, B., & Szylagyi, P. (1993). The effects of pubertal changes on body image and relations with peers of the opposite sex in adolescence. *Journal of Adolescence, 16*(4), 421–438.

Roeser, R. W. & Peck, S. C. (2009). An education in awareness: Self, motivation, and self-regulated learning in contemplative perspective. *Educational Psychology, 44*(2),119–136. doi:10.1080/00461520902832376.

Roeser, R. W., Vanderwolf, K., & Strobel, K. R. (2001). On the relation between social-emotional and school functioning during early adolescence: Preliminary findings from Dutch and American samples. *Journal of School Psychology, 39*(2), 111–139. doi:10.1016/S0022-4405(01)00060-7.

Romeo, R. D. (2010). Adolescence: A central event in shaping stress reactivity. *Developmental Psychobiology, 52*(3), 244–253. Retrieved from http://search.proquest.com/docview/622188805?accountid=14971.

Romero, L. M., & Butler, L. K. (2007). Endocrinology of stress. *International Journal of Comparative Psychology, 20*(2–3), 89–95. Retrieved from http://search.proquest.com/docview/622173660?accountid=14971.

Sapolsky, R. M. (1999). Glucocorticoids, stress and their adverse neurological effects: Relevance to aging. *Experimental Gerontology, 34*(6), 721–732.

Sapolsky, R. M. (2004). *Why zebras don't get ulcers* (3rd ed.). New York, NY: W. H. Freeman.

Schonert-Reichl, K., Oberle, E., Lawlor, M. S., Abbott, D., & Thomson, K. (2015). Enhancing cognitive and social-emotional development through a simple-to-administer mindfulness-based school program for elementary school children: A randomized control trial. *Developmental Psychology, 51*, 52–66.

Sebastian, C., Viding, E., Williams, K. D., & Blakemore, S. J. (2009). Social brain development and the affective consequences of ostracism in adolescence. *Brain and Cognition, 72*, 134–145. doi:10.1016/j.bandc.2009.06.008.

Segal Z. V., Williams J. M. G., & Teasdale J. D. (2002). Mindfulness-based cognitive therapy for depression: A new approach to preventing relapse. New York: Guilford.

Semple, R. J., Lee, J., Rosa, D., & Miller, L. F. (2010). A randomized trial of mindfulness-based cognitive therapy for children: Promoting mindful attention to enhance social-emotional resiliency in children. *Journal of Child and Family Studies, 19*, 218–229.

Shapiro, S. L., & Brown, K. W. (2007). *The relation of mindfulness enhancement to increases in empathy in a mindfulness-based stress reduction program* (Unpublished data). Santa Clara University.

Sibinga, E., Kerrigan, D., Stewart, M., Johnson, K., Magyari, T., & Ellen, J. (2011). Mindfulness-based stress reduction for urban youth. *Journal of Alternative and Complementary Medicine, 17*(3), 213–218. doi:10.1089/acm.2009.0605.

Silk, J. S., Siegel, G. J., Whalen, D. J., Ostapenko, L. J., Ladoucer, C. D., & Dahl, R. E. (2009). Pubertal changes in emotional information processing: Pupillary, behavioral, and subjective evidence during emotional work identification. *Development and Psychopathology, 21*, 7–26. doi:10.1017/S0954579409000029.

Sim, T. N., & Koh, S. F. (2003). A domain conceptualization of adolescent susceptibility to peer pressure. *Journal of Research on Adolescence, 13*, 57–80. Retrieved from http://search.proquest.com/docview/619995613?accountid=14971.

Spear, L. P. (2000). The adolescent brain and age-related behavioral manifestations. *Neuroscience and Biobehavioral Reviews, 24*, 417–463. Retrieved from http://search.proquest.com/docview/619536120?accountid=14971.

Spear, L. P. (2009). Heightened stress responsivity and emotional reactivity during pubertal maturation: Implications for psychopathology. *Development and Psychopathology, 21*, 87–97. doi:10.1017/S0954579409000066.

Steinberg, L. (2008). A social neuroscience perspective on adolescent risk-taking. *Developmental Review, 28*, 78–106.

Steinberg, L. (2014). *Age of opportunity: Lessons from the new science of adolescence*. Boston, MA: Houghton-Mifflin.

Stroud, L., Foster, E., Papandonatos, G., Handwerger, K., Granger, D., Kivlighan, K., & Niaura, R. (2009). Stress response and the adolescent transition: Performance versus peer rejection stressors. *Development and Psychopathology, 21*(1), 47–68. doi:10.1017/S0954579409000042.

Sumter, S. R., Bokhorsta, C. L., Miersa, A. C., Van Pelt, J., & Westenberg, P. M. (2010). Age and puberty differences in stress responses during a public speaking task: Do adolescents grow more sensitive to social evaluation? *Psychoneuroendocrinology, 35*, 1510–1516. doi:10.1016/j.psyneuen.2010.05.004.

Tan, L., & Martin, G. (2013). Taming the adolescent mind: preliminary report of a mindfulness-based psychological intervention for adolescents with clinical heterogeneous mental health diagnoses. *Clinical Child Psychology and Psychiatry, 18*(2), 300–312. doi:10.1177/1359104512455182.

Tang, Y., Ma, Y., Fan, Y., Feng, H., Wang, J., Feng, S., … Fan, M. (2009). Central and autonomic nervous system interaction is altered by short-term meditation. *PNAS Proceedings of the National Academy of Sciences of the United States of America, 106*(22), 8865–8870. doi:10.1073/pnas.0904031106.

Tapper, K., Shaw, C., Ilsley, J., Hill, A. J., Bond, F. W., & Moore, L. (2008). Exploratory randomized controlled trial of a mindfulness-based weight loss intervention for women. *Appetite, 52*, 396–404. doi:10.1016/j.appet.2008.11.012.

Thomas, K.M., Drevets, W.C., Whalen, P.J., Eccard, C.H., Dahl, R. E., Ryan, N.D., & Casey, B. J. (2001). Amygdala response to facial expressions in children and adults. *Biological Psychiatry, 49,* 309–316. doi:10.1016/S0006-3223(00)01066-0.

Tomb, M., & Hunter, L. (2004). Prevention of anxiety in children and adolescents in a school setting: The role of school-based practitioners. *Children & Schools, 26*(2), 87–101.

U.S. Public Health Service. (2000). *Report of the Surgeon's General's Conference on Children's Mental Health: A national action agenda.* Washington, DC: Department of Health and Human Services.

van den Hurk, P. A., Giommi, F., Gielen, S. C., Speckens, A. E., & Barendregt, H. P. (2010). Greater efficiency in attentional processing related to mindfulness meditation. *The Quarterly Journal of Experimental Psychology, 63*(6), 1168–1180. doi:10.1080/17470210903249365.

Watson, D., Clark, L. A., & Tellegen, A. (1988). Development and validation of brief measures of positive and negative affect: The PANAS scales. *Journal of Personality and Social Psychology, 54,* 1063–1071.

Weissberg, R. P., & O'Brien, M. U. (2004). What works in school-based social and emotional learning programs for positive youth development. *The ANNALS of the American Academy of Political and Social Science, 591,* 86–97. doi:10.1177/0002716203260093.

Ystgaard, M. (1997). Life stress, social support and psychological distress in late adolescence. *Social Psychiatry and Psychiatric Epidemiology, 32*(5), 277–283. Retrieved from http://search.proquest.com/docview/619085436?accountid=14971

Zeidan, F., Johnson, S. K., Diamond, B. J., David, Z., & Goolkasian, P. (2010). Mindfulness meditation improves cognition: Evidence of brief mental training. *Consciousness and Cognition, 19,* 597–605. doi:10.1016/j.concog.2010.03.014.

Zelazo, P. D., & Cunningham, W. (2007). Executive function: Mechanisms underlying emotion regulation. In J. Gross (Ed.), *Handbook of emotion regulation* (pp. 135–158). New York, NY: Guilford.

Zoogman, S., Goldberg, S. B., Hoyt, W. T., & Miller, S. (2015). Mindfulness interventions with youth: A meta-analysis. *Mindfulness, 6,* 290–302.

Zylowska, L., Ackerman, D., Yang, M., Futrell, J., Horton, N., Hale, T., … Smalley, S. (2008). Mindfulness meditation training in adults and adolescents with ADHD: A feasibility study. *Journal of Attention Disorders, 11,* 737–746.

Index

K.A. Schonert-Reichl, R.W. Roeser (eds.), *Handbook of Mindfulness in Education*, Mindfulness in Behavioral Health, DOI 10.1007/978-1-4939-3506-2

T

U

V

W